AF540816

PHARMACEUTICAL TECHNOLOGY

ENCYCLOPAEDIA OF PHARMACEUTICAL TECHNOLOGY

Vol. 1
PHARMACEUTICAL TECHNOLOGY

By
Dr. G.P. Garg
&
Dr. M. Prakash

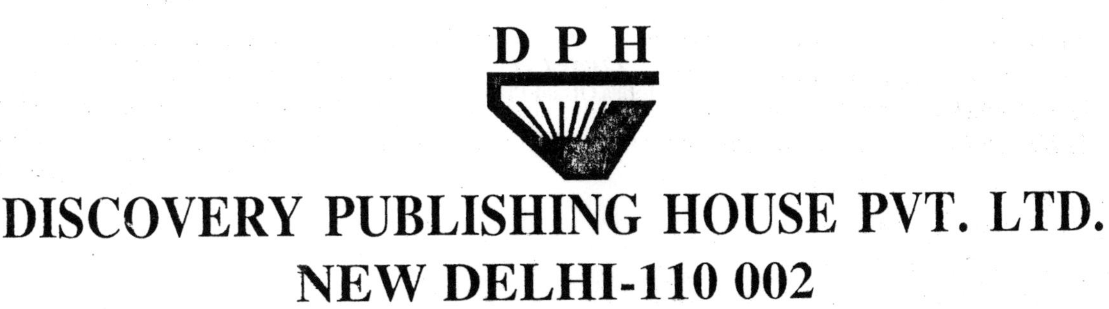

DISCOVERY PUBLISHING HOUSE PVT. LTD.
NEW DELHI-110 002

First Published-2010

ISBN: 978-81-8356-595-0 (Set)

Published by:
DISCOVERY PUBLISHING HOUSE PVT. LTD.
4831/24, Ansari Road, Prahlad Street
Darya Ganj, New Delhi-110002 (India)
Phone: 23279245, 43764432 • Fax: 91-11-23253475
E-mail: parul.wasan@gmail.com • dphbooks@rediffmail.com
web: www.discoverypublishinggroup.com

Printed at
Mehra Offset Press

Preface

The present title "Encyclopaedia of Pharmaceutical Technology" has been written for those in the pharmaceutical research and those responsible for the education and training in pharmaceutical science and technology of graduate and undergraduate students. Medicine is an ever changing science. As new research and clinical experience broaden our knowledge, changes in treatment and drug therapy are required. This branch of life science has progressed enormously in recent years and the significant advances in therapeutics and an understanding of the need to optimize during delivery in the body have brought about an increased awareness of the valuable role played by the dosage forms. This statement is as true as it was back in ninteenth century and perhaps more so, given the increasing emphasis being placed on discovery, development, and use of large molecular entities as therapeutic and diagnostic agents. Development of these abilities requires an integration of knowledge, skills, attitudes, and values that can be acquired only through structured learning process including independent study, hands on practice and the availability of advanced literature. This tittle has designed to meet such needs of learners in the health professions.

In the last two decades, the pharmaceutical industry has experimented and successfully adopted several integrated and multidisciplinary approaches in the research areas of dring compound screening, toxicological evaluation, and pharmaceutical product development. The book is written in a concise style that facilitates an in-depth level of understanding of the essential concepts. The objectives of the present title are three folds: (i) to serve as a useful tool to help guide scientists in research and development by outlining the theory and successful practice of in vitro - in vivo correlation, (ii) to help formulators apply the tool in designing and developing prototypes that enable selection of clinical formulations, and (iii) to help formulate strategy(ies) for product life-cycle management.

To make the work more comprehensive and informative, the author has consulted many authoritative books, research journals, abstracts, monographs etc., so there can be no claim to originality except in the manner of treatment.

The author expresses his thanks to his friends and colleagues whose continue inspirations have initiated him to bring out this book.

The author expresses his gratitude to Mr. Wasan and staff of M/s Discovery Publishing House Pvt. Ltd. for their whole hearted co-operation in the publication of this book.

Author

Preface

Editor

Contents

1

INTRODUCTION

Pharmaceutical substances form the backbone of modern medicinal therapy. Most traditional pharmaceuticals are low molecular weight organic chemicals. Although some (e.g. aspirin) were originally isolated from biological sources, most are now manufactured by direct chemical synthesis. Two types of manufacturing company thus comprise the '*traditional*' pharmaceutical sector: the chemical synthesis plants, which manufacture the raw chemical ingredients in bulk quantities, and the finished product pharmaceutical facilities, which purchase these raw bulk ingredients, formulate them into final pharmaceutical products, and supply these products to the end user.

Table 1.1 Some traditional pharmaceutical substances that are generally produced by direct chemical synthesis

Drug	*Molecular formula*	*Molecular mass*	*Therapeutic indication*
Acetaminophen (paracetamol)	$C_8H_9NO_2$	151.16	Analgesic
Ketamine	$C_{13}H_{16}C/NO$	237.74	Anaesthetic
Levamisole	$C_{11}H_{12}N_2S$	204.31	Anthelmintic
Diazoxide	C_8H_7C/N_2O_2S	230.7	Antihypertensive
Acyclovir	$C_8H_{11}N_5O_3$	225.2	Antiviral agent
Zidovudine	$C_{10}H_{13}N_5O_4$	267.2	Antiviral agent
Dexamethasone	$C_{22}H_{29}FO_5$	392.5	Anti-inflammatory and immuno-suppressive agent
Misoprostol	$C_{22}H_{38}O_5$	382.5	Anti-ulcer agent
Cimetidine	$C_{10}H_{16}N_6$	252.3	Anti-ulcer agent

In addition to chemical-based drugs, a range of pharmaceutical substances (e.g. hormones and blood products) are produced by/extracted from biological sources. In some instances, categorizing pharmaceuticals as products of biotechnology or chemical synthesis becomes somewhat artificial. For example, certain semi-synthetic antibiotics are produced by chemical modification of natural antibiotics produced by fermentation technology.

BIOPHARMACEUTICALS AND PHARMACEUTICAL BIOTECHNOLOGY

Terms such as '*biologic*', '*biopharmaceutical*' and 'products of pharmaceutical biotechnology' or '*biotechnology medicines*' have now become an accepted part of the pharmaceutical literature. However, these terms are sometimes used interchangeably and can mean different things to different people.

Table 1.2 Some pharmaceuticals that were traditionally obtained by direct extraction from biological source material. Many of the protein-based pharmaceuticals mentioned are now also produced by genetic engineering

Substance	*Medical application*
Blood products (e.g. coagulation factors)	Treatment of blood disorders such as haemophilia A or B
Vaccines	Vaccination against various diseases
Antibodies	Passive immunization against various diseases
Insulin	Treatment of diabetes mellitus
Enzymes	Thrombolytic agents, digestive aids, debriding agents (i.e. cleansing of wounds)
Antibiotics	Treatment against various infections agents
Plant extracts (e.g. alkaloids)	Various, including pain relief

Although it might be assumed that 'biologic' refers to any pharmaceutical product produced by biotechnological endeavour, its definition is more limited. In pharmaceutical circles, 'biologic' generally refers to medicinal products derived from blood, as well as vaccines, toxins and allergen products. 'Biotechnology' has a much broader and long-established meaning. Essentially, it refers to the use of biological systems (e.g. cells or tissues) or biological molecules (e.g. enzymes or antibodies) for/in the manufacture of commercial products.

The term '*biopharmaceutical*' was first used in the 1980s and came to describe a class of therapeutic proteins produced by modern biotechnological techniques, specifically via genetic engineering or, in the case of monoclonal antibodies, by hybridoma technology. Although the majority of biopharmaceuticals or biotechnology products now approved or in development are proteins produced via genetic engineering, these terms now also encompass nucleic-acid-based, i.e. deoxyribonucleic acid (DNA)- or ribonucleic acid (RNA)-based products, and whole-cell-based products.

History of the Pharmaceutical Industry

The pharmaceutical industry, as we now know it, is barely 60 years old. From very modest beginnings, it has grown rapidly, reaching an estimated value of US$100 billion by the mid 1980s. Its current value is likely double or more this figure. There are well in excess of 10 000 pharmaceutical companies in existence, although only about 100 of these can claim to be of true international significance. These companies manufacture in excess of 5000 individual pharmaceutical substances used routinely in medicine.

The first stages of development of the modern pharmaceutical industry can be traced back to the turn of the twentieth century. At that time (apart from folk cures), the medical community had at their disposal only four drugs that were effective in treating specific diseases:

1. Digitalis (extracted from foxglove) was known to stimulate heart muscle and, hence, was used to treat various heart conditions.
2. Quinine, obtained from the barks/roots of a plant (*Cinchona* genus), was used to treat malaria.
3. Pecacuanha (active ingredient is a mixture of alkaloids), used for treating dysentery, was obtained from the bark/roots of the plant genus *Cephaelis*.
4. Mercury, for the treatment of syphilis.

This lack of appropriate, safe and effective medicines contributed in no small way to the low life expectancy characteristic of those times.

Developments in biology (particularly the growing realization of the microbiological basis of many diseases), as well as a developing appreciation of the principles of organic chemistry, helped underpin future innovation in the fledgling pharmaceutical industry. The successful synthesis of various artificial dyes, which proved to be therapeutically useful, led to the formation of pharmaceutical/chemical companies such as Bayer and Hoechst in the late 1800s. Scientists at Bayer, for example, succeeded in synthesizing aspirin in 1895. Despite these early advances, it was not until the 1930s that the pharmaceutical industry began to develop in earnest. The initial landmark discovery of this era was probably the discovery, and chemical synthesis, of the sulfa drugs. These are a group of related molecules derived from the red dye *prontosil rubrum*. These drugs proved effective in the treatment of a wide variety of bacterial infections. Although it was first used therapeutically in the early 1920s, large-scale industrial production of insulin also commenced in the 1930s. The medical success of these drugs gave new emphasis to the pharmaceutical industry, which was boosted further by the commencement of industrial-scale penicillin manufacture in the early 1940s. Around this time, many of the current leading pharmaceutical companies (or their forerunners) were founded. Examples include Ciba Geigy, Eli Lilly, Wellcome, Glaxo and Roche. Over the next two to three decades, these companies developed drugs such as tetracyclines, corticosteroids, oral contraceptives, antidepressants and many more. Most of these pharmaceutical substances are manufactured by direct chemical synthesis.

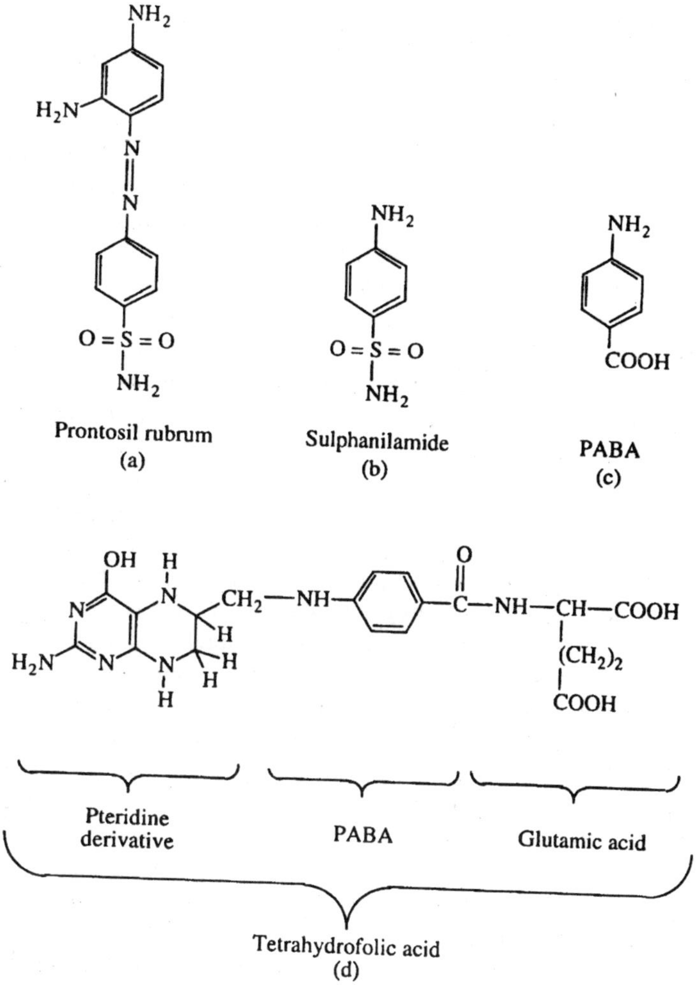

Prontosil rubrum (a) Sulphanilamide (b) PABA (c)

Pteridine derivative PABA Glutamic acid

Tetrahydrofolic acid (d)

Fig. 1.1. Sulfa drugs and their mode of action.

Age of Biopharmaceuticals

Biomedical research continues to broaden our understanding of the molecular mechanisms underlining both health and disease. Research undertaken since the 1950s has pinpointed a host of proteins produced naturally in the body that have obvious therapeutic applications. Examples include the interferons and interleukins (which regulate the immune response), growth factors, such as erythropoietin (EPO; which stimulates red blood cell production), and neurotrophic factors (which regulate the development and maintenance of neural tissue). Although the pharmaceutical potential of these regulatory molecules was generally appreciated, their widespread medical application was in most cases rendered impractical due to the tiny quantities in which they were naturally produced. The advent of recombinant DNA technology (genetic engineering) and monoclonal antibody technology (hybridoma technology) overcame many such difficulties, and marked the beginning of a new era of the pharmaceutical sciences. Recombinant DNA technology has had a fourfold positive impact upon the production of pharmaceutically important proteins:

1. *It overcomes the problem of source availability.* Many proteins of therapeutic potential are produced naturally in the body in minute quantities. Examples include interferons, interleukins and colony-stimulating factors (CSFs). This rendered impractical their direct extraction from native source material in quantities sufficient to meet likely clinical demand. Recombinant production allows the manufacture of any protein in whatever quantity it is required.
2. *It overcomes problems of product safety.* Direct extraction of product from some native biological sources has, in the past, led to the unwitting transmission of disease. Examples include the transmission of blood-borne pathogens such as hepatitis B and C and human immunodeficiency virus (HIV) via infected blood products and the transmission of Creutzfeldt–Jakob disease to persons receiving human growth hormone (GH) preparations derived from human pituitaries.
3. *It provides an alternative to direct extraction from inappropriate/dangerous source material.* A number of therapeutic proteins have traditionally been extracted from human urine. Follicle-stimulating hormone (FSH), the fertility hormone, for example, is obtained from the urine of post-menopausal women, and a related hormone, human chorionic gonadotrophin (hCG), is extracted from the urine of pregnant women. Urine is not considered a particularly desirable source of pharmaceutical products. Although several products obtained from this source remain on the market, recombinant forms have now also been approved. Other potential biopharmaceuticals are produced naturally in downright dangerous sources. Ancrod, for example, is a protein displaying anti-coagulant activity and, hence, is of potential clinical use. It is, however, produced naturally by the Malaysian pit viper. Although retrieval by milking snake venom is possible, and indeed may be quite an exciting procedure, recombinant production in less dangerous organisms, such as *Escherichia coli* or *Saccharomycese cerevisiae*, would be considered preferable by most.
4. *It facilitates the generation of engineered therapeutic proteins displaying some clinical advantage over the native protein product.* Techniques such as site-directed mutagenesis facilitate the logical introduction of predefined changes in a protein's amino acid sequence. Such changes can be as minimal as the insertion, deletion or alteration of a single amino acid residue, or can be more substantial (e.g. the alteration/deletion of an entire domain, or the generation of a novel hybrid protein). Such changes can be made for a number of reasons, and several engineered products have now gained marketing approval.

Despite the undoubted advantages of recombinant production, it remains the case that many protein-based products extracted directly from native source material remain on the market. In certain circumstances, direct extraction of native source material can prove equally/more attractive than recombinant production. This may be for an economic reason if, for example, the protein is produced in very large quantities by the native source and is easy to extract/purify, e.g. human serum albumin (HSA). Also, some blood factor preparations purified from donor blood actually contain several different blood factors and, hence, can be used to treat several haemophilia patient types. Recombinant blood factor preparations, on the other hand, contain but a single blood factor and, hence, can be used to treat only one haemophilia type.

The advent of genetic engineering and monoclonal antibody technology underpinned the establishment of literally hundreds of start-up biopharmaceutical (biotechnology) companies in the late 1970s and early 1980s. The bulk of these companies were founded in the USA, with smaller numbers of start-ups emanating from Europe and other world regions.

Many of these fledgling companies were founded by academics/technical experts who sought to take commercial advantage of developments in the biotechnological arena. These companies were largely financed by speculative monies attracted by the hype associated with the establishment of the modern biotech era. Although most of these early companies displayed significant technical expertise, the vast majority lacked experience in the practicalities of the drug development process. Most of the well-established large pharmaceutical companies, on the other hand, were slow to invest heavily in biotech research and development. However, as the actual and potential therapeutic significance of biopharmaceuticals became evident, many of these companies did diversify into this area. Most either purchased small, established biopharmaceutical concerns or formed strategic alliances with them. An example was the long-term alliance formed by Genentech and the well-established pharmaceutical company Eli Lilly. Genentech developed recombinant human insulin, which was then marketed by Eli Lilly under the trade name Humulin. The merger of biotech capability with pharmaceutical experience helped accelerate development of the biopharmaceutical sector.

Many of the earlier biopharmaceutical companies no longer exist. The overall level of speculative finance available was not sufficient to sustain them all long term (it can take 6–10 years and US$800 million to develop a single drug). Furthermore, the promise and hype of biotechnology sometimes exceeded its ability actually to deliver a final product. Some biopharmaceutical substances showed little efficacy in treating their target condition, and/or exhibited unacceptable side effects. Mergers and acquisitions also led to the disappearance of several biopharmaceutical concerns.

BIOPHARMACEUTICALS: CURRENT STATUS AND FUTURE PROSPECTS

Approximately one in every four new drugs now coming on the market is a biopharmaceutical. By mid 2006, some 160 biopharmaceutical products had gained marketing approval in the USA and/or EU. Collectively, these represent a global biopharmaceutical market in the region of US$35 billion, and the market value is estimated to surpass US$50 billion by 2010. The products include a range of hormones, blood factors and thrombolytic agents, as well as vaccines and monoclonal antibodies. All but two are protein-based therapeutic agents. The exceptions are two nucleic-acid-based products: 'Vitravene', an antisense oligonucleotide, and 'Macugen', an aptamer. Many additional nucleic-acid-based products for use in gene therapy or antisense technology are in clinical trials, although the range of technical difficulties that still beset this class of therapeutics will ensure that protein-based products will overwhelmingly predominate for the foreseeable future.

Many of the initial biopharmaceuticals approved were simple replacement proteins (e.g. blood factors and human insulin). The ability to alter the amino acid sequence of a protein logically coupled to an increased understanding of the relationship between protein structure and function has facilitated the more recent introduction of several engineered therapeutic proteins. Thus far, the vast majority of approved recombinant proteins have been produced in the bacterium *E. coli*, the yeast *S. cerevisiae* or in animal cell lines (most notably Chinese hamster ovary (CHO) cells or baby hamster kidney (BHK) cells.

Although most biopharmaceuticals approved to date are intended for human use, a number of products destined for veterinary application have also come on the market. One early such example is that of recombinant bovine GH (Somatotrophin), which was approved in the USA in the early 1990s and used to increase milk yields from dairy cattle. Additional examples of approved veterinary biopharmaceuticals include a range of recombinant vaccines and an interferon-based product.

At least 1000 potential biopharmaceuticals are currently being evaluated in clinical trials, although the majority of these are in early stage trials. Vaccines and monoclonal antibody-based products represent the two biggest product categories. Regulatory factors (e.g. hormones and cytokines) and gene therapy and antisense-based products also represent significant groupings. Although most protein-based products likely to gain marketing approval over the next 2–3 years will be produced in engineered *E. coli*, *S. cerevisiae* or animal cell lines, some products now in clinical trials are being produced in the milk of transgenic animals. Additionally, plant-based transgenic expression systems may potentially come to the fore, particularly for the production of oral vaccines.

Interestingly, the first generic biopharmaceuticals are already entering the market. Patent protection for many first-generation biopharmaceuticals (including recombinant human GH (rhGH), insulin, EPO, interferon-α (IFN-α) and granulocyte-CSF (G-CSF)) has now/is now coming to an end. Most of these drugs command an overall annual market value in excess of US$1 billion, rendering them attractive potential products for many biotechnology/pharmaceutical companies. Companies already/soon producing generic biopharmaceuticals include Biopartners (Switzerland), Genemedix (UK), Sicor and Ivax (USA), Congene and Microbix (Canada) and BioGenerix (Germany). Genemedix, for example, secured approval for sale of a recombinant CSF in China in 2001 and is also commencing the manufacture of recombinant EPO. Sicor currently markets hGH and IFN-α in eastern Europe and various developing nations. A generic hGH also gained approval in both Europe and the USA in 2006.

To date (mid 2006), no gene-therapy-based product has thus far been approved for general medical use in the EU or USA, although one such product has been approved in China. Although gene therapy trials were initiated as far back as 1989, the results have been disappointing. Many technical difficulties remain in relation to, for example, gene delivery and regulation of expression. Product effectiveness was not apparent in the majority of trials undertaken and safety concerns have been raised in several trials.

Only one antisense-based product has been approved to date (in 1998) and, although several such antisense agents continue to be clinically evaluated, it is unlikely that a large number of such products will be approved over the next 3–4 years. Aptamers represent an additional emerging class of nucleic-acid-based therapeutic. These are short DNA- or RNA-based sequences that adopt a specific three-dimensional structure, enabling them to bind (and thereby inhibit) specific target molecules. One such product (Macugen) has been approved to date. RNA interference (RNAi) represents a yet additional mechanism of achieving downregulation of gene expression. It shares many characteristics with antisense technology and, like antisense, provides a potential means of treating medical conditions triggered or exacerbated by the inappropriate overexpression of specific gene products. Despite the disappointing results thus far generated by nucleic-acid-based products, future technical advances will almost certainly ensure the approval of gene therapy and antisense-based products in the intermediate to longer term future.

Technological developments in areas such as genomics, proteomics and high-throughput screening are also beginning to impact significantly upon the early stages of drug development. By linking changes in gene/protein expression to various disease states, for example, these technologies will identify new drug targets for such diseases. Many/most such targets will themselves be proteins, and drugs will be designed/developed specifically to interact with. They may be protein based or (more often) low molecular mass ligands. Additional future innovations likely to impact upon pharmaceutical biotechnology include the development of alternative product production systems, alternative methods of delivery and the development of engineered cell-based therapies, particularly stem cell therapy. As mentioned previously, protein-based biotechnology products produced to date are produced in either microbial or in animal cell lines. Work continues on the production of such products in transgenic-based production systems, specifically either transgenic plants or animals. Virtually all therapeutic proteins must enter the blood in order to promote a therapeutic effect. Such products must usually be administered parenterally. However, research continues on the development of non-parenteral routes which may prove more convenient, less costly and obtain improved patient compliance. Alternative potential delivery routes include transdermal, nasal, oral and bucal approaches, although most progress to date has been recorded with pulmonary-based delivery systems. An inhaled insulin product was approved in 2006 for the treatment of type I and II diabetes. A small number of whole-cell-based therapeutic products have also been approved to date. All contain mature, fully differentiated cells extracted from a native biological source. Improved techniques now allow the harvest of embryonic and, indeed, adult stem cells, bringing the development of stem-cell-based drugs one step closer. However, the use of stem cells to replace human cells or even entire tissues/organs remains a long term goal. Overall, therefore, products of pharmaceutical biotechnology play an important role in the clinic and are likely to assume an even greater relative importance in the future.

2

BUFFERS, BUFFERING AGENTS, AND IONIC EQUILIBRIA

It is well known that many drugs are unstable when exposed to certain acidic or basic conditions, and such information is routinely gathered during the preformulation stage of development. When such instabilities are identified, one tool of the formulation sciences is to include a buffering agent (or agents) in the dosage form with the hope that such excipients will impart sufficient stability to enable the formulation. The properties that enable buffering agents to function as such is derived from their qualities as weak acids or bases, and have their roots in their respective ionic equilibria.

AUTOIONIZATION OF WATER

Even the purest grade of water contains low concentrations of ions that can be detected by means of appropriate conductivity measurements. These ions arise from the transfer of a proton from a water molecule to another:

$$H_2O + H_2O \leftrightarrow H_3O^+ + OH^- \qquad ...(1)$$

In Eq. (1), H_3O^+ is known as the *hydronium ion*, and OH^- is known as the *hydroxide ion*. This reaction is reversible, and the reactants are known to proceed only slightly on to the products. Approximating the activity of the various species by their concentrations, one can write the equilibrium constant for this reaction as

$$K_C = \frac{[H_3O^+][OH^-]}{[H_2O]^2} \qquad ...(2)$$

In aqueous solutions, the concentration of water is effectively a constant (55.55 M), and so Eq. (2) simplifies to:

$$K_W = [H_3O^+][OH^-] \qquad ...(3)$$

K_W is known as the *autoionization constant* of water, and is sometimes identified as the *ion product* of water. The magnitude of KW is very small, being equal to 1.007×10^{-14} at a temperature of 25°C.

For the sake of convenience, Sorensen proposed the "p" scale, where numbers such as K_W would be expressed as the negative of their base 10 logarithms. The value of pK_W would then be calculated as

$$pK_W = -\log(K_W) \qquad ...(4)$$

and would have a value equal to 13.997 at 25°C. Defining pH as

$$pH = -\log[H_3O+] \qquad ...(5)$$

and

$$pOH = -\log[OH^-] \qquad ...(6)$$

then Eq. (3) can then be expressed as

$$pK_W = pH + pOH \qquad ...(7)$$

The autoionization of water is an endothermic reaction, so K_W increases as the temperature is increased.

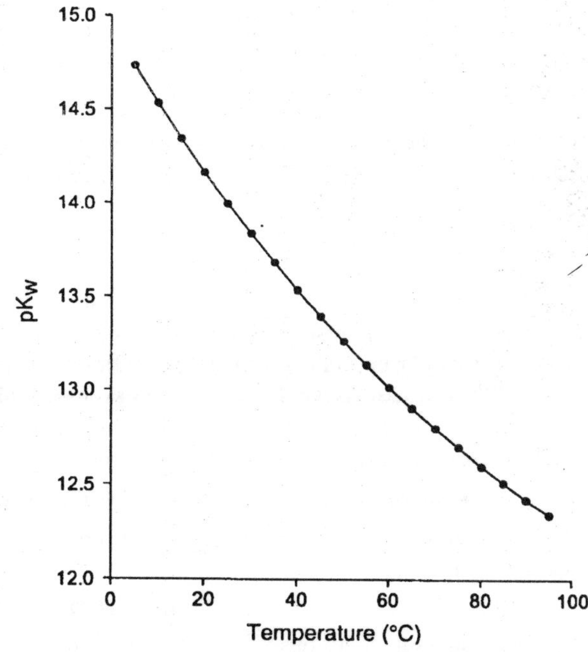

Fig. 2.1. Temperature dependence of the autoionization constant of water.

Ionic Equilibria of Acidic and Basic Substances

Of the numerous definitions of acids and bases that have been employed over the years, the 1923 definitions of J. N. Bronsted and T. M. Lowry have proven to be the most useful for discussions of ionic equilibria in aqueous systems. According to the Bronsted–Lowry model, an *acid* is a substance capable of donating a proton to another substance, such as water:

$$HA + H_2O \leftrightarrow H_3O^+ + A^- \qquad ...(8)$$

The acidic substance (HA) that originally donated the proton becomes the *conjugate base* (A^-) of that substance, because the conjugate base could conceivably accept a proton from an even stronger acid than the original substance. One can write the equilibrium constant expression corresponding to Eq. (8) as

$$K_C = \frac{[H_3O^+][A^-]}{[HA][H_2O]^2} \qquad ...(9)$$

But because $[H_2O]$ is a constant, one can collect the constants on the left-hand side of the equation to derive the acid *ionization constant* expression:

$$K_A = \frac{[H_3O^+][A^-]}{[HA]} \qquad ...(10)$$

And, of course, one can define pKA as

$$pK_A = -\log(K_A) \qquad ...(11)$$

A strong acid is a substance that reacts completely with water, so that the acid ionization constant defined in Eq. (10) or (11) is effectively infinite. This situation can only be achieved if the conjugate base of the strong acid is very weak. A weak acid will be characterized by an acid ionization constant that is considerably less than unity, so that the position of equilibrium in the reaction represented in Eq. (8) favors the existence of unreacted free acid.

A discussion of the ionic equilibria associated with basic substances parallels that just made for acidic substances. A base is a substance capable of accepting a proton donated by another substance, such as water:

$$B + H_2O \leftrightarrow BH^+ + OH^- \qquad ...(12)$$

The basic substance (B) that originally accepted the proton becomes the conjugate acid (BH^+) of that substance, because the conjugate acid could conceivably donate a proton to an even stronger base than the original substance. The equilibrium constant expression corresponding to Eq. (12) is:

$$K_C = \frac{[BH^+][OH^-]}{[B][H_2O]} \quad ...(13)$$

Because $[H_2O]$ is a constant, the constants are collected on the left-hand side of the equation to derive the *base ionization constant* expression:

$$K_B = \frac{[BH^+][OH^-]}{[B]} \quad ...(14)$$

pK_B is defined as

$$pK_B = -\log(K_B) \quad ...(15)$$

A strong base is a substance that reacts completely with water, so that the base ionization constant defined in Eq. (14) or (15) is effectively infinite. This situation can only be realized if the conjugate acid of the strong base is very weak. A weak base will be characterized by a base ionization constant that is considerably less than unity, so that the position of equilibrium in the reaction represented in Eq. (12) favors the existence of unreacted free base.

Ionic Equilibria of Conjugate Acids and Bases

Once formed, the conjugate base of an acidic substance (i.e., the anion of that acid) is also capable of reacting with water:

$$A^- + H_2O \leftrightarrow HA + OH^- \quad ...(16)$$

Because aqueous solutions of anions are commonly prepared by the dissolution of a salt containing that anion, reactions of the type described by Eq. (16) are often termed hydrolysis reactions. Eq. (16) is necessarily characterized by its base ionization constant expression:

$$K_B = \frac{[HA][OH^-]}{[A^-]} \quad ...(17)$$

and a corresponding pK_B defined in the usual manner, but because

$$[OH^-] = K_W/H_3O^+] \quad ...(18)$$

it follows that

$$K_B = \frac{[HA]K_W}{[A^-][H_3O^+]} \quad ...(19)$$

Eq. (19) contains the right-hand side expression of Eq. (10), so one deduces that

$$K_B = K_W/K_A \quad ...(20)$$

or

$$K_W = K_A K_B \quad ...(21)$$

The same relation between ionization constants of a conjugate acid–base pair can be developed if one were to begin with the conjugate acid of a basic substance, so Eq. 21 is recognized as a general property of conjugate acid–base pairs.

Ionic Equilibria of Buffer Systems

A buffer can be defined as a solution that maintains an approximately equal pH value even if small amounts of acidic or basic substances are added. To function in this manner, a buffer solution will necessarily contain either an acid and its conjugate base, or a base and its conjugate acid.

The action of a buffer system can be understood through the use of a practical example. Consider acetic acid, for which $K_A = 1.82 \times 10^{-5}$ ($pK = 4.74$). The following pH values can be calculated (for solutions having a total acetate content of 1.0 M) using its acid ionization constant expression:

Acetic acid, [HA]	*Acetate ion, [A⁻]*	Calculated pH
0.4	0.6	4.92
0.5	0.5	4.74
0.6	0.4	4.56

When an acidic substance is added to a buffer system it would immediately react with the basic component, as a basic substance would react with the acidic component. One therefore concludes from the table that the addition of either 0.1 M acid or 0.1 M base to a buffer system consisting of 0.5 M acetic acid and 0.5 M acetate ion would cause the pH to change by only 0.18 pH units. This is to be contrasted with the pH changes that would result from the addition of 0.1 M acid to water (i.e., 7.0 to 1.0, for a change of 6.0 pH units), or from the addition of 0.1 M base to water (i.e., 13.0 to 1.0, also for a change of 6.0 pH units).

A very useful expression for describing the properties of buffer system can be derived from consideration of ionization constant expressions. For an acidic substance, Eq. (10) can be rearranged as

$$[H_3O^+] = \frac{K_A[A^-]}{[HA]} \qquad \ldots(22)$$

Taking the negative of the base 10 logarithms of the various quantities yields the relation known as the Henderson–Hasselbach equation:

$$pH = pK_A + \log\{[A^-]/[HA]\} \qquad \ldots(23)$$

Eq. (23) indicates that when the concentration of acid and its conjugate base are equal (i.e., [HA] = [A⁻]), then the pH of the solution will equal the pK_A value. Therefore, a buffer system is chosen so that the target pH is approximately equal to the pK_A value.Viewed in this light, a buffer system can be envisioned as a partially completed neutralization reaction

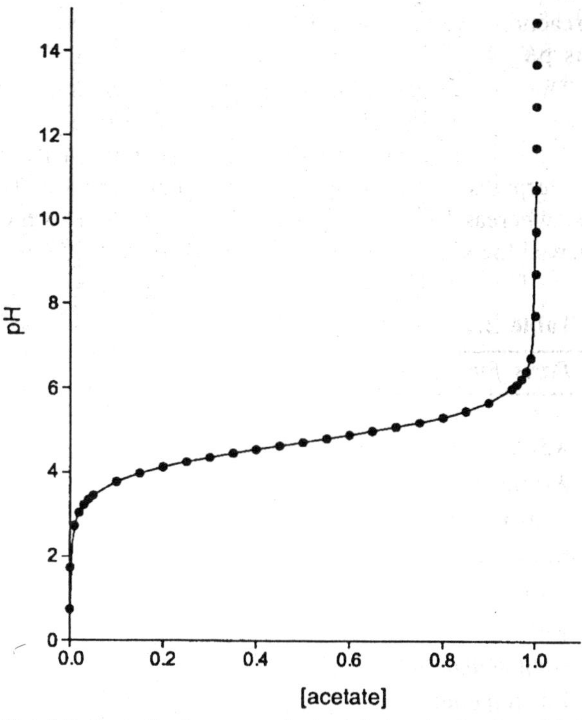

Fig. 2.2. Neutralization curve obtained during the titration of 1.0 M acetic acid, plotted as a function of the acetate ion concentration.

$$HA + OH^- \leftrightarrow A^- + H_2O \qquad \ldots(24)$$

where comparable amounts of HA and A⁻ are present in the solution. The buffer region within a neutralization reaction is shown in Fig. 2.2, where the horizontal region in the graph of anion concentration and observed pH reveals the buffer region of the system. For practical purposes, the buffer region would extend over [HA]/[A⁻] ratios of approximately 0.2 to 0.8.

Selection of an Appropriate Buffer System

The selection of a buffer system for use in a pharmaceutical dosage form is relatively straightforward. It is evident from the preceding discussion that the most important prerequisite for a buffer is the approximate equality of the pK_A value of the buffer with the intended optimal pH value for the formulation. Knowledge of the pH stability profile of a drug substance enables one to deduce the pH range for which formulation is desirable, and the basis for the most appropriate buffer system would be the weak acid or base whose pK_A or pK_B value was numerically equal to the midpoint of the pH range of stability.

There are, of course, other considerations that need to be monitored, such as compatibility with the drug substance. Boylan has provided a summary of the selection criteria for buffering agents:

1. The buffer must have adequate capacity in the desired pH range.
2. The buffer must be biologically safe for the intended use.
3. The buffer should have little or no deleterious effect on the stability of the final product.
4. The buffer should permit acceptable flavoring and coloring of the product.

A practical consequence of Eq. (23) is that as long as the concentration of a buffer is not overcome by reaction demands, a buffer system will exhibit adequate capacity within $\pm$ 1 pH unit with respect to its pK_A or pK_B value.

The second criterion from the preceding list restricts buffering agents to those deemed to be pharmaceutically acceptable. The use of buffering agents is most critical for parenteral formulations, and it has been noted over the years that phosphate, citrate, and acetate are most commonly used for such purposes. Ethanolamine and diethanolamine are also used to adjust pH and form their corresponding salts, whereas lysine and glycine are often used to buffer protein and peptide formulations. Akers has reviewed the scope of drug-excipient interactions in parenteral formulations and has provided an overview of the effect of buffers on drug substance stability.

Table 2.1. Acids and bases suitable for use as buffer systems in pharmaceutical products

Basis for buffering system	*pK_1*	*pK_2*	*pK_3*
Acetic acid	4.56	—	—
Adipic acid	5.03	4.26	—
Arginine	9.01	2.05	—
Benzoic acid	4.00	—	—
Boric acid	8.97	—	—
Carbonic acid	10.00	6.16	—
Citric acid	5.69	4.35	2.87
Diethanolamine	8.90	—	—
Ethanolamine	9.52	—	—
Ethylenediamine	9.89	7.08	—
Glutamic acid	9.59	4.20	—
Glycine	9.57	2.36	—
Lactic acid	3.66	—	—
Lysine	10.69	9.08	2.04
Maleic acid	5.83	1.75	—
Phosphoric acid	11.74	6.72	2.00
Tartaric acid	3.95	2.82	—
Triethanolamine	7.80	—	—
Tromethamine	8.09	—	—

Buffers in Pharmaceutical Systems

It is well known that the stability of many active pharmaceutical substances can be strongly dependent on the degree of acidity or basicity to which they are exposed, and that a change in pH can cause significant changes in the rate of degradation reactions. For such compounds, formulators commonly include a buffer system to ensure the stability of the drug substance either during the shelf life of the product, or during the period associated with its administration.

In addition, preformulation scientists routinely use buffer systems to set the pH of a medium in which they intend to perform experimentation. For instance, the pH stability profile of a drug substance is routinely obtained through the use of buffers, and the pH dependence of solubility is frequently measured using buffered systems. However, the possibility that the buffer system itself may influence or alter the results must be considered in these studies.

Stabilization of Drug Substances in Formulations by Buffers

As mentioned previously, the stability of parenteral formulations is often established through the use of buffer systems. The inclusion of a phosphate buffer in homatropine hydrobromide ophthalmic solution enabled formulators to fix the solution pH at 6.8, enabling the product to be lyophilized. This lyophilized product could be stored for extended periods without degradation. Tromethamine was found to effect a stabilizing effect on N-nitrosoureas (such as lomustine, carmustine, and tauromustine) in aqueous solutions. It has been reported that replacing succinate buffer with glycolate buffer improved the stability of lyophilized γ-interferon. In this work, it was found that the succinate buffer could crystallize in the frozen state, which limited its ability to maintain the appropriate pH, and therefore led to degradation. On the other hand, use of the glycolate buffer appeared to minimize the freeze-induced pH shifting, and the lyophilized product exhibited superior solid-state stability.

Table 2.2. Some of the buffer systems used to stabilize various parenteral products

Basis for buffering system	*Product trade name*
Acetic acid	Miacalcin injection
Benzoic acid	Valium injection
Citric acid	Aldomet injection
	Ceredase
	Cerezyme
	Duracillin A.S.
Diethanolamine	Bactrim IV
Glycine	Hep-B Gammagee
Lactic acid	Ergotrate maleate
	Fentenyl citrate and Droperidol
Maleic acid	Librium injection
Monoethanolamine	Terramycin solution
Phosphoric acid	Humegon
	Zantac injection Pregnyl
	Prolastin Synthroid
Tartaric acid	Compazine injection
	Methergine injection
	Priscoline injection
Tromethamine	Optiray

However, the use of buffers in parenterals is not always benign, and numerous instances have been summarized where buffers or other excipients have caused stability problems. For instance, the complexation of Ca(II) and Al(III) with phosphate buffer solutions has been studied at great length, as well as the kinetic characteristics of the subsequent precipitation of calcium and aluminum phosphate salts. The use of metal complexing excipients, such as citric acid or ethylenediaminetetraacetic acid, was found to be useful in delaying the onset of precipitation. The use of buffering agents in solid dose forms is not as widespread as the use in parenteral products. Nevertheless, the current Handbook of Pharmaceutical Excipients lists calcium carbonate, monobasic and dibasic sodium phosphate, sodium and potassium citrates, and tribasic calcium phosphate as potential buffering agents.

In one study, the effect of 11 different compounds representing various classes of buffering agents were studied with respect to their effect on the dissolution kinetics of aspirin from tablet formulations. It was found that buffering agents capable of reacting with acidic substances to evolve carbon dioxide (sodium bicarbonate, magnesium carbonate, or calcium carbonate) yielded the fastest dissolution rates, and hence were deduced to be more useful as tablet excipients. Less effective were water-soluble buffering agents (such as sodium ascorbate or sodium citrate), and least effective were water-insoluble buffering agents (such as magnesium oxide, magnesium trisilicate, dihydroxyaluminum aminoacetate, or aluminum hydroxide).

In another study, the kinetics of aspirin, salicylic acid, and salicyluric acid were followed upon oral administration of aspirin as either an unbuffered tablet or two buffered solutions. Significant differences in the absorption rates were observed, with the solution having 16 mEq of buffer being the fastest, the solution having 34 mEq of buffer being intermediate, and the unbuffered tablet being the slowest. These studies demonstrate that inclusion of a buffering agent in a tablet formulation of an acid-sensitive compound will lead to the generation of better dosage forms.

Use of Buffers to Study the pH Stability Profile of Drug Substances

The evaluation of the pH stability profile of a drug substance is an essential task within the scope of pre- formulation studies. Knowing the pH conditions under which a given compound will be stable is of vital importance to the chemists seeking to develop methods of synthesis, to analytical scientists seeking to develop methods for analysis, and to formulators seeking to develop a stable drug product. Typically, the preformulation scientist will prepare solutions of the drug substance in a variety of buffer systems, and will then determine the amount of drug substance remaining after a predefined storage period. However, for the information to be useful, the investigator will also need to verify that the buffer itself does not have an effect on the observed reactions.

The hydrolysis kinetics of vidarabine-5′-phosphate were studied at a variety of pH values that enabled the compound to exist as its protonated, neutral, and monoionized form. It was found that the hydrolysis reaction followed first-order kinetics at the five pH conditions tested, and that the buffer system used did not influence the reaction rates. The pH–rate profile suggested that even though the compound was most stabile over pH 9.0 to 9.5, the stability at pH 7.4 (i.e., physiological pH) was more than adequate for development of a parenteral formulation.

The degradation kinetics of phentolamine hydrochloride were studied over a pH range of 1.2 to 7.2 and in various glycol solutions. The kinetics were determined to be first order over all pH values studied, and a consideration of the ionization constant of the compound indicated that only the protonated form of the compound had been studied. At relatively low acidities, a pH-independent region (pH 3.1–4.9) was noted for the hydrolysis, and the kinetics were not affected by the concentration of buffer used. However, the degradation reaction was found to proceed at a much faster rate at a pH of 7.2, and a small dependence of rate constant on the concentration of phosphate in the buffer system was noted. Other examples where buffers were successfully used to study the pH stability of drug substances (and where little or no effect could be ascribed to the buffer system used) include the chemical stability of diisoxazolyl-naphthoquinone and metronidazole in aqueous solution. In another detailed study, the effect of pH, buffer species, medium ionic strength, and temperature on the stability of azetazolamide was studied.

There are probably as many instances where buffer catalysis exerts a strong influence on pH stability studies as where no such effect exists. For instance, the kinetics associated with the acid/base hydrolysis of ciclosidomine were found to be strongly affected by the concentration of buffer used to set the solution pH for each study. However, because a linear relationship was found between buffer concentration and observed first-order rate constant, the effect of pH on the degradation was assessed by extrapolating to zero buffer concentration. This information was used to deduce the buffer-independent pH–rate profile.

In another study on solutions of spironolactone, the concentration of buffer was found to exert a strong influence on the degradation rate constants. At the same time, the ionic strength of the medium did not appear to affect the rate constants. The decomposition pathway for aqueous solutions of batanopride hydrochloride was found to depend on the pH of the medium used for the study, although the concentration of buffer was found to exert catalytic effects.

To those beginning work in this field, the study reported by Zhou and Notari on the kinetics of ceftazidime degradation in aqueous solutions may be used as a study design template. First-order rate constants were determined for the hydrolysis of this compound at several pH values and at several temperatures. The kinetics were separated into buffer- independent and buffer-dependent contributions, and the temperature dependence in these was used to calculate the activation energy of the degradation via the Arrhenius equation. Ceftazidime hydrolysis rate constants were calculated as a function of pH, temperature, and buffer by combining the pH–rate expression with the buffer contributions calculated from the buffer catalytic constants and the temperature dependencies. These equations and their parameter values were able to calculate over 90% of the 104 experimentally determined rate constants with errors less than 10%.

Use of Buffers to Study the pH Dependence of Drug Substance Solubility

An evaluation of the effect of pH on the aqueous solubility of a drug substance is an essential component of preformulation research, and such work is usually conducted along with determinations of ionization constants, solubilization mechanisms, and dissolution rates. Methods for the determination of the solubility of pharmaceutical solids have been discussed at length, and a large number of pH–solubility profiles have been published in the 30 volumes of the Analytical Profiles series. A general treatment of the characteristics of the pH–solubility profiles of weak acids and bases is available.

When the pH conditions used for a given solubility determination are set through the use of buffers, the possible solubilization of the buffering systems must be established. For instance, no buffer effect was reported during the determination of the solubilities of trimethoprim and sulfamethoxazole at various pH values. On the other hand, correction for buffer effects was made during studies of some isoxazolyl-naphthoquinone derivatives.

With the continuing development of compounds exhibiting low degrees of intrinsic aqueous solubility, the combination of pH control and complexing agents in formulations has become important, and buffers play an important role in many of these formulations. A theoretical analysis of the synergistic effect observed in the combined systems has been developed and used to explain the solubilization noted for flavopiridol. In a subsequent work, the solubilization of this substance by pH control combined with cosolvents, surfactants, or complexing agents was investigated.

The combined effect of pH and surfactants on the dissolution of piroxicam has been reported. In this system, the dissolution rate and solubility of the drug substance could be well estimated by a simple additive model for the effect of pH and surfactant, where the total dissolved concentration equaled the summation of the amount of dissolved non-ionized substance, the amount of dissolved ionized substance, and the amount of substance solubilized in the surfactant micelles. It was suggested that the model developed in this work could be useful in establishing an in vitro–in vivo correlation for piroxicam.

An equilibrium-based model was proposed to characterize the drug–surfactant interactions observed in the system consisting of furbiprofen and polysorbate 80 in solutions of different pH. The model reflected both interactions and interdependence among all drug- containing species, namely, non-ionized drug in water, ionized drug in water, non-ionized drug in micelles, and ionized drug in micelles. The mathematical treatment also enabled modeling of the drug solubilization in the pH–surfactant solutions without requiring the use of inappropriate approximations. It was found that the solubility data estimated by the proposed model were more reliable when the surfactant concentration was high in the system. This finding confirmed that that consideration of interrelations and interdependence of all drug species in the various solutions was appropriate for this model. Buffers and buffering agents have been widely used for the stabilization of pharmaceutical formulations, and this aspect has proven to be especially important for parenteral products. Buffers and buffering agents have also been found to play a vitally important role during drug characterization studies, being vitally important to the conduct of solubility and drug stability studies. The range of pharmaceutically acceptable buffer systems spans all useful pH values, and it can be said that there is a buffer available for every intended purpose.

3

BIOPHARMACEUTICS

Biopharmaceutics is the study of the interrelationship of the physicochemical properties of the drug [*active pharmaceutical ingredient*, (API)] and the drug product (dosage form in which the drug is fabricated) based on the biological performance of the drug.

Biopharmaceutics also considers the impact of the various manufacturing methods and technologies on the intended performance of the drug product. Biopharmaceutics uses quantitative methods and theoretical models to evaluate the effect of the drug substance, dosage form, and routes of drug administration on the therapeutic requirements of the drug and drug product in a physiological environment.

Bioavailability is often used as a measure of the biological performance of the drug and is defined as a measure of the rate and extent (amount) to which the active ingredient or active moiety becomes available at the site of action. Bioavailability is also a measure of the rate and extent of therapeutically active drug that is systemically absorbed.

Biopharmaceutics allows for rational design of drug products to deliver the drug at a specific rate to the body in order to optimize the therapeutic effect and minimize any adverse effects. Biopharmaceutics is based on the physicochemical characteristics of the active drug substance, the desired drug product, and considerations of the anatomy and physiology of the human body. Inherent in the design of a suitable drug product is knowledge of the pharmacodynamics of the drug, including the desired onset time, duration, and intensity of clinical response, and the pharmacokinetics of the drug including absorption, distribution, elimination, and target drug concentration.

Thus, biopharmaceutics involves factors that influence the: (1) protection and stability of the drug within the drug product; (2) the rate of drug release from the drug product; (3) the rate of dissolution of the drug at the absorption site; and (4) the availability of the drug at its site of action.

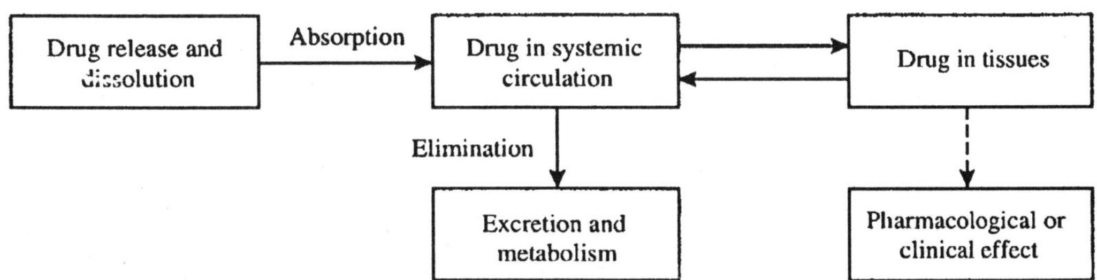

Fig. 3.1. Scheme demonstrating the dynamic relationships among the drug, the product, and pharmacologic effect.

Biopharmaceutic Considerations in Drug Product Design

Drugs are generally given to a patient as a manufactured drug product (finished dosage form) that includes the active drug and selected ingredients (excipients) that make up the dosage form. Common pharmaceutical dosage forms include liquids, tablets, capsules, injections, suppositories, transdermal systems, and topical drug products. The formulation and manufacture of a drug product requires a thorough understanding of the biopharmaceutics.

Each route of drug application presents special biopharmaceutic considerations in drug product design. Systemic drug absorption from an extravascular site is influenced by the anatomic and physiologic properties of the site and the physicochemical properties of the drug and the drug product. The anatomy, physiology, and the contents of the gastrointestinal tract (GI) are considered in the design of a drug product for oral administration. For example, considerations in the design of a vaginal tablet formulation for the treatment of a fungus infection include whether the ingredients are compatible with vaginal anatomy and physiology, whether the drug is systemically absorbed from the vagina and how the vaginal tablet is to be properly inserted and placed in the appropriate area for optimum efficacy. Requirements for an eye medication include pH, isotonicity, sterility, local irritation to the cornea, draining of the drug by tears, and concern for systemic drug absorption. An additional consideration might be the contact time of the medication with the cornea. Although, increased eye contact time might be achieved by an increase in viscosity of the ophthalmic solution, the patient may lose some visual acuity when a viscous product is administered. Biopharmaceutic considerations for a drugs administered by intramuscular injection include, local irritation, drug dissolution, and drug absorption from the injection site.

Biopharmaceutic studies may be performed using in vitro or in vivo methods. In vitro methods are useful to understand the physicochemical properties of the drug and drug product and to evaluate the quality of the manufacturing process. Ultimately, the drug must be studied in vivo, in humans to assess drug efficacy, including the pharmacodynamic, pharmacokinetic, therapeutic and toxic profiles. Drug dissolution, absorption, metabolism, and potential interaction with food and other components in the GI tract are major biopharmaceutic topics for research and regulatory considerations in drug development.

A drug given by intravenous administration is considered complete or 100% bioavailable because the drug is placed directly into the systemic circulation. By carefully choosing the route of drug administration and proper design of the drug product, drug bioavailability can be varied from rapid and complete systemic drug absorption to a slow, sustained rate of absorption or even virtually no absorption, depending on the therapeutic objective. Once the drug is systemically absorbed, normal physiologic processes for distribution and elimination occur, which usually is not influenced by the specific formulation of the drug. The rate of drug release from the product, and the rate of drug absorption, are important in determining the onset, intensity, and duration of drug action of the drug.

Rate-limiting Steps in Oral Drug Absorption

Systemic drug absorption from a drug product consists of a succession of rate processes. For solid oral, immediate release drug products (e.g., tablet, capsule), the rate processes include: (1) disintegration of the drug product and subsequent release of the drug; (2) dissolution of the drug in an aqueous environment; and (3) absorption across cell membranes into the systemic circulation. In the process of drug disintegration, dissolution, and absorption, the rate at which drug reaches the circulatory system is determined by the slowest step in the sequence.

The slowest step in a kinetic process is the rate- limiting step. Except for controlled release products, disintegration of a solid oral drug product is usually more rapid than drug dissolution and drug

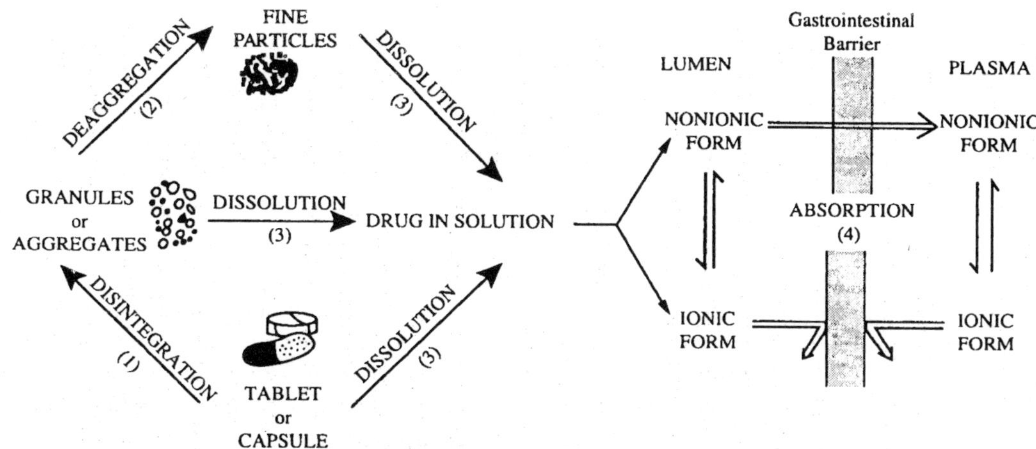

Fig. 3.2. Summary of processes involved following the oral administration of a drug in tablet or capsule form.

absorption. For drugs that have very poor aqueous solubility, the rate at which the drug dissolves (dissolution) is often the slowest step, and therefore exerts a rate-limiting effect on drug bioavailability. In contrast, for a drug that has a high aqueous solubility, the dissolution rate is rapid and the rate at which the drug crosses or permeates cell membranes is the slowest or rate-limiting step.

PHYSIOLOGIC FACTORS AFFECTING DRUG ABSORPTION

Passage of Drugs Across Cell Membranes

For systemic absorption, a drug must pass from the absorption site through or around one or more layers of cells to gain access into the general circulation. The permeability of a drug at the absorption site into the systemic circulation is intimately related to the molecular structure of the drug and the physical and biochemical properties of the cell membranes. For absorption into the cell, a drug must traverse the cell membrane. Transcellular absorption is the process of a drug movement across a cell. Some polar molecules may not be able to traverse the cell membrane, but instead, go through gaps or "*tight junctions*" between cells, a process known as *paracellular* drug absorption. Some drugs are probably absorbed by a mixed mechanism involving one or more processes.

Passive diffusion

Passive diffusion is the process by which molecules spontaneously diffuse from a region of higher concentration to a region of lower concentration. This process is passive because no external energy is expended. Drug molecules move randomly forward and back across a membrane. If the two regions have the same drug concentration, forward-moving drug molecules will be balanced by molecules moving back, resulting in no net transfer of drug. For a region that has a higher drug concentration, the number of forward-moving drug molecules will be higher than the number of backward-moving molecules, resulting in a transfer of molecules to the region with the lower drug concentration, as indicated by the big arrow. Flux is the rate of drug transfer and is represented by a vector to show its direction. Molecules tend to move randomly in all directions because molecules possess kinetic energy and constantly collide with each another in space. Only left and right molecule movements are shown in Fig. 3.3, because

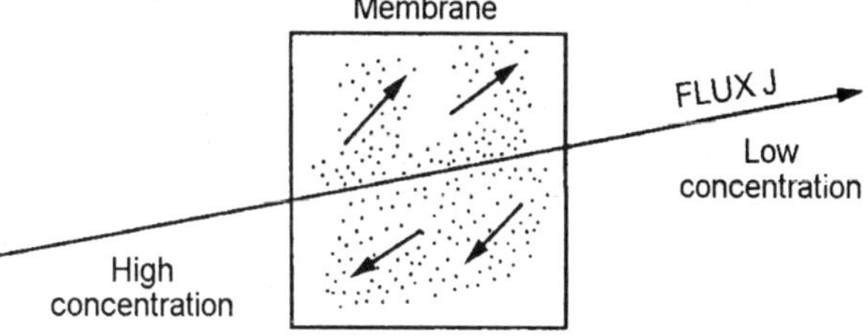

Fig. 3.3. Passive diffusion of molecules.

movement of molecules in other directions would not result in concentration changes because of the limitation of the container wall.

Passive diffusion is the major transmembrane process for most drugs. The driving force for passive diffusion is the difference in drug concentrations on either side of the cell membrane. According to Fick' s Law of Diffusion, drug molecules diffuse from a region of high drug concentration to a region of low drug concentration

$$dQ/dt = \{DAK/h\}(C_{GI} - C_p)$$

where dQ/dt = rate of diffusion; D = diffusion coefficient; K = partition coefficient; A = surface area of membrane; h = membrane thickness; and $C_{GI} - C_p$ = difference between the concentrations of drug in the GI tract and in the plasma.

Drug distributes rapidly into a large volume after entering the blood resulting in a very low plasma drug concentration with respect to the concentration at the site of drug administration. Drug is usually given in milligram doses, whereas plasma drug concentrations are often in the microgram per milliliter or nanogram per milliliter range. For drugs given orally, $C_{GI} > C_p$. A large concentration gradient is maintained driving drug molecules into the plasma from the GI tract.

As shown by Fick' s Law of Diffusion, lipid solubility of the drug and the surface area and the thickness of the membrane influence the rate of passive diffusion of drugs. The partition coefficient, *K*, represents the lipid–water partitioning of a drug. More lipid soluble drugs have larger *K* values that theoretically increase the rate of systemic drug absorption. In practice, drug absorption is influenced by other physical factors of the drug, limiting its practical application of *K*. The surface area of the membrane through which the drug is absorbed directly influences the rate of drug absorption. Drugs may be absorbed from most areas of the GI tract. However, the duodenal area of the small intestine shows the most rapid drug absorption due to such anatomic features as villi and microvilli, which provide a large surface area. These villi are not found in such numbers in other areas of the GI tract.

The membrane thickness, *h*, is a constant at the absorption site but may be altered by disease. Drugs usually diffuse very rapidly into tissues through capillary cell membranes in the vascular compartments. In the brain, the capillaries are densely lined with glial cells creating a thicker lipid barrier (blood–brain barrier) causing a drug to diffuse more slowly into brain. In certain disease states (e.g., meningitis) the cell membranes may be disrupted or become more permeable to drug diffusion.

Many drugs have lipophilic and hydrophilic substituents. More lipid soluble drug molecules traverse cell membranes more easily than less lipid-soluble (i.e., more water-soluble) molecules. For weak electrolyte drugs (i.e., weak acids, bases), the extent of ionization influences drug solubility and the rate of drug transport. Ionized drugs are more water soluble than non- ionized drugs which are more lipid soluble. The extent of ionization of a weak electrolyte depends on the pKa of the drug and the partition hypothesis (pH) of the medium in which the drug is dissolved. The Henderson and Hasselbalch equation describes the ratio of ionized (charged) to unionized form of the drug and is dependent on the pH conditions and the pKa of the drug:

$$\text{Ratio} = -\frac{(\text{salt})}{(\text{acid})} = \frac{(\text{A}^-}{(\text{HA})} = 10^{(\text{pH}-\text{pKa})}$$

For weak acids,

$$\text{Ratio} = -(\text{base})(\text{salt}) = (\text{RNH})2\ (\text{RNH}^{+3})$$
$$= 10^{(\text{pH}-\text{pKa})}$$

According to the pH, a weak acid (e.g., salicylic acid) should be rapidly absorbed from the stomach (pH 1.2) due to a favorable concentration gradient of the unionized (more lipid soluble) drug from the stomach to the blood, because practically all the drug in the blood compartment is dissociated (ionized) at pH 7.4. A weak base (e.g., quinidine) is highly ionized in acid pH and is poorly absorb from the stomach. Although many drugs obey by the pH, in practice, the major site of absorption of most drugs is usually in the small intestine (duodenum) due presence of a large surface area and high blood flow.

The drug concentration on either side of a membrane is also influenced by the affinity of the drug for a tissue component, which prevents the drug from freely moving back across the cell membrane. For example, drug that binds plasma or tissue proteins causes the drug to concentrate in that region. Dicumarol and sulfonamides strongly bind plasma proteins; whereas, chlordane, a lipid-soluble insecticide, partitions and concentrates into adipose (fat) tissue. Tetracycline forms a complex with calcium and concentrates in the bones and teeth. Drugs may concentrate in a tissue due to a specific uptake or active transport process. Such processes have been demonstrated for iodide in thyroid tissue, potassium in the intracellular water, and certain catecholamines in adrenergic storage sites.

Carrier-mediated transport

Theoretically, a lipophilic drug may pass through the cell or go around it. If drug has a low molecular weight and is lipophilic, the lipid cell membrane is not a barrier to drug diffusion and absorption. In the intestine, molecules smaller than 500 MW may be absorbed by paracellular drug absorption. Numerous specialized carrier-mediated transport systems are present in the body especially in the intestine for the absorption of ions and nutrients required by the body.

Active transport

Active transport is a carrier-mediated transmembrane process that is important for GI absorption of some drugs and also involved in the renal and biliary secretion of many drugs and metabolites. A carrier binds the drug to form a carrier-drug complex that shuttles the drug across the membrane and then dissociates the drug on the other side of the membrane. Active transport is an energy-consuming system characterized by the transport of drug against a concentration gradient, that is, from regions of low drug concentrations to regions of high concentrations. A drug may be actively transported, if the drug molecule structurally resembles a natural substrate that is actively transported. A few lipid-insoluble drugs that resemble natural physiologic metabolites (e.g., 5-fluorouracil) are absorbed from the GI tract by this process. Drugs of similar structure may compete for adsorption sites on the carrier. Because only a certain amount of carrier is available, the binding sites on the carrier may become saturated at high drug concentrations. In contrast, passive diffusion is not saturable.

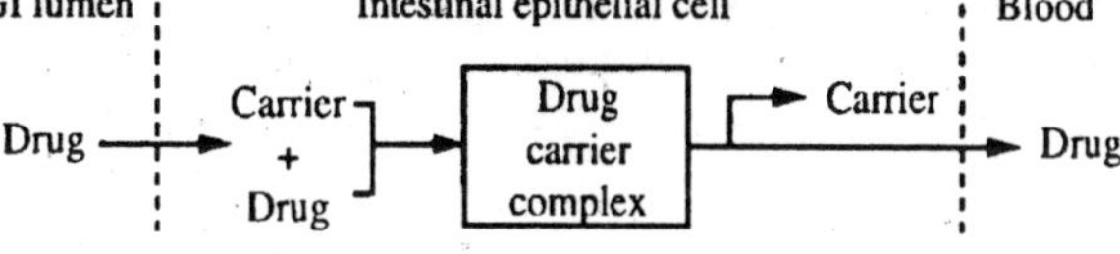

Fig. 3.4. Hypothetical carrier-mediated transport process.

Facilitated diffusion

Facilitated diffusion is a non- energy requiring, carrier-mediated transport system in which the drug moves along a concentration gradient (i.e., moves from a region of high drug concentration to a region of low drug concentration). Facilitated diffusion is saturable, structurally selective for the drug and shows competition kinetics for drugs of similar structure. Facilitated diffusion seems to play a very minor role in drug absorption.

Carrier-mediated intestinal transport

Various carrier mediated systems (transporters) are present at the intestinal brush border and basolateral membrane for the absorption of specific ions and nutrients essential for the body. Many drugs are absorbed by these carriers because of the structural similarity to natural substrates. An intestinal transmembrane protein, P-Glycoprotein (P-Gp) appears to reduce apparent intestinal epithelial cell permeability from lumen to blood for various lipophilic or cytotoxic drugs. Other transporters are present in the intestines. For example, many oral cephalosporins are absorbed through the amino acid transporter.

Vesicular transport

Vesicular transport is the process of engulfing particles or dissolved materials by the cell. Pinocytosis refers to the engulfment of small solutes or fluid, whereas phagocytosis refers to the engulfment of larger particles or macromolecules generally by macrophages. Endocytosis and exocytosis are the processes of moving macromolecules into and out of a cell, respectively.

During pinocytosis or phagocytosis, the cell membrane invaginates to surround the material, and then engulfs the material into the cell. Subsequently, the cell membrane containing the material forms a vesicle or vacuole within the cell. Vesicular transport is the proposed process for the absorption of orally administered sabin polio vaccine and various large proteins. An example of exocytosis is the transport of a protein such as insulin from insulin-producing cells of the pancreas into the extracellular space. The insulin molecules are first packaged into intracellular vesicles, which then fuse with the plasma membrane to release the insulin outside the cell.

Oral Drug Absorption

Physiologic Considerations

Drugs may be administered by various routes of administration. Except for intravenous drug administration, drugs are absorbed into the systemic circulation from the site of administration and are greatly affected by conditions at the administration site. Oral administration is the most common route of drug administration. Major physiologic processes in the GI system include secretion, digestion, and absorption. Secretion includes the transport of fluid, electrolytes, peptides, and proteins into the lumen of the alimentary canal. Enzymes in saliva and pancreatic secretions are involved in the digestion of carbohydrates and proteins. Other secretions such as mucus protect the linings of the lumen of the GI tract. Digestion is the breakdown of food constituents into smaller structures in preparation for absorption. Both drug and food constituents are mostly absorbed in the proximal area (duodenum) of the small intestinal. The process of absorption is the entry of constituents from the lumen of the gut into the body. Absorption may be considered as the net result of both lumen-to-blood and blood-to-lumen transport movements. Drugs administered orally pass through various parts of the enteral canal including the oral cavity, esophagus, and various parts of the GI tract. Residues eventually exit the body through the anus. Drugs may be absorbed by passive diffusion from all parts of the alimentary canal including sublingual, buccal, GI, and rectal absorption. For most drugs, the optimum site for drug absorption after oral administration is the upper portion of the small intestine or duodenum region. The unique anatomy of the duodenum provides an immense surface area for the drug to passively diffuse. In addition, the duodenal region is highly perfused with a network of capillaries, which helps to maintain a concentration gradient from the intestinal lumen and plasma circulation.

The total transit time, including gastric emptying, small intestinal transit, and colonic transit ranges from 0.4 to 5 days. Small intestine transit time (SITT) ranges from 3 to 4 h for most healthy subjects. If absorption is not completed by the time a drug leaves the small intestine, drug absorption may be erratic or incomplete. The small intestine is normally filled with digestive juices and liquids, keeping the lumen contents fluid. In contrast, the fluid in the colon is reabsorbed, and the lumen content in the colon is either semisolid or solid, making further drug dissolution erratic and difficult.

GI motility

Once the drug is given orally, the exact location and/or environment of the drug product within the GI tract is difficult to discern. GI motility tends to move the drug through the alimentary canal so that it may not stay at the absorption site. For drugs given orally, an anatomic absorption window may exist within the GI tract in which the drug is efficiently absorbed. Drugs contained in a non-biodegradable controlled-release dosage form must be completely released into this absorption window prior to the movement of the dosage form into the large bowel. The transit time of the drug in the GI tract depends upon the pharmacologic properties of the drug, type of dosage form, and various physiologic factors. Physiologic movement of the drug within the GI tract depends upon whether the alimentary canal contains recently ingested food or is in the fasted or interdigestive state.

Gastric emptying time

After oral administration, the swallowed drug rapidly reaches the stomach. Because the duodenum has the greatest capacity for the absorption of drugs from the GI tract, a delay in the gastric emptying time will slow the rate and possibly the extent of drug absorption from the duodenum, thereby prolonging the onset time for the drug. Drugs, such as penicillin, that are unstable in acid, may decompose if stomach emptying is delayed. Other drugs, (e.g., aspirin) may irritate the gastric mucosa during prolonged contact. Factors that tend to delay gastric emptying include consumption of meals high in fat, cold beverages, and anticholinergic drugs. Liquids and small particles less than 1 mm are generally not retained in the stomach. These small particles are believed to be emptied due to a slightly higher basal pressure in the stomach over the duodenum. Different constituents of a meal will empty from the stomach at different rates. For example, liquids are generally emptied faster than digested solids from the stomach. Large particles, including tablets and capsules, are delayed from emptying for 3–6 h by the presence of food in the stomach. Indigestible solids empty very slowly, probably during the inter- digestive phase, a phase in which food is not present and the stomach is less motile but periodically empties its content due to housekeeper wave contraction.

Intestinal motility

Normal peristaltic movements mix the contents of the duodenum, bringing the drug particles into intimate contact with the intestinal mucosal cells. The drug must have a sufficient time (residence time) at the absorption site for optimum absorption. In the case of high motility in the intestinal tract, as in diarrhea, the drug has a very brief residence time and less opportunity for adequate absorption.

Blood perfusion of the GI tract

The blood flow is important in carrying the absorbed drug from the absorption site to the systemic circulation. A large network of capillaries and lymphatic vessels perfuse the duodenal region and peritoneum. The splanchnic circulation receives about 28% of the cardiac output and is increased after meals. Drugs are absorbed from the small intestine into the mesenteric vessels which flows to the hepatic-portal vein and then to the liver prior to reaching the systemic circulation. Any decrease in mesenteric blood flow, as in the case of congestive heart failure, will decrease the rate of systemic drug absorption from the intestinal tract.

Some drugs may be absorbed into the lymphatic circulation through the lacteal or lymphatic vessels under the microvilli. Absorption of drugs through the lymphatic system bypasses the first-pass effect due to liver metabolism, because drug absorption through the hepatic portal vein is avoided. The lymphatics are important in the absorption of dietary lipids and may be partially responsible for the absorption for some lipophilic drugs such as bleomycin or aclarubicin which may dissolve in chylomicrons and be systemically absorbed via the lymphatic system.

Effect of food and other factors on GI drug absorption

Digested foods may affect intestinal pH and solubility of drugs. Food effects are not always predictable. The absorption of some antibiotics (e.g., penicillin, tetracycline) is decreased with food, whereas other drugs (e.g., griseofulvin) are better absorbed when given with food containing a high fat content. Food in the GI lumen stimulates the flow of bile. Bile contains bile acids. Bile acids are surfactants are involved in the digestion and solubilization of fats, and increases the solubility of fat-soluble drugs through micelle formation. For some basic drugs (e.g., cinnarizine) with limited aqueous solubility, the presence of food in the stomach stimulates hydrochloric acid secretion, which lowers the pH, causing more rapid dissolution of the drug and better absorption.

Generally, the bioavailability of drugs is better in patients in the fasted state and with a large volume of water. However, to reduce GI mucosal irritation, drugs such as erythromycin, iron salts, aspirin, and non-steroidal anti-inflammatory agents (NSAIDs) are given with food. The rate of absorption for these drugs may be reduced in the presence of food, but the extent of absorption may be the same. The drug dosage form may also be affected by food. For example, enteric-coated tablets may stay in the stomach for a longer period of time because food delays stomach emptying. If the enteric-coated tablet does not reach the duodenum rapidly, drug release and subsequent systemic drug absorption

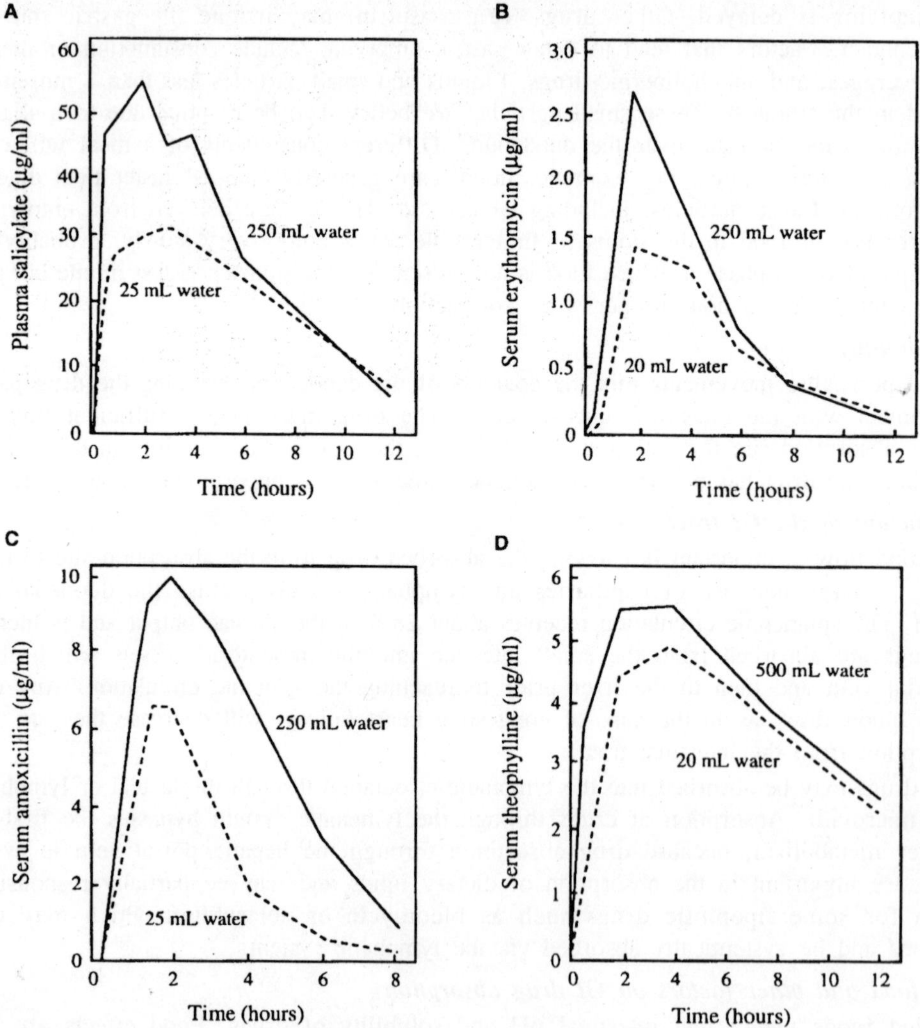

Fig. 3.5. Mean plasma or serum drug levels in healthy, fasting human volunteers who received single oral doses of aspirin tablets, erythromycin stearate capsules, and theophylline tablets, together with large.

are delayed. In contrast, enteric-coated beads or microparticles disperse in the stomach, are less affected by food, and demonstrate more consistent drug absorption from the duodenum.

Food may also affect the integrity of the dosage form, causing an alteration in the release rate of the drug. For example, theophylline bioavailability from Theo-24 controlled-release tablets is much more rapid when given to a subject in the fed rather than fasted state.

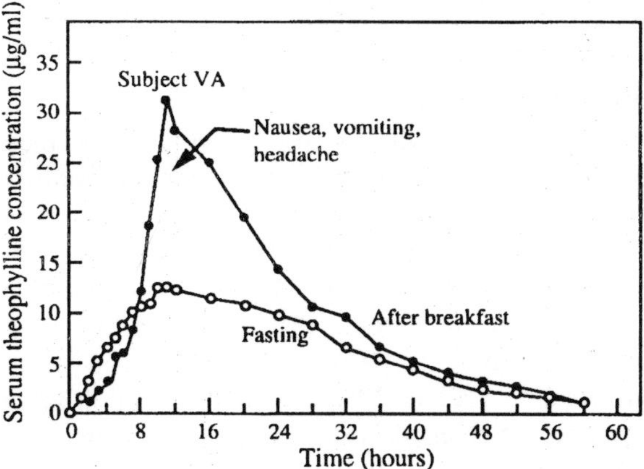

Fig. 3.6. Theophylline serum concentration in an individual subject after a single 1500 mg dose of Theo-24 taken during fasting, period during which this patient experienced nausea, repeated vomiting, or severe throbbing headache.

Some drugs, such as ranitidine, cimetidine, and dipyridamole, after oral administration produce a blood concentration curve consisting of two peaks. This double-peak phenomenon is generally observed after the administration of a single dose to fasted patients. The rationale for the double-peak phenomenon has been attributed to variability in stomach emptying, variable intestinal motility, presence of food, enterohepatic recycling, or failure of a tablet dosage form. For a drug with high water solubility, dissolution of the drug occurs in the stomach, and partial emptying of the drug into the duodenum will result in the first absorption peak. A delay in stomach emptying results in a second absorption peak as the remainder of the dose is emptied into the duodenum.

Diseases such as Crohn's disease that alter GI physiology and corrective surgery involving peptic ulcer, antrectomy with gastroduodenostomy and selective vagotomy may potentially affect drug absorption. Drug absorption may be unpredictable in many disease conditions. Drugs or nutrients or both may also affect the absorption of other drugs. For example, propantheline bromide is an anticholinergic drug that slows stomach emptying and motility of the small intestine and may reduce stomach acid secretion. Grapefruit juice was found to increase the plasma level of many drugs due to inhibition of their metabolism in the liver.

Pharmaceutical Factors Affecting Drug Bioavailability

Biopharmaceutic considerations in the design and manufacture of a drug product to deliver the active drug with the desired bioavailability characteristics include: (1) the type of drug product (e.g., solution, suspension; suppository); (2) the nature of the excipients in the drug product; (3) the physicochemical properties of the drug molecule; and (4) the route of drug administration.

Disintegration

Immediate release, solid oral drug products must rapidly disintegrate into small particles and release the drug. The United States Pharmacopoeia (USP) describes an official tablet disintegration test. The process of disintegration does not imply complete dissolution of the tablet and/or the drug. Complete disintegration is defined by the USP as "that state in which any residue of the tablet, except fragments of insoluble coating, remaining on the screen of the test apparatus in the soft mass have no palpably firm core." The USP provides specifications for uncoated tablets, plain coated tablets, enteric tablets, buccal tablets, and sublingual tablets. Exempted from USP disintegration tests are troches, tablets which are intended to be chewed, and drug products intended for sustained release or prolonged or repeat action. Disintegration tests allow for precise measurement of the formation of fragments, granules, or aggregates from solid dosage forms, but do not provide information on the dissolution rate of the active drug. The disintegration test serves as a component in the overall quality control of tablet manufacture.

Dissolution

Dissolution is the process by which a chemical or drug becomes dissolved in a solvent. In biologic systems, drug dissolution in an aqueous medium is an important prior condition of systemic absorption. The rate at which drugs with poor aqueous solubility dissolve from an intact or disintegrated solid dosage form in the GI tract often controls the rate of systemic absorption of the drug. Thus, dissolution tests are discriminating of formulation factors that may affect drug bioavailability.

As the drug particle dissolves, a saturated solution (stagnant layer) is formed at the immediate surface around the particle. The dissolved drug in the saturated solution gradually diffuses to the surrounding regions. The overall rate of drug dissolution may be described by the Noyes–Whitney equation which models drug dissolution in terms of the rate of drug diffusion from the surface to the bulk of the solution. In general, drug concentration at the surface is assumed to be the highest possible, i.e., the solubility of the drug in the dissolution medium. The drug concentration C is the homogeneous concentration in the bulk solution which is generally lower than that in the stagnant layer immediate to the surface of the solid. The decrease in concentration across the stagnant layer is called the diffusion gradient

$$dC/dt = DA(CS - C)h$$

where, dC/dt = rate of drug dissolution, D = diffusion rate constant, A = surface area of the particle, CS = drug concentration in the stagnant layer, C = drug concentration in the bulk solvent, and h = thickness of the stagnant layer.

The rate of dissolution, $(dC/dt) \times (1/A)$, is the amount of drug dissolved per unit area per time (e.g., g/cm^2 per min).

The Noyes–Whitney equation shows that dissolution rate is influenced by the physicochemical characteristics of the drug, the formulation, and the solvent. In addition, the temperature of the medium also affects drug solubility and dissolution rate.

Physicochemical Nature of the Drug

Solubility, pH, and Drug Absorption

The natural pH environment of the GI tract varies from acidic in the stomach to slightly alkaline in the small intestine. Drug solubility may be improved with the addition of acidic or basic excipients. Solubilization of aspirin, for example, may be increased by the addition of an alkaline buffer. Controlled release drug products are non-disintegrating dosage forms. Buffering agents may be added to slow or modify the release rate of a fast-dissolving drug in the formulation of a controlled release drug product. The buffering agent is released slowly rather than rapidly so that the drug does not dissolve immediately in the surrounding GI fluid. Intravenous drug solutions are difficult to prepare with drugs that have poor aqueous solubility. Drugs that are physically or chemically unstable may require special excipients, coating or manufacturing process to protect the drug from degradation.

Stability, pH, and Drug Absorption

The pH-stability profile is a plot of reaction rate constant for drug degradation versus pH and may help to predict if some of the drug will decompose in the GI tract. The stability of erythromycin is pH-dependent. In acidic medium, erythromycin decomposition occurs rapidly, whereas at neutral or alkaline pH the drug is relatively stable. Consequently, erythromycin tablets are enteric coated to protect against acid degradation in the stomach. In addition, less soluble erythromycin salts that are more stable in the stomach have been prepared.

Particle Size and Drug Absorption

The effective surface area of the drug is increased enormously by a reduction in the particle size. Because drug dissolution is thought to take place at the surface of the solute, the greater the surface area, the more rapid the rate of drug dissolution. The geometric shape of the drug particle also affects the surface area, and during dissolution the surface is constantly changing. In dissolution calculations, the solute particle is usually assumed to have retained its geometric shape.

Particle size and particle size distribution studies are important for drugs that have low water solubility. Particle size reduction by milling to a micronized form increased the absorption of low aqueous solubility drugs such as griseofulvin, nitrofurantoin, and many steroids. Smaller particle size results in an increase in the total surface area of the particles, enhances water penetration into the particles, and increases the dissolution rates. With poorly soluble drugs, a disintegrant may be added to the formulation to ensure rapid disintegration of the tablet and release of the particles.

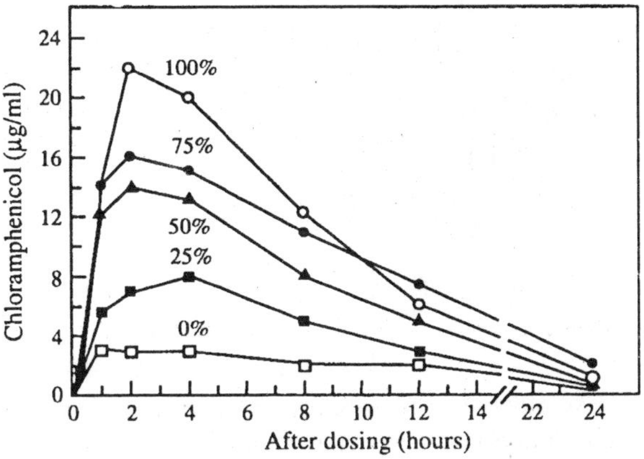

Fig. 3.7. Comparison of mean blood serum levels obtained with chloramphenicol palmitate suspensions containing varying ratios of α and β polymorphs, following single oral dose equivalent.

Polymorphic Crystals, Solvates, and Drug Absorption

Polymorphism refers to the arrangement of a drug in various crystal forms (polymorphs). Polymorphs have the same chemical structure but different physical properties, such as solubility, density, hardness, and compression characteristics. Some polymorphic crystals may have much lower aqueous solubility than the amorphous forms, causing a product to be incompletely absorbed. Chloramphenicol, for example, has several crystal forms, and when given orally as a suspension, the drug concentration in the body depended on the percentage of β-polymorph in the suspension. The β-form is more soluble and better absorbed. In general, the crystal form that has the lowest free energy is the most stable polymorph. Polymorphs that are metastable may convert to a more stable form over time. A crystal form change may cause problems in manufacturing the product. For example, a change in crystal structure of the drug may cause cracking in a tablet or even prevent a granulation to be compressed into a tablet requiring reformulation of the product. Some drugs interact with solvent during preparation to form a crystal called solvate. Water may form a special crystal with drugs called hydrates, for example, erythromycin forms different hydrates which may have quite different solubility compared to the anhydrous form of the drug. Ampicillin trihydrate, for example, was reported to be less absorbed than the anhydrous form of ampicillin due to faster dissolution of the latter.

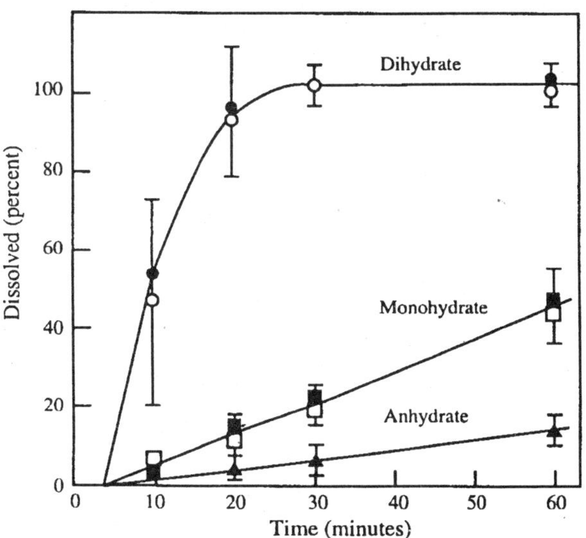

Fig. 3.8. Dissolution behavior of erythromycin dihydrate, monohydrate, and anhydrate in phosphate buffer at 37°C.

Table 3.1. Common excipients used in solid drug products

Excipient	*Property in dosage form*
Lactose	Diluent
Dibasic calcium phosphate	Diluent
Starch	Disintegrant, diluent
Microcrystalline cellulose	Disintegrant, diluent
Magnesium stearate	Lubricant
Stearic acid	Lubricant
Hydrogenated vegetable oil	Lubricant
Talc	Lubricant
Sucrose (solution)	Granulating agent
Polyvinyl pyrrolidone (solution)	Granulating agent
Hydroxypropylmethylcellulose	Tablet-coating agent
Titinium dioxide	Combined with dye as colored coating
Methylcellulose	Coating or granulating agent
Cellulose acetate phthalate	Enteric coating agent

Formulation Factors Affecting Drug Dissolution

Excipients are pharmacodynamically inactive substances that are added to a formulation to provide certain functional properties to the drug and dosage form. Excipients may be added to improve the compressibility of the active drug, stabilize the drug from degradation, decrease gastric irritation, control the rate of drug absorption from the absorption site, increase drug bioavailability, etc. For solid oral dosage forms such as compressed tablets, excipients may include: (1) diluent (e.g., lactose); (2) disintegrant (e.g., starch); (3) lubricant (e.g., magnesium stearate); and (4) other components such as binding and stabilizing agents. When improperly used in the formulation, excipients may alter drug bioavailability and possibly pharmacodynamic activity.

Table 3.2. Common excipients used in oral liquid drug products

Excipient	*Property in dosage form*
Sodium carboxymethylcellulose	Suspending agent
Tragacanth	Suspending agent
Sodium alginate	Suspending agent
Xanthan gum	Thixotropic suspending agent
Veegum	Thixotropic suspending agent
Sorbitol	Sweetener
Alcohol	Solubilizing agent, preservative
Propylene glycol	Solubilizing agent
Methyl propylparaben	Preservative
Sucrose	Sweetener
Polysorbates	Surfactant
Sesame oil	For emulsion vehicle
Corn oil	For emulsion vehicle

Excipients may affect the drug dissolution rate by altering the medium in which the drug is dissolving or by reacting with the drug itself. For example, suspending agents increase the viscosity of the drug vehicle, but may decrease the drug dissolution rate from the suspension. An excessive quantity of magnesium stearate (a hydrophobic lubricant) in the formulation may retard drug dissolution and slow the rate of drug absorption. The total amount of drug absorbed may also be reduced. To prevent this problem, the lubricant level should be decreased or a different lubricant selected. Sometimes, increasing the amount of disintegrant may overcome the retarding effect of lubricants on dissolution. However, with some poorly soluble drugs an increase in disintegrant level has little or no effect on drug dissolution because the fine drug particles are not wetted.

Excipients may enhance or diminish the rate and extent of systemic drug absorption. Excipients that increase the aqueous solubility of the drug generally increase the rate of drug dissolution and absorption. For example, sodium bicarbonate in the formulation may change the pH of themedium surrounding the active drug substance. Aspirin, a weak acid, in an alkaline medium will form a water-soluble salt in which the drug rapidly dissolves. This process is known as dissolution in a reactive medium. The solid drug dissolves rapidly in the reactive solvent surrounding the solid particle. As the dissolved drug molecules diffuse outward into the bulk solvent, the drug may precipitate out of solution with a very fine particle size. The small particles have enormous collective surface area and disperse and redissolve readily for more rapid absorption on contact with the mucosal surface.

Excipients may interact directly with the drug to form a water-soluble or water-insoluble complex. If tetracycline is formulated with calcium carbonate, an insoluble complex of calcium tetracycline is formed that has a slow rate of dissolution and poor absorption.

Excipients may increase the retention time of the drug in the GI tract and therefore increase the amount of drug absorbed. Excipients may act as carriers to increase drug diffusion across the intestinal wall. The addition of surface-active agents may increase wetting as well as solubility of drugs. In contrast, many excipients may retard drug dissolution and thus reduce drug absorption.

Shellac used as a tablet coating, upon aging, can slow the drug dissolution rate. Surfactants may affect drug dissolution in an unpredictable fashion. Low concentrations of surfactants lower the surface tension and increase the rate of drug dissolution, whereas higher concentrations of surfactants tend to form micelles with the drug and thus decrease the dissolution rate. High tablet compression without sufficient disintegrant may cause poor disintegration in vivo of a compressed tablet.

In Vitro Dissolution Testing

A dissolution test in vitro measures the rate and extent of dissolution of the drug in an aqueous medium in the presence of one or more excipients contained in the drug product. A potential bioavailability problem may be uncovered by a suitable dissolution method. The optimum dissolution testing conditions differ with each drug formulation. Different agitation rates, different medium (including different pH), and different dissolution apparatus should be tried to distinguish which dissolution method is optimum for the drug product and discriminating for drug formulation changes. The appropriate dissolution test condition for the drug product is then used to determine acceptable dissolution specifications.

The size and shape of the dissolution vessel may affect the rate and extent of dissolution. For example, the vessel may range in size from several milliliters to several liters. The shape may be round-bottomed or flat, so that the tablet might lie in a different position in different experiments. The amount of agitation and the nature of the stirrer affect the dissolution rate. Stirring rates must be controlled, and specifications differ between drug products. Low stirring rates (50–100 rpm) are more discriminating of formulation factors affecting dissolution than higher stirring rates. The temperature of the dissolution medium must be controlled and variations in temperature must be avoided. Most dissolution tests are performed at 37°C.

The nature of the dissolution medium, the solubility of the drug and the amount of drug in the dosage form will affect the dissolution test. The dissolution medium should not be saturated by the drug. Usually, a volume of medium larger than the amount of solvent needed to completely dissolve the drug is used in such tests. The usual volume of the medium is 500–1000 ml. Drugs that are not very water soluble may require use of a very-large-capacity vessel (up to 2000 ml) to observe significant dissolution. Sink conditions is a term referring to an excess volume of medium that allows the solid drug to continuously dissolve. If the drug solution becomes saturated, no further net drug dissolution will take place. According to the USP, "the quantity of medium used should be not less than three times that required to form a saturated solution of the drug substance."

Which medium is best is a matter of considerable controversy. The preferred dissolution medium in USP dissolution tests is deaerated water or if substantiated by the solubility characteristics of the drug or formulation, a buffered aqueous solution (typically pH 4–8) or dilute HCl may be used. The significance of dearation of the medium should be determined. Various investigators have used 0.1 *N* HCl, 0.01 N HCl, phosphate buffer, simulated gastric juice, water, and simulated intestinal juice, depending on the nature of the drug product and the location in the GI tract where the drug is expected to dissolve. No single apparatus and test can be used for all drug products. Each drug product must be tested individually with the dissolution test that best correlates to in vivo bioavailability.

The dissolution test usually states that a certain percentage of the labeled amount of drug in the drug product must dissolve within a specified period of time. In practice, the absolute amount of drug in the drug product may vary from tablet to tablet. Therefore, a number of tablets from each lot are usually tested to get a representative dissolution rate for the product. The USP provides several official (compendia) methods for carrying out dissolution tests of tablets, capsules and other special products such as transdermal preparations. The selection of a particular method for a drug is usually specified in the monograph for a particular drug product.

Bioavailability and Bioequivalence

Bioavailability and bioequivalence may be determined directly using plasma drug concentration vs. time profiles, urinary drug excretion studies, measurements of an acute pharmacologic effect, clinical studies, or in vitro studies. Bioavailability studies are performed for both approved active drug ingredients or therapeutic moieties not yet approved for marketing by the FDA. New formulations of active drug ingredients or therapeutic moieties must be approved, prior to marketing, by the FDA. In approving a drug product for marketing, the FDA must ensure that the drug product is safe and effective for its labeled indications for use. To ensure that the drug product meets all applicable standards of identity, strength, quality, and purity, the FDA requires bioavailability/pharmacokinetic studies and where necessary bioequivalence studies for all drug products.

For unmarketed drugs which do not have full New Drug Application (NDA) approval by the FDA, in vivo bioavailability studies must be performed on the drug formulation proposed for marketing. Essential pharmacokinetic parameters of the active drug ingredient or therapeutic moiety is also characterized. Essential pharmacokinetic parameters include the rate and extent of systemic absorption, elimination half-life, and rates of excretion and metabolism should be established after single- and multiple-dose administration. Data from these in vivo bioavailability studies are important to establish recommended dosage regimens and to support drug labeling.

In vivo bioavailability studies are performed also for new formulations of active drug ingredients or therapeutic moieties that have full NDA approval and are approved for marketing. The purpose of these studies is to determine the bioavailability and characterize the pharmacokinetics of the new formulation, new dosage form, or new salt or ester relative to a reference formulation. After the bioavailability and essential pharmacokinetic parameters of the active ingredient or therapeutic moiety are established, dosage regimens may be recommended in support of drug labeling.

Bioequivalent Drug Products

Bioequivalent drug products are pharmaceutical equivalents whose bioavailability (i.e., rate and extent of systemic drug absorption) does not show a significant difference when administered at the same molar dose of the therapeutic moiety under similar experimental conditions, either single or multiple dose. Some pharmaceutical equivalents or may be equivalent in the extent of their absorption but not in their rate of absorption and yet may be considered bioequivalent because such differences in the rate of absorption are intentional and are reflected in the labeling, are not essential to the attainment of effective body drug concentrations on chronic use, or are considered medically insignificant for the particular drug product studied.

Generic Drug Products

A generic drug product is considered bioequivalent to the reference listed drug product (generally the currently marketed, brand-name product with a full (NDA) approved by the FDA) if both products are pharmaceutical equivalents and its rate and extent of systemic drug absorption (bioavailability) do not show a statistically significant difference when administered in the same dose of the active ingredient, in the same chemical form, in a similar dosage form, by the same route of administration, and under the same experimental conditions.

Pharmaceutical equivalents are drug products that contain the same therapeutically active drug ingredient(s), same salt, ester, or chemical form; are of the same dosage form; and are identical in strength and concentration and route of administration. Pharmaceutical equivalents may differ in characteristics such as shape, scoring configuration, release mechanisms, packaging, and excipients (including colors, flavoring, preservatives).

Therapeutic equivalent drug products are pharmaceutical equivalents that can be expected to have the same clinical effect and safety profile when administered to patients under the same conditions specified in the labeling. Therapeutic equivalent drug products have the following criteria: (1) The products are safe and effective; (2) The products are pharmaceutical equivalents containing the same active drug ingredient in the same dosage form, given by the same route of administration, meet compendia or other applicable standards of strength, quality, purity, and identity and meet an acceptable in vitro standard; (3) The drug products are bioequivalent in that they do not present a known potential problem and are shown to meet an appropriate bioequivalence standard; (4) The drug products are adequately labeled; and 5) The drug products are manufactured in compliance with current good manufacturing practice (GMP) regulations.

The generic drug product requires an abbreviated new drug application (ANDA) for approval by the FDA and may be marketed after patent expiration of the reference listed drug product. The generic drug product must be a therapeutic equivalent to the Reference drug product but may differ in certain characteristics including shape, scoring configuration, packaging, and excipients (includes colors, flavors, preservatives, expiration date, and minor aspects of labeling).

Pharmaceutical alternatives are drug products that contain same therapeutic moiety but are different salts, esters or complexes (e.g., tetracycline hydrochloride versus tetracycline phosphate) or are different dosage forms (e.g., tablet versus capsule; immediate release dosage form versus controlled release dosage form) or strengths.

In summary, clinical studies are useful in determining the safety and efficacy of the drug product. Bioavailability studies are used to define the affect of changes in the physico chemical properties of the drug substance and the affect of the drug product (dosage form) on the pharmacokinetics of the drug; whereas, bioequivalence studies are used to compare the bioavailability of the same drug (same salt or ester) from various drug products. If the drug products are bioequivalent and therapeutically equivalent, then the clinical efficacy and safety profile of these drug products are assumed to be similar and may be substituted for each other.

Drug Product Performance In Vitro as a Measure of In Vivo Drug Bioavailability

The best measure of a drug product's performance is to give the drug product to human volunteers or patients and then determine the in vivo bioavailability of the drug using a pharmacokinetic or clinical study. For some well characterized drug products and for certain drug products where bioavailability is self-evident (e.g., sterile solutions for injection), in vivo bioavailability studies may be unnecessary. In these cases, the performance of the drug product in vitro is used as a surrogate to predict the in vivo drug bioavailability. Because these products have predictable in vivo performance as judged by the in vitro characterization of the drug and drug product, the FDA may waive the requirement for performing an in vivo bioavailability study.

Drug Products for which Bioavailability Is Self-Evident

Drug bioavailability from a true solution is generally considered self-evident. Thus, sterile solutions, lyophilized powders for reconstitution, opthalmic solutions do not need bioequivalence studies but still must be manufactured according to current GMPs. However, highly viscous solutions may have bioavailability problems due to slow diffusion of the active drug.

In Vitro–In Vivo Correlation (IVIVC)

In vitro bioavailability data may be used to predict the performance of a dosage provided that the dissolution method selected is appropriate for the solid oral dosage form and prior information has been collected showing that the dissolution method will result in optimum drug absorption from the drug product. In general, IVIVC is best for well absorbed drugs for which the dissolution rate is the rate-limiting step. Some drugs are poorly absorbed and dissolution is not predictive of absorption. The objectives of IVIVC are to use rate of dissolution as a discriminating (i.e., sensitive to changes in formulation or manufacturing process), as an aid in setting dissolution specifications. When properly applied, IVIVC may be used to facilitate the evaluation of drug products with manufacturing changes including minor changes in formulation, equipment, process, manufacturing site, and batch size.

Three levels of IVIVC are generally recognized by the FDA. Level A correlation is usually estimated by deconvolution followed by comparison of the fraction of drug absorbed to the fraction of drug dissolved. A correlation of this type is the highest level of correlation and best predictor of bioavailability from the dosage form. A Level A correlation is generally linear and represents a point-to-point relationship between in vitro dissolution rate and the in vivo input rate. The Level A correlation should predict the entire in vivo time course from the in vitro dissolution data. Level B correlation utilizes the principles of statistical moment analysis.

The mean in vitro dissolution time is compared to either the mean residence time or the mean in vivo dissolution time. Level B correlation, like Level A correlation, uses all of the in vitro and in vivo data but is not considered to be a point-to-point correlation and does not uniquely reflect the actual in vivo plasma level curve, since several different in vivo plasma level-time curves will produce similar residence times. A Level C correlation is the weakest IVIVC and establishes a single point relationship between a dissolution parameter (e.g., time for 50% of drug to dissolve, or percent drug dissolved in two hours, etc.) and a pharmacokinetic parameter (e.g., AUC, Cmax, Tmax). Level C correlation does not reflect the complete shape of the plasma drug concentration-time curve of dissolution profile.

Biopharmaceutics Classification System (BCS)

The FDA may waive the requirement for performing an in vivo bioavailability or bioequivalence study for certain immediate release solid oral drug products that meets very specific criteria, namely, the permeability, solubility, and dissolution of the drug. These characteristics include the in vitro dissolution of the drug product in various media, drug permeability information, and assuming ideal behavior of the drug product, drug dissolution and absorption in the GI tract. For regulatory purpose, drugs are classified according to BCS in accordance the solubility, permeability and dissolution characteristics of the drug.

This classification can be used as a basis for setting in vitro dissolution specifications and can also provide a basis for predicting the likelihood of achieving a successful in IVIVC. The solubility of a drug is determined by dissolving the highest unit dose of the drug in 250 ml of buffer adjusted between pH 1.0 and 8.0. A drug substance is considered highly soluble when the dose/solubility volume of solution are less than or equal to 250 ml. High-permeability drugs are generally those with an extent of absorption that is greater than 90%.

Solubility

An objective of the BCS approach is to determine the equilibrium solubility of a drug under approximate physiological conditions. For this purpose, determination of pH-solubility profiles over a pH range of 1–8 is suggested. Preferably eight or more pH conditions should be evaluated. Buffers that react with the drug should not be used. An acid or base titration method can also be used for determining drug solubility. The solubility class is determined by calculating what volume of an aqueous media is sufficient to dissolve the highest anticipated dose strength. A drug substance is considered highly soluble when the highest dose strength is soluble in 250 ml or less of aqueous media over the pH range of 1–8. The volume estimate of 250 ml is derived from typical bioequivalence study protocols that prescribe administration of a drug product to fasting human volunteers with a glass (8 ounces) of water.

Solution stability of a test drug in selected buffers (or pH conditions) should be documented using a validated stability-indicating assay. Data collected on both pH-solubility and pH-stability should be submitted in the biowaiver application along with information on the ionization characteristics, such as pKa(s), of a drug.

Determining Permeability Class

Studies of the extent of absorption in humans, or intestinal permeability methods, can be used to determine the permeability class membership of a drug. To be classified as highly permeable, a test drug should have an extent of absorption >90% in humans. Supportive information on permeability characteristics of the drug substance should also be derived from its physical–chemical properties (e.g., octanol : water partition coefficient).

Some methods to determine the permeability of a drug from the GI tract include: (1) in vivo intestinal perfusion studies in humans; (2) in vivo or in situ intestinal perfusion studies in animals; (3) in vitro permeation experiments using excised human or animal intestinal tissues; and 4) in vitro permeation experiments across a monolayer of cultured human intestinal cells. When using these methods, the experimental permeability data should correlate with the known extent-of-absorption data in humans.

Dissolution

The dissolution class is based on the in vitro dissolution rate of an immediate release drug product under specified test conditions and is intended to indicate rapid in vivo dissolution in relation to the average rate of gastric emptying in humans under fasting conditions. An immediate release drug product is considered rapidly dissolving when not less than 85% of the label amount of drug substance dissolves within 30 min using the USP apparatus I at 100 rpm or apparatus II at 50 rpm in a voluume of 900 ml or less in each of the following media: (1) acidic media such as 0.1 N HCl or Simulated Gastric Fluid USP without enzymes; (2) a pH 4.5 buffer; and (3) a pH 6.8 buffer or Simulated Intestinal Fluid USP without enzymes.

Biowaivers

In addition to routine quality control tests, comparative dissolution tests have been used to waive bioequivalence requirements (biowaivers) for lower strengths of a dosage form. The drug products containing the lower dose strengths should be compositionally proportional or qualitatively the same as the higher dose strengths and have the same release mechanism. Biowaivers are generally provided for multiple strengths after approval of a bioequivalence study performed on one strength, using the following criteria: For multiple strengths of IR products with linear kinetics, the bioequivalence study may be performed at the highest strength and waivers of in vivo studies may be granted on lower strengths, based on an adequate dissolution test, provided the lower strengths are proportionately similar in composition. Similar may also be interpreted to mean that the different strengths of the products are within the scope of changes permitted under the category "Components and Composition," discussed in the SUPAC-IR guidance.

Scale-up and Postapproval Changes (SUPAC)

After a drug product is approved for marketing by the FDA, the manufacturer may want to make a manufacturing change. The pharmaceutical industry, academia and the FDA developed a series of guidances for the industry that discuss scale-up and postapproval changes, generally termed, SUPAC guidances. The FDA SUPAC guidances are for manufacturers of approved drug products who want to change (1) a component and composition of the drug: product; (2) the batch size; (3) the manufacturing site; (4) the manufacturing process or equipment; and/or (5) packaging. These guidances describe various levels of postapproval changes according to whether the change is likely to impact on the quality and performance of the drug product. The level of change as classified by the FDA as to the likelihood that a change in the drug product might affect the quality of the product.

4

Pharmaceutical Bioassay

Some *Fusarium* mycotoxins and the metabolites of filamentous fungi and molds occur naturally in a variety of feeds, foodstuffs, crops, vegetables, fruits, water, and plants. Ingestion of the contaminative feeds, foodstuffs, crops, vegetables, fruits, water, and plants can produce health problems, such as reduced growth, anorexia, induced emesis, enhanced proliferation of estrogen-responsive tumor cells, human cervical cancer, and premature initial breast development in humans and animals. Among the common toxins, verrucarin A, T2-toxin, roridin A, deoxynivalenol (DON), zearalenone (ZEN), fumonisin B1 (FB1), moniliformin (MON), microcystin-LR (MCLR), and the toxins from *Bacillus thuringiensis* provide a worldwide threat to humans and animals. Based on these facts that the lactose-utilizing yeast *Kluyveromyces marxianus* exhibits well-characterized β-galactosidase activity and has chromogenic substrates, the toxicants interfering with any cellular function required for induction and expression of β-galactosidase gene can suppress β-galactosidase activity, DON and fumonisin B can inhibit cell growth, the dehydrogenase ensurveyed enzymes involved in mitochondrial functions can be inhibited by the toxicants, in axenic culture the melanin precursor overproducer mutant strain of the ciliate *Tetrahymena thermophila* can be grown to high concentration, in protecting plants from the hazardous effects of xenobiotics glutathione S-transferase (GST) and glutathione peroxidase (GPX) can play essential roles, colorimetric yeast assay, ciliate *T. thermophila* assay, MTT assay, mortality and frass production assay, and *Lepidium sativum* assay are established.

Bioassay for Detecting Toxicity of Toxins from a Microorganism

Colorimetric Yeast Assay for Detecting Trichothecene Mycotoxins

To 50 mL of liquid medium, a single-cell colony of *K. marxianus* GK1005 (maintained routinely and grown on 1% (w/v) yeast extract, 1% (w/v) bacteriological peptone, and 2% (w/v) glucose (YPD), solidified when required with 2% (w/v) agar) on agar plate is transfered to prepare cultures that are incubated for 16 h at 35°C and 200 rpm in a rotary incubator. At 560 nm, the absorbance is measured to determine cell density, which is calibrated by direct hemocytometer counts. Mycotoxins containing sample is dissolved in spectroscopic grade methanol to make stock solutions typically at 0.1 mg/mL. Cetyl trimethyl ammonium bromide, polymyxin B sulphate, and polymyxin B nonapeptide are dissolved in water, filter-sterilized, and kept no more than a day as stock solutions. 5-Bromo-4-chloro-3-indolyl-P-D-galactopyranoside (X-gal) is dissolved in dimethylformamide (DMF) at 100 mg/mL and stored at -20°C in the dark, and before each assay, it is immediately diluted in aqueous DMF (2 parts water : 3 parts DMF) to prepare a working solution of 20-mg/mL X-gal assay. Before use *o*-nitrophenyl-β-D-galactopyranoside (ONPGal) is immediately dissolved in water at 4 mg/mL and subsequently discarded. Before use, MTT is dissolved in phosphate-buffered solution (PBS) and filter-sterilized to prepare a 5-

mg/mL stock solution. In the wells of a microtiter plate (sterile, flat-bottomed), 136 μL of growth medium consisted of 1% (w/v) yeast extract, 1% (w/v) bacteriological peptone, and 50-mM glucose—"YPD-50" are mixed with polymyxin B sulphate to give a final assay concentration of 15 μg/mL, to which 8 μL of stock solution of mycotoxin containing sample or methanol (controls) and 16 μL of yeast inoculum are successively added to give an initial assay cell density of approximately 2 × 10^8 cells/mL. Blank wells contain 152 μL of medium and 8 μL of methanol. The plate is mixed, sealed with a plate sealer, and incubated at 35°C for the duration of the assay, during which cell density is regularly monitored at 560 nm. After about 10 h, the control (mycotoxin-free) cultures reach the stationary phase; the activity of β-galactosidase or mitochondrial (MTT-cleavage) in the cultures is assayed.

To each well of the microtiter plate, 5 μL of sodium dodecyl sulfate (SDS) (0.1%, w/v) and 3 μL of chloroform are added to permeabilize the cells. For *in vivo* experiments and experiments examining the effects of different carbon sources, 1 μL of 100-mg/mL X-gal in DMF are added to each well. For examining the effects of altering glucose concentration and inoculum cell density, 5 μL of 20-mg/mL X-gal in DMF are added to each well. For methanol and ethanol toxicity experiments and the standardized bioassay, 8 μL of 20-mg/mL X-gal in aqueous DMF are added. After mixing the contents in the wells, the plates are incubated at 35°C for a maximum of 30 min. Using a test filter at 666 nm and a reference filter at 560 nm, the plates are read. β-Galactosidase activity is expressed as product formation (A_{666}-A_{560}), as a function of cell density (A_{560}) as well.

After the addition of 16 μL of MTT in PBS to each well and statically incubated at 35°C for 4 h, the medium is displaced by 200 μL of dimethyl sulfate (DMSO). Thorough mixing and dissolution the MTT-cleavage product is pipeted repeatedly. Using a test filter at 560 nm and a reference filter at 666 nm, the plates are read.

Into 50 mL of the solution consisting of 1% yeast extract, 1% bacteriological peptone, and 50-mM lactose, a single colony of *K. marxianus* GK1005 is inoculated and then incubated for 16 h at 35°C and 200 rpm in an orbital shaker. Into each of two universal bottles 10 mL of the samples of the culture are transferred, and then 0.2 mL of chloroform and 0.1 mL of SDS (0.1%, w/v) are added. To permeabilize the cells, to one bottle 20 μL of X-gal (100 mg/mL in DMF) are added, and to the other bottle 20 μL of DMF are added. In an orbital shaker, both bottles are incubated at 35°C and 200 rpm until in the bottle containing X-gal visible indigo precipitate is formed, of which the absorption spectrum is determined with DMF control sample as a reference.

Ciliate *T. thermophila* Assay for Detecting Trichothecene Mycotoxins

The phenotype characteristics of *T. thermophila* strain BI3840 are amicronucleated (amc), pigment producing (pig), and resistant to 25 μg/mL of cycloheximide (cy-r) and mating type IV. The PP210 medium consists of aqueous solution of proteose peptone (2%, w/v), supplemented with 10 μM of $FeCl_3$, 250 μg/mL of streptomycin sulphate, and penicillin G. Mycotoxins containing samples are dissolved in propyleneglycol or acetonitrile to make stock solutions at 5 mg/mL. *T. thermophila* strain BI3840 are grown axenically in PP210 medium for 24 h and maintained constantly at 28 ± 1°C. Then the exponential phase cellular suspensions are distributed in microtiter plates (100 μL/well). According to the required final concentration, different dilutions of the stock solutions of mycotoxins containing samples in PP210 medium are added into the cultures (100 μL/well). To each 100 μl/well of *T. thermophila* strain BI3840 culture, 100 μl/well of PP210 medium without a mycotoxin containing sample is added to obtain one type of control, and 100 μl/well of PP210 medium plus the highest concentration of the corresponding solvent added to obtain another type of control. In all cases, the microtiter plates are incubated at 28 ± 1°C for 48 h and the wells with a dark-brown pigmentation are considered as the positive growth wells.

MTT Assay for Detecting Fusarium Mycotoxins

Caco-2, C5-O, V79 cells, and Chinese hamster ovary (CHO)-K1 cells (in DMEM/F-12) at passage numbers between 30 and 50, and HepG2 cells (in Minimum Essential Medium) at passage numbers between 80 and 100, are grown as monolayers in 80-cm^2 culture flasks, which are harvested when they reach 80% confluence to maintain exponential growth.

Using trypsin ethylenediaminetetraacetic acid (EDTA) (0.25% trypsin and 1-mM EDTA · 4Na), the cell monolayers in exponential growth are harvested and after repeated pipetting the single-cell suspensions are obtained. To 96 well plates, the single cell suspensions (1×10^2 to 5×10^4 cells per 200 μL medium/ well) are added by serial dilution. The medium are supplemented with 1.5-g/L sodium bicarbonate, 0.11-g/L sodium pyruvate, 1% nonessential amino acid, 25-mM HEPES, 100 U of penicillin/mL, 100 μg of streptomycin/mL, 25 ng of amphotericin B/mL, and 10% fetal bovine serum). Caco-2, C5-O, HepG2 (1×10^4 cells/100-μL medium), CHO-K1, and V79 (5×10^3 cells/100-μL medium) are seeded to each well of the 96 well plates and incubated in a humidified atmosphere of 5% CO_2 at 37°C for 24 h. A mycotoxin containing sample in 100 μL of medium is added from high to low concentration to the wells and adjusted to final concentration needed. MTT is dissolved in PBS (5-mg/mL final concentration), filtered (0.22-μm filter), and stored in the amber vials at 4°C for a month. After 48-h and 72-h incubation, to each well, 25 μL of MTT solution is added and incubated in a humidified atmosphere of 5% CO_2 at 37°C for 4 h. At the end of the incubation period, the media are discarded using a suction pump. The extraction buffer of 20% (w/v) SDS in a solution of 50% DMF in demineralized water (50:50, v/v) is prepared at pH 4.7 and filtered (0.22-μm filter). The buffer in 100 μL of 20% (w/v) of SDS is extracted and added into each well to solubilize formazan crystals, and the plates are shaked at 37°C overnight. The absorbance is measured at 570 nm with 690 nm as a reference wavelength. The positive control contains an adjusted seeding cell number in the log phase, of which the culture medium contains 0.1% ethanol.

Mortality and Frass Production Assay for Detecting Toxicity of Bacterial Strains

B. thuringiensis subsp. *tenebrionis* and the six unidentified strains of *B. thuringiensis,* labeled A30, A299, A311, A409, A410, and A429, are grown on nutrient agar buffered with an equimolar concentration of KH_2PO_4 (50 mM, pH 7.0) at 30°C for 5 days. The bacterial culture consists of vegetative cells, sporangia, spores, and crystals. These stages are lyophilized and stored at –20°C. The spore-crystal suspensions of each strain with 1:1 in the spore : crystal ratio are used in the toxicity assays. The concentration of extractable proteins (the final protein solution is referred to as extractable protein) is determined and adjusted to a given concentration of protein in the crystal-spore mixture. Spore-crystal mixtures are suspended in Triton X-100 solution (0.01%, v/v) and washed three times by centrifugation at 22°C and 11750 g for 3 min. To extract the proteins, the final pellet in a putatively selective crystal solubilizing buffer (40.5-mM Na_2CO_3, 0.5-mM phenylmethylsulfonylfluoride, 0.1-mM dithiothreitol, pH 10.0) is solubilized at 42°C by incubating for 2 h and vortexing every 30 min. The suspension is centrifuged (22°C, 11750 g, 3 min), and the supernatant is assayed for total protein with bovine serum albumin as the standard. The laboratory cultures of plants are periodically supplemented with pest insects to maintain hybrid vigor. The colony is reared in an incubator at 24°C under the light for 16 h and at 16°C in the darkness for 8 h. Abundant food is placed in plastic petri dishes (100 mm in diameter) with moist filter paper that contains 10 adults, the plastic petri dishes are incubated, and the number of frass pellets on filter paper is counted daily for 3 days.

Adult mortality and modified frass production assays are used to measure the toxicity of the extractable proteins of the bacterial strains against plants. The modified frass production assay is regarded as a rapid method to determine the specificity of numerous bacterial strains toxins against pest insect. The food cylinders (6 mm in length, 36 mm in diameter, 10 cylinders/plate) of optimum medium for insect feeding are cut from foliage homogenate supplemented with agar. The cylinders are dipped into distilled water containing different concentration of the extractable proteins, agitated for 5 s, air-dried, and then coated with test spore-crystal suspensions. The concentration of extractable proteins is 75-, 150-, 225-, and 300-μg protein/mL with distilled water as a control. Three to eight days after eclosion, starved adults are collected and added to the diet in petri dishes (15 × 100 mm diameter) containing moistened filter paper (15 adult insects per plate per dose). In the mortality assay, insects are fed at 25°C in darkness for 8 days. Mortality is monitored daily, and the LC_{50} for each test strain is calculated by probit analysis. In the frass assay, insects are fed for 6 days. The total number of frass pellets is calculated.

L. sativum Assay for Detecting Microcystin Toxicity

Toxic *Microcystis aeruginosa* PCC 7806 is cultured, and sufficient aeration is provided for culture mixing and air supply. From the freeze-dried cells, toxin is extracted by 70% aqueous methanol and determined using the protein phosphatase inhibition assay from the difference in the change in absorbance at 410 nm. With 5% H_2O_2 for 5 min, the seeds of *L. sativum* are surface sterilized, washed three times with sterile water for 10 min, left in fresh water overnight to germinate, and then transferred to nutrient medium containing 6.5% N, 2.7% P, 13% K, 7% Ca, 2.2% Mg, 7.5% S, 0.15% Fe, 0.024% Mn, 0.0024% B, 0.005% Zn, 0.002% Cu, and 0.001% Mo in 0.8% agar. The container (12 seeds/container) is cultured at 27°C under continuous light (20 photons/m^2/s). Before pouring, either 1- or 10-μg/L microcystin-LR (MCLR) toxin extracts are added to the medium. The fresh weights, root, and leaf lengths are measured daily in 2 days. GST and GPX activities are determined in 3 days.

The stems and roots of 10 plants from each of three containers from each group are prepared for 30% homogenate of plant material in buffer (0.01-M Tris-HCl pH 7.8, 7.5-mM PMSF, 2.5-mM EDTA, 325-μM bestatin, 3.5-μM E-64, 2.5-μM leupeptin, and 0.75-μM aprotinin). The homogenate is centrifuged at 4°C and 12,000 g in a benchtop centrifuge for 2 h, and the supernatant is stored at — 80°C for the GST and GPX assay.

In the GST assay, to the supernatant fluid, a cocktail containing 0.1-M potassium phosphate (pH 6.5), 30-mM 1-chloro-2,4-dinitrobenzene and 20-mM glutathione are added and measured immediately at 340 nm for 4 min. In the GPX assay, to the supernatant fluid, a cocktail of 0.1-mM potassium phosphate buffer (pH 7), glutathione reductase (4 ng/μL final), 10-mM glutathione, 30-mM EDTA, and 1-mM NADPH is added. The reaction is initated by adding cumene hydroperoxide and measured immediately at 340 nm for 3 min.

Toxicity Bioassay for Chemicals

Environmental chemical contaminants as toxic agents may be suspended in air, absorbed in suspended particulate matter (SPM) and foods, and dissolved in water, and thus, they may result in several toxic effects such as DNA damage, decline in lung function, imbalance of immune function, activation of aryl hydrocarbon receptor (AhR), abnormal reproduction, and urinary bladder injuries. Lux-Fluoro assay is developed on specific lesions for cells induced by DNA damaging chemicals may lead to cell death or induce an error-prone repair pathway leading to mutagenesis and cancer induction. Based on the air-liquid interface culture (ALIC) of the human alveolar type II cell line (A459) and culture of spleen cells obtained from BALB/c mice producing IgM after pokeweed mitogen (PWM) stimulation, ALIC-based assay and PWM-induced IgM assay are established. Exposure to extremely low concentrations of 2,3,7,8-tetrachlorodibenzo-p-dioxin (TCDD) results in activation of AhR and the induction of expression of a battery of genes, green fluorescent protein (GFP)-based cell assay is established. In Reproductive Assessment by Continuous Breeding (RACB) protocol, differential follicle counts can provide a sensitive means of estimating the extent of ovarian toxicity in females exposed to xenobiotics. Based on these facts that urinary bladder injuries induced by repeated oral administration of pharmaceuticals may be epithelial ulceration with edema and hemorrhage in the lamina propria and muscle layer of the urinary bladder, environmental chemical contaminants disrupt mammalian peptide signal transduction pathway via the interaction with the endocrine system in humans and various wildlife species and the cellular production of GFP is a function of nitrate concentration, uroepithelial cell assay, mating efficiency assay, and Pnar-gfp assay are established and can be used in bioassays.

Lux-Fluoro Assay for Detecting Combined Genotoxicity and Cytotoxicity of Chemicals

The plasmid pPLS-1 (DSM10333), the genotoxicity sensing reporter component of the test panel, which carries the luxCDABFE genes downstream of a strong SOS- dependent promoter is constructed. The plasmid pGFPuv that carries the optimized "cycle 3" variant of GFP in frame with the lacZ initiation codon is the cytotoxicity sensing reporter component of the test panel. According to the modified "Hanahan" procedure, pPLS-1 and pGFPuv are used to transform the strain *S. typhimurium* TA1535 (ATCC: *S. choleraesuis* subsp. *choleraesuis* strain TA1535). For selecting plasmid carrying cells, the bacteria are cultured at 37°C in NB-medium supplemented with 50-μg/mL ampicillin. The DNA damaging agents containing sample are dissolved in distilled water at high concentration and diluted for the test. Each well of White LB96P-CMP Mikro Lumat Plates with a transparent bottom contains 10 μL of the solvent or different concentration of the test sample. The agar plate containing a single colony of bacteria, 10 mL of NB-medium with 50-μg/mL ampicillin, is shaken on a rotary shaker at 37°C for 16 h. Then the dilution (1:50) of bacteria in fresh warm NB-medium containing 50-μg/mL ampicillin are incubated at 37°C until the absorbance at 600 nm (A_{600}) reaches 0.2–0.3. Aliquots of 90 μL of this culture are added to each well, the microplate is covered with a gas-permeable self-adhesive seal and placed into the temperature-controlled microplate reader. The absorbance, luminescence, and fluorescence of the culture is successively and repeatedly determined by the programmed measurement cycle at 30°C for up to 8 h of continuous incubation with a duration of about 10 min per measurement cycle (total of 50 cycles). The measurement cycle of each well includes 120-s shaking, 0.2-s luminescence measurement without filter, 0.1-s absorbance measurement (490 nm, 20 nm bandwidth), and 0.1-s fluorescence measurement (excitation at 405 nm, emission at 510 nm).

ALIC-Based Assay for Detecting Toxicity of Chemicals in SPM

A549 cells and Hep G2 cells cultured in DMEM supplemented with 10% fetal bovine serum, 20-mM hydroxyethylpiperazine-N′-2-ethanesulfonic acid, peni cillin (100 U/mL), streptomycin (100 μg/mL), amphotericin B (0.25 μg/mL), and 1.0% non-essential amino acid solution (only for Hep G2 cells) are subcultivated using 0.25% trypsin and 0.02% EDTA in PBS. After collection by trypsinization A549 cells are seeded at 1.0×10^5 cells/cm^2 onto the membrane culture insert precoated with a 0.03% type collagen solution. Initially, to both the apical (Ap) and the BL sides, the medium is added. Using a phase contrast microscope, the formation of the cell sheet is assessed. The evaluation of the development of tight junctions in the cell layers with a Millicell-ERS is performed based on the measurement of trans-epithelium electrical resistance (TEER). Until the TEER shows constant and saturated values (45–50 Ωcm^2 without the blank value of the membrane itself), the culture medium of A549 cells in the Ap side is removed and the ALIC is started. The chemical-free SPM samples are sterilized by ethylene oxide gas (EOG) performed with a commercially available sterilization system. After being measured carefully with a digital weighting machine, the EOG-sterilized SPM samples are loaded directly to the Ap side of an A549 cell layer in ALIC. In 12 well plates, A549 and Hep G2 cells are seeded at 1.0×10^5 cells/cm^2, cultured, and used after they reach confluence. In the preparation of the extracts of the SPM samples, the suspension of 24 mg of each sample and 200 μL of DMSO is sonicated for 15 min and centrifuged for 10 min at 15,000 rpm, and the supernatant is diluted with culture medium to adjust the final concentration of DMSO in the culture medium 0.5% and the highest concentration of SPM in the culture medium 600-μg-SPM/ mL-culture medium, which corresponds to the cell-surface-area-based load of the 158-μg-SPM/cm^2-cell surface.

The suspension of an SPM sample in 100 mL of CH_2Cl_2 is sonicated for 15 min and filtered with a membrane that has a 0.1-μm pore size, the filtrate is evaporated, and the residue is resolved in acetonitrile. The concentration of the chemicals in the SPM extracts is determined using a multicolumn high-performance liquid chromatography (HPLC)/spectrofluorometer/computer system. According to $EQ = S([PAH]_1EF_1 + ... + [PAH]_nEF_n)$, the chemically derived induction equivalent (EQ) is calculated to standardize the biological effect of the chemical on the EROD capacity of the Hep G2 cells.

After 48 h of exposure of SPM, each culture is rinsed twice with PBS, and to the Ap and BL sides, 500 μL and 1.5 mL of the substrate solution of acid phosphatase is added, respectively. For the monolayer culture, 1 mL of AP solution is added, the 12 well plates are incubated at 37°C for 2 h, the absorbance is measured at 405 nm with the value of cell-free well as control, and the cell survivability is calculated by referencing a predetermined calibration curve.

A549 and Hep G2 cells are cultured in 12 well plates, washed twice with PBS, and loaded with 10-μM 7-ethoxyresorufin in the presence of 10-μM dicumarol in culture medium. After 1 h of incubation, the fluorescence intensity is measured (530-nm excitation wavelength, 585-nm emission wavelength) to detect the formed resorufin. The intensity is calibrated to the resorufin concentration using a standard curve.

PWM-Induced IgM Assay for Detecting the Toxicity of Chemicals

The toxicants containing sample are dissolved in Ca, Mg-free PBS or DMSO, or the vehicle solvent (10 μL each). Spleen cells are aseptically removed from BALB/ cAnN mice (8–9 weeks old), washed in Hanks' balanced salt solution supplemented with 10-mM HEPES buffer (pH 7.4), and diluted by RPMI 1640 medium containing 10% heat-inactivated fetal bovine serum, 2-mM glutamine, 0.4-M sodium pyruvate, 20-mM mercaptoethanol, non-essential amino acids, and antibiotics to prepare suspensions of 10^6 cells/mL. Cells are cultivated in a 24-well culture plate under 5% CO_2-air and the presence of PWM at 37°C for 2 to 6 days, supplemented with chemical toxicants containing a sample at the beginning of the culture. A total of 700 μL of culture media and residual cells in 300 μL of media are used for total IgM assay and cell proliferation assay, respectively.

The 96-well microtiter immunoplates are precoated overnight at 4°C with 100 μL of rabbit anti-mouse IgM antibody (IgG) in PBS (pH 7.4), washed with PBS containing 0.05% Tween 20, and blocked overnight at 4°C with 150 μL of PBS containing 1% BSA. Each well is washed with PBS; into each well, 100-μL aliquots of culture media mentioned above (usually 11-fold diluted media) or reference mouse serum or standard mouse IgM diluted with 1% BSA-PBS are added, left at room temperature for 60 min, washed, and incubated; and 100-μL aliquots of horseraddish peroxidase-conjugated goat antimouse IgG in PBS are added. Sixty minutes later, to each well, 150-μL aliquots of substrate solutions containing 0.4% o-phenylenediamine and 0.01% hydrogen peroxide in 0.1-M citrate–0.2-M phosphate buffer are added and incubated. Fifteen minutes later, 50 μl of H_2SO_4 (0.5 M) is added to terminate the enzyme reaction. Using a microplate reader the optical density at 490 nm of each well is read.

After the addition of 30 μL of TetraColar One reagent, 300 μL of media mentioned above are incubated under 5% CO_2-air at 37°C for 2 h. The optical density at 450 nm of the media containing the water-soluble tetrazolium salt produced by the enzyme reaction is read, and the cell number in cultures is measured by the modification (WST-8 method) of the MTT assay for mitochondrial dehydrogenase activity in viable cells.

GFP-Based Cell Assay for Detecting the Toxicity of TCDD and Related Chemicals

By excising the 1846 base-pair (bp) Hind III fragment from the plasmid pGudLuc1.1, pGreen1.1 is created. pGreen1.1 contains the 480-bp dioxin-responsive domain from the mouse CYP1A1 gene inserted upstream of the mouse mammary tumor virus (MMTV) promoter, confers dioxin responsiveness upon the MMTV promoter and adjacent reporter gene, and is inserted into the Hind III site immediately upstream of the enhanced GFP reporter gene in the plasmid pEGFP-1.

Plates of the mouse hepatoma (Hepa1c1c7, approximately 80% confluent) cells maintained in αMEM containing 10% fetal bovine serum are transfected with the construct pGreen1.1 (20 μg) using polybrene, grown for 24 h, split 1 to 10, and replated into selective media. After growth for 4 weeks, resistant clones are isolated and screened for the EGFP assay. H1G1.1c3 cells and DMSO (1% maximum final concentration) or TCDD (1 nM in DMSO) are cultured in 6-well culture plates at 37°C for 24 h, harvested by scraping into lysis buffer (50-mM NaH_2PO_4, 10-mM Tris-HCl pH 8, 200-mM NaCl), and lysed by repeated passage through a 27-gauge needle. The medium is centrifuged, and the fluorescence of an aliquot of the supernatant is determined (460-nm excitation wavelength, 510-nm emission wavelength). In the microtiter plate analysis of EGFP, the intact cells are plated into 96-well tissue culture dishes at 7.5×10^4 cells/well and allowed to attach for 24 h. The selective media are then changed to 100 μL of nonselective media containing the test chemical or DMSO (1% final solvent concentration). EGFP levels of the intact cells in the nonselective media are measured (at the indicated time points, 485-nm excitation wavelength, 515-nm emission wavelength). To normalize results between experiments, the instrument fluorescence gain setting is adjusted so that the level of EGFP induction by 1-nM TCDD produces a relative fluorescence of 9000 relative fluorescence units (RFUs). To photograph the cells, after growth on 25-mm round cover slips for 24 h and treated with DMSO or a 1-nM TCDD containing sample for 48 h, H1G1.1c3 cells are replaced into PBS. Cell fluorescence is visualized at a 490-nm excitation filter and 535-nm emission filter.

Recombinant mouse hepatoma (H1L1.1c2) cells grown in 24-well microplates are incubated with DMSO (10 μL/mL) and a TCDD containing sample in DMSO or its related chemical containing sample in DMSO at 37°C for 4 h; luciferase activity of cells in each well is determined and normalized to sample protein concentration using fluorescamine with bovine serum albumin as the standard.

The complementary pair of 5′ -GAT-CTG-GCTCTTCTCACGCAACTCCG-3′ and 5′-GATCCGGAGTTGCGTGAGAAGAGCCA-3′ (corresponding to the AhR binding site of DRE3 and designated as the DRE oligonucleotide) is radio- labeled with [γ^{12}P]ATP (6000 Ci/mmol). Gel retardation analysis of cytosolic AhR complexes transformed *in vitro* with a TCDD containing sample (20 nM) or related chemical containing sample is performed and protein–DNA complexes are visualized. The amount of [^{32}P]-labeled DRE in the induced protein–DNA complex is determined.

RACB Protocol for Detecting Ovarian Toxicity of Xenobiotics

RACB protocol consists of Task 1 (initial dose-setting study), Task 2 (continuous breeding phase), Task 3 (crossover mating trial), and Task 4 (F_1 offspring dose). In Task 2, control (n = 40 animals/sex) and up to three treatment groups (n = 20 animals/sex) are implicated. In Task 2, F_0 (parental) rodents are exposed to a chemical containing sample during a 7-day premating period, randomly assigned to a mating pair, and treated with the same chemical containing sample and dose throughout a 98-day period of continual cohabitation (during which multiple litters are born). To encourage immediate remating, in early pregnancies, neonates are removed from the dam within 12 h. The principal toxicity in Task 2 is aberrant reproductive performance in F_0 rodents as indicated by alterations in the number of litters per breeding pair or neonatal body weight and sex ratio. If a positive toxicity is observed in Task 2, Task 3 should be performed to determine whether males or females are more sensitive. For this phase, both male and female high-dose F_0 mice are paired to control F0 mice of the opposite sex, and reproductive performance is compared to determine the affected sex (es). If a negative toxicity is observed in Task 2, Task 3 is omitted. After 98 days, breeding pairs are separated and continuously treated until the F_1 generation is delivered and weaned. In Task 4 the F_1 offspring of Task 2 parents are dosed until 74 ± 10 days of age, at which time male and female animals from the same treatment group but different litters are mated (n = 20 /sex/group) to generate F_2 litters. The F_1 offspring have been exposed to the chemical as gametes and as young adults during prenatal and post-natal development.

Ovaries from Task 1 (approximately 50 days old), F_0 parents from negative Task 2 (approximately 215 days old) or from Task 3 (approximately 240 days old), or F_1 offspring from Task 4 (approximately 120 days old) are removed at necropsy, trimmed of fat, fixed by immersion in Bouin's solution for 12 to 24 h, and transferred to 70% ethanol for storage and transport. An intact ovary from each animal is dehydrated in graded alcohols and xylene, embedded in a longitudinal orientation in separate paraffin blocks, and sectioned serially at 6 μm (approximately 400 sections per ovary). To each slide (approximately 40 slides per ovary), two rows of five sections retained in sequence are applied and stained with hematoxylin and eosin. Counts of ovaries from 10 mice per group are gathered. Ovaries are available from only 5 to 6 treated animals in F_1 offspring from two Task 4 EGME assays and from 9 treated animals from Task 2 oxalic acid study. To produce an equal number of control tissues for analysis from untreated animals of the same studies, the ovaries are also chosen randomly. Beginning with the first section of the first slide, sections from each ovary are examined. At least from the third or fourth section (a distance of 18 to 24 μm into the ovary), follicles are encountered and then categorized and enumerated. Differential counts from every tenth section or approximately 40 sections per ovary are made.

The ovarian follicles are categorized to small, growing, and antral ones by (1) the relative cross-sectional diameter of the follicle as measured from the outer margins of the granulosa cell layers, (2) the number of granulosa cell layers, and (3) the nature of the antral space. Small follicles, approximately 20 μm in mean diameters, consist of an isolated oocyte or an oocyte surrounded by a partial or unbroken, single layer of granulosa cells. Growing follicles, 20 to 70 μm, have an oocyte surrounded by a multilayered, solid mantle of granulosa cells. Antral follicles, more than 70 μm, are characterized by a central oocyte and fluid-filled space bordered by hundreds of layered granulosa cells. Each counting session is limited to no more than 3 h to limit fatigue.

Uroepithelial Cell Assay for Detecting Urotoxicity of Chemicals

Male beagle dogs (31 months old) are individually housed at 23 ± 2°C and a relative humidity of 60 ± 20% with a 12-h light/dark cycle. The dogs from a control group are anesthetized by sodium pentobarbital (25 mg/kg, i.v.) and killed by exsanguination. The bladder is aseptically excised, then lengthwise incised, and washed three times with the Krebs solution containing 110-mM NaCl, 5.8-mM KCl, 25-mM $NaHCO_3$, 1.2-mM KH_2PO_4, 2.0-mM $CaCl_2$, 1.2-mM $MgSO_4$, and 11.1-mM glucose (pH 7.4) at 4°C. After removal of excess fatty tissues, the bladder is transferred, mucosal side down, to a metal rack with 10 sharp metal pins along each edge, placed in 4°C Krebs solution, and the smooth muscle layer is carefully removed. The tissue is stretched, mucosal side up, across the metal pins on a 10 × 10/cm² plate, incubated in the minimum essential medium (MEM) containing 1% (v/v) penicillin/streptomycin/fungizon (PSF), 2.5-mg/mL dispase, and 20-mM MEM/ PSF/dispase solution (pH 7.4) at 4°C for 24 h, the MEM/PSF/dispase solution is aspirated, the stripped mucosa is transferred to a sterile 150-mm culture dish, and uroepithelial cells are scraped from the connective tissues with cell scrapers, which are suspended in 20 mL of trypsin-EDTA (0.25% trypsin and 1-mM EDTA·4Na) and incubated at 37°C for 30 min. Later, the single cell suspension is diluted with MEM containing 1% PSF, 5% FBS, and 20-mM MEM/PSF/FBS solution (pH 7.4) to 50 mL, spun down at 4°C, and centrifuged (1000 g, 5 min). The supernatant is aspirated to prepare the suspension of the cells in 50 mL of MEM/PSF/FBS solution. The cells are then rewashed in 50 mL of the keratinocyte-SFM medium and resuspended at 6.0–7.0 × 10^5 cells/mL.

By mixing 5 mg of type IV collagen, 100 μL of glacial acetic acid, and 50 mL of distilled water, the collagen solution is prepared, kept overnight at 4°C, sterilized with a 0.22-μm bottle top filter, and stored at 4°C. The keratinocyte medium is added to both chambers and incubated at 37°C for 2 h. Before use, the collagen solution is diluted 1:9 with 10-mM Na_2CO_3-HCl (pH 9.0), of which 500 μL is added to each apical chamber after aspirating the keratinocyte medium and incubated at 37°C for 1 h. Before plating, the collagen solution is aspirated, 0.5 mL of the cell suspension is added to the apical chamber, and 1.5 mL of keratinocyte medium is added to the basal chamber. After incubation at 37°C for 3 days, when the transepithelial electric resistance (TER) reaches levels of approximately 1000 Ωcm^2 or higher, the apical and basal media are aspirated and replaced with 0.5 and 1.5 mL of the keratinocyte medium containing 1-mM $CaCl_2$ (KM/Ca solution), respectively, and TER is measured. Before use, by immersing in 70% ethanol, the electrodes are sterilized and washed with sterile PBS, and Ωcm^2 are calculated.

Cultured cells on a 12-mm transwell filter are fixed in 2% glutaraldehyde of 0.1-M phosphate buffer (pH 7.4), rinsed with 8.2% sucrose, postfixed in 1% OsO_4 of the buffer, dehydrated with alcohol, and embedded in epoxy resin. For light microscopic examination, the semi-thin sections are stained with 1% toluidine blue. To observe cells with a transmission electron microscope, ultrathin sections are stained with uranyl acetate and lead citrate. For immunofluorescence staining, the cultured cells on a 12-mm transwell filter are successively fixed with HISTO-CHOICE at room temperature for 1 min and acidic methanol (95% methanol and 5% glacial acetic acid) at –20°C for 15 min, then incubated successively with anti-ZO-1 rabbit polyclonal antibody diluted 1 : 50 with PBS for 1 h and FITC-conjugated donkey antirabbit IgG diluted 1:40 with PBS for 30 min, or incubated successively with anti-E-cadherin mouse monoclonal antibody 1:100 with PBS and FITC-conjugated goat antimouse IgG diluted 1:10 with PBS. To observe cells with a confocal laser scanning microscope, the cells are washed three times for 5 min with PBS, the cell-grown transwell filters are cut, transferred to a slide glass, and mounted with the mounting medium.

After plating on a 12-mm transwell filter, TERs are monitored for 20 days, during which the medium is replaced every 3 days. When TER reaches 10,000 Ωcm^2 or more, the cultured cells are observed and their ZO-1 and E-cadherin are checked. Validating this culture system in the examination of the effects of cytochalasin-B on TER and ZO-1, cytochalasin-B is first dissolved in DMSO, diluted with the KM/Ca solution to make concentration of 1.6 μM (final DMSO concentration, 0.08%), 4 μM (final DMSO concentration, 0.2%), and 10 μM (final DMSO concentration, 0.5%), and sterilized with a 0.22-μm membrane filter. TER is measured 0, 1, 2, 4, 8, 24, and 48 h after exposure, and immunofluorescence for ZO-1 is observed 48 h after exposure, with DMSO diluted 1 : 200 with KM/Ca solution serving as a negative control solution.

Mating Efficiency Assay for Detecting Toxicity of Endocrine Disruptors

In the pheromone signaling pathway experiment, yeast *Saccharomyces cerevisiae* strains W303A (MATa; ade2, his3, trp1, ura3) with pSL307 plasmid fused to the FUS1-lacZ are cultured in SD medium (0.67% yeast nitrogen base and 2% glucose/ L) supplemented with adenine, l-histidine, and l-tryptophan at 30°C overnight. To fresh YPD medium (10 g of Bacto-yeast extract, 20 g of Bacto-peptone/L, and 2% glucose) or SD medium one tenth of the overnight culture is transferred, incubated at 30°C for 3 h, and the cultures that are adjusted at the logarithmic phase (OD = 0.8–1.0) of growth are harvested and subsequently used at 30°C.

W303A and W303A with fused plasmid pSL307 are incubated in YPD or SD medium for 60 min with or without test compound, harvested, washed three times with distilled water, and incubated in fresh YPD or SD medium with 5-mM α factor for 120 min to observe shmoo formation. Using a β-galactosidase activity assay, the pheromone response pathway in the W303A strain with pSL307 fused to the FUS1-lacZ reporter gene is quantified. Yeast cells are centrifuged at 3000 g, pellets are washed twice in distilled water, resuspended in 1.0 mL of Z buffer (21.5-g $Na_2HPO_4 \cdot 12H_2O$, 6.2-g $NaH_2PO_4 \cdot 2H_2O$, 0.75-g KCl, 0.246-g $MgSO_4 \cdot 7H_2O$, 2.7- mL β-mercaptoethanol/l, pH 7.0) with glass beads, with which three drops of chloroform and two drops of 0.1% SDS are mixed by ortex mixing, and incubated at 28°C for 5 min. After the addition of 0.2 mL of 4-mg/mL *p*-nitrophenyl-β-D-galactopyranoside at 28°C, the reaction is started, and by the addition of 0.5 mL of 1-M Na_2CO_3, the reaction is stopped. On removal of the cells by centrifugation, the superant is measured at 420 nm. In the mating efficiency assay, the diluted W303A strain is treated with the solution of test chemicals in YPD medium for 60 min and spread on both SD and YPD media. The colony-forming units (CFUs) of W303A strain on YPD medium are incubated for 2–3 days to give the cardinal number of mating efficiency. Simultaneously, the 144-3A strain (MATa; ura3, leu2, his4) is incubated on YPD medium for 60 min and streaked with diluted W303A strain on SD medium. Conjugated diploid 144-3A strain/W303A strain on SD medium complements the auxotrophy of each haploid cell.

Pnar-gfp Assay for Detecting Carcinogenic Toxicity of Nitrate

Escherichia coli DH5α (Φ80dlacZΔM15 recA endA gyrA thi hsdR supE relA deoRΔ [lacZYA-argF]), pUC18 (for routine cloning procedures), pCRII (for TA cloning of PCR products), pGreen-TIR containing the gfp gene, and pMV4 containing the narG promoter are used. Minimal medium (pH 7.0) contains 3.9-mM KH_2PO_4, 6.1-mM K_2HPO_4, 1.5-mM $(NH_4)_2SO_4$, 0.2-mM $MgSO_4 \cdot 7H_2O$, 22.4-μM $MnSO_4 \cdot 4H_2O$, 0.9-μM $FeSO_4 \cdot 4H_2O$, 4.4-μM $CaCl_2 \cdot 2H_2O$, 400-mg/L casamino acids, 14.8-μM thiamine hydrochloride, and 22.2-mM glucose. LB medium (pH 7.5) contains 10-g/L bacto-tryptone, 5-g/L yeast extract, and 10-g/L NaCl. *E. coli* DH5α (pPNARGFP) cultures are supplemented with 100-μg/mL ampicillin. Primers J1 (5′-CATCGAATTCTCCTGTGGGAGCCT-3′) and J2 (5′-CTGGCATGCATTCACTTGCCGCCTT-3′) are designated for the amplification of the nar promoter. J1 contains an artificial GAATTC (EcoRI site) and anneals to nucleotides +3 to –23 in the nar region, where +1 is the first nucleotide of the start codon. J2 contains an artificial GCATGC (SphI site) and anneals to nucleotides –438 to –414. After purification using Qiagen Plasmid Midi Kits or Wizard Plus SV miniprep kits, the DNA sequence is determined by MWG Biotech. The whole bacterial cells are measured with an excitation wavelength of 480 nm (10-nm bandwidth) and an emission wavelength of 510 nm (5-nm bandwidth) on a fluorescence spectrometer. The nitrate-induced fluorescence image of *E. coli* DH5α (pPNARGFP) is obtained with a BP465-495 excitation filter and a Ba 520 emission filter on a fluorescence microscope equipped with epifluorescence optics. The measurements of optical density are performed on a spectrophotometer at 600 nm.

Antiviral and Anticancer Assay

The elucidation of the mechanisms of special enzymes provides the bases for highly specific and sensitive bioassays focused on the target enzymes and cells. The alkaline phosphatase (AP) enzyme in the human endometrial adenocarcinoma cell line is sensitive to estrogen stimulation. Selective inhibition of the lyase activity of DNA polymerase sensitizes cancer cells to DNA-damaging agents. The human immunodeficiency virus type-1 reverse transcriptase (HIV-1 RT) and protease play key roles in HIV replication. The overexpression of the P-glycoprotein can produce cancer cell multidrug resistance (MDR). The receptor phosphorylation may induce ligand-induced receptor tyrosine kinase activation. Based on these facts, the human breast cancer cell assay, the Ishikawa cell and rat assay, the RT–PCR and swine assay, the antitubercular and cytotoxic assay, the DNA polymerase β lyase assay, the HIV-1 protease and reverse transcriptase kinetic assay, the P-glycoprotein pump assay, and the kinase receptor activation (KIRA) assay are established and can be used in bioassays.

Human Breast Cancer Cell Assay for Detecting Anticancer Activity

Toxicity against brine shrimp *Artemia salina* nauplii is carried out in 96-well micro- plates using emetine hydrochloride as a positive control. The selection of human breast cancer cell lines (MCF-7, MCF-7/ADR, MT-1, and MDA-MB-435) provides cells with a variety of receptor types; for instance, MCF-7 cells express high levels of estrogen receptors, MCF-7/ADR cells are resistant to doxorubicin, MT-1 cells have low estrogen receptor levels, the MDA-MB435 cell line has no estrogen receptors. In the determination of inhibition of cell growth in 96-well microtitre plates, the MTT assay is used. The samples of test compounds in DMSO are diluted in medium so that the concentration of DMSO is more than 1% and does not affect cell growth. Overall, 180-μL aliquots of a cell suspension (1–2 × 10^4 cells/mL) are plated into microplate wells and incubated overnight at 37°C in air containing 5% CO_2, and 150 μL of the culture medium is replaced with 150 μL of fresh medium, to which 20 μL of the solution of the test sample in medium is added to give final concentrations in the plate of 10, 1, 0.1, 0.01, and 0.001 μg/mL. Control wells with medium only and a positive control with 5-fluorouracil are used in each test. After 96 h of the incubation, 150 μL of medium is replaced with 150 μL of fresh medium, to which 20 μL of the 5-mg/mL MTT solution is added. After incubation for 4 h, 180 μL of medium is replaced with 180 μL of DMSO and carefully mixed and then determined at 540 nm using an enzyme-linked immunosorbent assay (ELISA) multiwell spectrophotometer.

Ishikawa Cell and Rat Assay for Detecting Antiestrogens

The cells are grown in 96-well plates in estrogen-free medium (phenol red free, with charcoal-stripped calf serum) and contain test compounds and antiestrogens at concentrations that are varied over several log orders. For the antiestrogen assay, to the cells, a range of concentrations of samples are added concurrently with 1-nM antiestrogens. After grown for 3 days, to determine AP activity, the cells are frozen, defrosted, and incubated with p-nitrophenylphosphate at room temperature, and the hydrolysis product p-nitrophenol is measured kinetically at 405 nm.

The specificity of the antiestrogenic activity is determined by using ERα and ERβ in ER element (ERE)-transfected human choriocarcinoma JAR cells, which are transfected with plasmids containing a consensus ERE fused to a firefly luciferase reporter gene and separately with the expression vectors for either human ERα or human ERβ. JAR cells are routinely cultured in RPMI 1640 supplemented with 10% fetal bovine serum, 0.5% non-essential amino acids, and 1% PEST (100-U penicillin/mL and 100-μg streptomycin/mL). After seeded in six-well plates for 24 h, cells are transfected using the Mirus Trans IT reagent in a serum- and antibiotic-free mixture of phenol-red free OptiMEM with 0.1–0.4-μg pC × N2 human ERα or pC × N2 h-ERβ, and a 0.75-μg 3 × ERE-TATA-Luc reporter constructed by introducing an HpaI/BglII fragment containing 3 × ERE-TATA into SmaI/BglII of the pGL3-Luc basic vector. Medium is replaced with a phenol red-free RPMI containing 10% dextran-coated charcoal-treated calf serum and 0.5% non-essential amino acids. Twenty-four hours later, antiestrogens are added. Cells are incubated at 37°C in 5% CO_2 for 12 h, harvested in 10-mM Tris-HCl/10-mM EDTA/150-mM NaCl, and centrifuged at 4000 g for 4 min. The supernatant is removed, the cell pellets are lysed in Lysis Buffer 2, and luciferase activity is measured.

After the AP assay and washing three times with PBS, the Ishikawa cells are lysed using 1% Nonidet P-40 and 0.1% sodium dodecyl sulfate in the presence of protease inhibitors. Before the antibody incubation, proteins (25 μg/well) separated by SDS–PAGE on ice using 10% polyacrylamide gel are transferred to nitrocellulose membranes stained with Ponceau Red to ensure proper transfer. After blocking the membranes with 5% powdered milk in water, immunoblotting is performed. The blots are incubated with the ERα monoclonal antibody clone 6F11 overnight at 4°C. Using peroxidase-labeled horse antimouse secondary antibody and Chemiluminescence Reagent Plus, ERα is detected by Western blotting. Using a digital imaging analysis system, the intensity of the signal is analyzed. To normalize the amount of protein loaded in the gels, β-actin is used as an internal control. The uterotrophic assay is performed with stimulation in immature rats. Female SD rats (22 days old) are injected s.c. daily for 3 days with antiestrogens, control animals receive the vehicle (0.1-mL sesame oil), then animals are killed, and uteri are removed, dissected, blotted, and weighed. To determine whether antiestrogens have tissue-selective effects in cholesterol, uteri, and bone, ovariectomized female SD rats (250 g) are injected with antiestrogens s.c. for 35 days, and then killed by exsanguination under ether anesthesia. The total cholesterol concentration of the serum is determined by a commercial chromogenic assay. The uteri are dissected, weighed, fixed in formalin, and imbedded in paraffin to prepare for 5-μm sections. Using the Openlab image analysis system, endometrial luminal epithelium and glandular cell height are measured. The tibia free of extraneous tissue are histomorphometrically analyzed. The bones fixed in 70% ethanol are dehydrated in graded ethanol and cleared in toluene. Then the specimens are infiltrated with increasing concentrations of methymethacrylate (MMA) and embedded in MMA. After polymerization, MMA blocks are cut to size, sanded, and polished to the appropriate level to prepare 4–5-μm sections. The sections are mounted on gelatin-coated slides, stained with toluidine blue, and measured.

RT–PCR and Swine Assay for Detecting Anti-HEV Antibody

To choose seronegative pigs for inoculation, 75 SPF pigs (2 weeks old) are tested by ELISA for swine Hepatitis E virus (HEV) IgG antibodies. Before inoculation, the pigs are allowed to acclimate to the research facilities for 1 week. Tissues (liver, heart, pancreas, or skeletal muscle) and feces of HEV-infected SPF pigs are collected at 3–7, 14–20, and 27–55 days postinoculation (DPI) and are pooled and stored at –70°C for inoculation. Each inoculum is prepared as a tissue homogenate or fecal suspension (10%, w/v) in PBS and tested by a semiquantitative RT–PCR for swine HEV RNA. The positive control inoculum is a standard infectious pool of swine feces with a $10^{4.5}$ 50% pig infectious doses (PID_{50}) of swine HEV/mL.

Total RNA is extracted from 100 μL of each sample by TriZol reagent and tested by a nested PCR with primers located in the putative capsid gene (ORF2. In the first round PCR, the fragment of 404 base pairs (bps) with the forward primer F1 (5′-AGCTCCTGTACCTGATGTTGACTC-3′) and the reverse primer R1 (5′-CTACAGAGCGCCAGCCTTGATTGC-3′) is formed. In the second round PCR, the fragment of 266 bps with the forward primer F2 (5′-GCTCACGTCATCTGTCGCTGCTGG-3′) and the reverse primer R2 (5² -GGGCTGAACCAAAATCCTGACATC-3²) is formed. With R1 reverse primer and SuperScript II reverse transcriptase (GIBCO/BRL), total RNA is reverse transcribed at 42°C for 1 h and the resulting cDNA is amplified by PCR with ampliTaq Gold DNA polymerase. The PCR reaction is carried out for 39 cycles of denaturation at 94°C for 1 min, annealing at 52°C for 1 min, extension at 72°C for 1.5 min, and incubation at 72°C for 7 min. Overall, 10 μL of each round of PCR are mixed as the template. By gel electrophoresis, the amplified PCR products are examined. The virus titer of inocula is calculated and expressed as a genome equivalent (GE)/mL. After 7 to 21 days, serum samples of inoculated pigs are collected and tested by RT–PCR for swine HEV RNA. Anti-HEV IgG antibodies in swine sera are detected using a standardized ELISA. A purified 55-kDa truncated recombinant putative capsid protein of human HEV strain Sar-55 is used as the antigen that cross-reacts well with the swine HEV. Peroxidase-labeled goat antiswine IgG is used as the secondary antibody. Duplicates per serum sample are used.

Antitubercular and Cytotoxic Assay

Using the microtiter plate alamarblue technique, the antitubercular activity is assessed against a nonvirulent strain of *Mycobacterium tuberculosis* ($H_{37}Ra$). As positive controls, isoniazid and kanamycin sulfate exhibit MICs in the ranges of 0.29–0.66 and 3.5–8.5 μM, respectively. According to the sulforhodamine B procedure, cytotoxicity is determined. MCF-7 (human breast adenocarcinoma), HeLa (human cervical carcinoma), KB (human oral epidermoid carcinoma), and HT-29 (colorectal carcinoma) are used as the target cell lines. After exposure to test samples, cell viability is determined colorimetrically at 515 nm. Dose-response evaluations yield a concentration mediating a 50% cytotoxic response (IC_{50}).

DNA Polymerase β Lyase Assay

Using terminal deoxynucleotidyltransferase + [α-^{32}P] ddATP, a 36-nucleotide oligodeoxyribonucleotide containing uridine at position 21 is labeled at its 3′-end and the product is subjected to 20% denaturing polyacrylamide gel electrophoresis for purification. Using autoradiography, the interesting band is visualized and excised. By heating to 70°C for 3 min and then slow cooling to 25°C, the DNA substrate is annealed to its complementary strand. To 200 μL of 354-nM [α-^{32}P]-labeled double-stranded oligodeoxynucleotide with uridine at position 21, 10-mM Hepes-KOH (pH 7.4), 5-mM $MgCl_2$, 50-mM KCl, 10-mg/mL bovine serum albumin, 2.4U of uracil-DNA glycosylase, and 3U of AP endonuclease are added, incubated at 37°C for 20 min, and an apurinic (AP) site is created in the [α-^{32}P]-labeled double-stranded oligodeoxynucleotide. To 5 μL of the above reaction mixture, the test samples and 0.172 U of rat DNA polymerase β are added. After incubation at room temperature for 30 min, the reaction is terminated by adding 0.5-M $NaBH_4$ (50-mM final concentration) and incubated at room temperature for 10 min. The reaction products are incubated at 70–80°C for another 20 min, separated on a 20% denaturing polyacrylamide gel, and visualized by autoradiography.

A total of 200 μL of culture samples containing approximately 1.0×10^4 A549 cells (maintained in Kaighn's modification of Ham's F12 medium (F12K) with 2-mM L-glutamine supplemented with 1.5-g/L sodium bicarbonate and 10% fetal bovine serum at 37°C in air containing 5% CO_2) are placed in each well of 96-well culture plates, treated with test samples, and incubated at 37°C for 48 h in air containing 5% CO_2. In the determination of cytotoxicity, the culture medium is replaced with 15 μL of 5-mg/mL MTT per well, the samples are incubated at 37°C for 4 h in air containing 5% CO_2, 200 μL of DMSO is added, and the OD_{570} value is obtained using a microplate reader.

HIV-1 Protease and Reverse Transcriptase Kinetic Assay

To the wells of a streptavidinecoated microtiter plate containing 20 μL of test sample solution and 4 ng of the HIV-1 RT in 20 μL of lysis buffer, 20 μL of the reaction mixture containing a homogenous template/primer hybrid ($(rA)_n(dT)_{15}$, 750 mA_{260nm}/mL final concentration) and a triphosphate substrate (dUTP/dTTP, 10-μM final concentration) are added. After the reaction is carried out at 37°C for 1 h, 200 μL of anti-digoxigenin-peroxide solution and ABTS [2,2–azino-bis- (3- ethyl benzothiazoline-6-sulfonic acid) diammonium salt] substrate are added for the coloring reaction. The absorbance of each well is measured at 405 nm with the reference wavelength at 490 nm and nevirapine as the reference compound. Using the same procedure mentioned above, except for the concentration of the enzyme solution (1 ng of the HIV-1 RT), the incubation time (30, 52, 80, 105, 130 min), and various concentrations of either the template/primer (1500, 750, 187.5 mA_{260nm}/mL) or the triphosphate substrate (20, 15, 10, 5, 2.5 mM) in the presence of the inhibitor, the enzyme kinetic assay is also performed. With a slight modified procedure to that mentioned above, the HIV-1 protease assay is performed. To the mixture of 1μL of the solution of test compound in DMSO and 10.5 μL of the substrate solution (His-Lys-Ala-Arg-Val-Leu-(p-NO_2)-Phe-Glu-Ala-Nle-Ser-NH_2, 0.1 mg/mL in HIV-1 protease assay buffer), 0.5 μL of the recombinant protease solution (0.3 mg/mL) is added and incubated at 37°C for 15 min, the reaction is stopped by the addition of 1.2 μL of 10% trifluoroacetic acid, and the reaction mixture is diluted with 20 μL of water. The hydrolysate and the remaining substrate are quantitatively analyzed by HPLC [column, Inertsil ODS-3 (4.6 × 150 mm), a linear gradient of CH_3CN (15% to 40%) in 0.1% TFA, an injection volume of 20 μL, and a flow rate of 1.0 mL/min, detection at 280 nm]. The hydrolysate and substrate are eluted at 8.61 and 10.84 min, respectively.

P-Glycoprotein Pump Assay

MCF-7R cells (human breast adenocarcinoma cell line, resistant to adriamycin) maintained at 37°C in humidified atmospheric air containing 5% CO_2 in nutrient mixture (F10/HAM, contains L-glutamine, with 10% fetal calf serum, 1% non-essential amino acids, 60-μg/mL tylosin, and 1% antibiotic/antimycotic solution) are seeded in the wells of 96-well tissue microtiter culture plates at 3 × 10^4 cells in 200 μL of medium per well, incubated at 37°C for 24 h in a humidified atmospheric air containing 5% CO_2, and the medium is replaced with fresh medium containing 0.3-μM rhodamine 6 G together with samples. To thorough mixing of 50 μL of each of these prepared mixtures, 450 μL of fresh medium containing 0.3-μM rhodamine 6 G is added. After incubation of the test compound, reserpine (positive control) or rhodamine alone (negative control) is added and the plates are incubated at 37°C for another 3 h. Then the cells are washed twice with 200 μL of ice-cold PBS and trypsinized with 100 μL of phenol-red free trypsin solution for 15 min, which is then transferred onto empty wells. Overall, 100 μL of 4% SDS in PBS is added and the plates are shaken for 2 h to solubilize the cells and release rhodamine 6 G, which is determined by measuring the fluorescence of the dye at excitation and emission wavelengths of 530 /25 and 590 /35 nm, respectively.

On Lab-Tek chamber slides, MCF-7R cells are seeded at 5 × 10^4 cells per chamber and incubated at 37°C for 24 h in a humidified atmospheric air containing 5% CO_2, and the medium is replaced with fresh medium containing 0.3-μM rhodamine 6 G with or without 50-μM reserpine, with 100-μg/mL samples in separate chambers of the slide. The cells are incubated at 37°C for another 3 h and imaged using fluorescence microscopy with a 510–560-nm band-pass excitation filter and a 590-nm long-pass emission filter set.

KIRA Assay

There are two different approaches using the KIRA format. The first approach, IGF-I KIRA, uses adherent MCF-7 cells derived from a human breast adenocarcinoma expressing an endogenous IGF-I receptor to measure the bioactivity of IGF-I. MCF-7 cells are seeded in each well of a flat-bottomed 96-well culture plate and incubated overnight, the supernatants are decanted, and the plates are lightly blotted on paper towels. To each well, the medium containing either experimental samples or the recombinant IGF-I standards are added. The cells are exposed to ligand for 15 min, the super natants are decanted, and the plates are blotted. After addition of lysis buffer containing Triton X-100, sodium orthovanadate, and a cock-tail of protease inhibitors, the crude lysates are generated and then transferred to an ELISA plate coated overnight with a 3B7 antibody (5.0 mg/mL) and blocked with 0.5% BSA. After removal of unbound material, the degree of receptor tyrosine phosphorylation is quantified with biotinylated anti-phosphotyrosine monoclonal antibody followed by HRP-conjugated dextranstreptavidin, and visualized with the development of a tetramethyl benzidine (TMB) substrate. The absorbance is determined at 450 nm with a 650-nm reference wavelength.

The second approach, N-terminal polypeptide D (gD)·trkA KIRA using CHO cells stably transfected with a recombinant human trkA receptor with an gD flag, is developed to measure the bioactivity of NGF. A polypeptide flag is cloned onto the N-terminus or C-terminus of the full-length recombinant human receptor stably transfected into CHO cells. A 26-amino-acid polypeptide derived from HSV gD as a capture reagent in the ELISA phase of the KIRA and a mAb 3C8 antibody as the capture antibody are used.

Hepatoxicity and Hepatoprotective Assay

Mitochondrial proliferation of the chemicals related to hepatocellular carcinomas and their hepatocarcinogenecity are important factors for health. The renal adenocarcinomagenecity, hepatic adenoma, and carcinomagenecity induced by chemicals can promote the formation of preneoplastic foci in rats or mice. The clonal growth of glutathione-S-transferase (GST-P) enzyme-altered foci and the histopathological change in the liver of rats or mice may relate to liver carcinogenesis of chemicals. In the liver injury induced by chemicals, such as CCl_4, Bacillus Calmette Guerin (BCG), and lipopolysaccharide (LPS), the activities of protein, glucose 6-phosphatase, amidopyrine *N*-demethylase, and aniline hydroxylase; the levels of hepatic triglycerides and lipid peroxidation; the concentrations of nitric oxide (NO), content of malondialdehyde (MDA), and superoxide dismutate (SOD); and the viability of thymocytes can be changed significantly. In the hepatocarcinogenesis induced by chemicals such as chloral hydrate, the body weight of B6C3F1 mice can be decreased significantly. Proliferation factor (PF) and hepatocyte growth factor (HGF) are involved in liver regeneration cascade and TGF-β-induced growth inhibition of CCL-64 cells; thus, PFs present in the partially hepatectomized rat serum can serve as an index of liver regeneration cascade and two cytokines (HGF and HGF) may result in an additive effect on proliferation. Based on these facts, the GST-P enzyme-altered foci assay, partial hepatectomy assay, hepatoprotective assay, immunological assay, body-weight-based liver tumor incidence assay, hepatocyte primary culture assay, and CCL-64 cell growth assay are established.

GST-P Enzyme-Altered Foci Assay

According to the required levels (0%, 0.03%, 0.1%, and 0.3%), the test chemical is incorporated into an irradiated (6.0 kGy) powder diet MF. The stability of 0.1%, 0.03%, 0.5%, and 5.0% chemical in the prepared diets is previously confirmed for 6 weeks at room temperature. Male F344/DuCrj rats (5 week old) are given an approximately 1-week quarantine/acclimation period to monitor health conditions and body weights. The normal rats (6 week old) are randomly divided into 8 groups (18 rats each for groups 1–5, 9 rats each for groups 6–8). The rats of groups 1–5 receive an injection of the initiator N-nitrosodiethylamine (200-mg/kg body weight, i.p.). The rats of groups 6–8 receive an injection of the vehicle. Two weeks later, the rats receive an injection of the test chemical at the desirable dose for a suitable treating period.

Three weeks after beginning the experiment, all rats are given two-thirds partial hepatectomy. At week 8, all surviving rats are killed under ether anesthesia and their organs in the thoracic and abdominal cavities are examined macroscopically. Their livers are immediately excised and weighed to calculate the liver-to-body-weight ratio. For the 4–5-mm thick sections, the cranial and caudal parts of the right lateral lobe and the caudal part of the caudate lobe of all surviving rats are fixed in 10% buffered formalin solution, embedded in paraffin wax, sectioned, and stained immunohistochemically for glutathione S-transferase analysis (GST-P, ABC method). All GST-P positive hepatocytic foci larger than 0.2 mm in diameter (the lowest limit for reliable evaluation) are measured using a color image processor, and the numbers and areas (foci/cm^2) of the liver section are calculated. By microscopic analysis, BrdU-positive labeling indices (LIs) are quantified by randomly counting the number of positive nuclei per 1000 hepatocytes or number per unit area (mm^2) in sections stained immunohistochemically for BrdU.

Partial Hepatectomy Assay

Male F344 rats (30 days old) acclimated for 4 weeks before the experiment are randomly divided into 3 groups. At week 0, the rats receive a single i.p. injection of the solution of N-nitrosodiethylamine (200 mg/kg) in 0.9% saline. Two weeks later, the rats receive daily gavage administration of corn oil or 0.1-mmol/kg test chemical in a corn oil vehicle through the remainder of the 8-week study. At week 3, all rats receive a partial hepatectomy. The rats are given food and water, and lighting is set on a 12-h light/dark cycle. On days 23, 26, 28, 47, and 56, at least five rats from each group are sacrificed by aortic exsanguination. Whole livers are removed, and the tissues are fixed in 10% neutral-buffered formalin, embedded in paraffin, serially sectioned at 5 μm, and mounted on microscope slides. Formalin-fixed sections are stained with hematoxylin and eosin to perform histopathological examination.

Hepatoprotective Assay

To induce liver injury, CF rats (150–200 g) and Swiss albino mice (20–30 g) of either sex are administered orally CCl_4 diluted with liquid paraffin. The animals of the vehicle control group are orally administered an equal volume of liquid paraffin. In hepatoprotective studies, four suitable doses of test compound and two standard doses of silymarin (25 and 50 mg/kg, p.o.) are fed to a respective group of rats 48 h, 24 h, and 2 h before and 6 h after CCl_4 (0.5 μL/kg, p.o.) intoxication. From the orbital sinus of all animals, blood is collected 18 h after CCl4 intoxication for glutamic-pyruvic transaminase (GPT), glutamic oxaloacetic transaminase (GOT), and bilirubin analysis. In the posttreatment studies, the same doses of test compound and silymarin as mentioned for hepatoprotective studies are fed to rats 6 h, 24 h, and 48 h after CCl_4 (0.5 mL/kg, p.o.) intoxication. From all animals blood is collected 2 h after the last dose of test compound administration for GOT, GPT, and bilirubin analysis. The test compound and silymarin (50 mg/kg, p.o.) are fed to two different groups of rats at 48 h, 24 h, and 2 h before and 6 h after CCl_4 (100 μl/kg, p.o.) intoxication, with the remaining two groups served as CCl_4 and vehicle control. Eighteen hours after CCl_4 intoxication, all animals of the four groups are fasted overnight and killed by decapitation. Livers are immediately excised and divided into two parts for preparing homogenate (10%, w/v), among which one part is homogenized in isotonic sucrose (0.25 M) for determining protein and glucose 6-phosphatase activity, and for preparing microsomes by calcium precipitation to determine amidopyrine N-demethylase and aniline hydroxylase activities with spectrophotometric methods, in which NADPH is used instead of the NADPH generating system, and another part is homogenized in isotonic PBS (0.01 M, pH 7.2, 0.15-M NaCl) for determining hepatic triglycerides and lipid peroxidation. The hepatoprotective activity is expressed as hepatoprotective percentage H and calculated by $H = [1 - (T - V)/(C - V)] \times 100$, wherein T is mean value of drug and CCl_4, C is mean value of CCl_4 alone, and V is the mean value of control-treated animals. In the determination of acute toxicity, different groups of mice (each ten) are fed with different doses of test compound, with one group with the same number of mice served as control. The animals are observed continuously for 1 h and then hourly for 4 h for any gross behavioral changes and further up to 72 h for any mortality.

Immunological Assay

A suspension of 2.5 mg of BCG (viable bacilli) in 0.2 mL of saline is injected via the tail vein into each mouse, and 10 days later a solution of 7.5 μg of LPS in 0.2 mL of saline is injected. The mice are anesthetized with ether, sacrificed by cervical dislocation 16 h after LPS injection, and trunk blood is collected into heparinized tubes (50 U/mL) and centrifuged at 4°C and 1500 rpm for 10 min. Serum is aspirated and stored at –70°C until assayed as described below. The liver is also removed and stored at –70°C until required.

For the *in vivo* experiment, the mice are equally divided into 5 groups randomly, including normal, model control, and test compound groups (3 different doses). Mice in test compound groups receive suitable doses using an 18-gauge stainless steel animal feeding needle for 10 days before LPS injection. Mice in the normal and model control groups are fed the same volume of vehicle only. For the *in vitro* experiment, the Kupffer cells isolated from normal and BCG priming rats are divided into 7 groups randomly, including control cells, cells added with LPS (5 μg/mL) alone, and cells added with LPS (5 μg/mL) and the test compound.

The liver of normal rat is initially perfused through the portal vein with D-Hank's until blood free and finally by recirculation with Hank's containing 0.5-g/L collagenase IV until the vessels are digested (up to 20 min). The liver is scraped using a cell scraper, filtered by a 100-μM filter, and stirred in Hank's containing 2.5-g/L pronase and 0.05-g/L DNase at 37°C for 20 min. After three times of centrifugation and washing at 4°C and 300 g for 10 min in Gey's balanced salt solution (GBSS), the cells are centrifuged in an 180-g/L Nycodenz gradient at 2500 g for 20 min. Kupffer cells are carefully sucked by cusp-straws at the pearl layer inderphase. The purified Kupffer cell fractions are finally collected by centrifugal elutriation. The Kupffer cells are washed with Hanks' and resuspended in RPMI 1640 medium containing antibiotics (100-U/mL penicillin, 100-mg/mL streptomycin), 2-mM glutamine, and 10% fetal calf serum. Overall, 1-mL aliquots containing 1×10^6 cells are added to 24-well culture plates. The cells are incubated for 60 min in a humidified atmosphere containing 5% CO_2 at 37°C. Nonadherent cells are removed, and adherent cells are washed twice with PBS. To observe the direct effect, the cells at a density of 1 x 10^6/mL are incubated with different concentrations of test compound. The cells (1×10^6/well) are cultured for 48 h with 5-μg/mL LPS, the supernatants are collected, and the concentrations of TNF-α and NO are measured.

According to the *in vitro* liver injury model, BCG-induced Kupffer cells are isolated from the livers of the rats injected via the tail vein with 3 mg of BCG 10 days before, and hepatocytes are isolated from the normal rats. The hepatocytes (1×10^9/mL), different concentrations of test compound, and BCG-induced Kupffer cells (1×10^6/well) are cocultured for 48 h with 5-μg/mL LPS and the supernatants are collected. In a 96-well plate, 100 μL of cell culture supernatant and 100 μL of Griess reagent (10-g/L sulfanilamide and 1-g/L N-1-naphthylethylenediamine dihydrochloride in 2.5% phosphoric acid) are incubated at room temperature for 10 min. Absorbance at 540 nm is measured. The nitrite concentration is calculated by comparing samples with standard solutions of sodium nitrite produced in the culture medium.

Livers are thawed, weighed, homogenized with Tris-HCl (5 mM containing 2-mM EDTA, pH 7.4), and centrifuged (1000 g, 10 min, 4°C), and MDA and SOD in the supernatant are immediately analyzed. MDA in liver tissue is determined by the thiobarbituric acid method. The assay for total SOD is based on its ability to inhibit the oxidation of oxyamine by the xanthine–xanthine oxidase system. The absorbance of the red nitrite produced by the oxidation of oxyamine is determined at 550 nm. Thymocytes (2×10^6/well) from mice are cultured for 48 h in 96-well plates containing RPMI 1640 medium supplemented with 5-μg/mL concanavalin A and 0.1 mL of collected supernatant. Three hours before the termination of the culture, cells are pulsed with MTT stock (in sterile PBS, 5 mg/mL, stored in the dark at 4°C for up to 1 week, before use immediately filtered, 0.22 μm, to remove any formazan precipitate, 20 μL/well), returned to 37°C, and incubated for another 3 h. The plates are centrifuged at 1000 g for 10 min to form cell pellets and MTT formazan products. The supernatant is carefully aspirated without disturbing the pellets, and formazan is solubilized by adding isopropanol (100 μL of isopropanol : 200 μL of supernatant). Insoluble material is then removed by centrifugation at 1000 g for 10 min. The solubilized formazan in isopropanol is collected and distributed into 12-well flat-bottom ELASA plates at a final volume of 100 μL/well. Plates are read at 570 nm within 1 h of adding isopropanol.

Body Weight-Based Liver Tumor Incidence Assay

Addition to extra groups for high and low outliers, the B6C3F1 mice (at the 9-week age point) are assigned to 1 of 17 consecutive weight groups ranging from 20 to 57.5 g in 2.5-g intervals. Each weight group of mice developing a liver tumor is sorted for the calculation of the relative tumor risk. The mice with hepatocellular adenoma, carcinoma, or hepatoblastoma are designated as positive or otherwise designated as negative. The process is repeated for each age point to 68 weeks.

Approximately 4-, 5-, and 6-week-old male B6C3F1/Nctr BR mice are used at receipt, the initiation of controlled feeding, and on the first day of dosing, respectively. During the studies, the health of the mice is monitored. The dose for groups of 120 male mice receiving the solution of chloral hydrate in distilled water is 0, 25, 50, or 100 mg/kg (all at 5 mL/kg), 5 days per week for 104 to 105 weeks, each of which is divided into two dietary groups of 60 mice, and the vehicle controls received distilled water only. The *ad libitum* fed mice are fed available *ad libitum*, and the dietary controlled mice are fed in measured daily amounts. All mice have water available *ad libitum*. At the 71-week age point, 12 mice of each diet/dose group are euthanized for pathological and biochemical evaluation. At the 110-week age point, the remaining 48 mice of each diet/dose group are fasted overnight before necropsy. Among them the mice with liver tumors refer to mice bearing single or multiple hepatocellular adenomas, hepatocellular carcinomas, and/or hepatoblastomas.

From week 21, the weight dataset of the first experimental group is imported with the preceding week's dataset as a reference. According to the predefined sort criteria (including whether the weight value for the previous week is outside either the 5% or the 12% confidence limits of the idealized weight curve or whether the mouse gains or loses weight in the preceding week), each mouse weight from the dataset is sorted into its appropriate weight group and assigned either the corresponding *ad libitum* or the weight-reduced tumor risk value from the tumor risk tables. The resulting tumor risk dataset in the appropriate week's column of a new table is stored and proceeded to the next week's dataset. According to all weekly datasets from 21 to 68 weeks, the mean tumor risk for each mouse in the dataset is calculated, the survival time for each mouse is imported, and the Poly-3 weighting time at risk factor (a_{ij}) for each mouse is calculated. The mean (cumulative) tumor risk dataset is sorted into 2% incremental percentage tumor risk groups, and the corresponding a_{ij} value for each mouse is assigned into the appropriate tumor risk group. This procedure can be adapted to sort individual data for each week rather than the means of all 48 weeks. The resulting tumor risk group table is used to calculate the mean tumor risk estimate and standard deviation of the experimental group to predict the survival-adjusted liver tumor rate, over all liver tumor rates and the number of animals bearing tumors.

Hepatocyte Primary Culture Assay

On anesthetic male SD rats (225–250 g) with sodium pentobarbital (65 mg/kg i.p), tracheotomy is performed. A catheter is flushed with heparin (200 U/mL) to prevent blood clotting of PE 240 polyethylene tubing that is insertcd into the trachea to facilitate the respiration. By inserting PE 50 polyethylene tubing, the right femoral artery and vein of the rats are cannulated, and the rats are infused with 0.5-mL saline containing 1-mg/mL sodium pentobarbital/100-g body weight/h through the vein by a Syringe Infusion Pump to supplement fluid loss and maintain the anesthetic level. On the abdomen posteriorly from the xiphoid process of the sternum, a 3-cm median-line incision, which is sutured with two layers of the muscle and skin, is made. Using surgical silk (size 0), left lateral and median liver lobes are ligated and given the partial hepatectomy (2/3 PHX). At various time points after PHX, the diaphragm is cut, and within 2 min from the right ventricle of the heart, a blood sample (5–10 mL per rat) is drawn and centrifuged (2500 g, 20 min) for collecting plasma. In the preparation of serum, the blood is allowed to clot on ice for 10 min, then spun down, with the serum of non-PHX rats as 0 h control. For sham-operated rats, the liver is manipulated without PHX.

In the liver perfusion, the male SD rat (300 g) is anesthetized with sodium pentobarbital (65 mg/kg, i.p.). By surgical silk an 18 G, 1.25-in (32 mm) i.v. catheter is used as the portal vein catheter tie to the vein. Through a catheter inserted into the inferior vena cava via the right atrium of the heart, the perfusion buffer is drained. The liver is perfused with 400 mL of nonrecycled oxygenated Ca^{2+}-Mg^{2+} free Dulbecco's PBS (DPBS, 2.68-mM KCl, 1.47-mM KH_2PO_4, 136.9-mM NaCl, 8.1-mM Na_2HPO_4, pH 7.4) containing 0.49-mM EDTA to reduce Ca^{2+} in the liver tissue, with 100 mL of DPBS without EDTA to wash out the EDTA in the system and with 100 mL of recycled oxygenated collagenase/Swim's 77 (0.25 mg/mL) with 5-mM Ca^{2+} for 10–15 min. Upon finishing perfusion, the liver is rinsed thoroughly with 10–20 mL of sterile DMEM. The liver is transferred into a sterile petri dish containing fresh medium. Using two forceps, the liver capsule membrane is slit, which is gently shaken and the cells are released into the medium. Two Spectra/ Mesh N filters (70 μm, 40 μm,

Spectrum) are used to filter the isolated liver cells to remove tissue chunks and cell debris. The cell suspension is filtered by low-speed differential centrifugation (300 g, 3 min, 4°C) for further purification. By aspiration the supernatant is discarded, the cell pellet is gently mixed with fresh medium, and the centrifugation procedure is repeated three times. Using the trypan blue exclusion method, viable cell concentration and percentage of nonhepatocytes is determined. In the purification of hepatocyte, 20 μL of trypan blue (0.4%) are added into 20 μL of cell suspension (dilution factor = 2), which is mixed and loaded onto the hemocytometer. All corner squares (64 squares/chamber) of the two chambers are counted (128 squares total; each square is 1 nL, 128 nL $\times$ 7.813 = 1 μL). Viable cells/μL = viable cells per 128 squares $\times$ 7.813 $\times$ 2. The final concentration is the average value of three separate countings. Viability (%) = viable cells/(viable + dead cells) $\times$ 100%. Nonhepatocyte (%) = non hepatocyte/total cells $\times$ 100%.

Each well of six-well plates is coated with 20 μL of the solution of rat tail collagen (0.8-mg/mL double distilled H2O with 0.1% acetic acid) and allowed to dry. To the well approximately 2 mL of DMEM/F-12 (supplemented with 25-mM sodium bicarbonate, 10-mM HEPES, 100-U/mL penicillin G, and 0.1-mg/mL streptomycin) is added. To each well the suspension of viable cells (final cell concentration, 100,000 cells/mL) are seeded and constantly mixed by agitation. The plates are incubated at 37°C overnight. When the attachment reaches the end, the medium is changed, mildly shaken, and aspirated. The wells are rinsed with 1 mL of medium and aspirated. From three randomly selected wells in the culture, the counts of the viable tarting-cell-number are calculated. Serum or plasma samples in 2 mL of fresh medium (10%) are added to wells, to which heparin (35-U/mL final) is added to prevent the medium from clotting during the culture. Cells grown in serum-free medium and in serum-free medium plus 100-ng/mL EGF and 20-mU/mL insulin are used as the negative and positive control, respectively.

The medium is changed by aspiration at 24 h with no rinse. To each well, fresh medium with serum or plasma and other additives are added. At the end of 48 h, culture-attached hepatocytes are harvested and counted. The medium in each well is aspirated, serum or plasma-containing wells are rinsed once with saline and aspirated to wash off various plasma proteins. Overall, 400 μL of trypsin-EDTA is added to each well. The plate is covered and in the incubator for approximately 1 min and checked. The trypsin digestion is assessed. The plate is immediately placed on ice, and the serum of SD rats (40 μL, final concentration 10%) is added into each well to inhibit further trypsin digestion of the cells (440 μL total volume per well). On ice and using a pasteur pipet, the cells are gently blown from the bottom of the well. After all cells are lifted, the cell suspension is transferred into a 1.5-mL Eppendorf tube and kept on ice for an immediate counting with no centrifugation or trypsin removal. In a plate (dilution factor = 1.25) 40 μL of cells and 10 μL of 0.4% trypan blue are mixed and loaded onto the hemocytometer.

CCL-64 Cell Growth Assay

Serial dilutions of test samples are prepared on 96-well flat-bottomed microplates with 100 μL of CM per well. Before the assay, to activate latent TGF-B, the samples are transiently acidified by first adding HCl to pH 2 and subsequently neutralizing with NaOH. CCL-644 cells (Mv-1-Lu) grown in RPMI 1640 supplemented with 10% FCS, 2-mM L-glutamine, and 40-μg/mL gentamicin (Complete medium, CM) are seeded at 1 $\times$ 10^4 cells/well and grown for 24 h in a total volume of 0.2-mL CM. After 20 h, the cells are pulsed for 4 h with 1 μCi/well of [methyl-^{3}H]thymidine and harvested with a Micromate 196 cell harvester. The concentration of TGF-β in the sample is determined by the growth inhibition caused by the sample, compared with a standard curve obtained by testing serial dilutions of porcine TGF-β. When the assay is used to measure HGF, the concentration is determined by this cytokine's ability to reverse the growth inhibitory effect of 350 pg/mL of TGF-β.

ANTI-INFLAMMATORY ASSAY

In the development of serious diseases, inflammatory is frequently involved. The development of inflammatory events may be induced by chemicals such as glucocorticoid; are regulated by endogenous factors such as tumor necrosis factor alpha (TNFα), enzymes and proteins such as copper and zinc-superoxide dismutase (SOD1), proinflammatory peptide substance P (SP), RGD peptides, interleukin-4 (IL-4), IL-10, interferon γ (IFN-γ), cyclooxygenase-1 (COX-1), cyclooxygenase-2 (COX-2), 5-lipoxygenase (5-LOX), macrophage inflammatory protein (MIP) -1R, glucocorticoid regulated protein CD163, FK506 binding protein 51 (FKBP51), and monocyte chemoattractant protein-1 (MCP-1); implicated by cytokine such as interleukin-1 (IL-1); and mediated by adhesions such as fibrous adhesions and cell adhesions resulting from the receptor, such as $\alpha_{II}\beta_{III}$, human glucocorticoid receptor and chemokine receptors (CCR5), and banding. Based on these facts, the adhesion formation assay; human peripheral blood mononuclear cell (PBMC) proliferation assay; COX-1, COX-2, and 5-LOX assay; CCR5 re-ceptor binding assay; tissue binding affinity assay; G93A-SOD1 transgenic mice assay; mitogen-activated protein kinases (MAPK) p44 (ERK1) and p42 (ERK2) assay; ELA4.NOB-1/cytotoxic T lymphocyte line (CTLL) cell assay; and FKBP51 mRNA assay; and Xylene-induced ear edema assay are established.

Adhesion Formation Assay

For assessment of the neurokinin 1 receptor antagonist (NK-1RA) on peritoneal adhesion formation, a laparotomy is performed through a midline incision, and four ischemic buttons, spaced 1 cm apart, are created on both sides of the parietal peritoneum by grasping 5 mm of peritoneum with a hemostat and ligating the base of the segment with a 4-0 silk suture. To assess the effects of NK-1RA on adhesion formation, peritoneal adhesions are induced in 42 male Wistar rats (200–250 g) that are randomized to experimental groups receiving the specific non-peptide NK-1RA, the test compound, or vehicle. In the initial study, the rats in the experimental group receive a 0.2-mL i.p. injection of 25-mg/kg NK-1RA twice a day for 2 days. At the time of surgery, 1 ml of a 0.75-mg/mL test compound is given as a peritoneal lavage, and the rats then received i.p. injection for 7 days. Control rats are similarly injected/lavaged with sterile vehicle. This experiment is repeated with 10-mg/kg NK-1RA per day. At day 7, all the rats are killed and the adhesions are quantified in a blinded fashion. Each rat receives a percent adhesion score based on the number of ischemic buttons with attached adhesions.

For assessment of NK-1RA on peritoneal tissue plasminogen activator (tPA) and PAI-1 expression and activity, the temporal expression pattern of tPA and PAI-1 mRNA in peritoneal tissue collected from a 0.5-cm radius of the ischemic buttons are determined by RT–PCR analysis at days 0, 1, 3, and 7 after surgery. Based on the results, the effects of NK-1RA administration on tPA and PAI-1 mRNA and protein levels are determined at postoperative day 1 in pedtoneal tissue and fluid by RT–PCR analysis and bioassay, respectively. The rats receive 5.0-mg/kg NK-1RA or vehicle per day. Control samples are collected from 6 nonoperated rats. All samples are immediately frozen in liquid nitrogen and stored at –80°C until used. Total RNA is isolated from 50 mg of peritoneal tissue with the SV Total RNA Isolation System, and RT–PCR is conducted with the Gene-Amp RNA PCR System. To amplify tPA and PAI-1, the 28 cycles of 95°C, 60°C, and 72°C for 30 s each are used. In the amplification of tPA, the primer sets of 5′-TCTGACTTCGTCTGCCAGTG-3′ (sense) and 5′-GAG-GCCTTGGATGTGG TAAA-3′ (antisense) are used. In the amplification of PAI-1, the primer sets of 5′- ATCAACGACT GGGTGGAGAG-3′ (sense) and 5′-AGCCTGGTCATGTTGCTCTT-3′ (antisense) are used. Overall, 15 μL of PCR products are subjected to electrophoresis on 2% agarose gels containing 0.03-μg/mL ethidium bromide, and the quantitative level of the transcript is determined by scanned photographs of gels. Levels of mRNA expression are normalized to GAPDH, a constitutively expressed gene that does not vary among treatment groups.

Using the corresponding kits, the total levels of tPA and PAI-1 in peritoneal fluid samples are measured. From 12 vehicle-administered, 12 NK-1RA-administered (10.0 mg/kg per day), and 12 nonoperated control rats, peritoneal fluid is collected in 5-mM citrate and 0.1-M acetate for assessment of fibrinolytic activity caused by tPA activation of plasminogen. Overall, 1.0 μL of peritoneal fluid samples are run on 10% SDS polyaerylamide gels containing 0.1% gelatin and 0.002% plasminogen. After electrophoresis the gels are washed twice in 2%Triton X-100 and incubated overnight at 37°C in 0.1-M glycine (pH 8.3). The gels are stained with a 0.25% Coomassie blue solution, and PA activity is visualized as clear bands produced by plasmin lysis of gelatin. Determining the contribution of serine pro- teases, a 10-mM serine protease inhibitor, PMSF, is added to the developing buffer. In the identification of the zones of lysis corresponding to tPA activity, tPA and/or uPA are immunoprecipitated from peritoneal fluid samples. To the mixture of 10 μL of peritoneal fluid and 10 μL of buffer containing 40-mM phosphate, 1-M NaCl, 0.2% SDS, 2% Igepal CA-630, and 1% deoxycholate (pH 7.5), 1 μg of tPA and/or uPA antibodies are added and incubated at 4°C overnight. To each sample, 10 μL of a 50% UltraLink protein A/G slurry is added and incubated overnight at 4°C. Samples are centrifuged at 4°C and 16,000 g for 1 min, and the supematant (50%) is analyzed by zymography for comparison with human recombinant tPA and uPA standards.

PBMC Proliferation Assay

On removal of plasma the heparinized human peripheral blood from 60 mL of healthy donors is centrifuged (4°C, 2000 g, 10 min), and the blood cells are diluted with PBS and centrifuged (1500 g, 30 min). After removal of red blood cells, the PBMC cell layers are collected, washed with cold distilled water and 10 x Hanks' buffer saline solution, and resuspended (2×10^6 cells/mL) in RPMI-1640 medium supplemented with 2% fetal calf serum, 100-U/mL penicillin, and 100-μg/mL streptomycin. In the determination of the lymphoproliferation, 100 μL of the PBMC suspension is deposited into a 96-well flat-bottomed plate with or without 5-μg/mL phytohemagglutinin (PHA, with cyclosporin as a positive control), into which solutions of various concentrations of test compounds are added, the plates are incubated at 37°C for 3 days in humidified atmospheric air containing 5% CO_2, tritiated thymidine is added, incubated for another 16 h, and the cells are harvested on glass fiber filters using an automatic harvester and measured with a scintillation counting. In the determination of cell viability, approximately 2×10^5 T cells with or without PHA are cultured with 0.1% DMSO, solutions of various concentrations of test compounds are added, the plates are incubated for 3 days, the viable cell numbers are counted using a microscope with a hemocytometer following staining by trypan blue, and the percentage of viable cells is calculated. To analyze the cell cycle, 1 mL of the PBMC suspension is added into a 6-well flat-bottomed plate with or without 5-μg/mL PHA, 25 μg/mL of each test compound is added, the plates are incubated at 37°C for 3 days in humidified atmospheric air containing 5% CO_2, the medium is centrifuged, and the cells are harvested, washed with PBS, and fixed in 70% ethanol at −20°C for 30 min. DNA is then stained with 4-μg/mL propidium iodide containing 100-μg/mL ribonuclease A. Flow cytometric analysis is conducted.

After incubation with PHA alone or in combination with solutions of varying concentrations of test compounds for 3 days, the medium is centrifuged, and PBMC (2×10^5 cells/well) supernatants are collected to quantify the concentrations of IL-2, IL-4, IL-10, and IFN-γ by means of enzyme immunoassays. After stimulation with or without PHA and coculture with 25-μg/mL, each compound for 18 h, the collected PBMC cells (5×10^6) are subjected to lysis with RNA-Beek and centrifuged, the supernatants are extracted with a phenol-chloroform mixture, and the extracted RNA is precipitated with isopropanol, pelleted by centrifugation, and redissolved in diethyl pyrocarbonate (DEPC)-treated H_2O. The concentration of the extracted RNA is measured using the optical density at 260 nm. In the synthesis of the first-strand cDNA, 1-μg aliquots of RNA are reverse- transcribed. The mixture of 1-

μg RNA in 12.5 μL of DEPC-treated H2O and 20-μM oligodeoxythymidine (oligo dT) 18 is heated at 72°C for 2 min, and then quick-chilled on ice. To this mixture, 5.5 μL of concentrated synthesis buffer (50-mM Tris-HCl, pH 8.3, 75-mM KCl, 3-mM MgCl2, 0.5-mM deoxynucleotides triphosphates (dNTPs), and 1 U ribonuclease inhibitor), and 10 U of moloney murine leukemia virus reverse transcriptase are added. The reaction mixture is incubated at 42°C for 1 h and then at 94°C for 5 min. To the reaction mixture, 80 μL of DEPC-treated H2O is added and the mixture is stored at –20°C for use in the PCR. To 5 μL of the first-strand cDNA, 0.6-μM primers, 1.25-U Taq polymerase, 10-μL reaction buffer (2-mM Tri-HCl, pH 8.0, 0.01-mM EDTA, 0.1-mM dithiothreitol, 0.1% Triton X-100, 5% glycerol, and 1.5-mM $MgCl_2$) and 15.75 μL of water are added and the total volume is 25 μL. According to the air thermocycler, a denaturing temperature of 94°C for 45 s, annealing temperature of 58°C for 45 s, and elongation temperature of 72°C for 1 min for the first 25 cycles, and finally 72°C for 10 min, PCR is carried out and the amplified product is run on 1.8% agarose gels.

COX-1, COX-2, and 5-LOX Assay

For the COX-1 and COX-2 assay, the diluted solution of the test compound is incubated with COX-1 or COX-2 according to the standard method and then the enzyme reaction is initiated by the addition of [1-^{14}C] -arachidonic acid. From the incubation mediate, prostaglandin E_2 and prostaglandin D_2 (PED_2) are extracted to measure radioactivity. Indomethacin is used as a positive control. For the 5-LOX assay, the inhibitory activity of the test compound is evaluated. The test compound is incubated with 5-LOX (46 μg of protein) at 24°C for 10 min, and then the enzyme reaction is initiated by the addition of [1-^{14}C] -arachidonic acid (50 nCi). After 5 min, 4-M formic acid is added to terminate the enzyme reaction. Indomethacin is used as a positive control.

CCR5 Receptor Binding Assay

In the determination of chemokine receptor (CCR5) binding activity, a 96-well scintillation proximity assay (SPA) format and CHO cells overexpress-ing the human CCR5 receptor are used. From the CHO cells, MIP-1α and membranes are obtained, and after ^{125}I labeling, the former is converted into [^{125}I]-human MIP-1α. The solution of the test compound, 12.5% aqueous DMSO, 12 μg of membranes, 0.17-nM [^{125}I] -MIP-1α, 0.25 mg of Wheat Germ Agglutinin-SPA beads, and assay buffer (50-mM HEPES, 1-mM $CaCl_2$, 1-mM $MgCl_2$, 1% BSA, and a protease inhibitor cocktail), is incubated at room temperature for 5 h with shaking. The beads are settled for 2 h, and the total binding is measured via the radioactivity test. In the presence of 1-μM recombinant human MIP-1α, the nonspecific binding is defined. A IC_{50} of 2.7 nM of human MIP-1α is used as a reference.

Tissue Binding Affinity Assay

In hydrophobic teflon bags, the test compound and blood monocytes isolated from pooled buffycoats at a density of 2×10^8-cells/mL McCoy's medium supplemented with 20% fetal calf serum are cultured for 2 days. The monocytes are washed with cold PBS (pH 7.4), incubated with BSA (1%) at 4°C for 30 min, washed with PBS, incubated with monoclonal antibody anti-CD163 (5–10 μg/mL) at 4°C for 45 min, washed with PBS, and incubated with FITC-labeled secondary antibody goat-antimouse IgG1 in 1% BSA at 4°C for 30 min. At the last 3 min of the incubation, Propidium iodide is added to determine cell viability and to exclude dead cells using activated cell sorter (FACS) analysis (488 nm, 250 mW, logarithmic amplification).

Human lung cancer-free tissue from patients with bronchial carcinomas and receiving no glucocorticoids for the last 4 weeks before surgery is immediately washed with Krebs-Ringer-HEPES buffer (118-mM NaCl, 4.84-mM KCl, 1.2-mM KH_2PO_4, 2.43-mM $MgSO_4$, 2.44-mM $CaCl_2 \cdot 2H_2O$, and 10-mM HEPES, pH 7.4) and sliced into pieces of 1 mm^3 or deeply frozen immediately in liquid nitrogen and stored at –70°C.

The frozen human lung tissue is pulverized and homogenized in three aliquots buffer solution A (10-mM TRIS, 10-mM $NaMoO_4$, 30-mM NaCl, 10% glycerol, 4-mM DTT, 5-mM dichlorvos, and 1-mM Complete) with an Ultra Turrax mixer in an ice bath and then centrifuged at 4°C and 105,000 g for 1 h to prepare glucocorticoid receptors (30–60 fmol/mg cytosol). The receptor binding experiments are performed according to the standard method. The radiochemical purity of the labeled glucocorticoid is determined by HPLC, TLC, and scintillation counting.

G93A-SOD1 Transgenic Mice Assay

EOC-20 cells are grown in 75-cm^2 cell culture flasks with DMEM supplemented with 10% fetal calf serum and 20% L292 fibroblast-conditioned medium, transferred into 24-well cell culture plates, treated with the solution of test compound in DMSO or DMSO vehicle alone (1% final volume) for 30 min, and challenged with TNFα for 24 h. The culture medium is collected and assayed for determining the IC_{50} of the test compound that suppresses TNFα-induced NO_2^- by 50% via the determination of NO_2. The medium is removed, and DMEM lacking the phenol red indicator is added. To each well, MTS reagent [3-(4,5-dimethylthiazol-2-yl)-5-(3- carboxymethonyphenol) -2- (4-sulfophenyl) -2H-tetrazolium, inner salt] is added and incubated at 37°C for 30–45 min. The aliquots of media are collected and evaluated spectrophotometrically at 540 nm. The MTS solution prepared for the blank is incubated in the absence of cells. Viability is calculated as the ratio of OD540 in test compound-treated wells, relative to the same variable measured in wells treated with approximately 25-μM (typically 20 ng/mL) TNFa alone, after subtraction of the blank.

Transgenic mice expressing high copy numbers of human mutant G93A-SOD1 are maintained in the hemizygous state by mating G93A males with B6SJL-TGN females. The mice are fed *ad libitum* standard AIN93G diets or the same diets formulated with nordihydroguaiaretic acid at 2500 ppm; at 90 days of age, drug administration is started to demonstrate motor weakness and fine limb tremors. At 90 days, 100 days of age, and subsequent 5-day intervals, mice are placed on a horizontal rod rotating at 1 rpm every 10 s until they fall from the rod; the mice that are no longer able to right themselves within 10 s of being placed on their sides are killed.

Using TRI reagent, total RNA is collected from the spinal cords of non-transgenic control and G93A+ transgenic mice. In the presence of avian myeloblastosis virus (AMV) RT using oligo(dT)15 to prime the reaction, 5 μg of RNA samples are reverse transcribed. On completion, each reaction mixture is diluted with a TE buffer (10-mM Tris, 1-mM EDTA, pH 8.0) to a final volume of 50 μL. PCR amplification of a 309-bp 5LOX gene product is accomplished with Taq DNA polymerase, using the buffer and final concentrations of 1.5-mM $MgCl_2$, 0.2-mM dNTP, and 0.3-μM primer (5′-GGCACCGACGACTACATCTAC-3′ , forward and 5′-CAATTTTG-CACGTCCATCCC-3′, reverse), of which the final volumes are 50 μL. A 353-bp PCR product of the β-actin primer (5′-CGGCCAGGTCATCACTATTG-3′, forward and ACT-CCTGCTTGCTGATCCAC-3′, reverse) is used as the normalization control. The optimal cycling conditions of PCR amplification of a 309-bp 5LOX gene product are at 94°C for 2 min, one cycle; at 94°C for 1 min, at 56°C for 1 min, and at 72°C for 1 min for 27 cycles; and at 72°C for 7 min, one cycle. The conditions for β-actin primers are the same as mentioned above, except that the annealing temperature is 54°C and performing 24 cycles. From each reaction, 25 μL of samples are collected, electrophoresed in 2% agarose/TBE [tris/borate/EDTA buffer (0.09-M Tris, 0.09-M borate, 0.002-M EDTA)] gels for 1.5 h, stained with ethidium bromide, and photographed with a Nucleo Vision imaging system. SL-29 fibroblast lysate is used as the positive control for 5LOX Western blots. On 4–20% gradient polyacrylamide gels, the electrophoresis is performed and the bands are visualized with chemiluminescence detection reagents. In the solution of 50-mM Tris-HCl (pH 6.8), 0.3-M NaCl, 1% [3-mercaptoethanol, 1-mM phenylmethylsulfonyl fluoride, and 5-liM leupeptin, the spinal cord samples are homogenized and centrifuged (4°C, 30,000 g, 5 min). The supernanants are boiled for 10 min and centrifuged at 30,000 g and 4°C for 30 min, and the supernatants are dialyzed overnight against 50-mM Tris-HCl. From the heat-soluble fraction of total spinal cord lysate, microtubule-associated tau protein (C-tau) is cleaved and measured by sandwich ELISA, using affinity-purified monoclonal antibody 12B2 In immunohistochemical experiments, the terminally anesthetized mice are successively perfused transcardially with PBS (pH 7.4) and 4% paraformaldehyde in 0.1-M phosphate buffer. The spinal cord is collected, and the lumbar L5 region is processed for paraffin embedding. Serial cross sections of 5 μM thickness of the L5 spinal cord region are prepared for immunostain with antibodies to glial GFAP. In the absence of primary antibody, negative immunohistochemical controls are treated in the same way. GFAP-labeled sections are counterstained with hematoxylin.

MAPK p44 (ERK1) and p42 (ERK2) Assay

By RT–PCR from PMA-treated THP-1 cells, cDNA encoding CCR2B is isolated and subcloned into the expression vector pXMT3-neo, which contains an adenovirus late promoter and neo- and DHFR-selectable markers. After transfection with pXMT3-neo-CCR2B, selection with G418, amplification with methotrexate, and clone of CHO DUK-X cells, the resultant CHO-CCR2B cell line is cultured with modified MEMα (without ribonucleosides and deoxyribonucleosides) containing Glutamax-I, 100-U/mL penicillin, 100-μg/mL streptomycin, 10% (v/v) dialyzed FBS, and 80-nM methotrexate. Parental CHO cells are cultured with original MEMα containing 100-U/mL penicillin, 100-μg/mL streptomycin, and 10% (v/v) FBS, split twice per week by incubation for 5 min with an enzyme-free cell dissociation buffer, and reseeded at a density of 1–2 × 10^4 cells/cm^2. Before an assay, the cells are seeded in methotrexate at 2 × 10^4 cells/well in flat-bottomed 96-well tissue culture plates, allowed to attach for 6 h, washed with 250-μL/well PBS, and incubated overnight in methotrexate containing endotoxin-free BSA (0.1%, w/v).

After preincubation of 60 μL of 20-nM MCP-1 with 60 μL of 0.4–1.8-μg/mL mAb at 37°C for 30 min, 50 μL of the MCP-1-mAb solution is added. The cells are preincubated at 37°C for 45 min with the solution of test compound in 50 μL of serum-free medium. After the addition of 50 μL of 20-nM MCP-1, the cells are incubated at 37°C for 5 min, the medium is replaced by 100-μL/well methanol equilibrated at –20°C, incubated at –20°C for another 20 min, and then washed three times with PBS containing Triton X-100 (0.1%, w/v). The cells are incubated with H_2O_2 (0.6%, v/v) in washing buffer for 20 min and washed as above, by which the activity of endogenous peroxidase is quenched. By adding a 250 μL/well assay buffer (washing buffer containing fraction V BSA, 5%, w/v) and incubating at room temperature for 1 h, the nonspecific binding sites are blocked. Then, the solution is replaced by a 100-μL/well monoclonal anti-phospho-ERK antibody (1 μg/mL in assay buffer). After incubating at 37°C for 1 h and washing three times with washing buffer, to the plate, a 100-μL/well goat-antimouse-IgG coupled with horseradish peroxidase (0.5 μg/mL in assay buffer) is added. After incubation at room temperature for 1 h and the plate is washed six times with washing buffer, 100 μL/well of tetramethylbenzidine is added. After color development for 10–30 min, the reaction is stopped by adding 50 μL of 2-M H_2SO_4 and the plates are read at 450 nm.

ELA4.NOB-1/CTLL Cell Assay

The ELA4.NOB-1 cells and CTLL cells maintained in RPMI 1640 containing 2-mM glutamine, 40-μg/mL gentamicin, and 100-U/mL penicillin, are transferred into a tissue culture medium (TCM) containing 5% heatinactivated fetal calf serum (FCS) and 10% FCS and recombinant human L-2 (100 U/mL), respectively. Cell lines are centrifuged (room temperature, 400 g, 1 min) and washed twice in fresh TCM supplemented with 10% FCS by resuspension and centrifugation. By enumeration using trypan blue (0.4%, w/v) in saline, ELA4.NOB-1 and CTLL cells are adjusted to 1 × 10^6 and 4 × 10^4 viable cells/mL, respectively. To 96-well round- bottom microtiter plates containing 100 μL of cytokine (control) or test compound, 50 μL aliquots of each cell suspension are placed. After incubation in air containing 5% CO_2 at 37°C for 24 h, the cells are treated with 50 μL of 2-μCi/mL tritiated thymidine, incubated for another 24 h, harvested onto printed filtermats that are dried at 30°C for 1 h and heat sealed into sample bags containing 4.5 mL of β-scintillant, and the radioactivity (cpm) is measured.

To each well containing 100-μL aliquots of the standard dilutions, 50 μL of ELA4.NOB-1 and 50 μL of CTLL cell suspensions are added. Using human recombinant IL-2 (0.025–1.6 U/mL) or test compound, the integrity of CTLL responses in the absence of ELA4.NOB-1 cells is measured. Human recombinant IL-1ra (0.1–100 ng/mL), ultrapure natural human TGF-β1 (0.01–10 ng/mL), and test compound are tested on ELA4.NOB-1 and CTLL cocultures in a similar way, generating standard dose response curves for these cytokines. In the tests of the effects of IL-1ra and TGF-β1 on IL-1 induced activity in the coculture bioassay and on IL-2 induced CTLL proliferation, serial dilutions of IL-1β (0.78–50 pg/mL), IL-2 (0.025–1.6 U/mL), IL-1ra (1–100 ng/mL), TGF-β1 (0.01–10 ng/mL), and test compound in TCM supplemented with 10% FCS are used. Overall, 50-μL aliquots of each dilution of IL-1ra and IL-1β are dispensed and pipetted into 96-well microtiter plates, respectively, and 50 μL of the suspension of ELA4.NOB-1 and CTLL cells are aliquoted into each well, incubated, and treated with ^{3}H-thymidine as described above; similar assays are set up for IL-1ra and IL-2, for TGF-β1 and IL-1β, and for TGF-β1 and IL-2.

FKBP51 mRNA Assay

Within a 2-week period between 9 and 10 h by venapuncture, the blood of nine healthy controls without a history of GC medication (37 years old) and one GC hyposensitive patient harboring one nonfunctional GC receptor allele and resulting in a net functional GC receptor expression of approximately 50% is collected in sodium heparin tubes, and centrifuged, and the isolated PBMC are washed twice with RPMI 1640 and resuspended in assay medium consisting of RPMI 1640 supplemented with 4-mM L-glutamine, 100-U/mL penicillin, 100-μg/mL streptomycin, and 10% dextran-coated charcoal steroid-stripped fetal calf serum at 0.5×10^6 cells/mL. Overall, 1-mL aliquots of the PBMC suspension are added onto 24-well plates and incubated overnight at 37°C in humidified atmospheric air containing 5% CO_2. To the medium, dexamethasone (DXM) or the test compound is added and incubated for another 24 h to isolate RNA. For activation of PBMC, 0.1-mL aliquots of 0.5×10^5 cells are added onto a 96-well round-bottom plate and incubated with 1.5-μg/mL etanus toxoid for 9 h. Seventy two hours later, DXM is added. Then 96 h later, RNA is isolated. In a simultaneous control experiment, 78 h later, 1μCi ^{3}H-thymidine is added, the cells are harvested, and incorporated radioactivity is determined.

For purification of PBMC subsets, cells are isolated, washed twice, resuspended in PBS at 1×10^7 cells/mL, incubated at room temperature for 30 min with phycoerythrin labeled primary antibodies (mouse-antihuman CD20, CD4, CD8, or CD14), and washed twice with PBS. The PBMC is resuspended in PBS at 1×10^8 cells/mL, incubated at 4°C for 30 min and labeled with goat-anti-mouse IgG, and washed and resuspended in 0.5 mL of PBS. The labeled and unlabeled PBMC are separated, resuspended in assay medium, divided into 0.1-mL aliquots onto a 96-well round-bottom plate, and incubated overnight. To the wells, DXM is added and incubated for another 24 h to isolate RNA.

For real-time PCR performed on the LightCycler, after the isolation by use of the TriPure reagent and reverse transcription by use of MMLV-RT RNase H Minus of RNA, the synthesized cDNA is diluted 20–40 times in ddH_2O. To calculate the relative expression level of the genes of interest, the relative expression level of the housekeeping gene β_2-microglobulin (β_2m) in each sample is determined. Real-time PCR is performed in 10-μL medium containing 5.0 μL of diluted cDNA (0.5 pmol/μL each primer), 10% either DNA master SYBR-green I solution (for the FKBP51 and β_2m PCR) or DNA hotstart mixture (for the FKBP12, FKBP13, FKBP22, FKBP25, FKBP52, and Cyp40 PCR), and an optimal concentration of $MgCl_2$ (4-mM β_2m PCR, 3-mM FKBP51 PCR). The mixture is denatured at 95°C for 30 s and 10 min for DNA Master I kit and Fast Start kit, respectively, and subjected to up to 40 amplification cycles: denaturing 15 s at 95°C, annealing 10 s at 56°C for β_2m or at 67°C for FKBP51, and elongation 30 s at 72°C. A single measurement of fluorescence is taken after each elongation step at 82°C.

Xylene-Induced Ear Edema Assay

Male Kunming mice (about 25 g) are randomly divided into three groups of 12 mice, namely the test group, vehicle control group, and positive control group. The mice in the vehicle control group are administrated orally a suspension of Aspirin in CMC at a dosage of 20 mg/kg, and a concentration of 0.3 mg/mL, whereas the mice in the test group are administrated orally a suspension of test compound in CMC at a dosage of 20 mg/kg, 4.0 mg/kg, and 0.8 mg/kg, and a concentration of 2.0 mg/mL, 0.4 mg/mL, and 0.08 mg/mL. Thirty minutes later, 0.03 mL of xylene is applied to both the anterior and the posterior surfaces of the right ear. The left ear is considered a control. Two hours after xylene application, the mice are killed and both ears are removed. Using a cork borer with a diameter of 7 mm, several circular sections are taken and weighed. The increase in weight caused by the irritant is measured through subtracting the weight of the untreated left ear section from that of the treated right ear section.

Thrombus-Related Assay

A series of events such as the platelet aggregation, fibrinogenesis, fibrin adhesion, fibrin aggregation, and vascular inner wall injury are implicated in the thrombosis. Thus the thrombosis, antithrombosis, and thrombolysis may relate to antiplatelet aggregation, chemical- and electrical-induced blood vessel injury, thread-induced fibrin or platelet adhesion, euglobulin clot lysis time, fibrinolytic area, and reduction of thrombus mass.

Antiplatelet Aggregation Assay

Platelet-rich plasma is prepared by centrifugation of normal rabbit blood anticoagulation with sodium citrate at a final concentration of 3.8%. The platelet counts are adjusted to $2 \times 10^5/\mu L$ by the addition of autologous plasma. Platelet aggregation tests are conducted in an aggregometer using the standard turbidimetric technique. The agonists used may be either the usual platelet-activating factor (PAF, final concentration 10^{-5}–10^{-7} M) and adenosine diphosphate (ADP, final concentration 10^{-5}–10^{-7} M) or thrombin and collagen. The effects of the tested compound on PAF or ADP-induced platelet aggregation are observed. The maximal rate of the platelet aggregation (Am%) is represented by the peak height of the aggregation curve.

Ferric Chloride-Induced Thrombosis Assay

After overnight fasting, male SD rats (320–38 0 g) are administered orally water (blank control), test compound (15, 30, 60 mg/kg), and aspirin (positive control, 30 mg/kg), and they are anesthetized with urethane (1.5 g/kg i.p.) at 90 min after the oral administration. The experiments are carried out according to the modified method described by Kurz et al. The left common carotid artery is isolated carefully, and a plastic sheet is placed under the vessel to separate it from the surrounding tissue. The surface of carotid artery is covered with a 4 × 0.5-cm cotton sheet saturated with 300 μL of $FeCl_3$ solution (25%, w/v) for 15 min. Then, the injured carotid artery segment (0.6 cm) is cut off, from which the formed thrombus is taken out. After drying for 24 h at room temperature in a dehumidifier, the dried weight of the thrombus is measured.

Electrical Stimulation-Induced Arterial Thrombosis Assay

After overnight fasting, male SD rats (250–350 g) are anesthetized with urethane (1.5 g/kg, i.p.). The left carotid artery is isolated carefully. A plastic sheet is placed under the vessel to separate it from the surrounding tissue. Thrombus formation is induced with the modified Hladovec method. The holder incorporates two electrodes, and the temperature sensor is fixed under the exposed carotid artery. Then, the rats are administered intravenously by NS (blank control), test compound (5, 10, 20 mg/kg), and aspirin (4 mg/kg), respectively. After 5 min, a current of 3 mA is delivered for 3 min. With thrombus formation, the temperature of carotid blood is abruptly decreased. The occlusion time (OT) is measured through the temperature sensor and timer on the electric thrombosis stimulator. The rate of thrombosis inhibition is calculated according to as follows: thrombosis inhibition (%) = $(A_1 - A)/A \times 100\%$, where A is the OT of the control group and A_1 is the OT of agent groups.

Thread-Induced Thrombosis Assay

Male SD rats (320–380 g) are treated with water (blank control), test compound (15, 30, 60, 120 mg/kg), and aspirin (positive control, 30 mg/kg, b.i.d. for 2.5 d i.g.) and anesthetized by intraperitoneal injection of urethane (1.5 g/kg) at 75 min after the last dose. The arteriovenous shunt operation is carried out as the method described by Umetsu and Sanai. The left jugular vein and the right carotid artery are annulated with a 4-cm-long polyethylene tube (o.d. 1 mm) with heparin (50 U/kg) injection intravenously for anticoagulation. These catheters are connected to the ends of a 15-cm-long polyethylene tube (o.d. 2 mm) containing a 5-cm-long suture silk thread (no. 4) measured wet weight. At 120 min after the last treatment, the blood flowing through the shunt is confirmed for 15 min. The silk thread with thrombus is gently removed and measured immediately for the wet gross weight. The thrombus wet weight is determined by subtracting the premeasured silk wet weight from the gross weight. The rate of thrombosis inhibition is calculated as follows: thrombosis inhibition (%) = $(A - A_1)/A \times 100\%$, where A is the thrombus wet weight of the control (water) and A_1 is the weight after treatment with the agents.

Euglobulin Clot Lysis Time (ECLT) Assay

The rabbit euglobulin clots are prepared according to a published method. Plasma diluted at 1:20 in distilled water is precipitated at pH 5.7 with acetic acid (0.25%). After 30 min at 4°C, the suspension is centrifuged at 2000 g for 15 min and the precipitate is resuspended to the initial plasma volume with 50-mM sodium barbiturate buffer (pH 7.8, containing 1.66-mM $CaCl_2$, 0.68-mM $MgCl_2$, and 93.96- mM NaCl). To the rabbit euglobulin clots, NS (blank control), UK (positive control), or test compound is added and the ECLT or time to clot lysis is determined in a 96-well microtiter plate.

Fibrinolytic Area Assay

The fibrinogen–agarose mixture is prepared and coagulated with thrombin in plastic dishes according to a published procedure. The fibrinogen–agarose mixture is prepared by mixing equal volumes of 0.3% of rabbit fibrinogen and 0.95% of agarose solutions, both dissolved in 50-mM sodium barbiturate buffer (pH 7.8). The fibrinogen–agarose mixture is coagulated with 100 mL of thrombin (100 U/mL) in plastic dishes (90 mm diameter × 1 mm depth). After 30 min at 4°C, an adequate number of wells, 5 mm in diameter, are perforated. To determine fibrinolytic activity, 30 μL of NS (blank control), UK (positive control), or test compound is added to the corresponding well. The plate is incubated, and areas of lysis are quantified by lysis area.

Thrombolytic Assay

Male Wistar rats (200–300 g) are anesthetized with pentobarbital sodium (80.0 mg/ kg, i.p.). The right carotid artery and left jugular vein of the animals are separated. To the glass tube containing 1.0 mL of blood obtained from the right carotid artery of the rat, a stainless steel filament helix (15 circles; 15 mm × 1.0 mm) is added immediately. Fifteen minutes later, the helix with thrombus is carefully taken out and weighed. It is then put into a polyethylene tube that is filled with heparin sodium (50-U/mL NS), and one end is inserted into the left jugular vein. Heparin sodium is injected via the other end of the polyethylene tube as the anticoagulant, after which the test compound is injected. The blood is circulated through the polyethylene tube for 90 min, after which the helix is taken out and weighed. The reduction of thrombus mass is recorded.

Immunomodulating Assay

Immunomodulation not only relates to a series of physiologic and pathologic phenomena, but also it can be estimated by related reaction cells, such as mast cells, DCs and NK cells, and level of cell factors such as interleukin, interferon, tumor necrosis factor, and transforming growth factor. Based on those facts, the rat mast cell and rabbit aortic assay, dendritic cell assay, lymphoid organ assay, IFN-γ assay, anti-rHuEPO NAb assay, and chemotaxic assay are established.

Rat Mast Cell and Rabbit Aortic Assay

The ice-cold PBS (10 mL, 137-mM NaCl, 2.68-mM KCl, 0.91-mM $CaCl_2$, 8.1-mM Na_2PO_4, 1.47-mM KH_2PO_4, 0.91-mM $MgCl_2$, 5.6-mM glucose, and 20.0-mM HEPES) is injected (i.p.) into male Wistar rats (200–250 g). Approximately 90–120 s later, PBS is collected and peritoneal is subsequently washed by 5 mL and 10 mL of PBS. The washing PBS are also collected and combined with first PBS, followed by centrifugation (200 g, 5 min, 4°C). After washing twice with PBS, the pellet is resuspended into 10 mL of PBS. From the rat, peritoneal lavage mast cells are isolated.

Preincubation of 1.8 mL of mast cell suspensions are carried out at 37°C for 10 min, and 0.1 mL of test compound is added to stimulate the mast cells, which are cooled in ice to terminate histamine release. After centrifugation (100 g, 10 min, 4°C), to the supernatant and the pellet, an equal volume of 0.8-M $HClO_4$ and twice volume of 0.4-M $HClO_4$ are added, respectively. A mixture of 125 μL of 5-M NaOH, 0.4 g of NaCl, and 2.5 mL of n-butanol is added to 1-mL solution of test compound, the mixture is centrifuged (200 g, 1 min, room temperature) and separated. The upper organic phase is mixed with 2 mL of 0.1-M NaOH saturated with NaCl and centrifuged (200 g, 1 min, room temperature), and the procedure is repeated, of which the upper organic phase is mixed with 2 mL of 0.1-M HCl and 7.6 mL of n-heptane. The lower aqueous phase (1 mL) is mixed with 0.1 mL of 10-M NaOH. By incubation with 0.1 mL of o-phthalaldehyde (10-mg/mL methanol) at room temperature for 4 min to perform the histamine-o-phthalaldehyde conjugation, and by addition of 0.6 mL of 3-M HCl to terminate the conjugation. The fluorescence of histamine-o-phthalaldehyde conjugate is assessed at 450 nm with emission excitated at 360 nm.

The thoracic aorta of male Japanese White rabbits (3–3.5 kg) is cut into helical strips (approximately 4 mm wide and 20 mm long), and the endothelium is removed by gently rubbing the endothelial surface with cotton pellets. In 1 mL of organ bath containing the modified Krebs–Ringer–bicarbonate solution (120-mM NaCl, 4.8-mM KCl, 1.2-mM $CaCl_2$, 1.3-mM $MgSO_4$, 25.2-mM $NaHCO_3$, 1.2-mM KH_2PO_4, 5.8-mM glucose), the strips are mounted and suspended. With a force-displacement transducer connected to a polygraph muscle, the tensions of the strips are recorded isometrically. A passive tension of 1 g is initially applied and the strips are equilibrated for 60 min, after which, 60-mM NaCl in the modified Krebs–Ringer–bicarbonate solution is replaced by equimolar KCl for precontraction of the strips. Reaching a steady level of the response, the experiment is started. Contractile response to histamine is normalized with that of high K^+.

Dendritic Cell (DC) Assay

Before being used either for DC culture or for preparing T cells, human peripheral blood mononuclear cells (PBMCs) isolated from freshly leukapheresed blood are centrifuged and cryopreserved in 90% autologous serum and 10% DMSO. By negative depletion and using anti-HLA-DR monoclonal antibody-conjugated paramagnetic beads from allogeneic PBMCs, enriched T cells are prepared. The cells possessing potential costimulatory function are removed from the PBMCs, as suspension each batch of which is tested for the presence of any remaining B cells, monocytes, and 80–90% T cells. Using cell-specific paramagnetic bead preparations and by biomagnetic separation of the stimulators, B cells and T cells are purified and the purity of each cell type is greater than 90%, as determined by flow cytometry.

The cryopreserved PBMCs are thawed in warm AIM-V medium, washed with PBS, and resuspended in Opti-MEM medium supplemented with 1% heat- inactivated autologous plasma to prepare (5–10) $\times 10^6$ cells/mL suspension. The suspension of 1×10^9 cells is transferred into T-75 culture flasks and cultured for 1 h, the nonadherent cells are resuspended, aspirated out, and stringently washed with cold PBS to remove loosely adherent cells. To each flask, 1.5×10^9 Opti-MEM medium containing 5% heat-inactivated autologous plasma, 500-U/mL rhGM-CSF, and 500-U/mL rhIL-4 are added and the adherent cells are incubated for 6 days. These DCs are then treated either with BCG alone or BCG plus IFN-γ for 24 h.

In the COSTIM bioassay, allogeneic T cells are thawed in warm AIM-V culture media, and washed with and resuspended in PBS at 1×10^5 DCs or 1×10^6 T cells/ mL. To each triplicate well of a U-bottom 96-well plate, 100 μL of 1×10^4 DCs and 100 μL of 1×10^5 allogeneic T cells are successively added, and with or without 0.005-μg/mL anti-CD3 monoclonal antibody, which is incubated at 37°C for 44 h in humidified atmospheric air containing 5% CO_2. A total of 0.5 μCi Tritiated (^{3}H)-thymidine in 50 μL of AIM-V is added to each well, cultured for the last 18 h, the cells are harvested, and the incorporated radioactivity is quantified. Before 1 h of adding T cells and anti-CD3, the sterile, azide-free, and low-endotoxin IgG1 monoclonal antibodies specific for CD54, CD80, CD86, and an isotype control (BD Pharmingen) are added to the DCs at 1 μg/well to observe the costimulatory molecule block. In the mixed lymphocyte reaction (MLR), the cryopreserved DCs (stimulators) and T cells (responders) are thawed in warm AIM-V media, washed with PBS, and resuspended in PBS at 1×10^5 DCs or 1×10^6 T cells/mL. To each well of a U-bottom 96-well plate, 100 μL of 1×10^4 DCs and 100 μL of 1×10^5 allogeneic T cells are successively added and incubated at 37°C for 6 days in humidified atmospheric air containing 5% CO_2. A total of 0.5 μCi Tritiated (^{3}H)-thymidine in 50 μL of AIM-V is added to each well, cultured for the last 18 h, the cells are harvested, and the incorporated radioactivity is quantified.

Lymphoid Organ Assay

After a 4-week acclimation period, male Wistar rats (4 weeks old, 225–250 g, housed in polypropylene cages in a environment-controlled room maintained at 22°C, 55% relative humidity, and a 12:12 h light/dark cycle) are allocated to six groups (n = 15–20 rats each). The untreated group is used as control (maintained on basal diet and sacrificed at weeks 4 and 30). During weeks 1 and 2, the DMBDD, DMBDD/PB, and DMBDD/2-AAF groups are sequentially treated with initiators DEN (N-nitrosodiethylamine, 100 mg/kg, i.p.), MNU (N-methyl-N-nitrosourea, 20 mg/kg, i.p., four times, two doses per week), and BBN (0.05% in drinking water during 2 weeks); during weeks 3 and 4, DHPN and DMH groups are sequentially treated with DHPN (0.1% in drinking water during 2 weeks) and DMH (1,2- dimethylhydrazine, 40 mg/kg, s.c., four times, two doses per week). At the end of the week 4, some animals of the DMBDD group are killed and the remainder is maintained on a basal diet until week 30. After the initiation, the DMBDD/PB and DMBDD/2-AAF groups are supplied with phenobarbital (PB, 0.05%) and 2- acetylaminofluorene (2-AAF, 0.01%) in the diet for 25 weeks, respectively. From the sixth week until week 30, two noninitiated groups receive PB or 2-AAF in the diet. At the week 4 or 30, all animals are killed under pentobarbital (45 mg/kg) anesthesia. The liver, kidneys, spleen, thymus, mesenteric lymph nodes, and bone marrow removed from all animals are fixed in buffered formalin for 48 h for tissue processing and histological analysis. Only at week 30 are the lung, small and large intestine, and Zymbal's gland examined. After removal of the liver, the kidneys, spleen, and thymus are weighed immediately. The spleen is cut in two halves for evaluation of cytokines and histological analysis, respectively. All removed organs are embedded in paraffin and stained with hematoxylin and eosin for histological analysis. The suspensions of spleen cells dispersed in a Petri dish containing RPMI-1640 culture medium are centrifuged; resuspended in RPMI-1640 culture medium supplemented with 20-mg/mL gentamycin, 2-mM glutamine, and 10% inactivated fetal calf serum; and washed twice by centrifugation at 1500 g for 10 min. To aliquots of 2×10^6 cells/mL (500 μL/well) in 24-well flat-bottom microtiter plates, RPMI-1640 (500 μL/well) or Concanavalin A (CON A-2.5 μAg/mL, 500 μL/well) or Staphylococcus aureus Cowan's strain 1 (SAC-1:5000, 500 μL/well) is added and the plates are incubated at 37°C for 72 h in humidified atmospheric air containing 5% CO_2. After incubation, the collected supernatants are stocked at –70°C for quantification of cytokines. CONA *in vitro* stimulated samples are used to quantify IL-2, IFN-γ, IL-10, and TGF-β1. SAC *in vitro* stimulated samples are used to quantify TNF-α and IL-12. Using ELISA kits, cytokine production, IL-2, IL-12, TNF-α, IFN-γ, and IL-10 levels are measured. Samples are acidified by 1-M HCl and measured by Quantikine antihuman TGF-h1 kit for detection of the TGF-h1 immunoreactive form.

IFN-γ Assay

Human myelomonocytic KG-1 cells (ATCCCCL246) are incubated with RPMI-1640 medium supplemented with 10% FCS, 100-μg/mL penicillin, and 100-μg/mL streptomycin at 37°C in air containing 5% CO_2. By expression of the corresponding cDNA in *E. coli* HuIL-18 and MuIL-18 are prepared and purified to homogeneity. Using Pfu DNA polymerase (at 95°C for 45 s; at 72°C for 3.5 min; 10 cycles and at 95°C for 45 s; at 68°C for 3.5 min; 35 cycles) MuIL-18R cDNA (1.7 kbp) are amplified from murine liver RNA by RT–PCR and cloned into pCRScript Cam SK (+) to synthesize 5´-AGAGGAACCACCCACAACGATCCT-3´ and 5´-TGAATAGGCACACGCAT-XGACCTCT-3´. With the EF-1 promoter of pEF-BOS vector, the dihydrofolate reductase unit of pSV2dhfr (ATCC 37146) and the backbone of pRc/CMV vector pREF-XN is constructed. IL-18R cDNA is ligated into *Xho*I/*Not*I sites of the vector to form MuIL-18R expression vector pRcEFM18R. KG-1 cells (1×10^7) are washed twice with RPMI-1640 medium and transfected with 50 mg of pRcEFM18R by electroporation. In the presence of 400-μg/mL G-418, the transformed cells are selected and cloned. The suspension of 2×10^6 cells, on which the receptor binding of ^{125}I-labeled MuIL-18 or HuIL-18 has been examined, in RPMI-1640 containing 0.1% NaN_3 and 100-mM HEPES (pH 7.2) is incubated at 4°C for 1 h with approximately 4 ng of ^{125}I-labeled MuIL-18 or HuIL-18. After the separation of unbound IL-18, the cell-bound ^{125}I count is determined. Subtracting the nonspecific binding measured from 3 μg of unlabeled cognate ligand, the specific binding of IL-18 is obtained. To prepare mice serum containing endogenous MuIL-18, C57BL/6 mice are treated with 500 μg of heat-killed *Propionibacterium acnes* for 1 week and challenged with 1 μg of lipopolysaccharide for 2 h to induce endotoxic shock. From the heart, under proper anesthetization, blood samples are taken to prepare sera. The MuIL-18R-expressing KG-1 cells are washed and resuspended at 5×10^5 cells/mL with RPMI-1640 medium for 2 days. The cells are adjusted to 1×10^6 cells/mL with RPMI-1640 containing 10% FCS, to which the indicated amounts of MuIL-18, HuIL-18, or serum sample are added. One day later, the culture supernatants are recovered and the quantitative analysis of the produced IFN-γ is performed by ELISA. The culture supernatant is incubated with mAb-IFN-γ-15. The bound IFN-γ is further incubated with mAb-IFN-γ-6 and detected with hydrogen peroxide and o-phenylenediamine.

Anti-rHuEPO NAb Assay

32D-EPOR cells are incubated at 37°C in humidified atmospheric air containing 5% CO_2 with RPMI 1640 supplemented with 15% heat-inactivated FBS, 2-mM l-glutamine, and penicillin/streptomycin (1%, v/v) mixture. The EPO-dependent cells are incubated in RPMI 1640 supplemented with 10 U/mL of rHuEPO. Via two to three subcultures a week, cell densities are maintained between 3×10^4

and 1 × 10^6 cells/mL. Up to 30 days after thawing, the old cells in the cryopreserved cells are discarded and a vial of frozen cells is thawed and expanded in culture.

In the cell proliferation assay, 32D-EPOR cells are incubated overnight, harvested, and washed twice with RPMI 1640 lacking rHuEPO by centrifugation (200–300 g). The supernatant is discarded, the cell pellet is resuspended in RPMI 1640, and the suspention is recentrifuged. The formed cell pellet is resuspended in RPMI 1640 and adjusted to 5 × 10^5 cells/mL. Cells are incubated at 37°C (humidified atmospheric air containing 5% CO_2, without rHuEPO) for 16–24 h, centrifuged, resuspended in fresh RPMI 1640, and counted. Overall, 100 μL of 2 × 10^4 staged 32D-EPOR cells and 100 μL of prepared testing sample are incubated at 37°C for 44 h in humidified atmospheric air containing 5% CO_2. The solution of 2-μCi [methyl-3H] thymidine diluted in 50 μL of RPMI 1640 is added to each well and incubated for 4 h. The contents of the plate are harvested, 25 μL of scintillation fluid are added, and the cells are counted.

All assay controls are prepared in a mixture of 5% human serum and 15% pooled rat serum. In anti-rHuEPO NAb assay, the background control (N) consisting of cells only is prepared by mixing 40 μL of pooled human serum with 240 μL of RPMI 1640 and 120 μL of pooled rat serum. The maximum growth control (M) consisting of cells and 1-ng/mL rHuEPO is prepared by mixing 40 μL of pooled human serum with 120 μL of rHuEPO at 6.67-ng/ml, 120 μL of RPMI 1640 and 120 μL of pooled rat serum. The neutralizing antibody positive control (P) consisting of cells, 1-ng/mL rHuEPO and 500-ng/mL positive control antibody is prepared by mixing 120 μL of RPMI 1640 with 120 μL of pooled rat serum. Samples are prepared by mixing 40 μL of individual donor serum with 120 μL of rHuEPO at 6.67 ng/mL, 120 μL of RPMI 1640, and 120 μL of pooled rat serum. Before addition to the cells, all controls and samples are preincubated at room temperature for at least 30 min.

Radial Assay of Chemotaxis

From stock sorocarp cultures of *D. discoideum* grown on agar plates, spores from strain v12 are harvested and heat-shocked at 45°C for 30 min. The suspension of the spores is mixed with a full loop of *E. coli* B/r, the 200-μL aliquots in new SM-agar plates are cultured at 22°C for 24 h, the cells are harvested and maintained vegetatively by shanking (200 rpm in Lpp medium, approximately 10^6 cells/mL), or the cells are starved by washing four times by centrifugation (3000 g, 30 s). The cells are shaken in 15-mM Tris-HCl (pH 7.0) for 2 h or 4 h; the latter is for routine chemotaxis assays. Chemotaxis of *D. discoideum* amoebae is performed on thin agar plates. Overall, 1 mL of 1.0% agarose in 15-mM Tris-HCl (pH 7.0) is added to each Petri plate and agitated to allow even spreading. The chemoattractants cAMP or folic acid are added to the agar with or without agonists before pouring plates. Chemotactically competent cells are centrifuged to form a viscous suspension and spotted on the agar plates. Each plate containing six aliquots of cells is covered, incubated at 22°C for 3 h, uncovered and placed on a heater to fix cells and dessicate the agar. As a measure of chemotactic efficiency, the initial spot diameters are subtracted from the diameters of visible rings or "halos" formed by outwardly migrating cells. During a period of 60 min with a playback time of 3 min, the individual halos on the agar plates are monitored. Proteins (20 μg/lane) are separated from whole cell lysates by polyacrylamide gel electrophoresis in 12% sodium dodecyl-sulphate polyacrylamide gels and transferred to nitrocellulose membranes in a mini-trans-blot cell using a buffer containing 25-mM Tris, 192-mM glycine (pH 8.3), and 20% methanol. Transfer is with 100 V for 40–60 min employing a frozen cooling unit. Using standard curves produced by running prestained Rainbow markers in parallel lanes, relative molecular weights are estimated. Nitrocellulose blots are blocked in 4% BSA at 4°C for 16 h, incubated for 1 h in 1/500 monoclonal anti-phosphotyrosine PT-66, and diluted by a 1/1000 dilution of peroxidase conjugated goat-antimouse IgG at room temperature for 1 h to detect the proteins containing phosphorylated tyrosine residues. Between each incubation, blots are washed three times for 5 min and immunoreactive bands are visualized using the chromogenic substrate diaminobenzidine HCl and 0.025% peroxide.

ESTROGEN ASSAY

After transfection, some cells become special fused cells such as the GAIA–DNA domain binding estrogen receptor yeast, the HELNa and HELNβ transfected cells, the yeast stably expresses human estrogen receptor β (hERβ), the yeast stably expresses human estrogen receptor α (hERα), and enhanced green fluorescent protein (yEGFP) in response to estrogens α (hERα). With the special characteristics and high response to estrogen stimulation, the mentioned cells and related substances are used for bioassays.

Yeast Oestrogen Assay

The yeast, of which the steroid-binding domain is fused by GAL4-VP16, is incubated with SC-medium without histidine at 30°C and 130 rpm overnight. By adding DMSO up to a final concentration of 15% (v/v), stock cultures are prepared from exponentially growing cultures and storéd in 0.5-mL aliquots at –80°C. Exponentially growing overnight, cultures are diluted with SC-medium to an OD_{600nm} of 0.75. To 10-mL aliquots 100 μL of DMSO (negative controls), 100 μL of 17β-estradiol in DMSO (positive controls), or 100 μL of test compound in DMSO are added, incubated at 30°C and 130 rpm for 2 h, diluted to five-fold volume and determined to get OD_{600nm}. To 200 μL of the test culture, 600 μL of Z-buffer (60-mM $Na_2HPO_4 \cdot 7H_2O$, 40-mM $NaH_2PO_4 \cdot H_2O$, 10-mM KCl, 1-mM $MgSO_4 \cdot 7H_2O$, 35-mM β-mercaptoethanol), 20-μL SDS solution (3.5 mM), and 50 μL of chloroform are added, carefully mixed, and pre-incubated at 28°C for 5 min, and then 200 μL of o-nitrophenyl-β-D-galactopyranoside in Z-buffer (13.3 mM) are added to initiate the enzyme reaction. The cultures are incubated at 28°C until a signifi- cant yellow color develops. For 17β-estradiol-induced positive controls, the yellow color occurs within 20 min. For test chemical-induced assays, the yellow color occurs after 120 min. To the cultures, 500 μL of Na_2CO_3 (1M) is added to stop the reaction, the cell debris is pelleted by centrifugation (25,500 g, 15 min), and the Ex_{420nm} of the supernatants is determined. The β-galactosidase activity of the test cultures is calculated according to u[μ mol/min] = Cs/t·V·ODs, wherein t = incubation time (min) of the enzyme reaction, V = volume (0.2 cm^3) of the used test culture aliquot, ODs = OD_{600nm} of test culture, Cs = concentration of o-nitrophenyl-β-D-galactopyranoside (μM) in the reaction supermatant calculated according to Cs (μM) = 10^6· [Exs-ExB] ∈N·d, wherein Exs = Ex_{420nm} of the enzyme reaction supernatant of test compound, ExB = Ex_{420nm} of the enzyme reaction supernatant of the blank control, $\in_N = \in$ for o-nitrophenyl-β-D-galactopyranoside in the enzyme assay reaction mixture (4666 × 10^3 cm^2/mole), and d = diameter of the cuvette (1 cm). EC_{50} are calculated from dose response curves obtained by fitting the data by $Y = D + [A - D]/[1 + (C/X)^B]$, wherein X = estrogen concentration in the test, Y = β-galactosidase activity, B = relative slope of the middle region of the curve as estimated from a linear/log regression of the linear part of the dose response curve, C = estrogen concentration at half maximal response, and D = minimum β-galactosidase activity. The relative β-galactosidase induction factor defined as the ratio of β-galactosidase activity in a chemical sample and in the corresponding negative control is used for test chemical sample screening results.

HELN α and HELN β Transfected Cell Assay

After incubation with 30 mg of C18 Oasis HLB batch for 10 min, 800 mL of every patient's serum are desteroided and centrifuged (13,000 g, 10 min) to separate the supernatant. To this stripped serum, a known amount of estradiol is added to obtain a set of estradiol standards with concentrations from 10^{-9} to 10^{-4} mM, and incubated for 4 h at 37°C to permit an equilibrium between free estrogens and estrogens bound to sex hormone-binding globulin. HeLa cells transfected with ERE-β Glob-Luc-SVNeo and pSG5-Puro-hERα or β, so-called HELNα and HELNβ, are selected by geneticin and puromycin at 1 mg/mL and 0.5 μg/mL, respectively. Luminescent and inducible clones are identified using photon-counting cameras. HELN Erα is cultured in 150-cm^2 plastic flasks in DMEM without phenol red, supplemented with 5% dextran-coated and charcoal-treated FCS, 0.25-μg/mL puromycin, and 0.5-mg/mL geneticin. To the culture medium, the aromatase inhibitor aminogluthetimide (AG) is added at a concentration of 50 μM. The cells are seeded in 96-well plates (3×10^4 cells per well) in the presence of DMEM without phenol red, supplemented with 3% dextran-coated and charcoal-treated FCS, 50-μM AG, and incubated for 8 h at 37°C. Culture medium is replaced by 100 μL of DMEM without phenol red, supplemented with 50-μM AG, to which 20 μL of human serum in triplicate is added.

Luciferase Assay

The p403- and p405-GPD yeast expression vectors and the p406-CYC1 yeast expression vector are used to express the human estrogen receptor α and β and construct the reporter plasmid, respectively. On the isolated mRNA of T47D human breast cancer cells and intestinal Caco-2 cells, cDNA is synthesized. Using the T47D cDNA, marathon uterus cDNA, and the human intestine cDNA by PCRs, full-length human estrogen receptor β (ERβ) cDNA is obtained. To perform the first PCR, 34.2 μL of ultra-pure water, 5 μL of 25-mM $MgCl_2$, 5 μL of Expand HF 10 × concentrated buffer (without $MgCl_2$), 0.8 μL of 25-mM dNTP mix, 1 μL of the enzyme mixture, 2 μL of the different cDNAs, and 2 μL of a primer mixture containing 10 μM of each primer are pipetted into a thin-walled PCR tube and (1) denature template 3 min at 95°C, (2) denature template 30 s at 94°C, (3) anneal primers 1 min at 60°C, (4) elongation 2 min at 72°C, (5) go to step (2) and repeat 35 times, (6) elongation 7 min at 72°C, and (7) for over 10°C. The second PCR is performed with the same conditions, but 2 μL of the first PCR mixture is used instead of 2 μL of the different cDNAs. The 5′- and 3′-primer, 5′-CGTCTAGAGCTGTTATCTCAAGACATGGATATAA-3′ and 5′-TAGGATCCGTCACTGAGA CTGTGGGTTCTG-3′, contains a restriction site for *XbaI* just before the ATG start codon and for *BamHI* just after the TGA stop codon, respectively. The full- length ERβ PCR product is isolated and ligated into a pGEM-T Easy Vector. The uterus/intestine human ERβ cDNA clone that fully corresponded to the ERβ sequence is cut out of the pGEM-T Easy plasmid with *XbaI* and *BamHI* and cloned into the corresponding *XbaI–BamHI* site of the p405-GPD-ERβ vector, which is used to transform Epicurian Coli XL-2 Blue Cells.

Yeast K20 is transfected with the p406-ERE2s2-CYC1-yEGFP reporter vector and integrated at the chromosomal location of the Uracil gene via homologous recombination to construct yeast hERα and hERβ cytosensors. The transformants are grown on MM/LH plates using PCR and Southern blot hybridization to select clones, in which the integration has occurred at the desired URA3 site with only a single copy of p406-ERE2s2-CYC1-yEGFP. This strain is transformed with the p403-GPD-Erα and the p405-GPD-ERβ, or both expression vectors and transformants are grown on MM/L, MM/H, or MM plates, respectively. The plate with selective MM/L, MM/H, or MM medium is inoculated with –80°C stock yeast ERα, ERβ, or ERα/β cytosensor (20% glycerol, v/v), respectively; incubated at 30°C for 24–48 h; and stored at 4°C. The day before the assay, a single colony of the yeast cytosensor is inoculated with 10 mL of the corresponding selective medium overnight at 30°C with vigorous orbital shaking at 225 g. At the late log phase, the yeast ERα, ERβ, and ERα/β cytosensor culture is diluted (1:10) in MM/L, (1:20) in MM/H, and (1:20) in MM, respectively. This minimal medium consists of a yeast nitrogen base without amino acids or ammonium sulphate (1.7 g/L), dextrose (20 g/L), and ammonium sulphate (5 g/L). The MM/L and MM/H medium are supplemented with L-leucine (60 mg/L) or L-histidine (2 mg/ L), respectively.

A total of 200-μL aliquots of the yeast culture are pipetted into each well of 96 well plates, and then 1 μL of ethanol or DMSO stock solution of test chemical is added to result in 0.5% final concentration. The plates are included for 4 h and 24 h, fluorescence at 485 nm and emission at 530 nm are measured directly, and the OD of the yeast culture at 630 nm is determined to check the toxicity of test chemical for yeast.

Green Fluorescent Protein Expression Assay

Aliquots of 2 mL of blank calf urine and 17β-estradiol (E2β, 1 ng/mL), diethylstilbestrol (DES, 1 ng/mL) and 17α-ethynylestradiol (EE2, 1 ng/mL), α-zearalanol (30 or 50 ng/mL) and mestranol (10 ng/mL), and spiked calf urine samples are adjusted to pH 4.8 and 20 μL of β-glucuronidase/arylsulfatase (3 U/mL) are added. The samples are deconjugated by enzyme at 37°C overnight, treated with 2 mL of 0.25-M sodium acetate buffer (pH 4.8) and subjected to solid phase extraction (SPE) on a C18 column conditioned previously with 2.5 mL of methanol and 2.5 mL of sodium acetate buffer. The column is successively washed with 1.5 mL of 10% (w/v) sodium carbonate solution, 3.0 mL of water, 1.5 mL of sodium acetate buffer (pH 4.8), 3.0 mL of water, and 2 mL of methanol/water (50/50 v/v). The column is air-dried and eluted with 4 mL of acetonitrile. The eluate is applied to an NH_2- column conditioned previously with 3.0 mL of acetonitrile. The acetonitrile eluate is evaporated to 2 mL by nitrogen gas stream, of which a 100-μL part (equivalent to 100-μL urine) is transferred to a 96-well plate and mixed with 50 μL of water and 2 μL of DMSO. The plate is dried overnight in a fume cupboard to remove the acetonitrile and screened on estrogenic activities with the yeast estrogen bioassay. In the same way, a reagent blank is prepared, using 2 mL of the 0.25-M sodium acetate buffer pH 4.8 instead of urine.

The yeast cytosensor (20% glycerol v/v) expressing the human estrogen receptor α (hERα) and yEGFP in response to estrogens is incubated in an agar plate containing the selective MM/L medium at 30°C for 24–48 h and then stored at 4°C. The day before the assay, a single colony of the yeast cytosensor is inoculated in 10 mL of selective MM/L medium overnight at 30°C with vigorous orbital shaking at 225 rpm. At the late log phase, the yeast ERα cytosensor is diluted in MM/L, giving an OD at 604 nm in the range of 0.07–0.13. For exposure in 96-well plates, aliquots of 200 μL of this diluted yeast culture are pipetted into each well, already containing the extracts of the urine samples. A E2β dose-response curve is included in each exposure experiment. Aliquots of 200 μL of the diluted yeast culture are pipetted into each well of a 96-well plate and exposed to different doses of E2βs performed through the addition of 2 μL of E2β stock solutions in DMSO. Each urine sample extract and each E2β stock is assayed. Exposure is performed for 0 h and 24 h. Fluorescence at these time intervals is measured directly using excitation at 485 nm and measuring emission at 530 nm. The densities of the yeast culture at these time intervals are also determined by measuring the OD at 630 nm to check whether a urine sample is toxic for yeast.

In the determination of the decision limit (CCα) and detection capability (CCβ) of the yeast estrogen bioassay, extracts of 20 blank calf urine, 20 spiked calf urine samples (E2β, DES and EE2 at 1 ng/mL, a-zearalanol at 30 or 50 ng/mL, and mestranol at 10 ng/mL), and a reagent blank are analyzed. After 24 h of exposure, the obtained fluorescence signals of the 20 blank urine samples, the 20 spiked urine samples, and a reagent blank are corrected for the signals obtained at 0 h (t_{24}-t_0). On three different days, the extracts of the blank urines and their corresponding spikes are prepared and analyzed in the yeast estrogen bioassay in three separate exposures. Within a time period of 10 days, these three sample treatments and exposures are performed. In another experiment, extracts of 20 blank urines and spikes of 50-ng zearalanol per mL urine are prepared in one day and are analyzed in the yeast estrogen bioassay in one exposure. In the context of EC Decision 2002/657, the mean signal of 20 blank calf urine samples plus 2.33 times the corresponding standard deviation is defined as the decision limit CCα (α = 1%), and the decision limit CCα plus 1.64 times the standard deviation of the signal of the spiked calf urine sample is defined as the detection capability CCβ (= 5%).

In the determination of the specificity of the yeast estrogen bioassay, three blank calf urine samples are spiked with a high dose of testosterone or progesterone (1000 ng/mL) and extracts are analyzed. In the determination of interference, these blank calf urine samples are spiked with a high dose of either testosterone or progesterone in combination with a low dose of estrogens (E2β, DES, and EE2 at 1 ng/mL, α-zearalanol at 50 ng/mL, and mestranol at 10 ng/mL).

ANTIMALARIAL ASSAY

The tremendous progress in the biology and the biochemistry of malaria parasites has led to the identification of drug targets that are both parasite specific and essential for parasite growth and survival, and some of them are now exploited in the mechanisms-based assays of various screening programs and determination of antimalarials' concentration such as plasmodium falciparum and murine P388 leukemia cell assay, histidine-rich protein II assay, anti-plasmodium activity assay, survival of Anopheles gambiae assay, chloroquine plus doxycycline assay, and plasmodium falciparum clone and dihydroartemisinin assay.

Plasmodium Falciparum and Murine P388 Leukemia Cell Assay

The required quantity of *P. falciparum* parasites maintained in a complete medium (RPMI-1640, 25-mM HEPES, 25-mM $NaHCO_3$, and 10% pooled human serum, with uninfected human red blood cells at 2.5% haematocrit) is introduced into flat-bottomed 96-well plates. The cell suspension (1% parasitaemia) is added to the plates (0.2 mL/well), which contains test compound in triplicate alongside untreated controls. The plates are shaken vigorously using a microculture plate shaker, and they are incubated at 37°C for 18 h under microaerophilic conditions. To each well, tritiating hypoxanthine with a specific activity of 14.1 Ci/mmol is added (0.5 μCi/well) and incubated at 37°C for another 24 h. The contents of the well are frozen at –30°C, unfrozen at 50°C, filtrated, and washed several times with water. The disks are dried and added to toluene scintillator in vials, and the radioactivity incorporated into parasites is estimated.

Test compounds inhibiting 75% or more of the parasite growth are systematically submitted to cytotoxicity tests. Murine P388 leukemia cells grown in RPMI 1640 medium containing 0.01-nM β-mercaptoethanol, 10-mM L-glutamine, 100-U/mL G-penicillin, 100-μg/mL streptomycin, 50-μg/mL gentamycin, and 50-μg/mL nystatine, supplemented with 10% fetal calf serum, are incubated in humidified atmospheric air containing 5% CO_2 at 37°C. The inoculum seed at 10^4 cells/mL (0.1 mL/well) is transferred into flat-bottomed 96-well plates containing serial concentrations of test compound, and the plates are incubated in the required atmosphere at 37°C for 72 h. Thereafter, cells are incubated at 37°C with a 0.02% solution of neutral red in 1/9 methanol/water (0.1 mL/well) for 1 h, washed with 1N PBS, and lyzed with 1% SDS. After a brief agitation, the plates are read at 540 nm to measure the absorbance of the extracted dye, and cell viability is expressed as the percentage of cells incorporating dye relative to the untreated controls and IC_{50} values are determined by the linear regression method.

Histidine-Rich Protein II Assay

The serial dilutions of complement-inactivated plasma samples, which are from uncomplicated falciparum malaria patients and a healthy volunteer treated with oral sodium artesunate (100 mg followed by 50 mg orally every 12 h for 5 days), are applied in two columns to 96-well microculture plates at 50 μL/well. The serial dilutions of spiked plasma are applied in two columns and added to each plate as controls. On each 96-well plate, five unknown samples plus the controls are tested; in addition, one plate with six serial dilutions of known drug concentrations covering the whole test range is also tested. According to the literature, the culture and ELISA procedures are performed. A total of 175-μL aliquots of the dilutions (0.1% parasite density, 1.7% hematocrit) of synchronized parasitized (clone W_2) blood samples from continuous culture are added to the plates (resulting in a total of 225 μL/well), with the frozen mixture of 1.05 mL of the remaining cell medium and 0.3 mL of drug-free plasma per plate as negative controls. Before being frozen- thawed, the plates are incubated at 37°C for 72 h in a candle jar or gas mixture (5% CO_2, 5% O_2, 90% N_2).

Antimalarial Activity Assay

The chloroquine resistant strain FcB1 of *P. falciparum* (50% inhibitory concentration [IC_{50}] of chloroquine = 62 ng/mL) maintained continuously in culture on human erythrocytes is used for the evaluation of antimalarial activities of test compounds. The semiautomated microdilution technique is modified to determine the *in vitro* antiplasmodial activity of test compounds. The serial medium dilutions of the stock solutions of test compounds in DMSO 10 mg/mL, of which the concentration never exceeds 0.1% and does not inhibit the parasite growth, are incubated with asynchronous parasite cultures (0.5% parasitemia and 1% final hematocrit) on 96-well plates at 37°C for 24 h and treated with [^{3}H] hypoxanthine (0.5 μCi/well) for 24 h. By comparison of the radioactivity incorporated into the treated culture with that in the control culture maintained on the same plate, the growth inhibition concentration for each test compound is defined. From the drug concentration-response curve, the IC_{50} is obtained and expressed as the mean determined from three independent experiments.

Survival of *Anopheles gambiae* Assay

Adults of laboratory-reared *An. gambiae* mosquitoes (from a colony established from wild gravid females. all mosquito life stages are maintained under semi-field conditions) are given 6% glucose solution on filter-paper wicks, water, and routine human bloodmeals three times per week. Three days after each bloodmeal inside the cages, which are kept in screen houses under ambient conditions, oviposition cups are used to collect eggs on the following day. Under semi-field conditions, the larvae for both the colony and the experiments are maintained on fish food and the plastic pans (25 × 20 × 14 cm) are filled with fresh water. In 30-cm cubic metal frame cages covered with mesh netting, approximately 100 pupae/cage and the test compound are for direct observation. *An. gambiae* mosquitoes are allowed to emerge, and evening observations of test compound feeding are conducted from 20:00 to 22:00 h, for which at intervals of 30 min, a flashlight is used. On a second night of observation, a mosquito net is placed over *Ricinus communis* in a screenhouse, under which a cup of water containing approximately 500 pupae is placed and emerging adults are allowed to feed on the test compound for 24 h. From 20:00 to 22:00 h in intervals of 30 min, on the following night, mosquitoes are observed until they are observed probing or feeding on the test compound.

For survival assay, mosquitoes are divided into regime groups. From the main mosquito colony, approximately 100 pupae per regime are harvested, transferred to plastic cups, and placed in cages and held in a screenhouse under ambient conditions. Each cage of mosquitoes has access to test compound sources; one group of mosquitoes has access to a cotton pad moistened with distilled water, representing negative controls; and another group of mosquitoes with neither test compound source nor water is used as an additional negative control. Dead mosquitoes are removed at 4-h intervals from 7:00 to 23:00 h until all die.

Chloroquine Assay

The blood samples (10 mL) from healthy volunteers who are on chloroquine (2 × 150-mg base weekly) and doxycycline (50 mg or 100 mg daily) malaria prophylaxis are centrifuged (1200 g, 10 min), and the plasma is separated and stored at –20°C. The chloroquine-sensitive FC27 strain of *P. falciparum* is used for the determination of antimalarial activity of each plasma sample. On microculture plates, the plasma samples are diluted twofold with drug-free serum and inoculated with a suspension of parasitized erthrocytes in culture medium. The drug susceptibility and minimum concentration of spiked drug that inhibits parasites, relative to control, from developing to schizonts is recorded. The maximum inhibitory dilution (MID) of the volunteers' samples containing a choroquine concentration and the minimum inhibitory concentration (MIC) observed in the sensitivity test are recorded. The chloroquine equivalent concentration in the prediluted volunteers' specimen is estimated by multiplying the MID by the MIC.

Plasmodium Falciparum Clone and Dihydroartemisinin (DHA) Assay

By centrifugation for 5 s, 50 μL of Affigel protein A (binding capacity of 20 mg of purified human immunoglobulin G[IgG]/mg of gel) is washed twice with PBS (pH 7.2, 50 μL), and the RPMI 1640 medium (50 μL) that is supplemented with 5.94-g/L HEPES and 2.1-g/L sodium bicarbonate, centrifuged to discarde the supernatant, and Affigel protein A gel is incubated with the plasma and serum (250 μL) spiked with dihydroartemisinin (DHA) or plasma from patients at room temperature for 30 min. The stock solution of DHA in 70% ethanol (1 mg/mL) is kept at –10°C for up to 1 month before use, which is further diluted in plasma or serum to give a working concentration (1.25 to 100 ng/mL). Affigel protein A-treated plasma (100 μL) and heat-inactivated serum (50 μL/ well) are transferred to row A and B of a flat-bottom plate, respectively. Using the heat-inactivated serum added through G into row B as the diluent for plasma or serum containing DHA, twofold serial dilutions are prepared. To row H, 50 μL of heat-inactivated control plasma or serum is added for parasitizing and nonparasitizing erythrocyte controls. To all wells for rows A to G and eight wells for row H, the suspension of 175 μL of malaria parasite-infected erythrocytes (W_2 clone; 0.5% parasitemia with 80% young rings at a 1.7% hematocrit) is added. To the remaining four wells of row H for nonparasitized controls, the similar suspension of uninfected erythrocytes is added. The microtiter plates are incubated at 37°C for 24 h and treated with 1 Ci/mmol [^{3}H] hypoxanthine by the addition of 25 μL of 0.5 μCi isotope solution to each well. The microtiter plates are incubated for another 18 to 20 h. Harvesting the contents of the plates, the particulate material of the water-lysed cell suspension is collected on glass-fiber filter paper by filtration, and the filter paper is dried in an oven and placed in a plastic bag, to which 10 mL of scintillation fluid is added and the plastic bag is then sealed. By counting in a liquid scintillation counter, the level of incorporation of [^{3}H] hypoxanthine by the malaria parasites is determined. Fresh whole blood is collected to heparinized tubes, and the plasma and buffy çoat are removed, and the erythrocytes are lysed and serially diluted (2- to 64-fold) with sterile water, of which 50-μL aliquots are diluted in 250 μL of plasma or medium spiked with DHA to give a final concentration of 50 ng/mL and a range of hemoglobin concentrations from 1.5 to 0.05 g%. The effect of hemolysate in both plasma and culture medium (RPMI 1640 medium with 15% heat-inactivated human serum) on the detection of DHA activity is examined. The final concentration of plasma and serum in each well is 30% and 15%, respectively, which is similar to that in the normal drug susceptibility test. In addition to testing hemolysates of normal erythrocytes, the plasma samples collected from patients with severe falciparum malaria before treatment with any antimalarial drugs can also be spiked with 50 ng of DHA/mL and subjected to the same bioassay.

Blood Pressure-related Assay

Blood pressure can be regulated by receptor, enzyme, endogerous substance, and cell, such as bradykinin B2-receptor, ACE, 5-Hydroxytryptamine, and endothelia cell. Based on these facts, the human plasma assay, pulmonary hypertension assay, coronary arteries (CA) constriction assay, MCAO and HSPG assay, and temperature assay in awake subjects are established.

Human Plasma Assay

The solution of test peptide is injected (i.v.) into adult male Wistar rats (housed in pairs, under a 12:12 h light/dark cycle, 0.4% NaCl rat chow, and water available *ad libitum*, after 3–5 days of adaptation to the facility, about 300 g) at a proper dose. The inactin (100 mg/kg, i.p.; sodium ethyl-(1-methyl-propyl) -malonylthio -urea) anesthetized rats are treated with atropine (2.4 mg/kg, s.c.), and their ganglions are blockaded with pentolinium (19.2 mg/kg, s.c.). Overall, 10-mg/kg captopril is administered i.v. acutely to the rats in the captopril group, and it inhibits fully the pressor effect of 60-ng/kg angiotensin I.

To assist ventilation, the trachea is intubated and both vagi are severed to block reflex bradycardia. Into the right femoral vein and carotid artery, catheters are inserted for the injection of test compound and other agonists and antagonists, and for monitoring arterial blood pressure and heart rate and for blood sampling, respectively, and blood pressure is monitored.

Responses, in terms of the increases in systolic (SBP) and diastolic (DBP) blood pressures, to test peptide and bradykinin are determined. After ganglion blockade with pentolinium (group GB) without or with added captopril (group GB+Cap), heart rate and plasma adrenaline and noradrenaline concentrations are determined. In some cases, the rats are not subjected to ganglion blockade and served as controls for animals in the GB group (control group).

To evaluate the contribution of bradykinin B2-receptor-mediated mechanisms, the selective bradykinin B2-receptor antagonist, HOE-140, is given to ganglion- blocked, the rats are captopril treated, and the increases in SBP, DBP, heart rate, and plasma adrenaline/noradrenaline induced by test peptide and bradykinin (group GB+Cap+HOE) are observed. To evaluate the contribution of AT1- receptor-mediated mechanisms, the selective AT1 receptor antagonist, losartan, is given to group GB rats before and after treatment with captopril (1 mg/kg, i.v.) and the increases in SBP, DBP, heart rate, and plasma adrenaline/noradrenaline induced by test peptide are observed.

For determining plasma adrenaline and noradrenaline arterially approximately 1 mL of blood is withdrawn via the carotid cannula at baseline (before injection of test peptide and bradykinin), at the peak of the SBP response, and after recovery from the response. Before each withdrawal, the rat is given a transfusion of approximately 1 mL of blood from a similarly prepared donor rat. The SBP peak is observed at 2–3 min after the injection of test peptide and at 1–2 min after the injection of bradykinin; blood sampling coincides with these intervals. Using HPLC and fluorimetric detection, plasma catecholamines are determined.

Pulmonary Hypertension Assay

The chest cavity of a mouse (10–20 weeks old, 22–30 g) anesthetized by pentobarbital sodium (80 mg/kg, i.p.) is opened, and the lungs are removed rapidly and placed in Krebs–Ringer bicarbonate solution (KRBS) containing 118.3-mM NaCl, 4.7-mM KCl, 1.2-mM $MgSO_4$, 1.2-mM KH_2PO_4, 2.5-mM $CaCl_2$, 25.0-mM Na_2CO_3, and 10.0-mM glucose, bubbled with 21% O_2. From the intrapulmonary artery (third to fourth generation, PA), rings (50–100 μm internal diameter, 2–3 mm long) are isolated using a dissection microscope. PA rings are mounted as ring preparations by threading two steel wires into the lumen and securing the wires to two supports, and they are placed in a small vessel wire myograph chamber. The support is attached to a micrometer for the control of ring circumference and to a force transducer for measurement of isometric tension, respectively. After removal of endothelial cells by gently rubbing the intraluminal surface with a steel wire, some vessels are successively perfused with 2-mL air bubbles and 2-mL of KRBS (perfusion pressure < 5 mm Hg), before being mounted in the chamber. In the chamber filled with KRBS (pH 7.35–7.45), bubbled with 21% O_2–5% CO_2–balance N_2, the whole preparation is kept at 37°C. To control oxygen tension over the superfusate, Plexiglas is used as a cover over the chamber. The temperature and PA tension are recorded. At initial tension of 0 mN (1 g = 4.905 mN), isolated murine PA rings in the chamber are allowed to equilibrate for 10–15 min, which are increased to 5 mN in 2.5-mN steps at 4- to 5-min intervals and held constant thereafter. Through preliminary experiments, the resting tension for maximal constrictor response is optimized, in which the resting tension levels of 2.5, 5, and 7.5 mN are compared. In the evaluation of vascular viability, after the treatment of PA with 60-mM KCl, the tension is determined. The PA is washed extensively with KRBS, successively exposed to U-46619 (0.01 μM, thromboxane A2 agonist) and 1-μM Ach, the resulting tension is recorded and stabilized for 5–10 min, and the agonists are washed out of the myograph chamber with KRBS.

Murine PA is isolated, placed in a confocal pressure myograph chamber, cannulated at both ends with glass micropipettes, and secured with a 12-0 nylon monofilament suture. To control transmural pressure, both cannulas are connected to a reservoir that can be raised or loared. In the chamber, PA is superfused at 37°C, constantly with KRBS, and gassed with 21%O_2–5%CO_2–balance N_2. To control oxygen tension over the superfusate, Plexiglas is used as a cover over the chamber. To the chamber, 0.1-mM dihydroethidum (DHE) is added, in which murine PA is incubated at 37°C for 45 min and then washed for 30 min. The reaction of ntracellular DHE and ROS produces a fluorescent oxidized product and PA images are scanned (480-nm-line argon laser, fluorescence 620 nm). Superoxide anion levels in isolated murine PA are measured by a lucigenin-enhanced chemiluminescence technique and scintillation counter, using a solution of 5-μM lucigenin in Krebs–HEPES buffer (10.0-mM HEPES acid, 135.3-mM NaCl, 4.7-mM KCl, 1.2-mM $MgSO_4$, 1.2-mM KH_2PO_4, 1.8-mM $CaCl_2$, 0.026-mM Na-EDTA, and 11.1-mM glucose), 1-mL total volume, after background chemiluminescence activity has stabilized for 5 min.

Coronary Arteries (CA) Constriction Assay

The left main coronary arteries (CA, 70–90 μm in diameter, 1-mm length) of a mouse are placed into a microvascular chamber, cannulated at both ends with glass micropipettes, and pressurized. By gently rubbing the intraluminal surface with a steel wire, the endothelial cells of some vessels are removed. The vascular intra-luminal pressure (Ptm) is measured by using a pressure transducer positioned at the level of vessel lumen. The vessels in the chamber are superfused constantly with recirculating Krebs–Ringer bicarbonate solution containing 118.3-mM NaCl, 4.7-mM KCl, 1.2-mM $MgSO_4$, 1.2-mM KH_2PO_4, 2.5-mM $CaCl_2$, 25.0-mM $NaHCO_3$, and 11.1-mM glucose, which is gassed with 16% O_2, 5% CO_2, and balance N_2 (pH 7.35–7.45), and maintained at 37°C. To control oxygen tension over the superfusate the chamber is covered by Plexiglas, through which port an oxygen electrode is passed into the superfusate and positioned near the vessel to provide continuous measurement of oxygen tension. The vascular intraluminal diameter (ID) is measured continuously. The oxygen tension, vascular ID, and Ptm are recorded. The isolated CA in the chamber is allowed to equilibrate 30 min at a Ptm of 10 mm Hg, which is increased to 60 mm Hg in 10-mm Hg steps at 5–7-min intervals and held constant thereafter. When Ptm is increased to 60 mm Hg (time 0), the ID is recorded (appointed to ID60, namely ID at Ptm = 60 mm Hg) and the measurement is continued throughout the experiment.

The superoxide anions produced in isolated murine CA are measured using a lucigenin (bis-*N*-methyacidinium nitrate)-enhanced chemiluminescence technique. After background has stabilized chemiluminescence activity for 5 min, CA is placed in the chemiluminometer containing 1 mL of 5-μM lucigenin buffer solution, photon emission is recorded continuously, and the chemiluminescence signal is recorded as relative light units per second (RLU/s).

Middle Cerebral Artery Occlusion (MCAO) Assay and Vascular Heparan Sulfate Proteoglycans (HSPG) Perlecan Assay

Male baboons are randomly divided into treatment and control groups. In the treatment groups the animals undergo MCAO for 1 h or 2 h, or 3 h MCAO with subsequent reperfusion for 1 h or 4 h, or 1.5 h MCAO with 24 h reperfusion. In the control groups, the animals do not undergo any preparation procedure or suffer from MCAO at surgical implantation and has sustained hemiparesis for 7 days. The animals are transcardially perfused with isosmotic heparinized perfusate, and their brain tissues are removed under thiopental Na and prepared for frozen and paraffin sections. The samples of normal and 50 μL of ischemic brain tissue or 100 μL of purified reagents are added to the recipient tissues consisting of unfixed 10-μm-thick normal basal ganglia sections mounted on microscope slides.

When proteases are added to the normal recipient tissues, PBS (pH 7.0) is the incubation buffer for type-7 bacterial collagenase. The solution of matrix metalloproteinases (MMPs) and urokinase/plasminogen in a buffer containing 90-mM NaCl, 5-mM KCl, 1.5-mM $MgCl_2$, 23-mM Na gluconate, 27-mM NaAc, 10-mM $CaCl_2$, and 40-mM $ZnCl_2$ (pH 7.4) is prepared. The solution of cathepsin B and L in 200-mM NaAc containing 8-mM dithiothreitol, 1-mM EDTA, and 2.7-mM L-cysteine (pH 6.0) is prepared. The mixture of 5-U/mL plasminogen and 5-U/mL uPA is incubated at 37°C for 1 h; 1-μg/mL Pro-MMP-2 or 1-μg/mL pro-MMP-9 is added and incubated for 1 h. The recipient sections are incubated with 100 μL of each mixture or buffer alone at 37°C for 5 h (collagenase) or 18 h (MMPs and cathepsins) and washed with PBS and fixed. From approximately 1.0-cm x 1.0-cm x 10-μm frozen sections, donor samples are derived. By centrifugation (300 g, 30 s) and repeated gentle pipetting, the mixture of 10 consecutive 10-μm sections of ischemic or normal basal ganglia is prepared. Overall, 50 μL of sample or PBS is added to the recipient sections, the mixture is incubated at 37°C for 18 h, and the recipient sections are washed with PBS and fixed in acetone or paraformaldehyde (PFA).

In the development of the specific antigens, the immunoperoxidase methods are used. At 4°C, the overnight incubation of acetone-fixed frozen sections in the presence of the primary antibody is followed by developing immunoperoxidase with 3,3´-diaminobenzidine tetrahydrochloride. At 4°C, the overnight deparaffination of acetone-fixed frozen sections in the presence of the primary antibody is also followed by developing immunoperoxidase with 3,3´-diaminobenzidine tetrahydrochloride. Incorporating dUTP into nuclear DNA is used as the evidence of nuclear DNA scission/repair, and at 2 h, MCAO defines the ischemic core and peripheral regions of cellular neuronal injury. PFA-fixed cryosections are subject to the DNA polymerase I method. All ischemic samples include ischemic core and ischemic peripheral regions. In the measurement of MMP-related activities, Gelatin zymography is performed with a modification to increase sensitivity . Protease activities are identified by incubation of the gels in buffer containing GM6001 or APMSF.

Temperature Assay in Awake Subjects

The male SD rats (250–325 g) are caused reversible ischemia with the intraluminal filament occlusion of the middle cerebral artery (MCA) and maintained anesthesia with 2% halothane and mixed gas of nitrous oxide and oxygen (60:40) by face mask. To expose the left carotid artery, a midline neck incision is made. The external carotid and pterygopalatine arteries are ligated with 5-0 silk. In the arterial wall, an incision is made. From the bifurcation of external and internal carotid arteries, a 4-0 heat blunted nylon suture of 18 mm is advanced. This distance reliably produces blockage of the origin of the MCA. The duration of occlusion for individual rats is varied to generate a range of ischemia durations for each experimental group. During surgery, the temporalis and brain temperature are monitored and maintained. During the period (4–5 h) of post-anesthetic recovery, the awake rats are kept on a pad maintained at 37.5°C. To verify the effect of this procedure on brain temperature, an indwelling radio telemetry thermister is implanted into the rat of the nonischemic group. After induction of anesthesia, the rat is placed in a stereotaxic head frame. A thermister probe is placed in the left parietal cortex (3 mm deep to dura and 1 mm anterior, 3 mm lateral to bregma). To secure the probe to the skull, a plastic cap is fitted using methylmethacrylate. After full recovery from the anesthesia, telemetered brain temperature is measured every 15 min. Temperatures are measured every 5 min for 24 h during a baseline period and 6 h after drug administration. After a drug treatment, some animals are placed on a heating pad for 2 h and their temperature is measured every 15 min. At

48 h and 72 h, the behavior of the rats is evaluated and classified to normal/abnormal according to a modified rodent examination scale. All obtundation/reduced exploration, forepaw retraction on tail lifting, asymmetric forepaw grasp, axial twist, forced circling, or death are defined as abnormal.

To correctly position the filament, 0.2 mL of 2% Evan's Blue in saline is injected into each rat via tail vein and circulated for 30 to 60 min, after which the rat is perfused transcardially with 100-mL normal saline, and the brain is removed and immediately examined. Each day, two rats of the control group and four or five rats of the drug treatment group are injected test compound dissolved in saline via tail vein at 30, 60, 75, 120, 240, or 360 min after initiating occlusion to assess therapeutic efficacy. To determine the effects of the test compound on blood gases, heart rate, and arterial blood pressure in separate groups, physiological determinations are performed. To observe the interaction between test compound and anesthesia, the determinations in awake or in anesthetized rats are performed. The ventral tail artery is cannulated with PE50 tubing for recording the arterial pressures and sampling arterial blood. Test compound is administered after the rat is stable for 30 min with no further adjustments needed to maintain homeostasis under 75– 90 mmHg steady-state mean arterial pressure (MAP) and minimal halothane. To obtain similar data from awake subject, tail artery catheters are implanted under halothane inhaled anesthesia. After implantation, the rat is allowed to recover and is lightly restrained. One hour after stopping the anesthesia, the cannula is attached to the transducer and vital signs are recorded for a 30-min baseline period. After the subject is shown to be stable for 30 min, the test compound is given. Blood pressures and blood gases are recorded every 10 min for 1 h and then hourly.

5

PROCESSING OF PHARMACEUTICALS

Corrosion, the degradation of a material's properties or mass over time because of environmental effects, is a costly reality that effects every industry. A study issued by the Federal Highway Administration (FHWA) in 2002 conservatively estimates the annual direct cost of corrosion in all U.S. industry sectors at US$276 billion. Costs associated with corrosion include cathodic/anodic protection; coatings; inhibitors; corrosion-resistant alloys and materials; and maintenance, repair, and depreciation of equipment. Indirect costs, such as lost productivity, environmental or product contamination, planning and design, and lost opportunities, can easily outpace direct costs by factors of two or more.

PHARMACEUTICAL EQUIPMENT

It is relatively easy to recognize the impact that corrosion has on chemical process industries (CPI). The FHWA indicates that annual direct costs for the refinery, chemical, petrochemical, paper, and food processing industries total US$13.5 billion. In the chemical and pharmaceutical sector alone, the conservative estimate given is that corrosion costs are roughly 8% of capital expenditures. The US$1.7 billion figure for this sector is very conservative because it does not include operating and maintenance costs. Corrosion within these industries ranges from mild (exposure of structures to atmospherical conditions) to very severe (strong acids, high temperatures, and halogen environments). Additionally, these industries use large quantities of water for not only chemical process, but for heating and cooling. The properties of water, a very mild corrodent, make it conducive to the electrochemical nature of corrosion processes. Acceptable performance of corrosion-resistant materials or systems can range from tens of years to weeks.

The control of corrosion in pharmaceutical product processes is largely managed through the use of stainless steel. Rust-free surfaces and cleanliness issues to prevent product contamination have been the primary corrosion concerns. Resistance to mildly aggressive cleaning solutions and saline solutions and the potential for under deposit or crevice corrosion present the most severe service conditions. The high standards of cleanliness necessary for pharmaceutical processes favor the mitigation of corrosion.

Corrosion Basics

The broadest definition of corrosion is the degradation of a material's properties or mass over time because of the effect of the environment. We can think of this in simpler terms by recognizing this process as the tendency for a material to return to its most thermodynamically stable state. For most metallic materials, this means the formation of oxides or sulfides, or other basic metallic compounds generally considered to be ores. For polymeric materials, the end result could be a variety of simple organic compounds. Only in vacuums or under inert atmospheres can corrosion processes be expected to halt entirely. In most cases, these processes are slow enough to afford useful and practical equipment life.

Corrosion is an electrochemical process and corrosion processes follow the basic laws of thermodynamics. Under controlled conditions, corrosion can be measured, repeated, and predicted. However, because corrosion takes place on an atomic level, corrosion can take place in an accelerated localized fashion, appear as uniform visible attack, or result in subsurface microscopical damage. Normal service environments can rapidly complicate these processes and mechanisms with such variables as pH, temperature, stress, surface finish, flow rates, etc. With the wide range of variables that can come into play, it should not be surprising that corrosion appears to be unpredictable at times.

Forms of Corrosion

Corrosion of metallic materials can take on many forms. Understanding and recognizing the basic forms of corrosion are necessary for developing a strategy for mitigation. These concepts can also be utilized in assessing non-metallic materials.

Uniform Corrosion

The simplest form of corrosion is "uniform" or "general" corrosion. This mode of corrosion is characterized by a uniform metal loss over the entire exposed surface. It is the most predictable and measurable form of corrosion. There are many sources of general corrosion data that list actual or typical rates of corrosion for many materials in common environments. Where data are not available, simple laboratory tests can be conducted to simulate process environments.

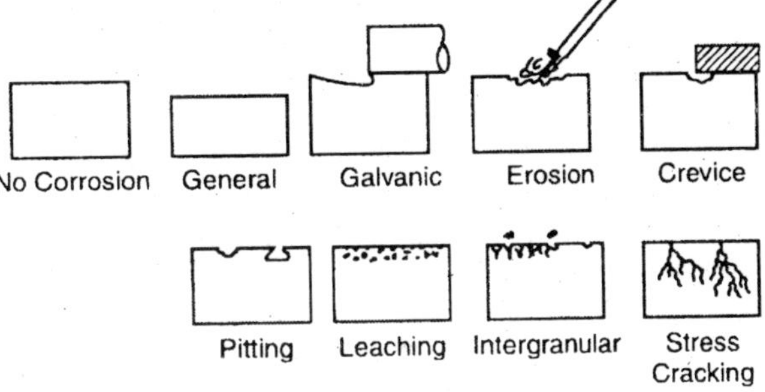

Fig. 5.1. Forms of corrosion.

The most common way to report uniform corrosion is in terms of metal thickness loss per unit of time, such as inches per year or millimeters per year. Because uniform corrosion is predictable, even moderately high corrosion rates can be tolerated provided a suitable monitoring and inspection system is utilized. For most chemical process systems, general corrosion rates of less than 2 mils per year (MPY) are acceptable. Rates between 2 and 20 MPY (1 mil = 0.001 in.) are routinely accepted as useful engineering materials. In severe environments, rates between 20 and 50 MPY may be economically justified. Rates exceeding 50 MPY are generally not acceptable. For pharmaceutical applications in particular, the rate of corrosion must be considered not only for the effect on equipment, but where the lost metal has gone. Product contamination can be of concern for other products as well, and when this is an issue, the selection of more corrosion-resistant materials is of utmost importance.

Galvanic Corrosion

When two different metallic materials are electrically connected and placed in a conductive solution, an electrical potential will exist. This potential difference will provide a stronger driving force for the dissolution of the less noble (more electrically negative) material. It will also reduce the tendency for the more noble material to dissolve.

Although the relative differences in potential will change from one environment to another, they remain fundamentally the same because the potential is related to the energy required to oxidize them to metal ions in the given environment. The precious metals of gold and platinum are at the high potential (more noble or cathodic) end of the series, whereas zinc and magnesium are at the low potential (less noble or anodic) end.

Erosion Corrosion

Erosion corrosion results in an increased rate of corrosion attack attributable to the velocity of a corrodent over the exposed surface. The movement of the corrodent can be associated with mechanical wear. The increased corrosion is usually related to the removal or damage of a protective surface film. The mechanism is usually identified by localized corrosion, which exhibits a pattern that follows the flow of the corrodent. Fretting corrosion is a specialized form of erosion corrosion where two metal surfaces are in contact and experience very slight relative motion that causes damage to one or both surfaces. Again, in the presence of a corrodent, the movement causes mechanical damage of the protective film, leading to localized corrosion. A second form of erosion corrosion is the case of cavitation. A type of corrosion familiar to pump impellers, this form of attack is caused by the formation and collapse of tiny vapor bubbles near a metallic surface in the presence of a corrodent. The protective surface film is again damaged, in this case by the high pressures caused by the collapse of the bubbles.

Pitting Corrosion

Pitting corrosion is in itself a corrosion mechanism, but is also a form of corrosion often associated with other types of corrosion mechanisms. It is characterized by a highly localized loss of metal. In the extreme case, a pit can appear as deep, tiny hole in an otherwise unaffected surface. The initiation of a pit is associated with the breakdown of the protective film on the metal surface. In cases where pit depths increase rapidly, the environment is usually such that no repair or repassivation of the protective layer can be accomplished. In situations where many shallow pits form, the environment is usually one where repassivation of the damaged film can be made, but initiation of new sites occurs on a regular basis. The localized nature of pitting attack can be associated with component geometry, the mechanics of the corrosion process, compositional inhomogeneity, or imperfection within the material itself. The growth of pits, once initiated, is closely related to another corrosion mechanism, crevice corrosion.

Crevice Corrosion

Crevice corrosion occurs in some environments because the nature of the environment within the crevice becomes more aggressive over time. There is little movement of the corrodent within a crevice. Over time, small changes in chemistry because of minor localized corrosion may become magnified because the solution is not being replenished by the bulk solution. As a result of a slow initial rate of the corrosion, the pH of the crevice environment may become more acidic, or detrimental ion species may concentrate. As a result of the low-flow condition, the crevice region may become depleted of oxygen, or preclude the replacement of reacted inhibitors.

Selective Leaching

Selective leaching is the process whereby a specific element is removed from an alloy because of an electrochemical interaction with the environment. Dezincification of brass alloys is the most familiar example of this type of corrosion. It occurs most commonly when there is exposure to soft waters and can be accelerated by high carbon dioxide concentrations and the presence of chloride ions. The result of this corrosion is the formation of a porous and usually brittle shadow of the original component. Other alloy systems are susceptible to this form of corrosion. Examples include the selective loss of aluminum in aluminum–copper alloys, and the loss of iron in cast iron–carbon steels.

Intergranular Corrosion

As the name suggests, this particular corrosion mechanism attacks those sites where individual grains within a metallic material touch each other. These boundaries are natural regions of higher energy because of the greater frequency of dislocations of atoms from the natural order of the material's structure. In addition, these regions also tend to act as sites for the formation of secondary phases, which are essentially small islands within the matrix that have a chemical composition different from the alloy itself. Depending on the corrodent and the alloy system, corrosion attack may initiate at these locations because of preferential attack of the secondary phase itself, or attack the surrounding matrix, which was locally dealloyed in forming the secondary phase. Either mechanism will result in the metallic surface being etched along the grain boundaries. As the attack progresses, individual grains are separated from the matrix and the surface layer becomes porous. In severe cases, the surface texture becomes grainy or powdery, leading to more rapid metal loss.

Stress Corrosion Cracking

The mechanism of stress corrosion cracking (SCC) is specific to certain alloys (or alloy systems) in specific environments. It is characterized by one or more crack fronts, which have developed as a result of a combination of the particular corrodent and tensile stresses. Depending on the alloy system and corrodent combination, the cracking can be either intergranular or transgranular. The rate of crack propagation can vary greatly and is affected by stress levels, temperature, and the concentration of the corrodent. In some severe combinations, such as type 304 stainless steel in a boiling magnesium chloride solution, extensive cracking can be generated in a matter of hours. In most industrial applications, the progress of SCC is, fortunately, at a much slower pace. However, because of the nature of the cracking, it is difficult to detect until extensive corrosion has already developed, which can lead to unexpected catastrophic failure. Alloy system and corrodent combinations that are known to exhibit SCC are fairly well documented and should be considered in initial design stages.

Apart from the SCC mechanism, stress can assist in other corrosion processes. Because this stress-assisted corrosion is related to tensile stresses, it is logical to expect that it will also accelerate the simple mechanical fatigue process. Corrosion fatigue is often difficult to differentiate from simple mechanical fatigue, but is recognized as a factor when the environment has been judged to have accelerated the normal fatigue process. Such systems can also have the effect of lowering the endurance limit such that fatigue will take place at a stress level wherein, without the environmental effect, fatigue failures would not be expected.

Corrosion Monitoring

The most common method of identifying and monitoring corrosion is visual inspection. Evidence of leakage, staining, or a change in surface appearance can be an indication that some type of corrosion is taking place. Experience with certain types of equipment and processes may help dictate inspection intervals and areas on which to focus the inspection. Records of vessel operation, maintenance, and repair can be helpful in establishing a pattern of performance that will improve predictability and minimize down time. In areas where general corrosion is the expected form, a simple ultrasonic thickness gage can be utilized to determine the extent of corrosion, based on baseline readings made at installation or previous inspections. The entire unit need not be examined. Attention can be focused on those areas most likely to corrode, such as liquid levels, mixing zones, or areas of high turbulence. Corrosion probes, which can be placed in process equipment or pipelines, can monitor corrosion conditions by measuring an actual corrosion current, or other process parameters known to be related to general corrosion rates. These data can be constantly monitored and recorded to predict equipment wear, or as an alert to upset conditions.

For detection of more localized corrosion, such as crevice corrosion or SCC, other ultrasonic inspection techniques may be useful. Baseline data generated at the time of installation will also be helpful in evaluating results. One benefit derived from this type of inspection technique is that it can often be conducted with little or no interference with production. Periodic planned visual inspection of equipment utilized under conditions likely to cause stress cracking is also an effective technique, especially when combined with non-destructive inspection techniques such as dye penetrant inspection. It may be necessary to remove coatings or insulation from the equipment surface to facilitate inspection.

Corrosion Processes and Mitigation

Electrochemical Nature of Corrosion

Corrosion, in its simplest definition, is the process of a material returning to the natural thermodynamic state. For most metallic materials, this means the formation of the oxides or sulfides that existed before being refined into useful engineering materials.

These changes are electrochemical reactions that follow the laws of thermodynamics. This concept aids in understanding why corrosion processes are time-dependent and temperature-dependent, and its application will indicate ways to mitigate corrosion. Corrosion reactions and rates are affected by ion and corrodent concentrations. One of the most basic corrosion reactions involves the oxidation of a pure metal when exposed to a strong acid. A familiar case is that of placing pure iron in hydrochloric acid. The resulting chemical reaction is quite obvious, with the solution beginning to bubble violently. The chemical reaction can be expressed as follows:

$$Fe + HCl \rightarrow FeCl_2 + H_2 \uparrow$$

The result of this reaction is evidenced by the gradual disappearance of the iron and the hydrogen bubbles rising rapidly to the surface. On an electro-chemical level, there is also an exchange of electrons taking place:

$$Fe + 2H^+ + Cl^{2-} \rightarrow Fe^{2+} + Cl^{2-} + H_2 \uparrow$$

The iron has been converted to an iron ion by giving up two electrons (oxidation), which were picked up by the hydrogen ions. By gaining electrons, the hydrogen ion was *reduced* and formed hydrogen gas. Note that the chlorine atom does not enter into the reaction itself. The transfer of electrons takes place on the metal's surface. Those locations where electrons are being given up are identified as "anodes." The sites where electrons are being absorbed are denoted as "cathodes." A difference in electrical potential exists between these two areas and a complete electrical circuit is developed. Negatively charged electrons flow in the direction of anode to cathode, and positively charged hydrogen ions in the solution move toward the cathode to complete the circuit. The faster the dissolution of the metal (rate of corrosion) is, the higher is the current flow. On a microscopical level, the sites of the anodes and cathodes can change locations on the surface. In fact, this is exactly what happens when general corrosion takes place, with the anodic areas moving uniformly over the metal's surface.

Anodic reactions in metallic corrosion are relatively simple. The reactions are always such that the metal is oxidized to a higher valence state. During general corrosion, this will result in the formation of metallic ions of all the alloying elements. Metals that are capable of exhibiting multiple valence states may go through several stages of oxidation during the corrosion process.

Cathodic reactions are more difficult to predict, but can be categorized into one of five different types of reduction reactions:

Hydrogen evolution

$$2H^+ + 2e \rightarrow H_2 \uparrow$$

Oxygen reduction in acids

$$O_2 + 4H^+ + 4e \rightarrow 2H_2O$$

Oxygen reduction–neutral solutions

$$O_2 + 2H_2O + 4e \rightarrow 4OH^-$$

Metal ion reduction

$$M^{3+} + e \rightarrow M^{2+}$$

Metal deposition

$$M^{2+} + 2e \rightarrow M$$

Cell Potentials

Understanding electrochemical behavior and the possible reactions can help in predicting the possibility and extent of corrosion. A reaction will only occur if there is a negative free energy change (ΔG). For electrochemical reactions, the free energy change is calculated from:

$$\Delta G = -nFE$$

where n is the number of electrons, F is Faraday's constant, and E is the cell potential.

Therefore for a given reaction to take place, the cell potential must be positive. The cell potential is taken as the difference between the two half-cell reactions, the one at the cathode minus the one at the anode. The half-cell potential exists because of the difference in the neutral state compared to the oxidized state, such as Fe/Fe^{2+}; or, at the cathode, the difference between the neutral state and the reduced state, as in H^+/H_2. These reduction–oxidation (redox) potentials are measured relative to a standard half-cell potential.

The larger this potential difference is, the greater is the driving force for the reaction. Whether corrosion does occur, and at what rate, is dependent on other factors. For corrosion to occur, there must be a current flow and a completed circuit, which is then governed by Ohm's law: $I = E/R$. The cell potential calculated here represents the peak value for the case of two independent reactions. If the resistance were infinite, the cell potential would remain as calculated but there would be no corrosion at all. The resistance in the circuit is dependent on a number of factors, including the resistivity of the media, surface films, and the metal itself. As current begins to flow, the potentials of both half-cell reactions move slightly toward each other. This change in potential is called polarization.

Once the corrosion current has been determined, the corrosion current density can be calculated by determining the surface area. However, polarization data can be more useful than just estimating corrosion rates. The extent of polarization can help predict the type and the severity of corrosion. As polarization increases, corrosion decreases. Polarization may be preferential to either the cathodic or anodic reactions. Understanding the influence of environmental changes on polarization can offer insights to controlling corrosion. For example, in the iron–hydrochloric acid example, hydrogen gas formation at the cathode can actually slow the reaction (increased circuit resistance) by blocking the access of hydrogen ions to the cathode site. This results in cathodic polarization and lowers the current flow and corrosion rate. If oxygen is bubbled through the solution, the hydrogen will be removed more rapidly by combining to form water and the corrosion rate increases significantly. Although this is an oversimplified view of the effects of oxygen, it does indicate that the degree of polarization can be affected by changes in the environment, either natural or induced.

Polarization

There are three basic causes of polarization. They are termed activation, concentration, and potential drop. Potential drop is the change in voltage associated with effects of the environment and the circuit between the anode and cathode sites. It includes the effects of the resistivity of the media, surface films, corrosion products, etc.

Activation polarization is because of a rate-controlling step within the corrosion reaction(s) at either the cathode or anode sites. An example of this can be seen with the H^+/H_2 conversion reaction. The first step of this process, $2H^+ + 2e \rightarrow 2H$, takes place at a rapid pace. The second part of this reaction, $2H \rightarrow H_2$, occurs more slowly and can become a rate-controlling factor.

Concentration polarization is the effect resulting from the excess of a species, which impedes the corrosion process, or from the depletion of a species critical to the progression of the corrosion process.

The earlier case with an excess concentration of hydrogen gas impeding the rate of reaction is an example of concentration polarization. Although, in this case, it occurred at the cathode, it can also develop at the anode.

Measuring Polarization

Although polarization always leads to lower rates of corrosion, identifying the effects of the environment on polarization of the corrosion circuit is useful in predicting corrosion behavior. It is possible to measure the corrosion current while the corrosion potential is varied. Most often, it is the anodic polarization behavior that is useful in understanding alloy systems in various environments. Anodic polarization tests can be conducted with relatively simple equipment and the scans themselves can be done in a short period of time. They are extremely useful in studying the active–passive behavior that many materials exhibit. As the name suggests, these materials can exhibit both a highly corrosion-resistant behavior or that of a material that corrodes actively, while in the same corrodent. Metals that commonly exhibit this type of behavior include iron, titanium, aluminum, chromium, and nickel. Alloys of these materials are also subject to this type of behavior.

Active–passive behavior is dependent on the material–corrodent combination and is a function of the anodic or cathodic polarization effects, which occur in that specific combination. In most situations where active–passive behavior occurs, there is a thin layer at the metal surface that is more resistant to the environment than the underlying metal. In stainless steels, this layer is composed of various chromium and/or nickel oxides, which exhibit substantially different electrochemical characteristics than the underlying alloy. If this resistant, or passive, layer is damaged while in an aggressive environment, active corrosion of the freshly exposed surface will occur. The damage to this layer can be either mechanical or electrochemical in nature.

The behavior of iron in nitric acid underscores the importance of recognizing the nature of passivity. Iron is resistant to corrosion in nitric acid at concentrations around 70%. Once passivated under these conditions, it can also exhibit low rates of corrosion as the nitric acid is diluted. However, if this passive film is disturbed, rapid corrosion will begin and repassivation is not possible until the nitric acid concentration is raised to a sufficient level.

Anodic Polarization

Active–passive behavior is schematically represented by the anodic polarization curve shown in Fig. 5.2. Starting at the base of the plot, the curve starts out with a gradually increasing current as expected. However, at point A, there is a dramatical polarizing effect, which drops the current to a point where corrosion is essentially halted. As the potential is increased further, there is little change in current flow until the next critical stage, point B, where a breakdown of the passive film occurs, and the corrosion current again begins to rise. Even with an established anodic polarization behavior, the performance of a material can vary greatly with relatively minor changes in the corrodent. Frame 1 illustrates the case where the anodic and cathodic polarization curves intersect much as in materials with no active–passive behavior. The anode is actively corroding at a high, but predictable, rate.

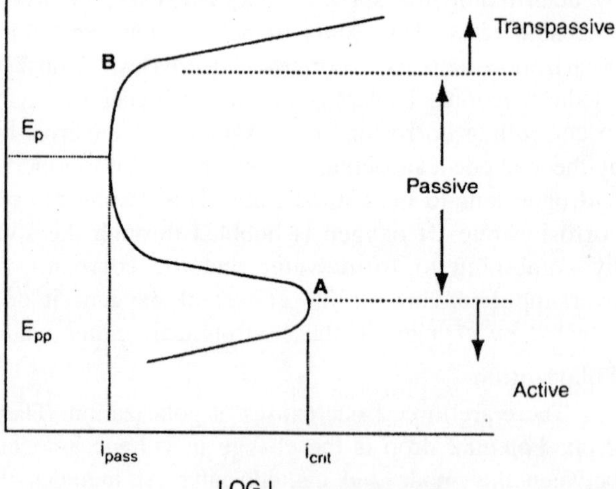

Fig. 5.2. Anodic polarization curve for a material exhibiting active-passive behavior.

Frame 2 represents the condition often found perplexing when using materials that exhibit active– passive behavior. With relatively minor changes within the system, the corrosion current could be very low as when the material is in the passive state, or very high when active corrosion begins.

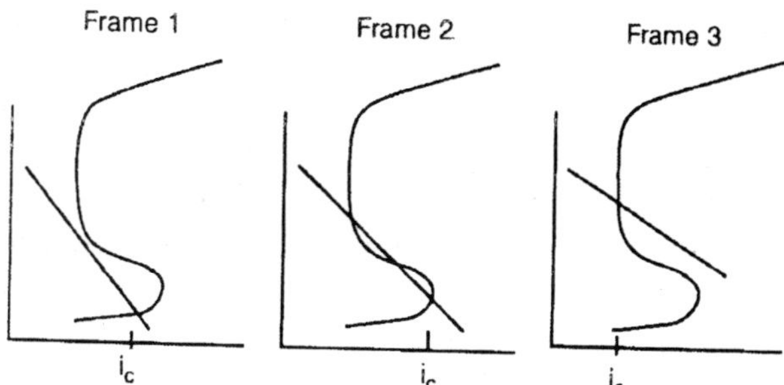

Fig. 5.3. Conditions within the corrosive environment can alter the cathodic polarization curve to create fluctuations between passive and active behavior.

Frame 3 typifies the condition sought after when using materials in the passive state. In this example, the cathodic polarization curve intersects only in the passive region, resulting in a stable and low corrosion current. This type of system can tolerate moderate upset conditions without the onset of accelerated corrosion.

Corrosion Mitigation

The basic principles outlined here can be applied to identified corrosion problems and can provide solutions or alternatives. Corrosion control in many forms and approaches is founded on these concepts.

The principle of cathodic or "sacrificial" protection is founded in the natural potential differentials between different metals. Zinc anodes are intentionally placed in electrical contact with steel structures so that, as they corrode, the steel is protected. In other systems, a current may be applied to the structure to be protected so as to cause the current to flow to an artificial anode. For similar reasons, it is desirable to build process systems out of the same materials. In systems where contact of dissimilar metals cannot be avoided, it is helpful to have the less noble material possess the largest surface area. By doing so, the corrosion current that is generated is distributed over a much greater area and slows the overall rate of penetration. In many such systems, it is also possible to electrically insulate one alloy network from the other.

Anodic protection finds its basis in the understanding of active–passive behavior. By increasing the potential of the component to be protected, it moves from an actively corroding situation to one where passivity can be induced. Such techniques can be quite cost-effective, but must be applied under well-controlled operating conditions because slight overprotection or underprotection can lead to accelerated rates of corrosion.

The types and varieties of inhibition systems are quite diverse, but also derive their fundamental logic from the principles reviewed here. Inhibitors slow corrosion by increasing polarization at either the anodic or cathodic reactions, or by increasing the electrical resistance of the media.

As an alternative to controlling the corrosion processes, the environmental conditions under which the system is operating may lend themselves to control. Temperature can have a significant influence on the corrosion process. This is not surprising because it is an electrochemical reaction and reaction rates do increase with increasing temperature. If reducing the temperature is not possible, then it may be possible to eliminate one or more corrodents present, which are not critical to the product process. Halogen ions can be particularly aggressive on many materials and are often present only as a contaminant. Careful control of the pH can also be employed in many processes. There are additional environmental influences on corrosion other than the corrodent itself.

The relative velocities between the component and the media can have a direct effect on the corrosion rate. In some instances, increasing the velocity of the corrodent over the surface of the metal will increase the corrosion rate. When concentration polarization occurs, the increased velocity of the media will disperse the concentrating species. However, with passive materials, increasing the velocity can actually result in lower corrosion rates. The surface finish of the component also has an impact on the mode and severity of the corrosion that can occur. Rough surfaces or tight crevices can facilitate the formation of concentration cells. Surface cleanliness can also be an issue with deposits or films acting as initiation sites. Biological growths can behave as deposits, or can change the underlying surface chemistry to promote corrosion.

One of the most common and cost-effective methods of preventing harmful corrosion is the selection of more corrosion-resistant materials. In addition to selecting the proper material, fabricating and finishing the equipment can have critical impact on performance. Variations within the metal surface on a microscopical level influence the corrosion process. Microstructural differences such as secondary phases or grain orientation will affect the way corrosion manifests itself. For corrosive environments where grain boundaries are attacked, the grain size of the material plays a significant role in how rapidly the material's properties deteriorate. Chemistry variations in the matrix of weld deposits are also factors that must be considered in some corrosive environments. The corrosion engineer can play a major role in system design, material selection, process or environmental control, and remediation. The focus of these efforts should not necessarily be the complete elimination or avoidance of corrosion, but rather the selection of the most cost- effective means of corrosion control and abatement.

Material Selection

The range and the availability of various types of engineering materials of construction continue to grow. As these materials improve, the benefits appear not only in terms of equipment reliability, but also processes pushed to more extreme conditions. These materials of construction can be generally classified as ferrous metals, non-ferrous metals, plastics, elastomers, and other non-metallics.

Ferrous Metals

This group of materials encompasses some of the most widely used construction materials as it includes steels and stainless steels. In pharmaceutical process applications, low-alloy steels are typically limited to structural uses and see little contact with product. Mild steels have been utilized successfully in stills, provided the oxygen content is maintained at very low levels. Tool and die steels may be used in areas where the product is dry and no corrosion is anticipated.

Steel and Stainless Steel

In areas where steels are in contact with the product or raw materials, stainless steels are often used as the workhorse. The production of stainless steel began in the early 1900s. The original efforts in this area were presumably based on the observation that chromium-plated steels parts were highly corrosion-resistant. The end result was the introduction of the ferritic *family* of stainless steels. The first documentation of the development of this class of steel began to appear in the 1920s.

Today, there are seven basic families of stainless steels with compositions that contain 11–33% chromium, 0–38% nickel, and 0–7% molybdenum as the major alloying elements. These families are:

- Ferritic
- Austenitic
- Precipitation-hardenable
- Superferritic
- Martensitic
- Duplex (ferritic–austenitic)
- Superaustenitic

Chromium is a metal that readily forms an oxide, which is transparent and happens to be extremely resistant to further degradation. As a further benefit to alloying with steel, it is less noble than iron and thus tends to form its oxide first. For exposure to mild, wet environments, the addition of about 11% chromium is sufficient to prevent "rusting" of steel components, hence the term "stainless."

Ferritic stainless steels are magnetic, have body-centered cubic atomic structures, and possess mechanical properties similar to carbon steel, although less ductile. These materials are historically known as "400" series stainless as they were identified with numbers beginning with 400 when the American Institute for Iron and Steel (AISI) had the authority to designate alloy compositions. Alloy identification is now formally handled by the Unified Numbering System (UNS), where stainless alloy identification numbers generally begin with "S" followed by a five-digit number. Ferritic stainless steels find little application in the pharmaceutical industry owing to their low level of corrosion resistance and strength. The corrosion resistance of the martensitic steels is again dependent solely on chromium, and because the carbon contents are generally higher than the ferritic alloys, they are less corrosion-resistant. Nevertheless, the combination of useful corrosion resistance in mild environments coupled with high strengths makes the martensitic stainless alloys candidates for cutting tools, molds, gears, shafts, and ball bearings.

Austenitic Stainless Steels

This family of stainless accounts for the widest usage of all the stainless steels. These materials are non-magnetic, have face-centered cubic structures, and possess mechanical properties similar to the mild steels, but with better formability. The AISI designation system identified the most common of these alloys with numbers beginning with 300 and resulted in the term 300 series stainless. Table 3 lists the chemical analyses of some standard austenitic stainless steels and compares them to a few materials from other families of materials. Once the corrosion resistance plateau in ferritic alloys of 18% chromium is reached, the addition of about 8% nickel is required to cause a transition from ferritic to austenitic. The primary benefit of this alloy addition is to achieve the austenitic structure, which, relative to the ferritics, is very tough, formable, and weldable. The added benefit, of course, is the improved corrosion resistance to mild corrodents. This includes adequate resistance to most foods, a wide range of organic chemicals, mild inorganic chemicals, and most natural environmental corrosion.

Nickel is used judiciously as an alloying element because its cost is substantially higher than chromium. However, type 304 is balanced near the austenite–ferrite boundary for another reason. Compositions similar to type 304 that are unable to form ferrite when solidifying after welding are prone to cracking during solidification and are more difficult to hot work. As a result, adding more nickel to the 18–8 composition offers little benefit from a corrosion standpoint and would be detrimental in other regards. The next major step in alloying additions comes from molybdenum. This element also provides excellent corrosion resistance in oxidizing environments, particularly in aqueous corrosion. It participates in strengthening the passive film, which forms on the stainless steel surface along with chromium and nickel. A significant benefit is realized with the addition of only about 2% molybdenum. Added directly to the 18–8 composition, the alloy would contain too much ferrite so it must be rebalanced. The resulting chemistry is roughly 16% chromium, 10% nickel, and 2% molybdenum, and is recognized as type 316 stainless.

Austenitic alloys also make use of the concept of stabilization. Stainless types 321 and 347 are versions of type 304 stabilized with titanium and niobium, respectively. These elements will preferentially combine with carbon that comes out of solid solution during weld solidification. Rather than a loss of corrosion resistance associated with formation of harmful chromium carbides, the carbides of titanium and niobium are not detrimental to corrosion resistance. The austenitic family of stainless also prompted another approach to avoiding the effects of chromium carbide precipitation. Because the amount of chromium that precipitated was proportional to the carbon content, lowering the carbon could prevent sensitization. Maintaining the carbon content to below about 0.035% vs. the usual 0.08% maximum will avoid the precipitation of harmful levels of chromium carbide. This discovery, along with improvements in melting technology, resulted in the development of the low-carbon version of many of these alloys. When first introduced, Extra Low Carbon (ELC) grades (i.e., 304L and 316L) required premiums on pricing because of higher production costs. This differential has essentially disappeared in the face of modern argon–oxygen decarburization (AOD) furnaces.

Argon–oxygen decarburization furnaces, utilized as a final refining stage in melting, are designed to permit the bubbling of the molten steel with oxygen, which facilitates the removal of carbon and sulfur. During this process, the exposed surface of the melt is protected with an inert argon atmosphere. This arrangement also permits bubbling with nitrogen gas, which will dissolve as atomic nitrogen into the steel. Nitrogen acts in a fashion similar to carbon by pinning slip planes, thus leading to higher-strength materials. Modern melting technology is also responsible for another trend in stainless metallurgy. At one time, the permissible chemistry ranges for alloying elements needed to be broad to accommodate inhomogeneity in electrical furnace melts, chemical analysis variations, and raw material quality. For example, the chromium range for type 304 was 8.0–10.0, and still heats were occasionally missed. With current technology, it is possible to maintain $\pm 3\sigma$ limits on chromium to 0.5% or better. The result is that alloys are currently being produced with 0.50–0.75% less of an alloying element than they were just 15 years ago.

Even with alloying additions such as molybdenum to improve localized corrosion resistance to halogens, the workhorse 304L and 316L alloys are susceptible to chloride SCC. This cracking mechanism manifests itself as branched, generally transgranular cracks that are so fine as to be virtually undetectable until it has progressed to catastrophical proportions. This mode of failure can occur when the austenitic alloy is under stress in the presence of halogen ions at temperatures above about 120°F. Studies by Copsen underscored the benefit of very low nickel contents, such as the ferritic stainless steels, or nickel levels in excess of about 20%. In fact, the nickel contents in these two alloys are in the range that tends to crack most quickly in chloride-bearing environments.

Duplex Stainless Steels

Stainless alloys that contain roughly equal amounts of austenite and ferrite are termed duplex stainless. This family of alloys grew out of one basic material originally identified as type 329. They are balanced to contain relatively high chromium contents, with only enough nickel and austenitizers to develop about 50% austenite. These alloys offer several useful advantages. First, their general corrosion resistance is typically slightly above that of 316L in most media. In addition, because the nickel content is held low, they offer very good resistance to chloride SCC. In combination with good corrosion resistance, duplex stainless alloys offer higher strengths than those typically found with austenitic steels. Table 4 compares some typical mechanical properties for common stainless and nickel alloys. Although more formable than the ferritic alloys, they are not as ductile as the austenitic family of alloys. Welding requires more care than with the austenitic alloys because of a greater tendency toward compositional segregation and sensitivity to weld heat input. Improper fabrication techniques can result in equipment that falls short of expectations for corrosion resistance and mechanical properties.

Superaustenitic

During the 1970s and into the 1980s, there was much attention focused on a family of stainless alloys, which came to be identified as superaustenitic. The foundation for the development of this class of materials was in the development of Carpenter no. 20 stainless, introduced in 1951. Consisting of 28% nickel and 19% chromium with additions of molybdenum and copper, this alloy was first produced as a cast material. 20Cb-3 Stainless became popular in the CPI as an intermediate step between type 316 stainless and the more highly alloyed nickel base materials. In particular, it was a cost-effective way to combat chloride SCC. Because of the high nickel content of 20Cb-3 Stainless, it received a nickel base alloy UNS designation as UNS N08020. However, because the major constituent is iron, it is truly a stainless steel. The superaustenitic term is derived from the fact this composition is so far from austenite–ferrite boundary that, unlike the 300 series stainless alloys, there is no chance of developing ferrite in this material.

The main approach to improving the pitting and crevice corrosion resistance of the basic 35% nickel, 19% chromium, and 2% molybdenum alloy was to increase the molybdenum content. Among the first of the newer alloys introduced was 904 L (UNS N08904), which boosted the molybdenum content to 4% and reduced the nickel content to 25%. The reduction in nickel content was beneficial as a cost-saving factor, with minimal loss of general corrosion resistance and sufficient resistance to chloride SCC. The next progression was to raise the molybdenum content to a higher level of 6% and to offset the tendency for the formation of sigma phase by the alloying addition of nitrogen. This concept was introduced with two alloys, 254SMO (UNS S31254) and AL-6XN (UNS N08367). The major benefit of the addition of nitrogen was the ability to produce these alloys in heavy product sections such as plate, bar, and forgings. An additional benefit was derived from alloying with nitrogen in terms of increased pitting resistance. A significant amount of work by a large body of researchers has demonstrated a relationship between pitting or crevice corrosion resistance and alloy content, which is approximated by:

$$Cr\% + 3{:}3^{*}Mo\% + 16^{*}N\%$$

where increasing values indicate increased resistance. A value in excess of approximately 33 is considered necessary for pitting and crevice resistance to ambient seawater.

Other Stainless

The precipitation-hardenable family of stainless alloys utilizes thermal treatment to intentionally precipitate phases, which cause a strengthening of the alloy. The precipitating phase is generated through an alloy addition of one or more of niobium, titanium, copper, molybdenum, or aluminum. The metallurgy is such that the material can be solution-treated (i.e., all alloying elements are in solid solution and the material is in its annealed or softest state). In this condition, the material can be machined, formed, and welded in the desired configuration. After fabrication, the unit is exposed to an elevated temperature cycle (aging), which precipitates the desired phases to cause an increase in mechanical properties.

As a class, these alloys offer high mechanical properties, although not as high as martensitic low-alloy steels, in combination with very useful corrosion resistance. On average, their general corrosion resistance is below that of type 304 stainless. The corrosion resistance of the PH 15-7 Mo and A-286 alloys approaches that of type 316. The martensitic and semi-austenitic pH grades are resistant to chloride cracking. These materials are susceptible to hydrogen embrittlement. In the pharmaceutical industry, these materials might find useful applications in valve components, bolting materials, or wear surfaces. The ability of the ferritic alloys to resist chloride SCC is one of their most useful features in terms of corrosion resistance. During the 1970s, developmental efforts were directed at producing ferritic materials that could also exhibit a high level of general and localized pitting resistance as well.

The first commercially significant alloy to meet this expectation was an alloy containing 26% chromium and 1% molybdenum. To obtain the desired corrosion resistance and acceptable fabrication characteristics, the material had to have very low interstitial element contents. To achieve these levels, the material was electron beam-refined under a vacuum, and was introduced as E-BRITE Alloy. Carbon plus nitrogen contents were maintained at levels below 0.020%.

Materials such as SEA-CURE (S43635) and 29-4C Alloy (S44735) represent the most recent developments in superferritic materials. These alloys do exhibit excellent localized corrosion resistance. Although the superferritic materials alloyed with some nickel have improved mechanical toughness and are less sensitive to contamination from interstitial elements, their availability is still limited to heat exchanger tubing with wall thicknesses below about 0.100 in. This is related to the formation of embrittling phase during cooling from annealing temperatures. Section thicknesses over these levels cannot be cooled sufficiently fast to avoid a loss of toughness.

Cast Stainless Steel

The discussion thus far has been devoted to examining the different families of stainless steel metallurgy. The alloys discussed were wrought materials (i.e., materials that are hot-worked following being cast into ingots). The practice of hot working steels improves the uniformity of their chemical, mechanical, and corrosion- resistant properties. These materials are suited for fabrication by bending and welding. Cast stainless steels can be divided into the same families as the wrought materials, except for the superferritics. Castings offer the particular advantage of being able to obtain complex shapes without extensive fabrication or machining. Cast alloys usually cost less per pound than the wrought counterpart because the hot working operations are avoided. Cast stainless steels can also have chemistry modifications to enhance properties that would otherwise render them unworkable as a wrought product. Heat-resistant cast alloys, such as HK, usually have high carbon and silicon contents, which improve elevated temperature strength considerably, but at the expense of room temperature toughness. The cast structure of such materials is also less resistant to thermal fatigue than the wrought material.

Although the compositions of the basic austenitic cast alloys are very similar to the wrought versions, the cast versions usually contain significant amounts of delta ferrite. As in the solidification of weld metal, ferrite is beneficial in reducing the tendency for the material to form cracks during solidification. The ferrite content in CF-8M can approach 20% and can readily attract a magnet. Although high ferrite contents are often not of concern, the ferrite can be attacked preferentially in some environments such as urea, nitric acid, and hydrochloric acid. The existence of significant amounts of ferrite is one form of segregation that can be encountered in cast stainless alloys. Because cooling rates are generally slow for cast components, other secondary phases can form. Chromium carbide precipitation is a particular concern for many of these materials and, under most circumstances, the casting should be solution- annealed prior to being placed in corrosive service.

Non-Ferrous Metals

Nickel Alloys

Nickel is very effective in improving the corrosion resistance of stainless steels and is also utilized as the base material for a number of specialty alloys. By definition, nickel alloys contain more nickel than any other constituent. Alloy 625 has been widely used throughout the CPI for its corrosion resistance to strong acids, including hydrochloric acid, and for its resistance to halogen attack. This material also has excellent high- temperature mechanical properties and is used in gas turbine applications. Another nickel base alloy more familiar to the pharmaceutical industry is alloy C-276. This alloy combines the general corrosion resistance advantages of nickel with the benefits of oxidation and localized corrosion resistance derived from chromium and molybdenum.

Nickel alloys are also austenitic, non-magnetic under all conditions, and possess formability similar to the austenitic stainless steels. The same welding techniques utilized for stainless alloys can be used for joining the nickel alloys.

Recent additions to the wide range of nickel alloys include materials designed to resist even more severe environments, such as hot halogenated acids, which are likely to induce crevice corrosion. Such materials include alloy 686, alloy 59, and alloy C-2000. These materials contain high levels of chromium (over 22%) and molybdenum (over 15%).

Other Non-Ferrous Materials

Other significant non-ferrous materials include copper, aluminum, and titanium, and their alloys. Copper is resistant to most neutral waters, including seawater, and to strong reducing acids. However, it is not resistant to oxidizing acids, amines, metal salts, and sulfur compounds, and is also sensitive to erosion from high velocities. Aluminum is useful in resisting atmospherical corrosion and neutral waters, but can corrode quickly in acids or bases. As such, copper and aluminum alloys are used sparingly in the CPI. Titanium offers a much broader range of corrosion resistance and its applications are similar to those of the superaustenitic stainless steels and some nickel alloys. It has good resistance to pitting and crevice corrosion. Titanium alloys offer good general corrosion resistance to a variety of oxidizing and reducing acids. Although titanium alloys can be fabricated by welding, the required procedures are best suited for shops geared for this type of work. Field fabrication and repair are possible, but do require specialized equipment and procedures.

Plastics

This is a huge general category of materials, which includes both thermoplastics and thermosetting polymers. Tabular data on the corrosion resistance of these materials in a wide range of environments are available from a variety of sources. Commonly used materials of construction in the CPI include polyvinyl chloride (PVC and CPVC), polyethylene, polypropylene, polystyrene, polycarbonate, polytetrafluoroethylene (PTFE), fiberglass composite materials, and a variety of epoxies used for coatings or adhesives. This class of materials can be a solution to handling a wide range of very aggressive chemicals, often resulting in a cost savings over more expensive metallic materials. However, some important differences between these materials and metals can limit their application. First, there is a maximum temperature limitation for these materials, which generally ranges from 120°F to 400°F. Many of these materials are limited to useful service temperatures below 200°F. Second, corrosion of these materials rarely occurs by direct material loss through a chemical reaction similar to that of metallic materials. The degradation of properties is usually the result of permeation by, or absorption of, the corrosive media. This attack can result in embrittlement, softening, blistering, crazing, swelling, dissolution, or some other loss of physical properties. Finally, the mechanical strength of this group of materials is generally lower than that of metal alloys. This can usually be accommodated through design, or with suitable exterior support structures.

Within the pharmaceutical industry, these materials are utilized for bulk acid storage at room temperature, storage of dry powders, piping of potable water, sewer lines, and wastewater treatment. The Food and Drug Administration (FDA) recognizes acceptable materials for food contact in the Code of Federal Regulations (CFR) 21 part 177.

Elastomers

Elastomers or rubbers are also available in a wide variety of chemistries starting with natural rubber and including neoprene, urethane, polyester, silicone, and fluoroelastomers. These materials are subject to the same types of degradation as the thermoplastic materials. Temperature limitations are similar, or perhaps slightly lower. The widest usage of these materials within the chemical process and pharmaceutical industries is for gasket and sealing applications, linings, flexible tubing, electrical insulation, and drive belts.

Other Non-metallics

Included in this category are materials such as concrete, chemical-resistant grouts, ceramics, and glass. These materials are highly resistant to chemical attack from most media normally encountered in the chemical process and pharmaceutical industries. In general, their usage is restricted as they tend to be brittle, have poor mechanical properties in tension, and are sensitive to thermal shock.

Chemical-resistant grouts and mortars and ceramic tile systems are very effective in providing cleanable surfaces, such as flooring and walls, and for containment. Ceramics are typically silicate-based materials, but there are also types produced from metallic oxides, nitrides, borides, and carbides. Although they generally have good corrosion resistance, they can be attacked by strong, hot alkalis and acidic fluoride media. The chemical-resistant grouts utilize inorganic binders, fillers, and a hardener. The exact formulation utilized must be based on the resistance to the environment to which it will be exposed.

Glassware and glass-lined equipment also offer excellent resistance to corrosion, similar to that of ceramic materials. In addition to the advantages of corrosion resistance, it also affords a very cleanable surface. Glass-lined vessels are used in the pharmaceutical industry for reactors, mixers, storage tanks, transfer piping, and high-purity water systems.

Equipment and Service Considerations

Welding

From an engineering standpoint, the ability to weld stainless steels with relative ease is a major advantage to their usefulness. Weld deposits, because they are cast structures, are subject to discussion regarding corrosion resistance similar to the cast materials. The chemistry of a weld deposit is likely to exhibit segregation and, depending on the alloy and the welding technique employed, may develop deleterious secondary phases in either the weld or heat-affected zone.

Two ways to address this concern have already been discussed. These involve the reduction of carbon content to low levels and the use of stabilizers to prevent chromium depletion. Either of these methods is typically used for components that are assembled in the field, because subjecting the fabricated unit to an annealing treatment is neither practical or desirable in most instances.

In many cases, a small decrease in the corrosion resistance of weldments is tolerable. When the environment is particularly severe for the alloy being used, the weld may be attacked preferentially. This condition can be exaggerated by the area effects of the more noble base metal compared to the small weld zone. An alternate approach for field welding is to select a higher alloy welding consumable so the weld deposit is more noble than the base metal. Preferential attack can also occur in the heat-affected zone of the base metal. This is typical of weldments made in standard type 304 where the carbon content will lead to chromium carbide precipitation. Of course, this condition cannot be avoided by using a different filler metal and the only remedy is a postweld anneal.

Aside from the actual weld deposit chemistry, welding techniques can have an influence on corrosion resistance. First and foremost, the area to be joined should be clean and free of dirt and grease. Carbonaceous materials will contaminate the weld deposit and will deplete chromium from the alloy. For a similar reason, carbon arc gouging or cutting should be avoided. Contamination from other metals should also be avoided. Although free iron will essentially be melted into the weld deposit unnoticed, rust can affect weldability. At best, it can lead to lack of fusion or porosity and, at worst, it may act as a preferential site for the onset of corrosion. Joint preparation should be accomplished using properly sharpened tooling, and wire brushing should be performed using stainless steel brushes.

Low-melting-point metals are of particular concern. Molten copper, zinc, or aluminum will attack the grain boundaries of austenitic alloys preferentially. Copper alloy clamps or fixtures used to hold work, whereas welding has been known to leave smears of metal that have subsequently caused cracking. Zinc from galvanized steel or paint primers has also been known to contaminate weld joints.

Full-penetration weld joints should also be made. This is a good practice from a strength and fatigue resistance standpoint, but is also a factor in avoiding corrosion. Unfused joints are sites likely to trap corrodents and corrosion products increasing the likelihood that oxygen or metal ion concentration cells are developed. This will generally mean that joints will have to be beveled if the thicknesses to be joined are in excess of 3/16 in. Beveling joints also insures that adequate filler metal will penetrate to the root in those instances where overalloying is desired.

Finally, the surface finish of the weld area should be similar to that of the base metal. Although a slightly higher roughness is usually unavoidable unless welding is followed by grinding to blend in the weld, minimizing roughness in the weld zone can be beneficial. Weld spatter should be removed by grinding. The weld slag from covered electrodes, which prevents oxidation of the metal during solidification, should be completely removed prior to making a second weld pass or placing the weld in service. Slag deposits on the surface will act as crevices in corrosive service. Removal of heat tints on the surface from bare wire or autogenous welding processes is preferred. In severe service, these areas may be attacked preferentially.

Passivation

Stainless steels offer useful resistance because they tend to exhibit passive corrosion behavior as a result of the formation of protective oxide films on the exposed surfaces. Under normal circumstances, stainless steels will readily form this protective layer immediately on exposure to oxygen. When this protective film is violated or fails to form, active corrosion can occur. Some fabrication processes can impede the reformation of this passive layer, and to insure that it is formed, stainless steels are subjected to "passivation" treatments. The most common passivation treatments involve exposing the metal to an oxidizing acid. Nitric and nitric–hydrofluoric acid mixtures comprise the predominant usage in stainless steel production. The nitric–hydrofluoric acid mixtures are more aggressive and are typically used to remove the oxide scales formed during thermal treatment. This "pickling" process provides two benefits. First, it removes the oxide scale and passivates the underlying metal surface. Second, because of its aggressive nature, the process will remove any chromium-depleted layer that may have formed as a result of the scale formation.

For passivation treatments other than scale removal following thermal treatment, less aggressive acid solutions are usually employed. The primary purpose of these treatments is to remove contaminants that may be on the component's surface and could prevent the formation of the oxide layer locally. The most common contaminant is imbedded or free iron particle from forming or machining tools. Mechanical polishing can be employed to provide a uniform surface finish and to remove these contaminants. The polishing materials should be used for stainless only as they can carry over small particulates from one part to the next. In addition, the work-hardened state of this fine particulate, even from a stainless vessel, can have a lower threshold for corrosion and act as an initiation site if not removed. A dilute (10%) solution of nitric acid is effective at removing free iron, or similar contaminants. For ferritic, martensitic, or precipitation-hardening grades, a nitric acid solution inhibited with sodium dichromate is used so as not to attack the stainless too aggressively. For the more resistant stainless alloys, phosphoric acid at 1% concentration and citric acid at 20% concentrations are also effective. Other commercially available chelating agents can be employed.

Electropolishing

Electropolishing is actually controlled corrosion, resulting in the uniform removal of the surface layer of metal. Electropolishing is not a passivation treatment, although the process does result in a passive surface. Proper electropolishing technique maintains the part in the electrochemically passive range whereas the passivated layer is only allowed to grow several atoms thick, at most. The electrolyte simultaneously promotes dissolution of this layer. The electropolishing process does remove surface impurities as is accomplished with passivation. During the cleaning and rinsing process following electropolishing, the material does passivate naturally on exposure to oxygen containing rinse water or air. No additional passivation procedure is required.

Electrolytes used for electropolishing are usually proprietary mixtures with contents that are not quantitatively revealed. Any electrolyte will typically have the ingredients to facilitate three different actions of the polishing process. These are: (1) a contaminant, which facilitates the breakdown of a passive film; (2) an oxidizer, which helps form a passivating film; and (3) a highly viscous constituent, which promotes the formation of a diffusion layer. The oxidizer and the contaminant assist in maintaining the part in a pseudo-passive state whereas the diffusion layer control is necessary to promote uniform metal loss. For electropolishing 316 L stainless, the electrolyte will often contain perchloric acid, which can provide both oxidizing power and a halide contaminant. Acetic anhydride may be used to control the diffusion layer. Stainless and higher nickel alloys might also use nitric acid, sulfuric acid, phosphoric acid, hydrogen peroxide, and methyl alcohol. Determining the ideal electrolyte ingredients is an important part of the process. Because this is an electrochemical process, other variables to be controlled include the voltage, current density, and solution temperature. Voltages that are too low can cause etching of the surface because of more rapid general corrosion; too high a voltage will result in pitting. Cathode design is important because it is imperative to distribute the current as uniformly as possible over the part's surface.

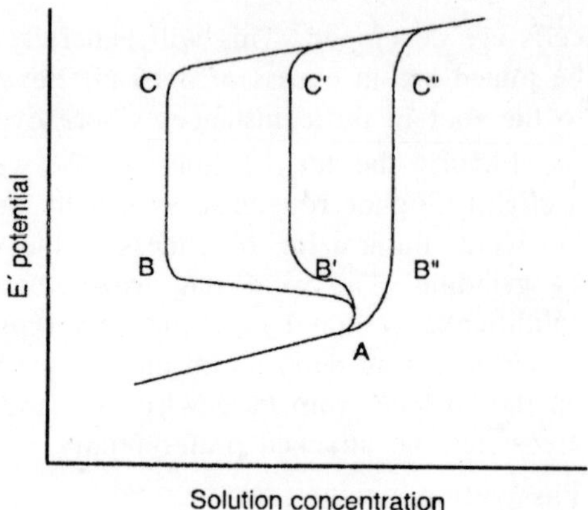

Fig. 5.4. Anodic polarization curve illustrating the unstable state created and maintained during electropolishing.

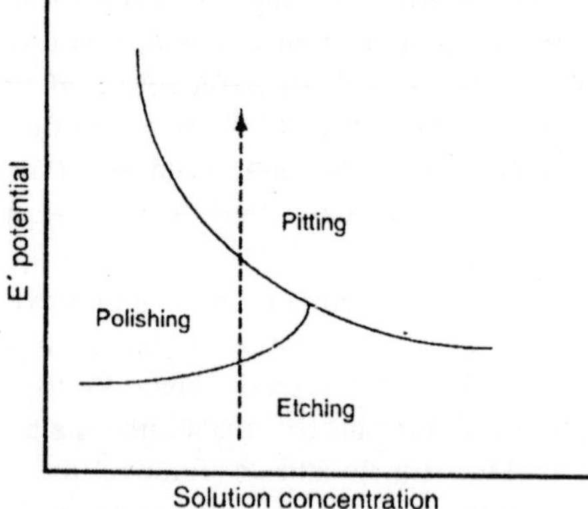

Fig. 5.5. Schematic diagram illustrating how, as electropolishing potential is increased, conditions may change from etching to polishing and, finally, to pitting.

Rouging

Rouging is a phenomenon of particular interest to the pharmaceutical industry. It is the presence of a surface layer of oxide found on stainless equipment or piping, typically handling high-purity water at temperatures above ambient. This includes stills, steam systems, purified water, and water for injection (WFI). The oxides can range in composition, degree of oxidation, color, texture, and adherence. Although generally shown to be innocuous, the mere presence of these deposits can raise concern.

The rouge itself is typically composed primarily of iron oxides or iron hydroxides, but because these are developing on stainless surfaces, they also contain oxides of chromium, nickel, and molybdenum as well. There are empirical data indicating that resistance to rouging increases with increasing Cr/Fe ratios in the passive layer, and/or the depth of the passive layer itself. Because electropolishing and passivation both increase the Cr/Fe ratio, application of these processes can increase resistance to rouging. Even with such treatments, the passive layer can break down because of the ionizing effect of high-purity water. The low oxygen content of these waters also slows the rate of repassivation and may cause the layer to linger in intermediate states of oxidation. Repeated cycles of this process result in the entrapment of various oxides in the passive layer, hence the wide variation in colors.

Removal of rouging can be accomplished mechanically, but is usually addressed by chemical cleaning. Repassivation treatments with nitric, phosphoric, citric, or other oxidizing acid solutions have been effective in removing or fully reoxidizing this layer. As with any chemical reaction, the process is time-dependent and can be influenced by temperature. For more resistant rouge patterns, reducing acids such as hydrofluoric or hydrochloric may be used in combination with a passivation treatment. The use of these acids in strong concentrations may etch the surface.

Potentiodynamic polarization studies have been conducted to measure the efficacy of passivation treatments. It has been shown that the breakdown (pitting) potential is raised by passivation or electropolishing techniques, which result in higher Cr/Fe ratios and increased depth of the passive layer. These potentials can be increased by as much as 50–100 mV over mechanically polished or pickled surfaces, and have been equated to increased resistance to rouging. Additionally, breakdown potentials of the 6% molybdenum alloy N08367 were shown to be 400 mV higher prior to enhancing passivation treatments, and another 50 mV higher following such treatments. Such studies would suggest that higher alloys such as N08367 or the C-276 type alloy are highly resistant to rouging.

This discussion provides for a fundamental understanding of corrosion and corrosion processes. It also offers an overview of both metallic and non-metallic materials utilized in the construction of pharmaceutical equipment and some of the special considerations in their application. Suppliers of materials and fabrication services are valuable resources of information and should be included in the design process. Because corrosion processes are often complex, the services of corrosion engineering professionals should be considered in the original design or performance analysis activities as part of an in-house team, or on a consulting basis.

Continuous Processing of Pharmaceuticals

In the pharmaceutical industry, production processes are traditionally based on batch-type procedures, whereas continuous processing has fewer applications. An important factor contributing to the limited introduction of continuous production is that it is especially suited for very-high-volume production capacities, whereas batch manufacturing allows more flexibility when smaller volumes of different products have to be manufactured (the most common situation for a pharmaceutical production site).

The batch concept offers the advantage that a well- defined and limited amount of product is being processed (characterized by the batch number) and, as a finished product, the entire batch can be accepted or rejected. In the case of a continuous production process, batch definition is less obvious and one has to look for an acceptable compromise related to this definition (e.g., the amount of product manufactured within a certain period).

Another major drawback of continuous production is related to the quality assurance of the manufactured goods, more specifically to the documentation of the production run: documentation of a continuous process emphasizes process control, whereas a batch process emphasizes recording. Therefore the recent advances of "process analytical techniques" (PATs) are of great importance for the further implementation of continuous production in the pharmaceutical industry.

However, despite its drawbacks, the implementation of a continuous process should definitely be considered by process engineers as there are some distinct advantages compared with batch processing: reduced capital investment, space saving, reduction of labor costs, ease of automation, and ease of scaling-up. Especially the reduction of scaling-up time is a major advantage as the production volume can be increased by simply extending the time the process is run.

To introduce successfully a continuous process, several factors are of major importance: it requires a robust process able to compensate for raw material variability; at steady-state conditions, a product of constant quality must be produced; the process should reach steady state quickly, allowing to process limited amounts of materials (during development and scaling-up) as well as to do full-scale production on the same equipment. Finally, it should be mentioned that the combination of continuous manufacturing and automation should make 24-hr "lights-out" operations possible.

Continuous Production of Solid Dosage Forms

Traditionally, the manufacturers of tablets and capsules have relied on individual unit operations as, very often, equipment was installed without attention being paid to the links between the different process steps. Recently, because of increasing labor costs and reduction on profit margins, facility design and production process had to be adapted using an integrated approach—with safety, reproducibility, improvement of productivity, and quality nowadays being the principal benefits of a well-designed automated facility. Automation and (semi) continuous production are only possible if large production capacities per drug are required, or if the company is operating on a campaign basis. A typical example is the Merck facility in Elkton. Raw materials are loaded into product holding hoppers on the third floor. This loading step is performed by operators and it is the only time throughout the manufacturing process that personnel are required to handle the materials. From this point, material flow is computer-controlled and accomplished by gravity or by pneumatic, belt, or bucket conveying systems. All hoppers are equipped with load cells to monitor and control the flow of materials through the process and to provide the information needed for mass balance and accountability.

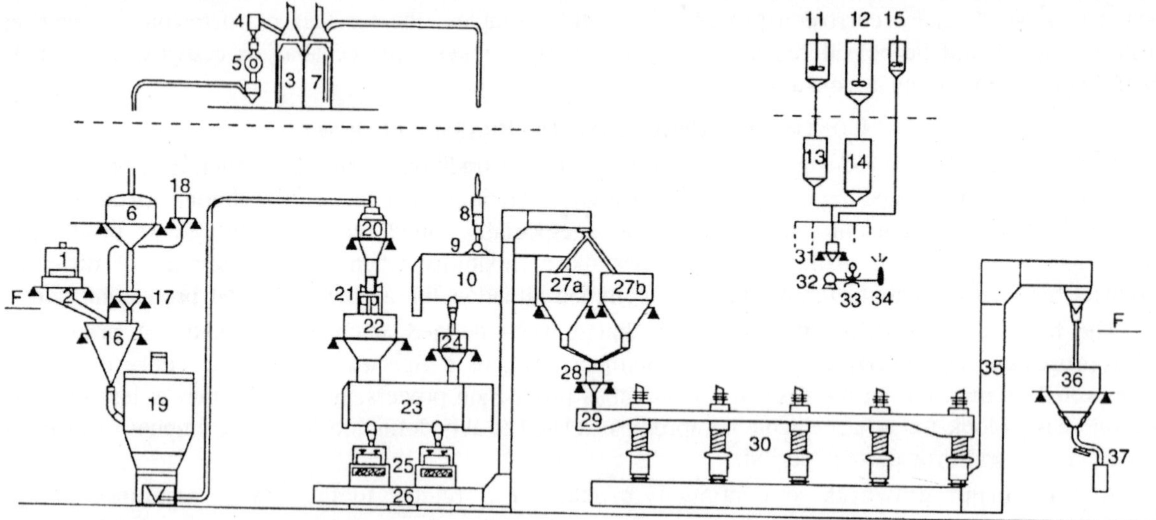

Fig. 5.6. Flow diagram of the continuous production line of Merck.

The ingredients are discharged in the proper weight proportions onto a ribbon blender located on the second floor. After mixing, the material is fed to the granulator by a weight belt feeder, which continuously weighs the material on a given length of belt and adjusts the speed of that belt to ensure that the material is fed to the granulator at a constant flow rate. The granulator is a "zigzag" blender and was selected because it can be incorporated in a continuous flow process. The zigzag blender continuously rotates to provide for complete blending of the powders and granulation solution (continuously sprayed onto the powder bed) and to transport the material through the granulator. After granulation, the material is discharged in a continuous throughput fluid bed dryer and followed by lubrication, compression, and film coating. The total throughput of granulation is about 5000 kg/16 hr day. Obviously, the film coating step is a batch process.

However, recently efforts have been made to develop a continuous coating system. The Böhle concept, although basically a batch-based granulation/ compression process, incorporates a continuous coating system with two independent coating drums connected to each other. Half of the coating solution is sprayed on the tablets in the first drum. Next, the cores are automatically transferred into the second drum, where the coating process is completed. After coating, the tablets are discharged from the coater through the discharge valve onto a conveying belt, which shuttles the tablets into a container feeding the automatic packaging line. It is claimed that a continuous coating procedure is possible as all tablets—without exception—are transferred from the first into the second drum, and from the second drum onto the belt. Hence, it is possible to combine the packaging machine directly with the coater in a continuous process. Most continuous applications for the production of solid dosage forms are used for granulation purposes and, according to Bonde, continuous granulation equipment can be divided in two groups: continuous fluid bed granulators and continuous mechanical granulators.

Most continuous fluid bed granulators have at least five functional zones (not necessarily mechanically separated from each other): the feed zone, mixing/preheating zone, spraying zone, drying/ cooling zone, and discharge zone. The product is transported in a given direction by vibrating the fluid bed or by a directed airflow using an air distribution plate. After the process air has passed through the fluidized product layer, it is filtered through stainless steel cartridge filters, enabling clean-in-place (CIP). As the batch size of a continuous process is not well defined, Leuenberger and Betz, Junker-Burgin, and Leuenberger developed a quasi-continuous production concept. This concept, developed in cooperation between the Institute of Pharmaceutical Technology, Glatt, and Hoffmann-La Roche, is based on the "semicontinuous" production of minibatches (subunits) in a specially designed high-shear mixer/granulator, connected to a continuous multicell-fluidized bed dryer. After granulation in a high-shear mixer, the moist granules are discharged from the granulator into the first cell of the multicell-fluidized bed dryer unit through a screen to avoid any lumps. The multicell dryer consists, in general, of three cells, so designed that in the first cell, the granules are dried at a high temperature (e.g., 60° C), whereas in the last cell, ambient air temperature and humidity are used to achieve equilibrium conditions. If required, more cells can be added. It is even possible to add an additional chamber for coating the granules. The system can be described as a series of minibatches passing like parcels through the compartments of dry mixing, granulation, and drying. Using a pneumatic transport system, each subunit is collected into the final container for further processing. This approach has the advantage that, conceptually, it can be viewed as a chain of existing unit processes; thus changing a commercial product from a conventional production to this Glatt Multicell production line can be considered as a minor change. According to needs, a "just-in-time production" of the desired batch size can be implemented. Leuenberger reported that Roche was able to produce a total batch size consisting of 600 minibatches. Within the continuous mechanical granulators, one needs to mention two important techniques: extrusion (wet granulation) and roller compaction (dry granulation).

Extrusion as a continuous granulation technique has already been described by Lindberg et al. using a Baker Perkins cooker extruder for the production of an effervescent granulation. Recently, the Warner- Lambert Company filed a patent application for a continuous granulation/dryer system using a twin-screw wet granulator/chopper device used for granulating the active ingredients and additives received from the liquid and powder feeders. At the outlet of the extruder, a belt conveyor continuously transports the wet granules to a microwave dryer and, finally, as a dry granule to a size reduction mill. Schroeder and Steffens presented a continuous granulation system using a modified "Planetwalzextruder," in combination with gas injection, to adjust the porosity of the granules and to improve the tableting properties.

Keleb et al. described the suitability of continuous twin-screw extrusion for the wet granulation of α-lactose monohydrate and concluded that it was a robust process offering a suitable alternative to high- shear granulation. The same authors proposed a cold extrusion process as a continuous single-step granulation and tableting process: extrudates (Ø 9 mm) were produced using extrusion, cut into tablets (thickness, 4 mm), and finally dried.

Another continuous wet granulator is the Nica Turbine mixer and granulator (Ivarson mixer) described by Bonde and Lindberg. This granulator contains a high-speed turbine used to disperse the powder. The granulation liquid is introduced from below and, because of the rotation of the turbine, breaks up into small droplets at the edge of the plate where they instantly mix with the powder, forming agglomerates. Product residence time in the granulation chamber is very short and the capacity is up to 360 kg/hr. As a dry granulation technique, roller compaction has to be considered as a simple continuous process able to convert powder into granules. The system comprises powder hoppers, feeding screws, a roller press, a mill, and, optionally, a recycling unit. A final technique presented for the continuous production of solid dosage forms is extrusion/spheronization—a technique producing spherical agglomerates of very uniform size. The process is based on low-pressure extrusion and shaping the moist, plastic extrudate into spheres in a spheronizer. These spheres (pellets) are, in most cases, coated after drying and filled into hard gelatin capsules or compressed into tablets. The system can be operated batchwise (using one spheronizer) or semicontinuous (using two spheronizers, which are alternately loaded with moist extrudate). Continuous spheronization is possible using two spheronizers in sequence, forming a cascade system or using a spheronizer with an overflow system. In this design, the finished most spherical pellets are discharged over the rim of the spheronizer because they will travel to the top ring-shaped. The load of the spheronizer is being maintained at a constant level by continuously feeding the outlet from the extruder into the spheronizer.

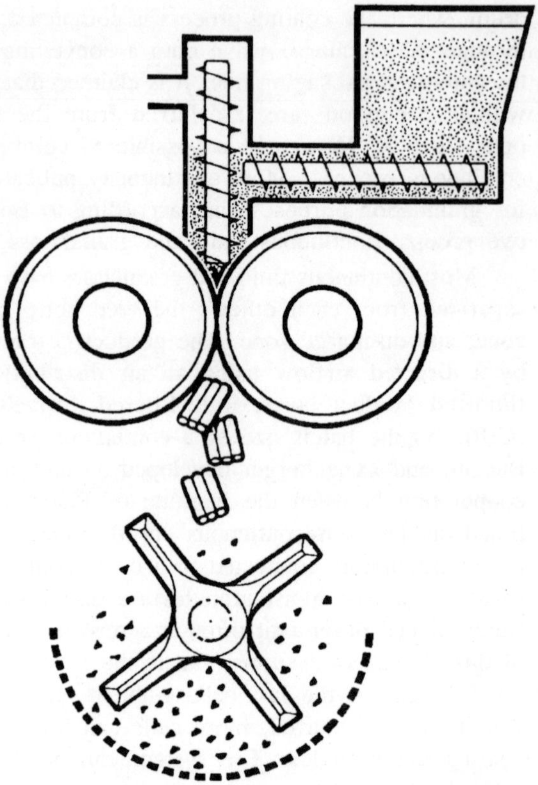

Fig. 5.7. Flow diagram of the roller compaction process.

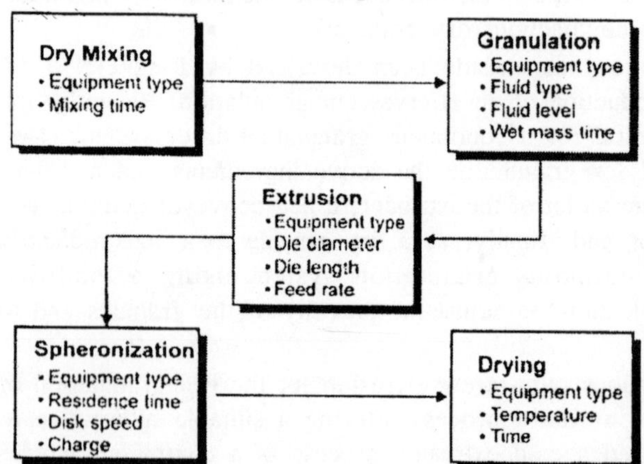

Fig. 5.8. Flow chart of the extrusion-spheronization process showing the process variables.

Continuous Production of Sterile Dosage Forms

Continuous processes offer many opportunities in this area and the increasing interest for continuous operations during sterile production has forced engineering departments and equipment builders to pay attention to specific problems (e.g., design and monitoring of input and output systems of sterile lines, leak tightness of the total system, etc.). However, how much customization and specific equipment engineering are required will be determined by the specific needs of each process and the required output.

Very often, integrated operations are used, combining the advantages of both batch and continuous processes. Therefore a parenteral production process may be broken down into discrete steps that have been grouped and linked into a larger, more efficient process. The preparation of vials (unpacking, washing, and depyrogenation) is performed in a continuous manner. Immediately thereafter, the containers are continuously transferred to the filling area. After filling, sterilization is done separately as a unique batchwise step. Finally, inspection and packaging are grouped into a continuous process, located in an area requiring less rigid environmental control.

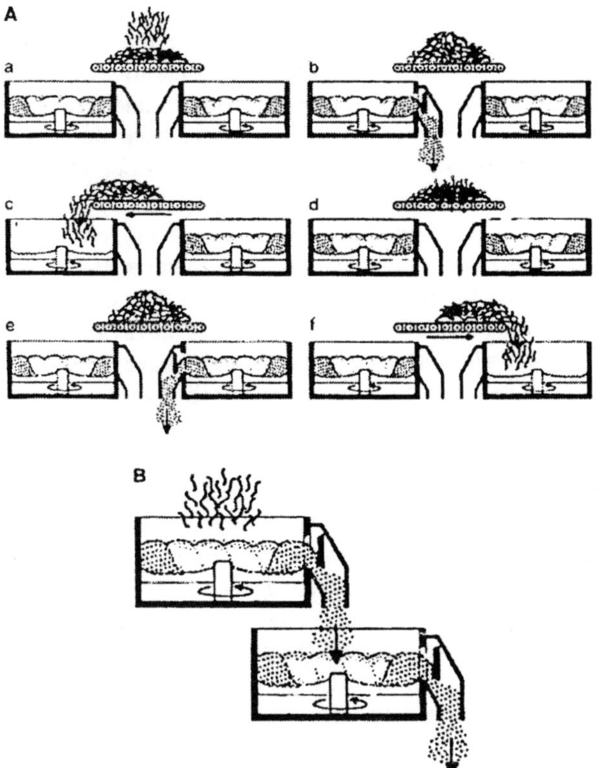

Fig. 5.9. (A) Spheronization process using two spheronizers in parallel. (B) Spheronization process using two spheronizers in sequence.

Blow–fill–seal (BFS) is today mainly used to produce pharmaceutical products and can be considered as a truly continuous process. It is an aseptic processing technique, forming in a continuous manner liquid-filled and sealed plastic containers out of molten extruded polymer granules. Because intermediate material-handling steps are eliminated, the potential for product contamination no longer exists. During the BFS process, polymer grains are continuously fed from a hopper into an extruder where the polymer is subjected to high temperature and pressure and becomes molten. It is then extruded into a mould to form the container. This container is shuttled to the filling station and, after filling, the containers are sealed. The liquid product is pumped to the BFS machine from a holding vessel and is sterilized by in-line filtration. Aseptic BFS machines are connected to clean-in-place (CIP) and steam-in-place (SIP) systems. Continuous sterilization has been used since the 1960s as part of integrated filling lines for glass containers and is becoming increasingly important, especially in the area of contract sterilization.

Continuous dry heat belt sterilization has been used for a long time in the pharmaceutical industry. In this case, glassware is loaded onto a bottle washer. After the glassware is washed and rinsed with purified water, it is placed on a moving belt that conveys the containers into a tunnel. The tunnel typically consists of a preheat zone (gradual increase of the glass temperature), a sterilization zone, and a cooling zone. Finally, the moving belt delivers the treated and cooled bottles to the filling line. The major advantages of this process are: container handling is limited to machine loading operation; after washing, the bottles are immediately processed, avoiding recontamination; and following dry heat sterilization and depyrogenization, the glass containers are sent immediately to the filling zone. Most popular are the laminar air flow (LAF) tunnels where a circulating air-stream is heated by electric elements and passed

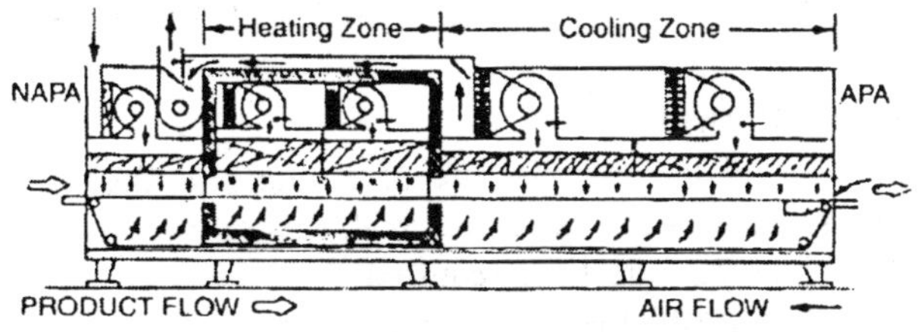

Fig. 5.10. Flow diagram of LAF continuous-belt tunnel for dry heat sterilization and depyrogenization.

through high-efficiency particulate air (HEPA) filters to minimize the risk of particle contamination. These metal frame HEPA filters and the steel mesh belt can withstand temperatures up to 400°C. Major improvements in tunnel design led to significant improvement of temperature distribution, improved heat transfer, lower processing times, and better control of particulate matter. Air temperature, air velocity sensors, belt speed recorders, heat regulation control, and temperature of cooling air are some of the common good manufacturing practice (GMP) features found on modern LAF tunnels.

Using continuous production lines, the transfer of materials into the sterile area is often challenging. When materials presterilized in a bag or container need to be introduced in the sterile interior of a barrier isolator, contamination at the outer surface of the bag or container is a concern. Therefore continuous transfer chambers using ultraviolet (UV) radiation (sterile pass-through) have been developed to facilitate the transport of presterilized components (stoppers, bags, etc.). UV radiation has been considered as it has little or no effect on material or package integrity, no residual chemicals are formed, cycle times are short, it requires minimal utilities, and the maintenance and operational costs are low. Recently, a new sterilization method was proposed using pulsed light for continuous surface sterilization. The sterilizing effect of pulsed light originates from its rich and broad UV spectrum and very high peak intensity of the light pulse. Unique bactericidal effects that are not seen when the same total energy is applied at low intensity over a longer period are obtained. This method is capable of in-line sterilization at a high throughput.

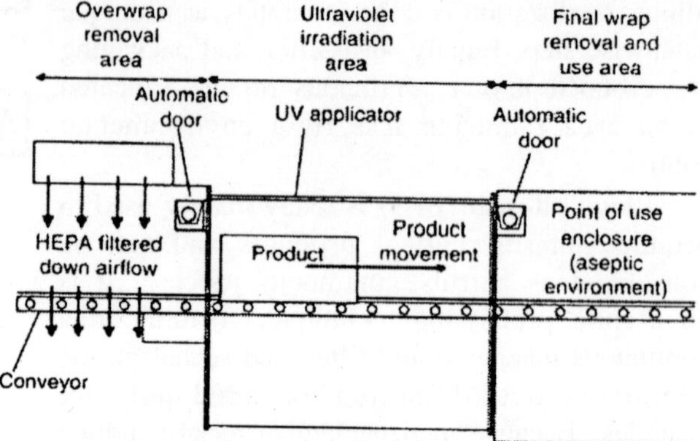

Fig. 5.11. Flow diagram of continuous transfer chamber for the production of sterile dosage forms.

In the domain of contract sterilization, continuous processing in cobalt-60 radiation facilities has proved to be economically competitive with other sterilization methods, especially in the area of medical devices and packaging. When using a continuous carrier irradiator as described by Masefield et al., the materials are loaded onto the carriers and introduced into the irradiation chamber on a timed sequence. The carriers make four passes around the source, stopping at each carrier position for a certain time before being shuttled to the next position. The throughput is a function of the radiation dose required, the density of the device, and the amount of radiation source installed. A possible alternative to radioisotope irradiators is the use of electron beam accelerators. Although having several advantages, they suffer from the limited penetration ability of electrons into the material. The development of machines generating X-rays with analogue penetration capacities of radioisotopes might, in the future, increase the role of electron beam sterilization for continuous applications.

Continuous Production of Semisolids

Continuous production of semisolids is most interesting in the manufacture of a single product in large quantities as batch productions of a large volume of semisolids are associated with several problems: very large mixers required, space required for their installation, long time required for cooling with a possible loss of homogeneity, and scaling-up or cleaning problems. On the contrary, continuous production equipment for semisolids is smaller, requiring less space, and usually produces a final product with a lower microbiological contamination.

During batch production, the individual components are weighed and separately added to the reactor, whereas in continuous production processes, the individual components are added using dosing pumps. A problem related to this procedure is that this type of dosing requires a constant volume and that small changes in temperature induce important changes in volume and, consequently, less precise dosing. The continuous production of very viscous products such as pastes remains difficult.

Although a lot of pharmaceutical production equipment is available that allows continuous processing (e.g., granulation during the production of solid dosage forms, sterilisation of vials), to date they are mainly used in batchwise production lines where only a number of steps are run continuously. Factors contributing to the limited implementation of fully continuous processes within the pharmaceutical industry (from raw materials to the packaged and labeled end product) are that the traditional concept of the batch definition has to be revised and the belief that batch processing offers more flexibility when several products are processed within the same plant. However, when developing a new production process the opportunities offered by continuous processing (ease of automation and less scale-up issues being the main advantages versus a batch process) should definitely be assessed.

6

Computers in Pharmaceutical Technology

The computer has become a very common tool in all areas of science and technology, and there seems to be no end in sight for future applications. With the proliferation of the Internet and the developments in computer technology and manufacturing, the ratio of price-to-performance of computers continues to decrease. This has resulted in the development of a number of computer applications. The field of pharmaceutical technology has also benefited from the use of computers and will continue to benefit as the professionals in the field gain more familiarity with computers. This chapter will discuss some examples of existing computer applications, the fundamentals of computer technology, and issues to be addressed when applying computers in pharmaceutical technology and assessing their future applications.

Computer Applications

Computers have been successfully utilized in pharmaceutical technology to improve productivity, collaborate with other professionals, and to provide solutions for time-consuming manual tasks. For purposes of discussion, the various computer applications are classified as follows:

1. Data and information management systems
2. Interactive voice response systems
3. Group collaboration tools
4. Document management and publishing systems
5. Internet-based applications and tools
6. Problem-solving applications
7. Communication aids
8. Laboratory automation
9. Process control
10. Computer-based training

Some computer applications are so complex that it is difficult to classify them into any one of the categories. Nevertheless, any complex computer application can be broken down into smaller parts, and each part may then be described under one of the classifications.

Data and Information Management Systems

The first computers were primarily used for computational purposes. As hardware prices dropped and computer storage technology developed, it became cost-effective to use computers for storing vast amounts of data and information in a variety of formats (e.g., text, numbers, audio, image, and video). Along with the advances in computer hardware, software development also advanced rapidly and resulted in the development of database management packages, such as Oracle, Sybase, and Microsoft Access. By using these packages, a number of computer-based systems can be developed in-house in order to organize data and information and then to query the data in a number of ways. An alternative would be to acquire commercially available systems that use these popular database packages. In either case, the challenge with these systems is to determine what type of information has to be stored in the database and how it can be retrieved in a number of ways. These systems, when designed properly and implemented with active user participation, minimize the paperwork and improve the productivity of personnel involved. Data and information management systems are usually built by the in-house data processing department or acquired from a vendor to meet the needs of users in a given organization. More often than not, the same data management system can be implemented differently in different organizations. A number of systems will be described in general terms in order to give the reader an idea of the available data management programs.

Material inventory system

This system maintains a running inventory of raw materials used in pharmaceutical manufacturing. It will be updated at regular intervals when new materials arrive, as well as when materials are drawn out. This system is useful in tracking existing inventory, lot numbers, and quantities of raw materials needed for manufacturing a product, as well as other pertinent information. Some systems also accommodate the need to reserve a certain lot of raw material for use in manufacturing a particular batch of the product to be used for a stability or clinical study.

Inventory report for GMP items

Description	Item #	Unit of measure	Lot #	Quantity
MICROCRYSTALLINE CELLULOSE NF/BP/DAB (AVICEL PH101/EMCOCEL)	Z00106	KGS	SP2359	50.00
MICROCRYSTALLINE CELLULOSE NF/BP/DAB (AVICEL PH102/EMCOCEL 90M)	Z00102	KGS	L00616	10.57
MICROCRYSTALLINE CELLULOSE NF/BP/DAB (AVICEL PH103)	Z00103	KGS	SP1029	9.70
MILLER FROCKS 5 SNAPS L CODE 1212	Z02204	CS	SP2059	1.00
MILLER FROCKS 5 SNAPS M CODE 1212	Z02205	CS	SP2060	1.00
MILLER FROCKS 5 SNAPS S CODE 1212	Z02206	CS	L00604	90.00

Fig. 6.1. Sample output from a material inventory system.

Formulation information system

This system can be used to store the information on raw materials that constitute a batch of a pharmaceutical bulk product. Typically, the lot numbers of the ingredient, the name of the ingredient, amount per dosage form, percent composition, weight of the batch, and the actual amount of each ingredient are stored in these systems. Other information, such as manufacturing summary, shipping history, and relevant storage information, is also stored. The system's greatest benefit is its different retrieval methods. For example, during product recalls, audits, or tracking an excipient problem, one might be interested in determining all the batches of products made using a particular lot of raw material. This system can also be used to archive the formulation information generated during formulation screening studies. Consequently, data collected in this fashion can be utilized for subsequent

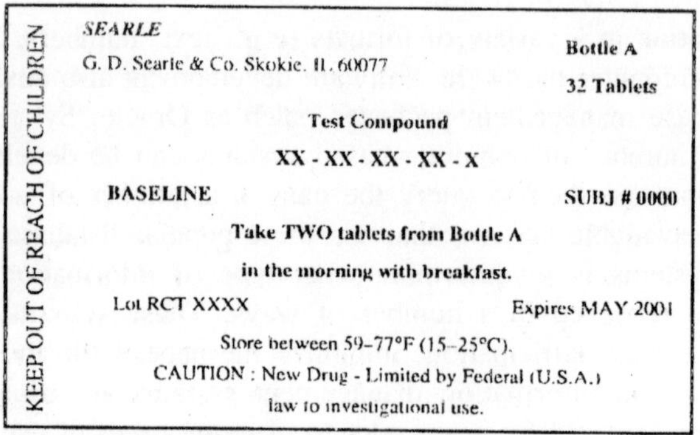

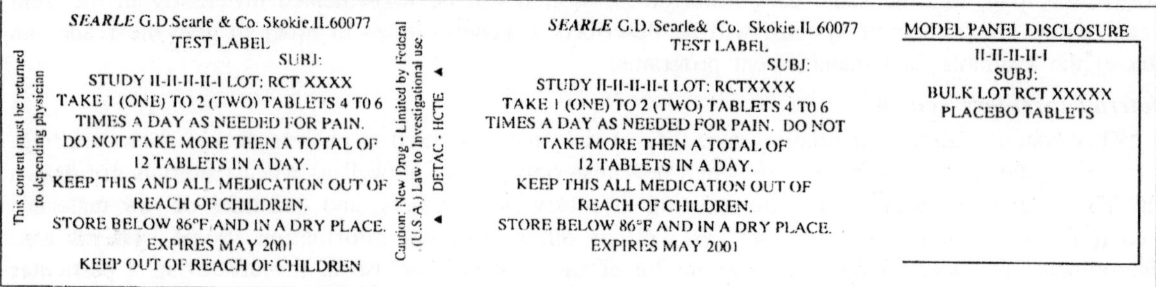

Fig. 6.2. Sample labels generated by a computer program.

statistical analysis. This system can also act as a repository of information that might be helpful in serving as a knowledge base to develop new formulations.

Clinical supplies inventory system

In pharmaceutical research and development (R&D), a number of clinical trials are conducted to determine the therapeutic effectiveness of potential new drugs and novel dosage forms of well-established drugs. In order to provide the necessary clinical supplies in a timely manner and to plan for the manufacture of needed supplies, clinical supplies inventory systems are used.

Clinical supplies labeling

The clinical pharmacy is often called upon to supply complex labeling requirements for investigational drugs used in clinical studies. Depending on the number of patients and investigators, several hundreds or even thousands of labels with randomized patient and investigator numbers are prepared. Well-designed computer programs eliminate the manual labor involved in hand-numbering each label. The computer also sorts the labels by investigators and treatment groups, and prints the labels accordingly.

Stability information systems

The pharmaceutical manufacturer conducts stability studies to develop stable dosage forms in a variety of packages and, in the process, generates vast amounts of data and information. Stability information systems are designed to organize these data and help retrieve the needed information to establish an expiration date for a product. The stability information is also submitted to the regulatory agencies, such as Food and Drug Administration (FDA), from time to time in support of investigational new drug applications (INDAs), new drug applications (NDAs), new dosage forms, abbreviated new drug applications (ANDAs), biological license applications (BLAs), and product license applications. When it is time to initiate a study, the computer is used to generate the stability calendar. Using this calendar and the protocol, the list of samples for chemical, physical observations, and microbiology

STABILITY PROTOCOL FOR A TABLET DOSAGE FORM PACKAGED IN ALUMINUM FOIL POUCH
STABILITY NO.: 20000

STORAGE CONDITION	CODE	****** EVALUATION PERIOD-WEEKS ******										
		0	8	13	26	39	52	78	104	156	208	260
+5°C	C		Ct	Ct	Ct	Ct	Ct	Ct	Ct	Ct	Cn1	Cn1
25°C-60% RH CL	NH	CP		CP	CP	CP	CP	CP	CP	CP	Cn	Cn
30°C-60% RH CL	XH			CP	CP	Cn1	CP	Cn				
40°C-75% RH CL	BH		CP	CP	CP	Cn						

Abbreviations :

P - Physical Tests Ct - Control Sample Cn - Contingency Sample S - Special Instructions

Analytical Tests: E - Exploratory test (For Internal Use Only)

C: 3, 10, 11, 17, 22

Compound for Assay: COMPOUND A Impurities or Degradation Products: COMPOUND B

Dissolution: IN GASTRIC FLUID

Physical Tests:

Appearance of tablet and package. Compare to control stored at 5 deg C. Hardness

Instructions:

ICH Study. Stored locally and testing at Contract labs.

Store the following number of samples counted as 1's : c = 100 P = 10 Ct = 10 Cn = 300 Cn1 = 20

Sample Cn (contingency samples).

A1 pouches are packaged in strips of 2×4's for a total of 8 pouches. Each pouch = 1's.

(3). ASSAY (10). DISINTEGRATION (11). DISSOLUTION (17). IMPURITIES OR DEGRADATION PRODUCTS (22). MOISTURE

Fig. 6.3. A sample stability protocol generated by using a computer program

analysis of a given time period is generated. The chemical analysis results and the physical observations are stored in a database for further retrieval. The data can also be presented in a graphic form, which makes it easy to review large amounts of data in a short time. Other programs that are used to carry out statistical analysis can access the required data from the stability database.

STABILITY CALENDAR FOR THE PROTOCOL 20000

NH – 0	10 – DEC – 1999
C – 8 BH – 8	4 – FEB – 2000
C – 13 NH – 13 XH – 13 BH – 13	10 – MAR – 2000
C – 26 NH – 26 XH – 26 BH – 26	9 – JUN – 2000
C – 39 NH – 39 XH – 39 BH – 39	8 – SEP – 2000
C – 52 NH – 52 XH – 52	8 – DEC – 2000
C – 78 NH – 78 XH – 78	8 – JUN – 2001
C – 104 NH – 104	7 – DEC – 2001
C – 156 NH – 156	6 – DEC – 2002
C – 208 NH – 208	5 – DEC – 2003
C – 260 NH – 260	3 – DEC – 2004

Fig. 6.4. A sample computer-generated stability calendar.

Analytical information systems

The analytical laboratory generates vast amounts of data and information while developing analytical methods, supporting product stability studies, and aiding formulation development. The analytical laboratory needs sample management in addition to the management of data it generates. The analytical systems help by providing lists of samples to be analyzed. These are sorted by project, laboratory location, etc. The system also generates reports of analysis, cumulative analytical data, and other types of reports needed by an organization.

Quality assurance information system

Several systems are used by the quality assurance unit to help carry out quality assurance functions. One such system helps the quality assurance function track information on chemical raw materials, package components, intermediate raw materials, and finished products. The information maintained in this system usually includes a lot number assigned in-house, name of manufacturer, date sampled, and type of release and release status. Using other systems, the quality assurance function compares the physical, chemical, and biological test data generated with the specifications established on products or package components and determines whether the product is released or rejected. Production personnel can access these systems online and determine the status of the materials they have produced or determine the status of raw materials to be used in production.

Interactive Voice Response (IVR) Systems

An IVR system is a specially configured personal computer that contains unique voice software that enables a sound-based interface between a user and the system via a telephone. On the most basic level, these systems let callers exchange information with a computer over the telephone without a human intermediary. Popular applications of IVR systems include banking by phone, flight scheduling, and shipment tracking. In the last five years, IVR systems have gained acceptance in the management of clinical trials. Some of the current uses include randomization of patients, drug supply inventory management, real-time patient enrollment status, and emergency code breaking in double blind clinical trials. These systems enable the conduct of clinical trials in multiple countries by providing customized voice prompts in various languages.

Group Collaboration Tools

The exponential growth in Internet technologies has allowed companies to set up private Internets, known as Intranets, for effective sharing of information and online meetings where the participants can see each other to collaborate on projects. These tools help to archive project documentation and provide capabilities for searching information across several projects with ease. Some current uses of these tools include collaboration between geographically distributed pharmaceutical R&D and manufacturing plants on process technology data and information.

Document Management and Publishing Systems

In the last 15 years, the size of a typical new drug application has grown from thousands of pages to several hundred thousand pages. To cope with this and to help speed up the submission process, a number of software tools have been developed. These tools provide control and access to documents in a collaborative environment and help publish electronic and paper copies of submissions.

Internet-Based Applications and Tools

Easy navigation of the Internet led to the development of software applications that use web pages for data collection, analysis, browsing, and reporting. As a result, it is becoming easier to deploy software that gathers patient enrollment status information and certain types of clinical trial data. In addition, a number of search tools have been developed that query information across several hundred million pages of information currently available on the Internet. Examples of these tools include Alta Vista, Excite, and HotBot.

Project Management Systems

The successful development of a new pharmaceutical product requires careful planning of various activities and resources, as well as tracking the project's progress. A small project is not difficult to monitor manually; however, multiple projects benefit from an automated tool to support the planning process as well as the monitoring of various activities. In addition, these systems will help develop "what if" scenarios for the resources in the new projects as well as help to terminate the projects. Several project management systems currently available on the market are designed to fulfill these needs. These systems are available for all types of computers—from personal computers to mainframes.

Problem-Solving Applications

The computer is an excellent tool for statistical analysis of data and for solving mathematical problems. Commercial software packages are generally used for statistical analysis. The scientist often works with the statistician to design an experiment and determine the most appropriate statistical method to analyze the collected data. Custom-designed software or commercial software that allows tailoring is generally used to solve mathematical problems.

Spreadsheet Software

This software is available commercially for almost all types of computers and is becoming a valuable tool to solve mathematical problems. The data are entered in the form of tables, the mathematical formulae are defined, and at the push of a button the answer is obtained. The user can easily modify the formula as well as add rows or columns of data and obtain the results easily and quickly. As such, this software enables the user to determine "what-if" scenarios for the problem at hand. It also is extremely valuable in helping the pharmacist compute percent composition and the amount of each ingredient necessary for preparing different strengths of dosage forms. In addition to providing the computational ability, the software also enables the user to prepare data and information in the form of tables and plots.

Expiry Date Prediction

Expiration dating, required on the label of a drug product by good manufacturing practices (GMPs), is arrived at by analysis of data collected on samples exposed to storage conditions defined in a stability protocol. The establishment of an expiry date has evolved from "eyeballing" the time–temperature plot on graph paper and drawing an approximate regression line, to the rigorous application of physical–chemical laws and sophisticated statistical analysis using computers. Using the speed and accuracy available from the computer and expert advice from a statistician, the pharmaceutical scientist can try various statistical models to fit the data and arrive at an optimal expiration date.

Pharmacokinetics

For a number of years, computers have been successfully utilized in pharmacokinetics to: (1) fit blood-level data to the appropriate model (single, two, or multiple compartments) and to calculate model parameters, such as absorption rate constant, elimination rate constant, half-life, and volume of distribution; (2) evaluate bioavailability parameters, such as peak plasma concentration, time of peak concentrations, and area under the concentration time curve obtainable from a blood-level curve; and (3) calculate dosage regimens in patients with renal failure.

Currently, the growing trend is to make use of physiologically–based pharmacokinetic models to study the behavior of drugs in animals and extrapolate the data to humans. In this context, computers will be of immense help in developing predictive models that might assist in the scale-up of animal data to humans and predicting the concentration of drugs in human body fluids.

Microcomputers are also used to systematize, speed up formulation, simplify manufacturing processes, and reduce the number of needed bioavailability studies through simulated models and plasma level predictions. Commercially available software packages, such as WINNONLIN, SAS, and other custom- designed programs, are generally used to solve the often complex mathematical formulae encountered in pharmacokinetic research and applications.

Communication Aids

The computer has become an excellent tool for communication. It can store information entered by one user and send a signal to another user who then reads the information. When several computers are connected through a network, users of one computer can send information to other users in the network almost instantaneously. This feature makes the computer a powerful and effective communication medium for organizations with various remote locations. Examples of communication aids are discussed below.

Electronic mail

With the proliferation of the Internet, electronic mail (e-mail) has become an integral part of browsers, such as Netscape Navigator and Microsoft Internet Explorer. At times, e-mail software is also bundled into other office automation software packages, such as word processing. This e-mail software allows users to send messages to other users (with e-mail accounts) anywhere on the Internet. In addition to sending mail messages to other users, the software allows the user to file, forward, reply, delete, and print messages sent by others. Most e-mail software packages allow attachment of files that contain text, graphics, video, or audio information. Electronic mail provides almost instantaneous communication to remote users, helps improve the productivity of firms operating on a worldwide basis, and improves communication with regulatory agencies.

Distributed information management systems

A pharmaceutical company with different geographic locations often has a need to communicate between locations in order to share data and information. Using the concept of distributed data processing, the company sets up a data processing center at each location and connects these centers by networks. In this setup, common data management systems running at each site make it easy for the company to work on the same project at several sites and funnel the information back and forth. For example, a company conducting toxicology or stability studies can consolidate the information at one site and use it for generating regulatory reports or for other purposes. In addition, these systems help transfer technology developed at one site to another site and allow access to data generated from other sites.

Laboratory Automation

Many laboratory instruments available on the market today contain built-in microprocessors that process data collected on samples and display or send the answer to a computer. In addition, they may have an interface that attaches to an external computer for processing the data generated by the instrument. With regard to experiments or analyses performed frequently, it is often desirable to interface the instrument to a computer to aid in the subsequent analysis of data. Some of the commonly encountered systems following.

Chromatography systems

The computer has become a valuable tool in automating chromatographic techniques, especially high- performance liquid chromatography (HPLC). Prior to automation, strip chart recorders were used to record the analog signals from an HPLC detector, and the calculations were done manually. In automated systems, the output from an HPLC detector is digitized through an analog-to-digital (A/D) converter, the digitized information is stored in the computer, and the data is analyzed to compute the final result. The inherent disadvantages associated with a strip- chart recorder are overcome in automation because the computer enables the analytical chemist to change calculation parameters (e.g., the base line, peak start, and peak end) as needed. As a result, the number of repeat analyses to be performed is minimized. The computer, utilized as a systems controller, is especially useful in applications that require techniques such as column switching and solvent gradients.

Automated dissolution systems

The application of computers to solid dosage form dissolution allows for nearly complete automation. Analyst intervention is limited to the analysis setup. The computer executes all other steps by controlling the system devices, such as the sampling pump and the spectrophotometer generally used for analysis.

Typically, a fraction of the sample solution is pumped into a spectrophotometer flow-through cell, where its absorbance is measured. The computer uses the absorbance reading to perform calculations and reports the analysis results in a tabular or graphic format. Sampling, analysis, quantitation, data handling, and reporting are all performed by the computer according to the analysis parameters specified before each run or included in a setup table. Automation has played a key role in the development of dissolution systems, which attempt to simulate changes in pH in the gastrointestinal tract or the presence of bile salts.

Microprocessor-based balances

Microprocessor-based balances are used in the pharmaceutical industry for automating a number of routine operations. Some organizations use these balances to automate the United States Pharmacopoeia (USP) weight variation test. In this application, the printer attached to the balance prints a hard copy of the individual weights of the dosage form as well as the average and standard deviation. The balances are also used in the toxicology and pathology laboratories to weigh animals or organs and then transmit the information to a central computer for further processing.

Process Control

Computerized process-control systems are used to measure process variables through sensors at predefined intervals, make appropriate decisions, and take appropriate actions to keep the process under control. In an open-loop process-control operation, the computer records sensor readings, compares readings against standards, and notifies human operators of needed actions to regulate devices. In more complex closed- loop process-control operations, the computer records the measurements, makes the comparisons with standards, and transmits signals to the regulating devices to make the necessary changes. The automation of process control is often limited by the availability of pharmaceutical processing equipment. To date, a number of companies have succeeded in implementing the process-control applications. Two examples are automated tableting and automated freeze-drying.

Automated tableting

Instrumented tablet presses with computer interfaces allow the pharmaceutical scientist to study the mechanism of compaction and the relationship of the mechanism to tablet-compaction properties and formulations. In addition, automated systems are useful to develop compression profiles for reference purposes, to control weight of tablets during development and production, and to monitor punch wear. This automation reduces the burden on personnel faced with the requirements of quality control. Merck Sharp and Dohme's major production facility in the United Kingdom is fully computerized to manufacture a high-volume tablet product as well as multiple-tablet products.

Automated freeze-drying

Pharmaceutical or biological products that are unstable in solution form are converted to a stable solid state using the freeze-drying technique and later reconstituted prior to administration to a patient. Freeze-dryer equipment manufacturers are now upgrading their equipment with automated control systems. Typically, the automated control system has a personal computer and a programmable logic controller. The personal computer is used to initiate the process, monitor the process, maintain recipes, and archive data. The programmable logic controller is used to control the freeze-drying, sterilization, and cleaning process by means of instructions downloaded from the personal computer.

The computer is useful in avoiding long freezing times since it is possible to monitor product temperature with ease, and eliminate the need for human operator intervention during transition from one freeze-drying phase to the other. The computer also helps in process documentation and in developing cost-effective freeze-drying profiles that should be useful in scaling up a product from the pilot plant to the production area.

Regulatory Issues Affecting Use of Computers

As previously described, the use of computers and computerized systems in the pharmaceutical industry is growing at a rapid rate. Some of the systems used in the industry range in complexity from the use of personal computers for performing simple tasks (word processing, e-mail, Internet access) to the use of powerful computers in process-control applications. In addition, to help eliminate or reduce paper usage, the pharmaceutical industry has implemented a number of electronic batch record systems in drug substance and product manufacturing to keep track of process documentation.

As the regulatory authority, FDA wants the computerized systems to be validated and requires manufacturers to comply with regulations that cover electronic records and signatures. The FDA's General Principles of Validation Guideline defines validation as establishing documented evidence that provides a high degree of assurance that a specific process will consistently produce a product meeting its predetermined specifications and quality attributes. This definition applies to computer systems as well as to the processes. To date, the industry has done a good job in validating computerized systems and is beginning to address the implications of electronic records/signature rule.

Future Trends

The computer provides solutions to problems that can be defined in a language it understands. Although the computer works faster than humans, it still lacks the human qualities of intuition, insight, and experience. A great deal of effort has been expended in the development of computer languages and software tools that allow for ease in writing programs and obtaining desired solutions. In spite of this, researchers still need programmers to translate their requirements to the computer; it is probably unrealistic at this time to assume that they can do away with programmers. The challenge facing scientists today is to determine ways in which to help non-experts accomplish sophisticated tasks with computers. In this regard, Internet technologies have helped a great deal by implementing simple to use and standardized navigation techniques for accessing and interacting with information on a personal computer. Any savvy Internet user can now buy airline tickets, shop for electronic items, and search the Internet for information on diseases, product specifications, etc. This trend will continue for the foreseeable future. Human genomics is another area that is beginning to benefit from the use of computers. Researchers have just begun amazing discoveries in this particular field. As more information on the human genome is discovered, we will begin to understand human diseases at a gene level, thus allowing researchers the opportunity to discover cures for deadly diseases.

7

SCREENING TECHNOLOGY

The need for new antibiotics is driven by the recent rise in the incidence of resistance to commonly used antibiotics. The emergence of multiple-drug resistance to community-acquired infections, such as those caused by *Streptococcus pneumoniae*, is particularly alarming due to the ease of transmission. Recent reports show that methicillin-resistant *Staphylococcus aureus*, the common cause of hospital-acquired infections, has also moved into the community.

SCREENING FOR *STREPTOCOCCUS PNEUMONIAE*

An approach to combat this situation is to discover and develop novel antibiotics with new mechanisms of action. Analysis of the recent genomic data from bacteria estimates that, of the thousands of genes in any given genome, only 250-300 genes are essential for bacterial life. This minimal gene set includes approximately 25 genes whose products are inhibited by the current arsenal of antibiotics. The potential for the discovery and development of new antibiotics is staggering, since only 10% of the possible targets have been exploited.

Cell wall biosynthesis is a target of many commonly used antibiotics. The unique nature of the cell wall allows specific inhibitors of this process to be used therapeutically with few side effects. Penicillins, the most commonly used antibiotics, inhibit cell wall biosynthesis by virtue of their interaction with the enzymes responsible for cross-linking peptidoglycan. Many enzymes in the cell wall biosynthetic pathway remain unexploited, including the cytosolic ligases responsible for the synthesis of the stem peptide precursor of peptidoglycan. Four enzymes, MurC, MurD, MurE, and MurF, in this pathway carry out nonribosomal peptide synthesis and are essential for cell wall- containing bacteria.

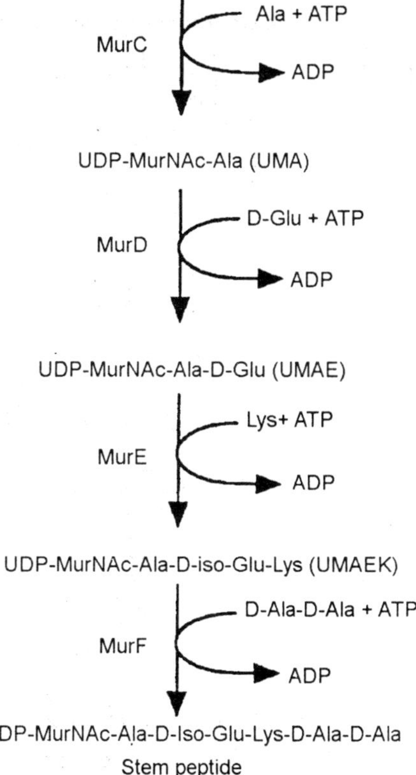

Fig. 7.1. Stem peptide biosynthetic pathway.

The MurD enzyme is a particularly attractive target for drug development since one of its substrates, D-glutamic acid, is not found in mammalian cells. The D-glutamic acid-binding site may be utilized to generate an active-site inhibitor specific for MurD. A competitive inhibitor with respect to D-glutamic acid would be expected to have less toxicity because of the absence of the D configuration in the host. With this rationale in mind, we set out to develop a high-throughput screen to search for *S. pneumoniae* MurD inhibitors.

The published assays for the Mur enzymes are not amenable to high- throughput screening. Radiolabeled substrates are commonly used to follow ligase reactions where the product is separated either by HPLC, activated- charcoal adsorption, or some other appropriate adsorbent. The separation of radiolabeled substrates from products is cumbersome and necessitates disposal of large amounts of radioactive waste from a high-throughput screen. ADP is a substrate for pyruvate kinase (PK), and the products from this reaction are substrates for lactate dehydrogenase (LDH). PK and LDH can be coupled to an ADP-generating reaction, such as the one catalyzed by MurD. The reaction progress can be monitored spectrophotometrically at 340 nm since LDH generates NAD from NADH, leading to a decrease in absorbance as ADP is produced. In spite of its attractiveness as a continuous assay, the PK/LDH coupled spectrophotometric assay suffers from low sensitivity and interference from natural products and some organic compounds.

We developed an alternative assay format using a coupled enzyme assay with MurD as the rate-limiting enzyme reaction and MurE and MurF as the coupling enzymes. The final product formed, stem peptide or UDP-MurNAc-pentapeptide, contained a pentapeptide that was found to be immunogenic, thus allowing the product to be detected in an ELISA. The rationale for using a coupled enzyme assay to generate stem peptide arose from the fact that the minimum epitope size for antibody recognition in proteins is six amino acids. We reasoned that the pentapeptide might be immunogenic, since it was close in length to the minimum of six amino acids and it contained three amino acids in the D configuration as well as an unusual isoglutamic acid linkage to lysine. We present here the results of developing a robust high-throughput MurD coupled enzyme assay with ELISA detection. The methodology presented here can be adapted to other enzyme systems to produce small-molecular-weight products that can be detected using ELISA.

Enzyme Assay Reagents

The substrate for MurD (UDP-MurNAc-L-Ala) and purified Mur enzymes were required to develop a coupled enzyme assay. None of the Mur enzymes or their substrates were available commercially, although purification procedures for the enzymes are reported as well as the enzymatic preparation of the MurD substrate, UDP-MurNAc-L-Ala (UMA). The other reagents for the coupled enzyme assay were all commercially available. Since our ultimate goal was to develop an antibacterial agent to combat *S. pneumoniae*, we cloned recombinant MurD and MurE from *S. pneumoniae*. Both enzymes contain a D-glutamic acid-binding site, the target we hoped to exploit. MurF, required as the last step in the coupling assay, was cloned from *Escherichia coli*. All enzymes were expressed and purified from *E. coli*.

Biosynthetic methods to produce the MurD substrate, UMA, are not suitable for making the large quantities required for a high-throughput screen. Methods for chemically synthesizing the substrate were therefore developed and scaled up so as to provide the multigram quantities required for the screen and its development.

Cloning of MurD, MurE, and MurF

The *mur*D and *mur*E genes from *S. pneumoniae* (*hex*) R6, as well as the *mur*F gene from *E. coli*, were amplified by PCR with primers containing convenient restriction sites for cloning into *E. coli* expression vectors. Upstream PCR primers to amplify these genes were designed around the ATG initiation codon, with *Bam*HI or *Eco*RI and *Nde*I restriction sites included for cloning purposes. These primers also contained sequences encoding a His_8 chelating peptide or purification tag, followed by a

Factor Xa cleavage site (IEGR) for removal of the His tag following purification. The downstream primers for all three genes spanned the stop codon and incorporated a *Bam*HI restriction site into the resulting fragment.

Primer pairs used for the amplification of the *S. pneumoniae mur*D gene, PS225 and PS226, were designed using the patented *mur*D gene sequence. Primers SPMUREEXP-1 and SPMUREEXP-2 used for the amplification of the *S. pneumoniae mur*E gene, were designed using the patented *mur*E gene sequence. The primer pair PS214 and PS215 was designed from the published *E. coli mur*F sequence using the ATG of the presynthetase enzyme.

Standard PCR reaction conditions were used with either *S. pneumoniae (hex)* R6 genomic DNA or genomic DNA isolated from *E. coli* K-12 as the template and AmpliTaq DNA polymerase for the enzyme. Resulting PCR products were washed, digested with *Nde*I and *Bam*HI and ligated to pET11a. Clones containing an insert of the correct size were sequenced in their entirety to verify that no errors were introduced by PCR. DNA sequencing was performed using PE-ABI Prism Dye Terminator Cycle Sequencing Ready Reaction fluorescent-based chemistry. Sequence data were collected on an ABI377 and analyzed using PE-ABI Sequence Analysis v.3.0 software. Data were edited using Sequencher v.3.0.

Expression of *E. coli* MurF and *S. pneumoniae* MurD and MurE

All proteins were expressed in *E. coli* using identical conditions. The expression plasmids were transformed into BL21DE3 cells. An isolated colony was used to inoculate 200 ml of TY broth with 100 μg/ml ampicillin. This culture was grown overnight at 30°C, with aeration. In the morning, the overnight culture was diluted 1/50 into 2 liters of fresh TY broth containing 100 μg/ml ampicillin. The culture was shifted to 37°C and the OD_{600} was monitored. At OD_{600} = 0.5–1.0, expression from the T7 promoter was induced by adding IPTG to a final concentration of 0.4 mM. After 3 hr, the cells were harvested by centrifugation at 12,000 X *g* for 10 min.

Purification of MurD, MurE, and MurF

High expression levels of soluble and active Mur enzymes in *E. coli* enabled the rapid purification of large amounts of enzyme for the high-throughput screen. Approximately 120 mg of purified Mur enzymes could be purified from each liter of expression culture.

E. coli expressing His-tagged Mur enzymes were lysed with lysozyme and sonication and the proteins purified by Ni^{2+}-IMAC. Typically, 4.0 ml (32 mg total protein) of *E. coli* supernatant was injected onto a 1.0 × 10 cm column of ToyoPearl AF-Chelate 650M equilibrated with 50 mM sodium phosphate, 1.0 M NaCl, pH 7.2 (buffer A). The column was eluted with a linear gradient of buffer A to 100% 50 mM sodium phosphate, 1.0 M NaCl, and 500mM imidazole, pH 7.2 (buffer B) over 12 column volumes. Each of the Mur enzymes eluted from the column with 35% buffer B and was pooled and dialyzed against 50 mM Tris, pH 8.1, at 4°C. The dialyzed protein was collected and stored at –20° C in 10% glycerol. MurE and MurF also contained 1 mM DTT to keep the protein reduced. All three enzymes were characterized by amino acid analysis, N-terminal sequencing, and mass spectrometry.

MurD Substrate

UDP-MurNAc-L-Ala (UMA) and UDP-MurNAc-L-Ala-D-Glu (UMAE) were synthesized as described for the stem peptide. The synthesis of UMA was conducted on a multigram scale to afford enough substrate to run a high-throughput screen or 600,000 assays.

Enzyme Assay

Since MurD was the primary target, it was made the rate-limiting step in the coupled enzyme assay and conditions were optimized for that catalytic reaction. The kinetic parameters were determined for MurD. The K_m for UMA and d-Glu guided the choice of substrate concentrations for the MurD reaction so the enzyme was optimally efficient. The kinetic parameters for the amino acid or dipeptide and tripeptide substrates for MurE and MurF were then determined under the optimal MurD conditions. We developed a sensitive HPLC assay system to follow each separate reaction and measure the amount of each intermediate in the coupled enzyme reactions. Measuring the amount of each intermediate verified that MurD was controlling the rate of product formation during the optimization of each coupled enzyme reaction. This empirical approach made efficient use of the enzymes and substrates while maintaining a kinetically robust assay for MurD.

HPLC Assay

The progression of the reaction catalyzed by MurD was monitored by HPLC. The reaction was quenched at various time points by adding an equal volume of 2% acetic acid and UMA and UMAE were separated by HPLC using a MetaChem Inertsil ODS-35 μm 4.6 × 250 mm column at a flow rate of 1.5 ml/min with detection at 263 nm. Buffer A was 50 mM NaH_2PO_4, pH 4.0, and buffer B was 9 volumes of buffer A and 1 volume of acetonitrile. The gradient used to separate all the UDP-MurNAc peptides consisted of a 3.3-min wash with 10% B after the sample was injected, followed by a 10-min gradient to 30% B, and then a sharper 13-min gradient to 90% B. The column was washed for 14 min with 90% B, followed by a 1 5-min equilibration with 10% B before injecting the next sample. UMA eluted at ~9 min, UMAE eluted at ~11 min, UDP-Mur-NAc-Ala-D-iso-Glu-Lys (UMAEK) at ~8 min, and stem peptide (UM-PP) at ~12 min. The HPLC assay was also used to assess the stability of the enzymes, substrates, and products as a function of time and storage conditions.

Optimization of the MurD Reaction

The MurD reaction conditions were optimized at 22°C with 50 μM UMA by varying the other reaction components using experimental design software by JMP. The pH and concentrations of the following components were varied within the ranges given: pH (7.0–8.8), Tris HCl (25–100 mM), $MgCl_2$ (3–50 μM), D-glutamate (50–510 μM), ATP (0.5–1.5 mM), BSA (0–100 μg/ml), and MurD (2.5–1000 ng/ml). Only $MgCl_2$, D-glutamate, and enzyme concentrations affected the reaction rate. The initial velocities (10- 20% product formation calculated by integrating both substrate and product peaks) were measured at various enzyme concentrations and found to be linear up to 5 ng!ml MurD. Initial velocity conditions were achieved with 3 ng/ml MurD for a 2-hr duration. A fixed-time assay of 2-hr duration accommodated the plate rotation times necessary for a high-throughput automated screen. The optimized conditions for the assay were 50 mM Tris, pH 7.7, 20 mM $MgCl_2$, 1.0 mM ATP, 400 μM D-glutamic acid, 50 μM UMA, 3 ng/ml

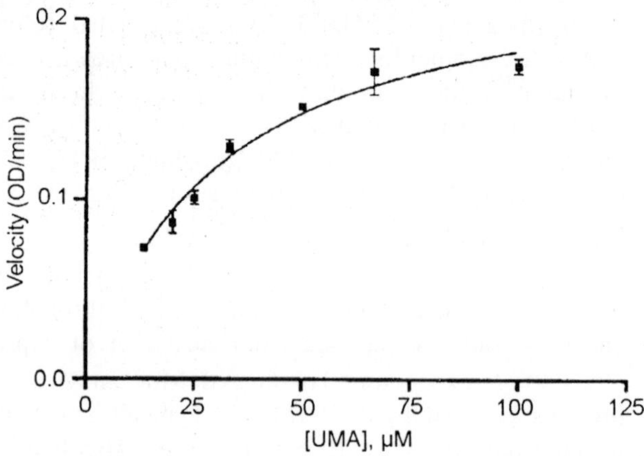

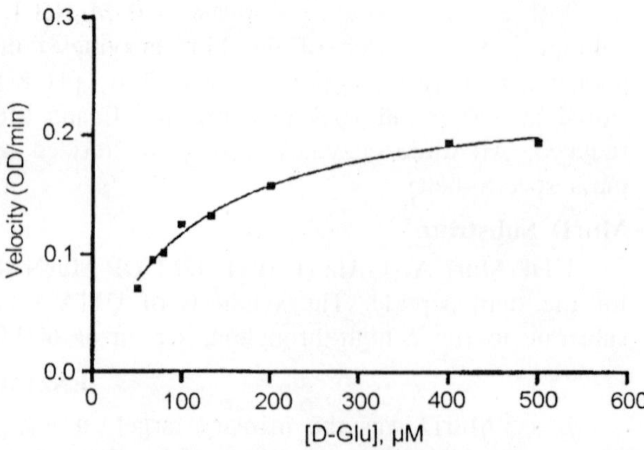

Fig. 7.2. Determination of S. pneumoniae MurD kinetic parameters.

MurD, and 100 μg/ml BSA. The HPLC system and an ADP coupling assay were used to measure the K_m of MurD for UMA and D-Glu, which were found to be 30 and 105 μM, respectively.

Coupled Enzyme Assay

The next step was to couple the MurD reaction to MurE and then MurF so as to produce stem peptide with a rate of formation dependent on MurD concentration. The reactions were followed using the HPLC system described above. MurD conditions were used to determine the saturating lysine concentration for the MurE reaction under initial velocity conditions for a 2-hr period. The presence of a reducing agent, such as DTT, was also examined, since MurE contains two cysteines, but no effect was observed on the rate of the reaction. With the optimal lysine concentration determined for the MurE reaction (2 mM), a coupled assay with MurD and MurE was then performed. The MurD conditions with 2 mM lysine were used and the MurE concentration was varied to give an initial velocity of UMAEK production equivalent to that of generating UMAE when MurD was used alone. The intermediate MurD product was absent in the HPLC, proving that MurE was in excess.

The MurF concentration required to drive the production of UM-PP, at the same initial velocities as UMAE when MurD was used alone, was determined in the presence of varied D-Ala-D-Ala concentrations, with MurD and E under the optimized conditions. The minimal D-Ala-D-Ala concentration (50 μM) required to saturate the system was chosen so as to give the same initial velocities.

The optimized MurD coupled enzyme reaction contained 50 mM Tris, pH 7.7, 20 mM $MgCl_2$, 1 mM ATP, 100 μg/ml BSA, 400 μM D-glutamic acid, 2 mM lysine, 50 μM D-Ala-D-Ala, 50 μM UMA, 3 ng/ml MurD, 15 ng/ml MurE, and 100 ng/ml MurF in 100 μL at 22°C. The reaction was started with the addition of UMA.

ELISA Detection of the Coupled Enzyme Reaction

ELISA Reagents

The first step in developing an ELISA to detect the stem peptide product of the coupled enzyme reaction was to determine if antibodies to the stem peptide could be raised in animals. Only small quantities of stem peptide could be isolated or prepared enzymatically, so we used the commercially available pentapeptide portion of the stem peptide as the hapten in the hopes of generating high-affinity antibodies that would cross-react with the stem peptide.

Pentapeptide (Ala-D-iso-Glu-Lys-D-Ala-D-Ala) was conjugated to Keyhole Limpet hemocyanin at a 220:1 ratio using glutaraldehyde and was used to immunize rabbits. A second conjugate, BSA-pentapeptide, was prepared for use in measuring the antibody titer as well as in the ELISA, so as to eliminate any cross-reactivity with anti-hemocyanin antibodies. BSA-pentapeptide was prepared in two steps by reacting BSA with glutaraldehyde followed by dialysis to remove residual glutaraldehyde. Glutaraldehyde-activated BSA was reacted with 15 equivalents of a blocked form of pentapeptide (Ala-D-iso-Glu-Lys(N-ε-OCF3)-D-Ala-D-Ala) followed by removal of the lysine-protecting group with three equivalents of LiOH in THF/water at pH 11 for 2 hr at room temperature, followed by neutralization to pH 7.0. This method ensured that pentapeptide was linked via the N-terminus, thus exposing the maximum amount of peptide for antibody recognition. The antibody produced by the rabbits was affinity purified using pentapeptide as a ligand, and then stored at 1 mg/ml in PBS with 10% glycerol and sodium azide at –20°C.

ELISA

A competitive ELISA was developed to detect stem peptide generated from the coupled enzyme reaction as well as to measure the cross-reactivity of the antibody with small peptides. BSA-pentapeptide (BSA-PP) was immobilized onto the wall of a microtiter plate. Samples or standards containing pentapeptide were then added, followed by rabbit antipentapeptide antibody. The amount of anti-

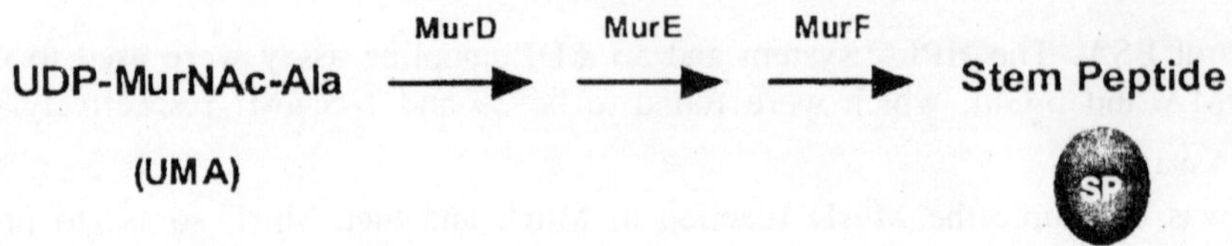

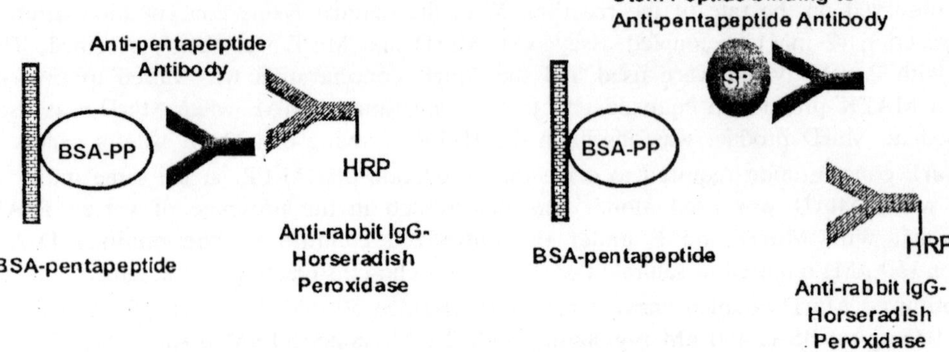

Fig. 7.3. Schematic of ELISA for stem peptide detection.

pentapeptide antibody bound to immobilized BSA-PP was visualized by adding a second anti-rabbit IgG antibody labeled with horseradish peroxidase. In the absence of free pentapeptide, maximum binding of the antibody was observed and gave a maximum OD reading after adding the peroxidase substrate. Molecules reactive with the antibody, such as stem peptide or pentapeptide fragments, bound to the anti-pentapeptide antibody and prevented it from binding to the immobilized BSA-PP, which resulted in a lower absorbance. The decrease in absorbance was proportional to the increase in the concentration of the competing species.

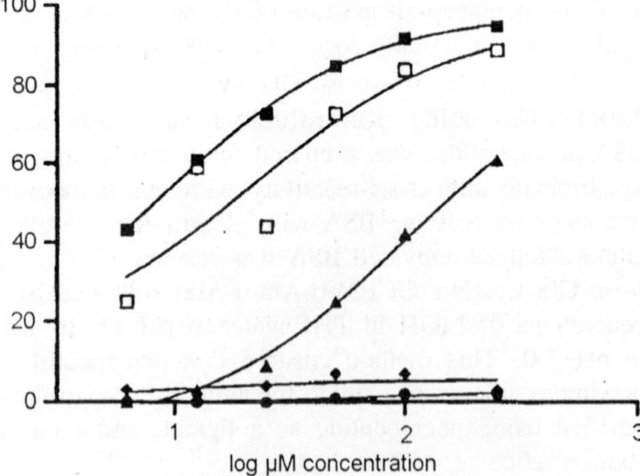

Fig. 7.4. Reactivity of the anti-pentapeptide antibody.

The results of a competitive ELISA with Ala-D-iso-Glu-Lys-D-Ala-D-Ala (pentapeptide), Lys-D-Ala-D-Ala, Ala-D-Ala-D-Ala, Ala-D-iso-Glu, Ala-D-iso-Glu-Lys, D-Ala-D-Ala, and Lys-D-Ala-D-Lac. The antibody reacted strongly with pentapeptide and Lys-D-Ala-D-Ala but weakly with Ala-D-Ala-D-Ala, suggesting that the immunogenic determinant of the pentapeptide to this antibody resides in the last three residues, Lys-D-Ala-D-Ala. The cross-reactivities of the pentapeptide and stem peptide in the competitive ELISA were virtually identical.

The MurD, E, and F coupled reaction was performed with and without enzymes and the amount of stem peptide generated was measured by HPLC and ELISA. The amount of product measured by both methods was the same.

These results validated the ELISA detection method for stem peptide. In addition, the other components of the enzyme reaction mixture were tested in the ELISA, and none cross-reacted with the antibody at concentrations used in the assay.

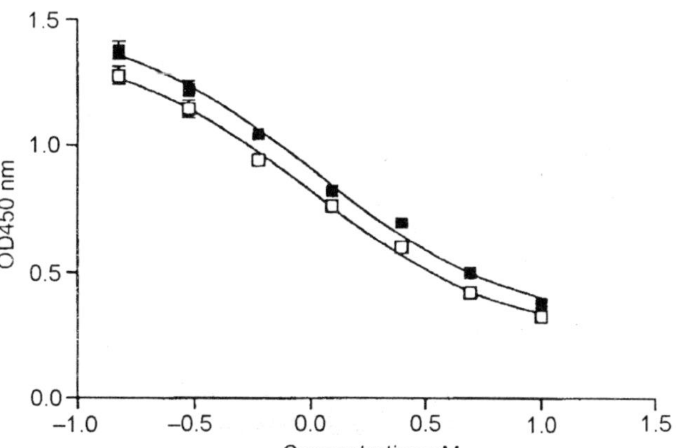

Fig. 7.5. Reactivity of the anti-pentapeptide antibody with stem peptide and pentapeptide.

High-Throughput Screen

The two-part protocol for the high-throughput screen is depicted in Figure 6. The first part involved the use of Titertek's Multidrop liquid dispenser to automate the addition of reagents for the coupled enzyme assay and quenching the reaction. Samples from the coupled enzyme assay were then transferred to a second liquid-dispensing system (MRD8) for running the ELISA to detect the product of the coupled enzyme assay. To ensure a high-quality run through the screen, stability studies were performed on the reagents and products used in the screen. Variability studies were performed using robots.

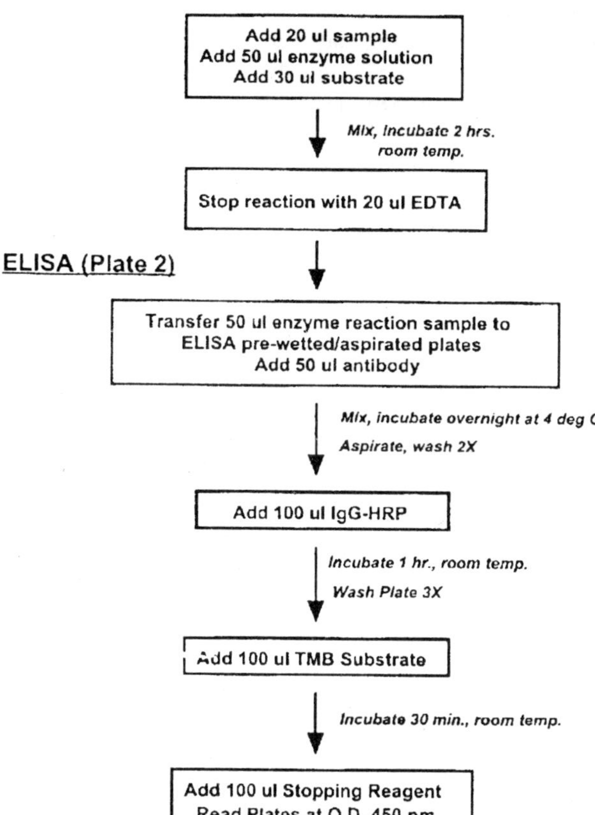

Fig. 7.6. Flow chart of the MurD ELISA-based high-throughput screen.

High-Throughput Screen

Compounds for testing were dissolved in 10% DMSO and diluted 1/20 in water to give a final stock concentration of 50 μM. A 20-μl aliquot of the compound stock was added to each well in a 96-well plate, followed by 50 μl of the enzyme solution. The reaction was started by adding 30 μl of 166.67 μM UMA to all wells. The final reaction well contained 50 mM Tris, pH 7.7, 20 mM $MgCl_2$, 1.0 mM ATP, 0.4 mM D-Glu, 2.0 mM Lys, 0.05 mM D-Ala-D-Ala, 3 ng/ml MurD, 15 ng/ml MurE, 100 ng/ml MurF, and 100 μg/ml BSA. The 96-well plates were either stacked or covered and incubated for 2 hr at room temperature. The reaction was stopped by adding 20 μl of 250 mM EDTA followed by mixing.

A 50-μl aliquot of the reaction was transferred to the ELISA plate, which had been prepared earlier using the following protocol. Each well of a plate (# 3590, Costar) was coated with 100 μl of 250 ng/ml BSA-pentapeptide in PBS overnight at 4°C. The plates were then washed three times with PBS-0.05% Tween 20 using 120 μl/well. The plates were blocked with 120 μl/well of Pierce Superblock for 3 hr at room temperature and then aspirated and dried in a vacuum oven at room temperature for 3 hr. The plates were stored in plastic bags containing desiccant at 4°C. Plates were soaked with 120 μl/well of PBS-0.05% Tween 20, 1% BSA in 0.02% Thimerosal, and then aspirated before use.

After adding the quenched enzyme reaction sample to the ELISA plate, 50 μl of a 25-ng/ml solution of affinity-purified pentapeptide antibody was added to each well, and the plates were allowed to incubate overnight at 4°C. Liquid was aspirated from the wells, followed by two 120-μl washes with PBS-0.05% Tween 20. After washing, each well received 100 μl of anti-rabbit IgG conjugated with horseradish peroxidase at a dilution, usually 1/10,000, sufficient to give an OD reading between 1.5 and 2.0 on plates reacted with antibody alone. The second antibody was incubated on the plate for 1 hr, washed three times with 120 μl of PBS-0.05% Tween 20, followed by TMB (3,3′,5,5′-tetramethylbenzidine) peroxidase substrate addition (100 μl of a 1:1 solution of TMB and peroxidase according to the protocol of Kirkegaard & Perry). After a 30-min incubation, 100 μl of 1 M phosphoric acid was added to stop the peroxidase reaction. The plates were read at 450 nm.

Reagent and Product Stability Studies

Stability studies on all the enzyme reaction components showed that the reagents were stable over an 8-hr period at room temperature and for months when stored at –20°C. Since the stem peptide enzyme reaction was performed one day and the ELISA the following day, the stability of the stem peptide product was measured using both HPLC and ELISA. There was no detectable change in the amount of stem peptide when measured immediately or when the enzyme reaction was stored overnight at 4°C. The anti-rabbit IgG-HRP conjugate, purchased from American Qualex, showed some instability after a week of using material from an opened vial. To circumvent this stability issue, a new vial was used each week after titering it to an OD of 1.5–2.0. The antibody was stable, as measured by its reactivity to pentapeptide, for at least 5 months when stored at 4°C in PBS with 0.02% sodium azide.

The effect of solvents such as DMSO, ethanol, and methanol, on the MurD coupled enzyme reaction and the ELISA was studied. The MurD enzyme reaction was run in the presence and absence of Mur enzymes to generate minimum and maximum signals. Final solvent concentrations up to 2% had no effect on the reaction when measured by either HPLC or in the ELISA.

Performance Validation

Multidrop liquid dispensers were used to add the enzyme solution to the compound plate, followed by the substrate, UMA, to start the reaction. The reaction was stopped by adding EDTA using Titertek's Multidrop liquid dispenser. The ELISA was automated using an eight- head MRD8. The instrument is designed specifically for ELISAs and allows washes, additions, and programmed timing of the various steps. Both the MRD8 and the Multidrop were calibrated each day prior to running the assay. This was done by dispensing 100 μl of wash containing a yellow dye and reading at 450 nm. If the coefficient of variation on either instrument was greater than 1.5%, then the instrument was calibrated and the validation repeated.

A two-plate, 3-day study was performed to measure the inter- and intraplate variation at the minimum, maximum, and 50% signals. The minimum signal was generated by letting the enzyme reaction proceed without inhibition so as to produce free stem peptide, which would compete with immobilized BSA-PP for antibody binding. The maximum signal was produced by omitting the enzymes from the MurD reaction so no stem peptide was produced, so as to give maximum antibody binding to immobilized BSA-PP. The 50% signal was made by adding 20 μl/well of 3 μM pentapeptide in the absence of Mur enzymes, to provide enough competing peptide to decrease antibody binding to the plate. Each plate had CVs of less than 5% with one or two exceptions where a plate contained a single high-value outlier. The CVs for the same signal on all plates on a single day were less than 10%, with the higher values arising from the outliers. The CVs for the means over the 3-day period were 10.05% for the minimum signal, 7.78% for the middle signal, and 4.45% for the maximum signal, which satisfied the criteria of less than 20% variation between days. No significant edge effects or drifts in signal across the plate were observed.

Evaluation of MurD Inhibitors

Hits from the screen were used to select related compounds for further testing from the Lilly collection of compounds. The HPLC assay was used to measure MurD inhibition and standard antimicrobial assays were carried out with *S. pneumoniae*, *Haemophilus influenzae* 76, *Staphylococcus aureus* 027, and *Moraxella catarrhalis* BC-1. A series of indole and phenoxypropyl amine derivatives with activity against MurD, were discovered that exhibited broad- spectrum antibacterial activity.

A high-throughput screen for *S. pneumoniae* MurD was developed that did not require radioactivity. The high expression levels of soluble active Mur enzymes in *E. coli* allowed large quantities of enzymes to be purified rapidly. The chemical synthesis of multigram quantities of the MurD substrate made the development and implementation of the screen possible. Assay conditions were optimized for the detection of MurD inhibitors, and the optimized assay was validated in high- throughput format. Stem peptide produced in the assay was dependent on MurD activity because MurE and MurF were present in excess. The immunogenicity of the pentapeptide portion of stem peptide allowed the stem peptide product of the coupled enzyme reaction to be detected using a competitive ELISA. A high-throughput screen employing this assay was used to screen a large library of compounds and natural products. The screen was reproducible and efficiently identified inhibitors of MurD. Inhibitors were verified with the HPLC assay and then tested for antibacterial activity with *S. pneumoniae*. Many of the inhibitors identified by the screen also exhibited antibacterial activity.

Screening for Parasiticides

Therapeutic Challenges of Parasites

All animals and plants are plagued by parasites. Although it is not commonly appreciated, more animal species can be called "*parasite*" than any other classification. Pathogens targeted for control are found in multiple protozoan, helminth, and insect phyla. This extraordinary diversity complicates antiparasitic chemotherapy, in which breadth of spectrum is a key attribute. The demand for broad spectrum provides one of the most difficult challenges for the discovery of commercially viable antiparasitic drugs. The challenge is made more difficult by the fact that parasites inhabit virtually every tissue of the host, requiring delivery of antiparasitic drugs to multiple target compartments. Evolution of resistance to these drugs by parasites is the rule rather than the exception and obviously makes matters worse. Resistance has been used to justify the search for new drugs and for nonchemotherapeutic methods of control. In agriculture, control of nematode and arthropod pests poses huge challenges, including resistance and environmental concerns

Although parasites are among the most prevalent pathogens of humans and their domesticated animals, relatively little attention is paid to them in either basic research or drug discovery programs. Reasons for this unfortunate status can be summarized as follows.

1. Human parasitoses occur primarily among the poor; there is little incentive for wealthy governments (which support most research) or pharmaceutical industries (which prosper by selling drugs at a profit) to invest in diseases of the poor. Although the enormous rise in opportunistic protozoal infections in AIDS patients stimulated research on parasites such as *Toxoplasma gondii* and *Cryptosporidium parvum*, the remarkable success of combination antiviral chemotherapy subsequently

Table 7.1. Examples of insect parasites

Order	*Examples*
	Phylum Arthropoda
Phthiraptera	Chewing and sucking lice
Hemiptera	Whiteflies, cinch bugs (plant pests)
Heteroptera	Kissing bugs (reduviids), bedbugs
Siphonoptera	Fleas
Diptera	Mosquitoes, biting flies
Arachnida	Ticks, mites

reduced the incidence of these infections. Not surprisingly, the impetus to discover new antiprotozoal compounds lessened. Recent efforts to stimulate public and private investment in malaria research involve a very small fraction of the funds devoted to other (Western) diseases, despite the fact that *Plasmodium falciparum* causes $>10^6$ deaths/year.

2. Helminth infections of humans are rarely immediately life-threatening. Competing health care demands in poor countries, including basic nutrition, sanitation, HIV infection and tuberculosis, dwarf the demand for better control of worms.
3. Veterinary diseases attract little government support for research. Animal health applications are typically cost-constrained by the economics of animal production. Consequently, the profit found in veterinary products is usually lower than in human pharmaceuticals, which draws industrial research investment away from animal health, including parasitology.

Current Status of Antiparasitic Drug Discovery

The relatively primitive condition of parasitology research threatens the survival of antiparasitic drug discovery in the continually evolving screening strategies of the pharmaceutical industry. All available antiparasitic drugs were initially discovered in screens that employed whole organisms, both target and host, in protocols pioneered by Ehrlich and perfected during the second era of discovery. Subsequent developments, including the paradigm known as drug design (era 3), required increasingly intensive investment in personnel training and equipment as well as in-depth knowledge of the target. Parasites compete poorly in terms of return on investment and state-of-the-art target knowledge.

Table 7.2. Eras of drug discovery

1. *Gleaning* from herbal medicine: the genesis of pharmacology (digitalis; salicylic acid—aspirin; morphine; quinine; artemisinin; reserpine; taxol). Ancient history–present.
2. *Screening* in whole animals or against whole organisms or cells in culture (Trypan red; arsphenamine; prontosil and sulfa drugs; penicillin and all other antibiotic classes; almost all antiparasitic drugs; most anticancer, antiviral, and antifungal agents). 1910–present.
3. *Drug design*, based on crystal structures of target incorporated with substrate or inhibitor (primarily for enzymes). More useful for lead optimization than for primary discovery. Can be configured to serve as electronic ("virtual") random screen. 1980s–present.
4. *Mechanism-based, high-throughput random screening*, utilizing isolated proteins (enzymes, receptors), cloned regulatory domains, or recombinant cells. Trend toward miniaturization and increasing throughput and automation. Mid-1980s–present.

The fourth era of discovery has seen a return to the paradigm of random screening that provided antiparasitic drugs in the preceding 80 years or so. However, instead of using whole animals, tissues, or cells, the new approach focuses on the discovery of compounds that interact specifically with a defined target. The development of a plethora of elegant systems for rapidly screening hundreds of thousands of compounds has revolutionized drug discovery in all therapeutic areas. Unfortunately, these systems are expensive to implement and operate and are typically located in a core facility of a company. Highly trained personnel are needed to design, implement, and run the screens.

Different formats are required for different targets, so a considerable investment may be required before screening can begin. Consequently, access to the screening facility and the associated expertise is limited by the perceived quality of the drug target and by the size of the market for which the drug is targeted. Parasitological drug targets are often difficult to validate (due to the scarcity of research), and animal health is not very competitive in terms of market size. Since it is not generally possible to routinely obtain large amounts of parasite tissue for target purification to support high-throughput screening (HTS), recombinant systems are absolutely required. Additional up-front investment is required to fit parasite targets into systems that can process tens of thousands of samples per week. Facing a future in which antiparasitic drug discovery could become extinct in the pharmaceutical industry, we sought to develop an alternative platform for parasiticide screening that would enable the field to keep pace with changing technology.

Basis for the Use of Recombinant Microbes in HTS

First Screen Employed Microbes

The onset of the second era of discovery can be traced to the decision by Ehrlich to screen a collection of industrial dyes for activity in mice infected with trypanosomes; the first screen was thus a search for an antiparasitic drug. This research eventually led to the discovery of arsenical treponemacides and then to the sulfa antibiotics, the first of which was Prontosil, based on industrial dyes. Later, recognition of the antibiotic activity of penicillin led to the widespread adoption of whole-bacteria screens to test both natural products and synthetic compounds for antibiotic activity. Consequently, the first HTS technology was based on simple assays of bacterial viability. The extension of this paradigm to other pathogens became the standard. It is worth noting that all antiparasitic drugs were either isolated from herbal remedies or discovered in relatively simple *in vivo* or *in vitro* screens.

Microbial Screens for Nonantibiotic Discovery

Further development of microbial-based screening platforms for nonantibiotic discovery programs was exemplified by the work of Hitchings and Elion. Focusing initially on the discovery of compounds that interrupted specific steps in purine metabolism, they developed a screening system based simply on the survival of *Lactobacillus casei*. Initial screening was done in medium that lacked purines. Compounds that inhibited growth of *L. casei* under this condition were retested in medium containing purines or purine precursors to determine if any could reverse the toxicity. Observation of reversal with a particular supplement pinpointed the site of inhibition. This represents perhaps the first example of what we have termed a *nutrient-dependent viability screen*. The approach was extended to screens for inhibitors of folate metabolism using *Enterococcusfaecium*, among many other examples, primarily by Japanese workers.

The key conceptual development in the paradigm established by Hitchings and Elion is that screens based on bacterial viability can discover compounds for nonantibiotic indications; their purine antimetabolites found clinical employment as anticancer drugs and immunosuppressive and antiviral agents. However, in this case, the drug targets were bacterial enzymes, which bear an unknown resemblance to the homologous enzyme in the target species. The extension of nutrient-dependent viability screening to specifically constructed recombinant microorganisms represents the next logical evolution of the paradigm. The principle of complementation of a bacterial mutation by functional expression of a homologous enzyme has been well established for many microorganisms. It is possible to construct a system in which viability of the recombinant microbe is dependent on the function of the foreign (drug target) protein under specific nutritional conditions.

Antiparasitic Drug Discovery Using Recombinant Microbes

Screens employing Escherichia coli

A screen using multiple complemented strains. An initial approach toward the use of recombinant microorganisms for antiparasitic drug discovery is found in the example of a key enzyme in glycolysis in the parasitic protozoan *Trypanosoma brucei*. A *T. brucei* gene encoding 6-phosphogluconate dehydrogenase (6-PGD) was cloned by complementation of a strain of *Escherichia coli* in which the homologous gene had been inactivated by mutation. The mutant could not utilize glucose as a sole carbon source, a trait that was reversed by expression of the parasite enzyme. A screen for inhibitors of parasite 6-PGD was proposed in which compounds would be screened for activity against the recombinant bacterial strain in the presence of glucose as the sole carbon source. Specificity of inhibition could be determined by testing active compounds against either wild-type bacteria or against the mutant complemented with the homologous human gene.

Nutrient-dependent viability screens for antiparasitic drugs. The approach proposed for 6-PGD relies on species-dependent differences in potency to identify active compounds. However, as a primary screen, it is often preferable to identify specific enzyme inhibitors that can be refined to achieve selectivity through medicinal chemistry. Thus, the recombinant microbe paradigm was further refined by the addition of nutrient-dependent viability as a screening variable. Practical application of this principle was first demonstrated by development of a screen for inhibitors of the rate-limiting step in glycolysis, phosphofructokinase (PFK), from the parasitic nematode *Haemonchus contortus*. A very similar strategy was simultaneously developed for another nematode enzyme that plays a crucial role in energy generation, phosphoenolpyruvate carboxykinase.

A strain of *E. coli* that carries mutations in the two loci that encode PFK (*pfk A*, *pfk B*) was used to clone by complementation a cDNA encoding PFK from *H. contortus*. The parent strain is unable to grow on media in which a hexose (conveniently, mannitol) is the sole carbon source. The transformed, complemented strain expresses fairly high levels of PFK enzyme activity compared to wild-type *E. coli*, and grows well (but slightly slower than wild-type *E. coli*) on mannitol (doubling times 1.5 versus 1.1 hr). To be consistent with modern screening formats and automated pipetting platforms, we configured a 96-well microtiter plate screen using the complemented strain of *E. coli*. Each well received an aliquot of minimal medium + mannitol and an inoculum of the complemented strain that provided linear growth for at least 24 hr. After overnight growth at 37°C, an aliquot of a solution of a viability dye, Alamar blue, was added to each well. Alamar blue is a redox-sensitive dye that has been widely used in viability assays for

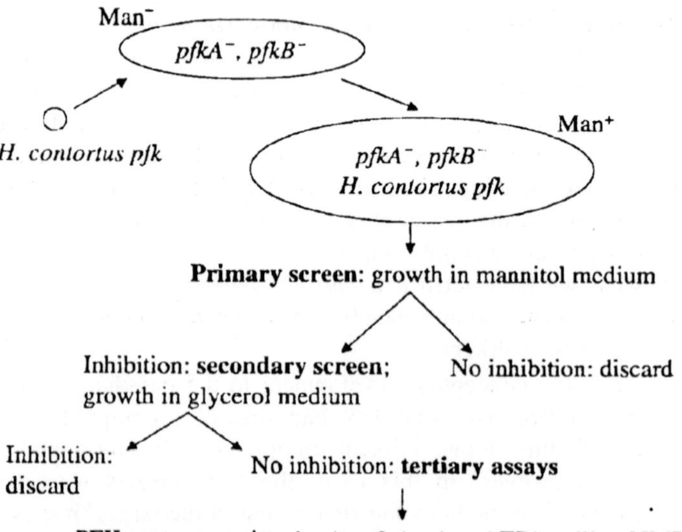

Fig. 7.7. Diagrammatic representation of screening stream for inhibitors of nematode phosphofructokinase.

mammalian cells and microbes. Wells in which cellular replication has occurred turn from blue to pink, depending on the extent of growth. The dye has both a visible and fluorescent spectrum, so that a correlation between absorbance or emission and viability can be drawn. However, it has been our experience that simple visual inspection of 96-well plates identifies wells that differ from control wells in color. In the PFK assay, inoculum size and time of incubation are chosen to allow a minimum of 10 doubling times. Wells are read within 1 hr of Alamar blue addition. Wells in which bacterial replication was minimal appear blue or purple and are easy to distinguish from the vast majority of pink wells, which contain innocuous compounds.

Active compounds were retested in medium containing glycerol as a carbon source. Glycerol does not require PFK for introduction into bacterial energy metabolism pathways. Compounds that were as toxic to the recombinant bacteria in the presence of glycerol as they were in mannitol could not be acting via inhibition of PFK. Conversely, compounds that are significantly more toxic in mannitol medium than in glycerol medium are candidate PFK inhibitors and are further characterized in tertiary assays.

Other examples. A number of additional parasiticide screens have been developed in *E. coli*. Much work has been done on hypoxanthine phosphoribosyl transferase (HPRT). The gene encoding this enzyme in *P. falciparum* was shown to complement purine metabolism mutants of *E. coli* and *Salmonella typhimurium*. Subsequent studies used HPRT-encoding genes from this parasite as well as those from the protozoan parasites, *Tritrichomonas foetus* and *Trypanosoma cruzi*, and the helminth *Schistosoma mansoni* to construct an assay for enzyme inhibitors. Inclusion of a recombinant strain of *E. coli* expressing human HPRT permitted the early determination of host– parasite selectivity. Later work converted the assay to a liquid format in 96-well microtiter plates, which is more compatible with modern HTS platforms. The assay is performed in a semidefined medium in which HPRT function is required for replication. The authors measured optical density after exposure to test compounds as an index of bacterial replication.

Another example of a recombinant, nutrient-dependent viability screen for a parasite enzyme is built on a bifunctional aldehyde dehydrogenase-alcohol dehydrogenase from *Entameoba histolytica* (EhADH2). A gene encoding this enzyme (*EhADH2*) was cloned by complementation of a strain of *E. coli* with a mutation in aldehyde dehydrogenase (*adhE*) gene. *E. histolytica* is an obligate anaerobe and requires EhADH2 for fermentation of glucose to ethanol. AdhE is necessary for anaerobic growth in *E. coli*, and *EhADH2* was identified by its ability to support growth of the *adhE*⁻ strain of *E. coli* in the absence of oxygen. Using O_2 as the discriminating nutrient, a screen was proposed for inhibitors of EhADH2 in which compounds are tested against the recombinant bacterium under anaerobiosis. Specific inhibition of this enzyme by active compounds can be shown by retesting them in the presence of O_2, as EhADH2 inhibitors will not be active in this case, while actives that do not target this enzyme should still be toxic. Many other parasite enzymes have been functionally expressed in strains of *E. coli* in complementation formats. Most examples are protozoal enzymes that function in glycolysis, including glucose phosphate isomerase from *Plasmodium falciparum*; phosphoglycerate kinase from *T. brucei*; triosephosphate isomerase from *Giardia lamblia*; and glucose 6-phosphate isomerase and enolase from *T. gondii*. In addition, inosine monophosphate dehydrogenase (IMPDH) from *T. foetus* has been expressed in a strain of *E. coli* in which the *IMPDH* gene was deleted. A cDNA encoding superoxide dismutase from *Leishmania donovani* was expressed in a strain of *E. coli* lacking superoxide dismutase (SOD) activity. Complementation was demonstrated by protection from paraquat toxicity in the recombinant strain; paraquat is a herbicide that is metabolized to a strongly oxidizing derivative. An additional example is malic enzyme from the nematode *H. contortus*, which has also been functionally expressed in *E. coli*.

Screens using Saccharomyces cerevisiae

The yeast *Saccharomyces cerevisae* is well known as a host for the expression of heterologous proteins. It is also exceptionally useful for nutrient-dependent viability screening, and is even more versatile than *E. coli*. Examples of the myriad ways in which genes encoding heterologous proteins can be functionally expressed in yeast for HTS are readily available. However, few applications for antiparasitic drug discovery have been described.

Perhaps the first yeast-based, high-throughput, nutrient-dependent viability screen for antiparasitic drugs was designed to discover inhibitors of nematode (*H. contortus*) ornithine decarboxylase (ODC). A strain of *S. cerevisiae* in which the ODC gene was deleted did not grow in the absence of exogenous polyamines, a defect corrected by expression of the nematode ODC gene. The *H. contortus* ODC gene was transcribed at a low level in this system, but still provided robust growth in polyamine-free medium. The screen was performed in 96-well microtiter plates. Each well was inoculated with 100 recombinant yeast in the presence of minimal medium and test compounds. After 48 hr at 30°C, plates received an aliquot of Alamar blue solution and were read as described above. Active compounds were retested in the presence of putrescine. Compounds that were candidate ODC inhibitors would not be toxic in the presence of putrescine, while compounds that acted against any other target were expected to demonstrate polyamine-independent toxicity.

Further modifications using the same strain of ODC^- *S. cerevisiae* reconstituted a bacterial/plant polyamine synthesis pathway in yeast. The ODC strain was transformed with plasmids encoding arginine decarboxylase and agmatine ureohydrolase, which conferred polyamine-independent growth on the recombinant microbe. A similar construction could be used to screen for inhibitors of the homologous enzymes from Apicomplexan protozoa, which synthesize polyamines through this pathway.

Of interest is a recently described yeast-based, nutrient-dependent viability screen for inhibitors of protozoal dihydrofolate reductase (DHFR). Anti-protozoal activity of DHFR inhibitors is well known, and $DHFR^-$ yeast complemented with the DHFR gene derived from the malaria parasite *P. falciparum* have been used to characterize the molecular pharmacology of resistance to the antimalarial DHFR inhibitors pyrimethamine and cycloguanil. The subsequent development of a screen was based on the demonstration that the protozoal enzymes could complement the mutation in yeast. The screen includes multiple strains of recombinant yeast, each transformed with and dependent on a different heterologous DHFR gene, including those from *P. falciparum*, *T. gondii*, *C. parvum*, *Pneumocystis carinii*, and *Homo sapiens*. As designed, all these recombinant strains are simultaneously exposed to test compounds in order to identify any with selective activity. The screen can be run in 96-well microtiter plates, with yeast replication measured by changes in optical density.

Other parasite proteins of interest have been functionally expressed in *S. cerevisiae*, including a transporter, pgh, thought to be at least partially responsible for resistance to certain quinoline-containing antimalarial drugs in *P. falciparum*. The gene encoding this transporter, *pfmdr1*, complements a pheromone transporter in*S. cerevisiae*, which has allowed preliminary analysis of its function in a heterologous system. Two other examples illustrate the variety of targets that can be studied in yeast. A *Schistosoma mansoni* gene encoding a sarcoplasmic endoreticulum Ca^{2+}-ATPase complemented a mutant strain of *S. cerevisiae*. The mutant strain lacked both yeast genes encoding homologs of this Ca^{2+} sequestration pump and could not grow on normal (low-Ca^{2+}) medium. In another example, the gene encoding an important trypanosomal glycosyltransferase was cloned by complementation in *S. cerevisiae*. In trypanosomes, many proteins are anchored to the cell membrane through glycosylphosphatidylinositol (GPI) anchors. The enzyme that donates a mannose residue for the synthesis of GPI and other purposes was cloned by complementation of a temperature-sensitive mutation in an essential yeast gene that is involved in protein glycosylation.

Considerations of Assay Design

Control of Level of Target Expression

Overexpression of a target enzyme in a recombinant screen would obviously make lead identification more difficult, simply because more of a compound would be needed to cause a detectable decrease in enzyme activity. In the PFK assay, enzyme activity was abundant in recombinant bacteria, but the assay was configured to make the rate of growth tightly dependent on available mannitol. Compounds that reduced mannitol catabolism were thus easily detectable. Conversely, the nematode ODC construct expressed in the yeast screen was present at very low levels. As relatively small amounts of polyamines are needed for cell growth, read-through transcription of the ODC gene behind a galactose-responsive (GAL) promoter provided sufficient amounts of the enzyme for robust yeast growth. Expression levels of different *HPRT* genes in *E. coli* had to be modified in order to permit comparative screening, and sulfanilide had to be added to the system to improve the sensitivity of detection of known DHRF inhibitors in some of the recombinant strains.

Assay Design

Endpoint

There are many ways to estimate microbial growth. The simplest is visual inspection of colonies growing on agar plates, though this method is difficult to adapt for HTS. There is a well-known correlation between cell density and optical density, which can be exploited in a 96-well microtiter plate format. Measurement of the incorporation of radioactive nutrients is an excellent quantitative method, but has fallen from favor due to concerns about spills and contamination. Finally, both spectrophotometric and fluorimetric assays are conveniently adapted to HTS formats, and Alamar blue is only one example of the tools available for this purpose. As mentioned, we have even found it convenient to use simple visual inspection of Alamar blue plates to identify wells of interest. However, quantification obtainable with a microplate reader is attractive in many settings.

Secondary testing

Many screens for antiparasitic drugs based on recombinant microorganisms are constructed to allow simultaneous evaluation of test compounds against the target enzyme from parasite and host. While this format is useful for small numbers of compounds, it makes screening large compound collections much more difficult. Instead, such collections should be initially screened against the recombinant microbe under nutrient conditions that isolate the parasite enzyme (e.g., in mannitol medium for PFK or polyamine-free medium for ODC). Active compounds in the primary screen can then be tested for specificity in one of two ways. One can ask for host:parasite selectivity at an early stage by testing against a recombinant microbe that is complemented with the host enzyme. Conversely, one can first ask for specificity of inhibition against the target enzyme by retesting against the parasite-complemented strain under nutrient conditions that do not require function of the parasite enzyme (glycerol medium for PFK or putrescine-supplemented medium for ODC). In this case, actives that do not interfere with the target protein will retain toxicity. Specific compounds will not be toxic under conditions in which the function of the target protein is not required.

The availability of medicinal chemistry resources can decide which approach to take; in the absence of chemistry, a specific enzyme inhibitor that does not distinguish between host and parasite has little value. If chemistry is available, however, identifying a specific enzyme inhibitor can lead to the discovery of parasite-selective compounds. Random screens that search for novel structures are based on the premise that discovery of a specific inhibitor is an extremely rare event, and so the nutrient-dependent viability format is more desirable for HTS.

Tertiary tests

Further testing of confirmed positives in the microbial screening phases, using nutrient dependence of toxicity as a variable, is required to determine if the candidate inhibits the target enzyme, and thus merits a medicinal chemistry program. In the PFK screen, for example, several glycolytic enzymes lie between the target (PFK) and the enzymatic entry of glycerol into energy metabolism. Candidate compounds could inhibit any of them. It is also possible that compounds could appear to be active by inhibiting the uptake of mannitol, but not glycerol. Therefore, actives were tested for inhibition of *H. contortus* PFK in enzyme assays employing whole-worm homogenates. In addition, we measured the response of *H. contortus* motility to exposure to actives, and correlated reductions in motility with reductions in worm ATP levels. In this secondary assay, neuroactive substances reduce motility without affecting ATP levels, while the two variables diminish in concert in the presence of metabolic poisons, such as a PFK inhibitor. Finally, whole, live *H. contortus* were exposed to candidate inhibitors in the presence of [^{13}C]glucose, with the distribution of glycolytic intermediates determined by NMR. One can predict that a PFK inhibitor will cause an accumulation of specific metabolic intermediates and a depletion of those formed downstream from PFK. The same approach can be used for candidate inhibitors of other glycolytic enzymes. Used together, these tests both confirm if specific inhibition of PFK has been attained, and document the consequences of that inhibition for parasite viability.

Similarly, candidate leads discovered in the ODC assay could act by inhibiting *H. contortus* ODC or yeast S-adenosylmethionine decarboxylase. A single confirmed positive was tested for inhibition of both enzymes in assays using extracts of the recombinant *S. cerevisiae*. The compound, stilbamidine isethionate, was shown in these experiments to inhibit S-adenosylmethionine decarboxylase, but not ODC, and no further work was done with it.

Test substances

Collections of synthetic compounds are easily screened in recombinant microbes. Fermentation extracts present more problems, since they may contain nutrients that reduce dependence on the target protein. It proved difficult to screen fermentation extracts in the ODC assay, since even trace amounts of poly-amines in the extract eliminate dependence on the parasite enzyme. Conversely, the PFK assay was compatible with fermentations. The suitability of fermentation extracts must be empirically determined in each case.

Risk/benefit analysis of recombinant microbe-based screens

The advantages of an HTS platform based on recombinant microbes are obvious for relatively small screening operations (e.g. parasiticide discovery). Two profound benefits for resource consumption are evident. A distinct financial and time advantage arises from the use of a single format for multiple, diverse targets. This limits the amount of training required for personnel in the screening laboratory, and also greatly reduces equipment expense, since the endpoint (microbial viability) is so easily measured. The second advantage is a reduction in downstream resources spent on nonspecific actives. The inclusion of the nutrient-dependent viability test (or testing against host and parasite targets in different recombinant strains) drastically limits the number of positives that require follow-up. For example, we found a single confirmed positive fermentation extract in the nematode PFK screen out of 40,000 tested; this extract reduced motility and ATP levels in *H. contortus* simultaneously, caused an accumulation of [^{13}C]glucose 6-phosphate in *H. contortus*, and inhibited nematode PFK in enzyme assays. Similarly, we found one confirmed candidate ODC inhibitor in a collection of 80,000 synthetic chemicals.

The unique benefit of recombinant microbes for screening is that target specificity is evaluated early in the process. Compounds that nonspecifically affect enzyme function (by sulfhydryl modification, cation chelation, alkylation, etc.) will not survive the comparative testing phase. The hit rate in our laboratories in these types of screens has been under 0.01%, which means that additional attention can be focused only on the most promising candidates. In contrast, screens that employ purified recombinant enzymes for HTS often have hit rates ≥2.5%. Further characterization of so many candidates requires a considerable effort in both biology and chemistry laboratories.

The biggest concern over the use of recombinant microbes is that microbial cell walls constitute a permeability barrier for test compounds. Enzyme inhibitors that cannot accumulate in bacterial or yeast cytoplasm will appear as false negatives in a screen. Permeability characteristics of *E. coli* and *S. cerevisiae* have not been rigorously described, so it is not possible to arrange for a different testing scheme for compounds with particularly unfavorable physical chemical properties. We have argued elsewhere that this concern is overstated. Missing some active compounds is of less concern than missing all of them by not running a screen.

Furthermore, compounds that have difficulty entering microbial cells may also have difficulty crossing lipid membranes in the parasite or host. Screens that use purified proteins demand no accounting for pharmaceutical properties in active compounds, and often identify "leads" with poor behavior in animals. Such leads can consume considerable amounts of chemistry and biology resources in follow-up work. Therefore, whether permeability concerns constitute a problem or an advantage for screens based on recombinant microbes is moot.

Undeniably, not all targets are suited for HTS in recombinant microbes. In our own experience, we found that we were unable to complement a PFK strain of *S. cerevisiae* with the cDNA encoding *H. contortus* PFK, despite the fact that it was functionally expressed in *E. coli*. Conversely, we initially attempted to construct an ODC screen using a strain of *E. coli* that was unable to synthesize polyamines. However, this strain required mutations in multiple genes in order to achieve the polyamine phenotype, and proved to be too leaky for routine screening. The ODC strain of *S. cerevisiae* was much better suited for HTS.

It must also be acknowledged that some targets are not suitable for screens that employ purified proteins. The most convenient assay for PFK activity requires the presence of several additional enzymes that link to generate a product that can be quantified by spectrophotometry. ODC enzyme activity is most commonly measured by trapping $[^{14}C]CO_2$ for quantification by scintillation spectrometry. Neither assay is well suited for current HTS formats. It would have been technically difficult to screen for inhibitors of either enzyme without the use of recombinant microorganisms.

Future Directions

The advantages of screens based on this paradigm are most evident for smaller- scale screening operations. However, their robust nature and ease of operation could make them attractive options for any screening laboratory. Expected developments in bioinformatics will only accentuate the benefits of the format.

Sequenced Genomes

The availability of complete genome sequences for *E. coli*, *S. cerevisiae*, and *C. elegans* provides an enormous advantage for the construction of specifically mutated strains. Furthermore, as noted above, HTS formats in *S. cerevisiae* have been developed for a variety of drug targets that have no yeast homolog. Screens can be devised for inhibitors of protein:-protein interactions, protein:DNA interactions, and protein:RNA interactions; alternative screening strategies for such purposes are not often apparent. These developments extend the utility of yeast as a screening tool far beyond the search for enzyme inhibitors, to include a variety of neurotransmitter receptors, ion channels, and transcriptional regulators. To date, antiparasitic drug discovery programs have not employed such novel strategies (at least publicly). It is not unreasonable to expect developments in this area in the future.

C. elegans as a Screening Tool

The free-living nematode *C. elegans* was the first metazoan organism to have its genome sequence defined. The utility of this organism for anthelmintic screening has been recognized for 20 years. Specific screens for anthelmintic as well as nonanthelmintic leads can be based on changes in behavior or survival of *C. elegans*. It is also well known that phenotypes caused by mutations in *C. elegans* genes can be complemented by homologous genes from other organisms, including humans.

However, there are as yet no public examples of the use of recombinant *C. elegans* for the discovery of anthelmintics. The potential of this system is illustrated by the use of *C. elegans* to confirm that a specific mutation in a gene encoding β-tubulin from the parasitic species *H. contortus* underlies the phenotype of benzimidazole resistance. It is to be expected that the enormous potential of *C. elegans* will be exploited in a variety of creative ways for anthelmintic discovery. Developments in genetic technology for the protozoan parasite *T. gondii* may likewise portend future benefits for the discovery of antiprotozoal drugs.

Screening for Inhibitors of Lipid Metabolism

In lipid metabolism, there is elegant balance in the levels of end-product lipids, and the enzymes and genes involved in their biosynthesis, as well as close cooperation with other metabolisms to maintain homeostasis. When the balance is lost, obesity or hyperlipidemia will develop, leading to a variety of serious diseases including atherosclerosis, hypertension, diabetes, functional depression of certain organs, and so on. Therefore, the control of lipid metabolism by drugs could lead to the prevention or treatment of these diseases.

Hypercholesterolemia involves heterogeneous disorders of lipid metabolism characterized by elevated levels of plasma total cholesterol and low-density lipoprotein (LDL)-derived cholesterol. It is definitively linked to increased morbidity and mortality due to myocardial infarction. Cholesterol enters the body in two ways; absorption from diet or endogenous biosynthesis. The interference of either process would provide an effective means of lowering plasma total cholesterol. 3-Hydroxy-3-methylglutaryl coenzyme A (HMG-CoA) reductase, a rate- limiting enzyme in the cholesterol biosynthetic pathway, was considered a promising target of inhibition, and in the 1970s, screening for inhibitors of this enzyme was carried out extensively. Eventually, the structurally related compounds compactin (ML236B) and mevinolin (monacolin K) were discovered from fungal culture broths as potent and specific inhibitors of HMG-CoA reductase. Since then, the derivatives, lovastatin and pravastatin, and mevinolin, have been used clinically for the treatment of hypercholesterolemia. Now, novel synthetic inhibitors of this enzyme, such as cerivastatin, are acknowledged as more effective agents.

Recent reports on clinical trials of pravastatin and simvastatin have shown a significant reduction in patient mortality rates for both hypercholesterolemic patients without known coronary heart disease and for those with existing coronary heart disease. These trials have established cholesterol-lowering agents as an effective treatment for coronary disease and have stimulated the search for new cholesterol-lowering agents with other mechanisms of action.

For the last 25 years, we have searched for new biologically active compounds of microbial origin, including a number of enzyme inhibitors. They are categorized into three classes on the basis of how they were discovered. The first class of compounds, cerulenin, herbimycin, lactacystin, and staurosporine, were originally discovered in assay systems nonspecified as enzyme inhibitors. Later studies on the mechanism of action revealed that they are enzyme inhibitors. The second class of compounds, arisugacins, pyripyropenes, and pepticinnamins, were discovered in direct assays using target enzymes themselves. So, it is necessary to test their specificity since they might inhibit other enzymes. The third class, diazaquinomycins, hymeglusin (1233A or F-244), phosalacine, and triacsins, were discovered in mechanism-based assays using intact mammalian cells or micoorganisms with specific functions. This kind of assay is expected to facilitate the discovery of highly specific enzyme inhibitors.

Table 7.3. Enzyme inhibitors of microbial origin

Compound	*Discovered as/in*	*Target enzyme*
Cerulenin	Antibiotic	Fatty acid synthase
Herbimycin	Herbicide	Tyrosine kinase
Pyripyropenes	Enzyme inhibitor	ACAT
Pepticinnamins	Enzyme inhibitor	Protein farnesyltransferase
Lactacystin	Inducer of neurite outgrowth	Proteasome
Hymeglusin	Mechanism-based screen	HMG-CoA synthase
Arisugacins	Enzyme inhibitor	Acetylcholine esterase
Staurosporine	Chemical screen	Protein kinases
Phosalacine	Mechanism-based screen	Glutamate synthase
Diazaquinomycins	Mechanism-based screen	Thymidylate synthase
Triacsins	Mechanism-based screen	Acyl-CoA synthetase

In this chapter, our recent experiences in screening for inhibitors of lipid metabolism are reviewed. We have concentrated on novel enzymes or proteins as a target of inhibition for drug discovery, and in some cases, established intricate assay systems even in the primary screens for drug discovery. The practical assay methods are also described.

New Target Enzymes and Proteins of Lipid Metabolism

We established a screening system for inhibitors of mevalonate biosynthesis from microbial metabolites by utilizing intact animal cells as a test organism. Microbial culture broths were screened whose cytotoxic effects were rescued by the addition of mevalonate to the cell culture medium, resulting in the discovery of fungal beta-lactone hymeglusin (1233A or F-244). Studying the mechanism of action revealed that hymeglusin inhibits HMG-CoA synthase specifically by modifying the active-site cysteine of the enzyme covalently. Second, although HMG-CoA reductase inhibitors have proved effective and clinically well tolerated, the enzyme steps after formation of farnesyl pyrophosphate in the cholesterol biosynthetic pathway are considered preferable as targets of inhibition, because a potentially dose-limiting toxicity might arise from the consequent reduced levels of essential isoprenoid precursors, the antioxidant ubiquinone, or the dolichols. Similarly, inhibiting enzymes after the formation of lanosterol has the potential to result in toxicity arising from the utilization of intermediates having the complete sterol ring system. Therefore, squalene synthase, squalene epoxidase, and lanosterol synthase (oxidosqualene cyclase) remain for further consideration as enzyme inhibition targets. Now, considerable effort has been directed toward screening for inhibitors of these enzymes. Glaxo and Merck researchers independently discovered a series of similar fungal metabolites, squalestatins and zaragozic acids, as potent inhibitors of squalene synthase, respectively. However, the inhibitors also have an ability to inhibit protein farnesyltransferase because both enzymes recruit farnesyl pyrophosphate as a common substrate [30], so specific inhibitors have been sought or chemically synthesized on the basis of squalestatin or zaragozic acid as a lead.

Third, acyl-CoA:cholesterol acyltransferase (ACAT), an enzyme that works after the formation of cholesterol, was considered a unique target of inhibition. ACAT catalyzes the synthesis of cholesteryl esters from cholesterol and long-chain fatty acyl-CoA. ACAT plays important roles in the body, for example, in the absorption of dietary cholesterol from the intestines, production of lipoprotein in liver and formation of foam cells from macrophages in arterial walls. Therefore, ACAT inhibition is expected not only to lower plasma cholesterol levels but also to have a direct effect at the arterial wall. A number of synthetic ACAT inhibitors such as ureas, imidazoles, and acyl amides have been developed. Several groups have searched for novel ACAT inhibitors of natural origin with structures different from the synthetic ones. We discovered purpactins, glisoprenins, terpendoles, and pyripyropenes from fungal culture broths.

Among the natural inhibitors so far reported, pyripyropenes show the most potent inhibitory activity against ACAT, and proved to be orally active in hamsters, reducing cholesterol absorption from intestines. Issues surrounding the toxic effect of ACAT inhibitors on the adrenal gland are pervasive. There has been no conclusive data as to whether the toxic effects on the adrenal gland are due to the mechanism of action of these drugs. However, certain synthetic inhibitors proved effective *in vivo* but had no effect on the adrenal gland. Furthermore, recent molecular biological studies have afforded new information about ACAT. Chang and co-workers succeeded in cloning cDNA for an ACAT gene from macrophages, now known as ACAT-1. ACAT-1 is ubiquitously expressed, and high-level expression is observed in sebaceous glands, steroidogenic tissues, and macrophages. ACAT-1-deficient transgenic mice were viable, fertile, and ostensibly healthy, with no evidence of adrenal dysfunction, indicating that the observed toxicity is not related to ACAT inhibition and that the loss of ACAT-1 is not incompatible with life. Furthermore, the knockout mice had a reduced ability to synthesize cholesteryl esters, but only in specific tissues, suggesting the presence of another ACAT. These findings have led to the discovery of ACAT-2, responsible for cholesterol esterification in the liver and intestine. Therefore, ACAT inhibitors need to be reevaluated for their specificity for ACAT-1 or -2 inhibition and toxicity to the adrenal gland.

More attention is now being paid to lipid metabolic pathways as promising targets of inhibition for the treatment of infectious diseases. An alternative mevalonate-independent (nonmevalonate) pathway has been defined specifically in some bacteria and malaria. *Mycobacterium tuberculosis*, the organism that causes tuberculosis, has unique cell wall lipids. An enzyme in lipid biosynthesis was found to be a target of isoniazid, an important first-line antituberculosis drug. Therefore, enzymes involved in these pathways are expected to make novel targets for antibacterial, antimalarial, and antituberculosis drugs.

Screening for Inhibitors of Diacylglycerol Acyltransferase

Triacylglycerol (TG) synthesis in mammals is important in many processes, including lactation, energy storage in fat and muscle, fat absorption in the intestine, and the assembly of lipoprotein particles in the liver and small intestine. Too much accumulation of TG in certain organs and tissues of the body causes fatty liver, obesity, and hypertriglyceridemia. Diacylglycerol acyltransferase (acyl-CoA:1,2-diacyl-*sn*-glycerol *O*-acyltransferase, abbreviated as DGAT) catalyzes the reaction of acyl residue transfer from acyl-CoA to diacyl-glycerol to form TG. The reaction is the final step of *de novo* triacylglycerol biosynthesis, and is the only pathway which is exclusively involved in triacylglycerol formation. Therefore, DGAT is considered a potential target of inhibition for control of such disorders. However, few DGAT inhibitors have been reported.

Screening Method

The enzyme DGAT has not been purified to date, probably because it is a hydrophobic and integral membrane protein. Therefore, DGAT activity was measured using rat liver microsomes as an enzyme source and radiolabeled palmitate as a substrate by the method of Mayorek and Bar-Tana with some modifications. The reaction mixture contains microsomal protein, BSA, [^{14}C]palmitoyl-CoA, $MgCl_2$, diisopropyl fluorophosphate, 1,2-dioleoyl-*sn*-glycerol, and a test sample in a total volume of 0.2 ml. After a 1 5-min incubation at 23° C, lipids are extracted and separated by thin-layer chromatography

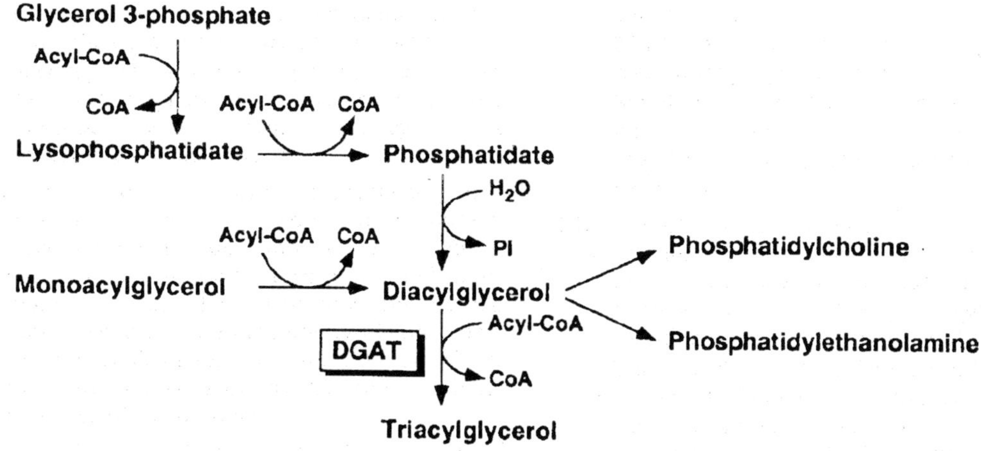

Fig. 7.8. Triacylglycerol biosynthetic pathway.

(TLC). The distribution of radioactivity on TLC is analyzed with a radioscanner to determine the amount of [^{14}C]TG. To investigate the specificity of DGAT inhibitors, synthesis of lipids including TG, phosphatidylcholine (PC), and phosphatidylethanolamine (PE) was measured in an intact cell assay using Raji cells by our established method. Raji cells are incubated in the presence of [^{14}C]oleic acid with or without a test sample in a total volume of 0.2 ml. After a 20-min incubation at 37°C, [^{14}C]oleic acid is incorporated mainly into PC, PE, and TG, which are extracted and separated by TLC. The distribution of radioactivity in these lipids on TLC is analyzed. If the sample inhibits DGAT activity specifically in Raji cells, incorporation of [^{14}C]oleic acid only into the TG fraction should be inhibited.

Inhibitors

About 15,000 samples, mostly microbial culture broths, were subjected to our screening program for DGAT inhibitors. Finally, we obtained amidepsines and roselipins from fungal strains, and xanthohumols from a plant extract as novel DGAT inhibitors.

Five amidepsines, A to E, were isolated from the culture broths of fungal strains FO-2942 and FO-5969, which were considered to belong to the genus *Humicola*. They are structurally related, with the common skeleton of tridepside gyrophoric acid. Many gyrophoric acid derivatives were isolated from lichens and amidepsine D was identical with 2,4-di-*O*-methylgyrophoric acid. However, the other amidepsines are a new type of compound having an amino acid (alanine or valine) attached to the skeleton. Two chalcones were isolated from extracts obtained by treatment of hop of *Humulus lupulus* (L.) with 70% methanol. One was identical with xanthohumol and the other, named xanthohumol B, was found to be a new compound. Very recently, four novel glycolipids, named roselipins, were isolated from the culture broth of *Gliocladium roseum* KF-1040, a marine isolate. They are composed of highly methylated fatty acid, hexose, and alditol moieties. The different terminal hydroxy residue of the alditol is bound to the carboxylic acid of the fatty acid to form the diastereoisomers of roselipins 1A and 1B, or roselipins 2A and 2B.

In the assay using rat liver microsomes, the compounds all inhibited DGAT activity in a dose-dependent manner, and amidepsines A, B, and D, and roselipins are potent, with IC_{50} values of 10–22 μM. In the intact Raji cell assay, amidepsine B showed inhibition of TG synthesis, but almost no effects on phosphatidylcholine and phosphatidylethanolamine syntheses, indicating that the drug inhibits DGAT activity in Raji cells specifically. Amidepsine D and xanthohumols also showed specific inhibition of DGAT to some extent. However, roselipins did not show selective TG inhibition, probably due to lack of permeability through the cell membrane.

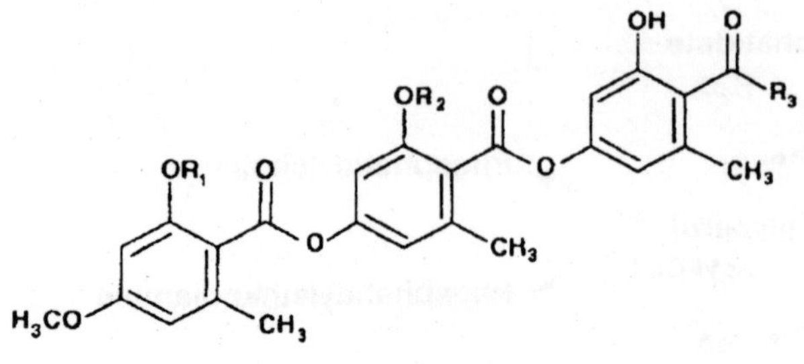

Amidepsine	$-R_1$	$-R_2$	$-R_3$
A	$-CH_3$	$-H$	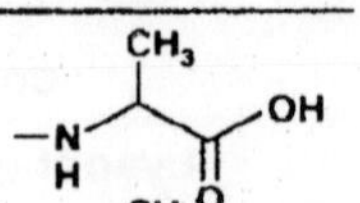 CH_3, $-N(H)$, OH, O
B	$-H$	$-H$	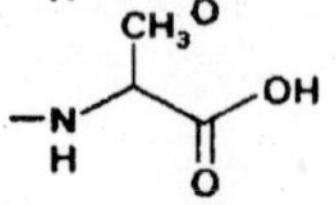 CH_3, $-N(H)$, OH, O
C	$-H$	$-H$	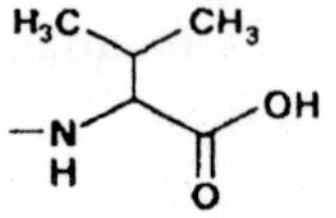 H_3C, CH_3, $-N(H)$, OH, O
D	$-CH_3$	$-H$	$-OH$
E	$-CH_3$	$-CH_3$	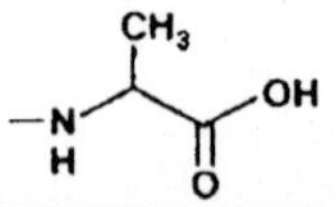 CH_3, $-N(H)$, OH, O

OR_1 O OR_2 O OH O R_3 CH_3 CH_3 CH_3 H_3CO

Amidepsines

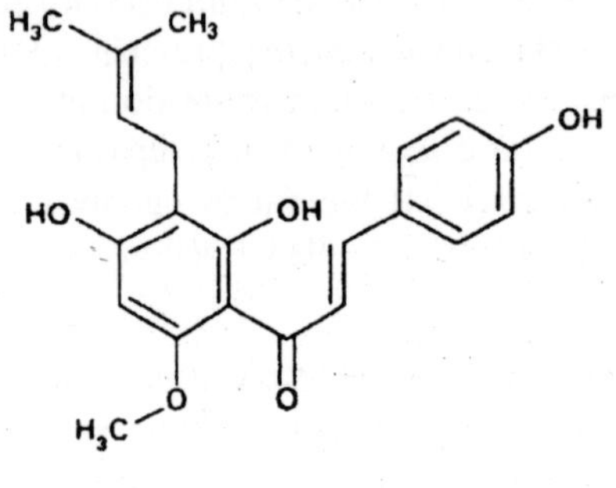

H_3C CH_3 OH HO OH H_3C O O

Xanthohumol

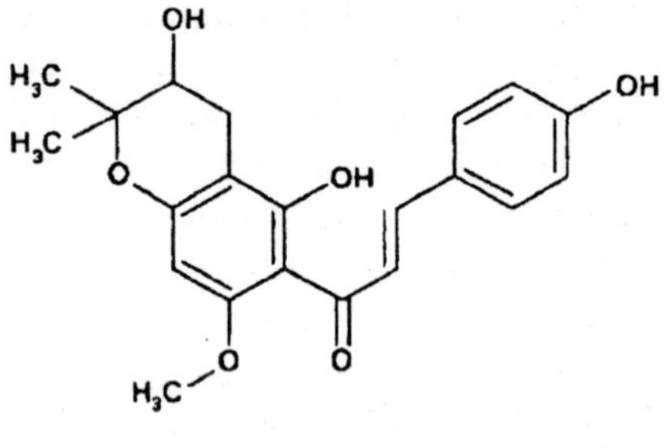

OH H_3C H_3C O OH OH H_3C O O

Xanthohumol B

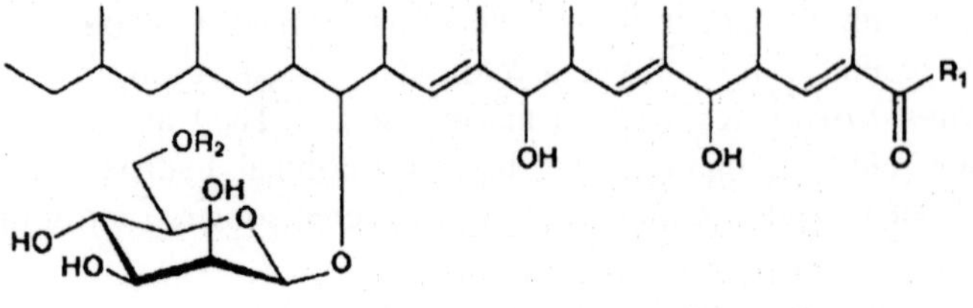

Roselipin	R_1	R_2
1A	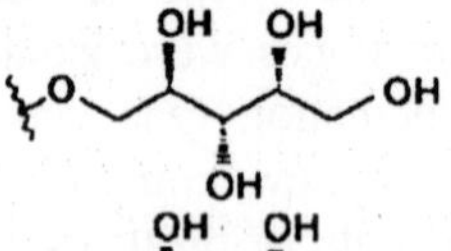 O, OH, OH, OH, OH	$-H$
1B	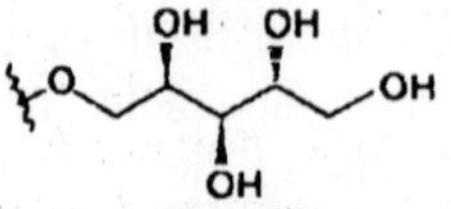 O, OH, OH, OH, OH	$-H$
2A	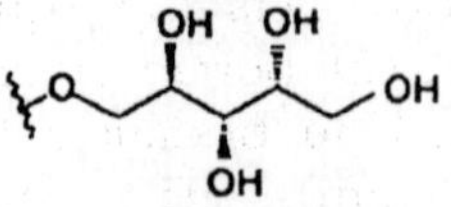 O, OH, OH, OH, OH	$-COCH_3$
2B	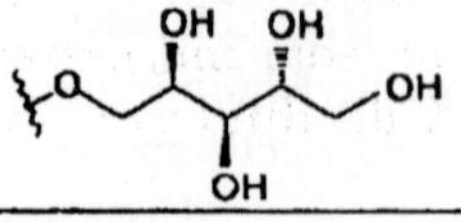 O, OH, OH, OH, OH	$-COCH_3$

R_1 OR_2 OH O HO HO O OH OH O

Roselipins

Fig. 7.9. Structures of DGAT inhibitors.

Table 7.4. Inhibition of triacylglycerol synthesis by DGAT inhibitors in assays using rat liver microsomes and intact raji cells

	Rat microsomes	*Raji cells*		
DGAT inhibitor	*TG*	*TG*	*PC*	*PE*
IC_{50} (μM)	IC_{50} (μM)	IC_{50} (μM)	IC_{50} (μM)	IC_{50} (μM)
AmidepsineA	10	16	>100	>100
Amidepsine B	19	3.4	>100	>100
Amidepsine C	52	17	52	>100
Amidepsine D	18	2.8	10	>100
Amidepsine E	124	91	100	100
Xanthohumol	50	21	>100	>100
XanthohumolB	190	34	>100	>100
Roselipin 1A	17	30	30	>30
Roselipin 1B	15	24	24	28
Roselipin 2A	22	20	20	20
Roselipin 2B	18	20	20	20

The DGAT enzyme has been known to exist for years, and a number of researchers have contributed to characterizing its biochemical properties. Recently, Farese and co-workers identified a gene encoding a mammalian DGAT. Interestingly, the translation of a full-length cDNA predicts an open reading frame encoding a 498-amino acid protein that is about 20% identical to mouse ACAT, with the most highly conserved region in the C terminus. From the predicted protein sequence, a potential *N*-linked glycosylation site, a putative tyrosine phophorylation site, and an active site serine residue also found in ACAT are shown. The protein has multiple hydrophobic domains and 6-12 possible transmembrane domains. Its mRNA expression was detected in every mammalian tissue, and the highest expression levels were found in the small intestine. These findings are consistent with a proposed role for DGAT in intestinal fat absorption. However, mRNA expression was relatively low in the livers of humans regardless of high DGAT activity, suggesting the existence of a second DGAT in livers. They established a DGAT expression system, and samples including our DGAT inhibitors are to be evaluated. Thus, further understanding of DGAT at a molecular level will help us search for DGAT inhibitors, leading to potential approaches for treating hypertriglyceridemia or obesity in humans.

Screening for Inhibitors of Cholesteryl Ester Transfer Protein

Cholesteryl ester transfer protein (CETP) promotes exchange and transfer of neutral lipids such as cholesteryl ester (CE) and TG between plasma lipoproteins. CETP is a very hydrophobic and heat-stable glycoprotein with an apparent molecular weight of 74 kDa as determined by SDS-PAGE analysis. The cDNA from human liver was cloned and sequenced. It encodes for a 476-amino acid protein (53 kDa), suggesting that the apparent higher molecular weight is due to the addition of carbohydrate residues by posttranslational modification.

Evidence has been accumulating of the importance of CETP in atherosclerosis: (1) CETP decreased the cholesterol concentration in high density lipoprotein (HDL) *in vitro* and *in vivo*; (2) rats and mice deficient in CETP activity have high plasma HDL and are resistant to atherosclerosis; (3) human subjects with a genetic deficiency of CETP have very high HDL and low LDL cholesterol levels and are resistant to atherosclerosis; (4) human CETP gene-introduced transgenic mice have a redistribution of cholesterol from HDL to LDL and exhibit a marked increase in susceptibility to diet-induced

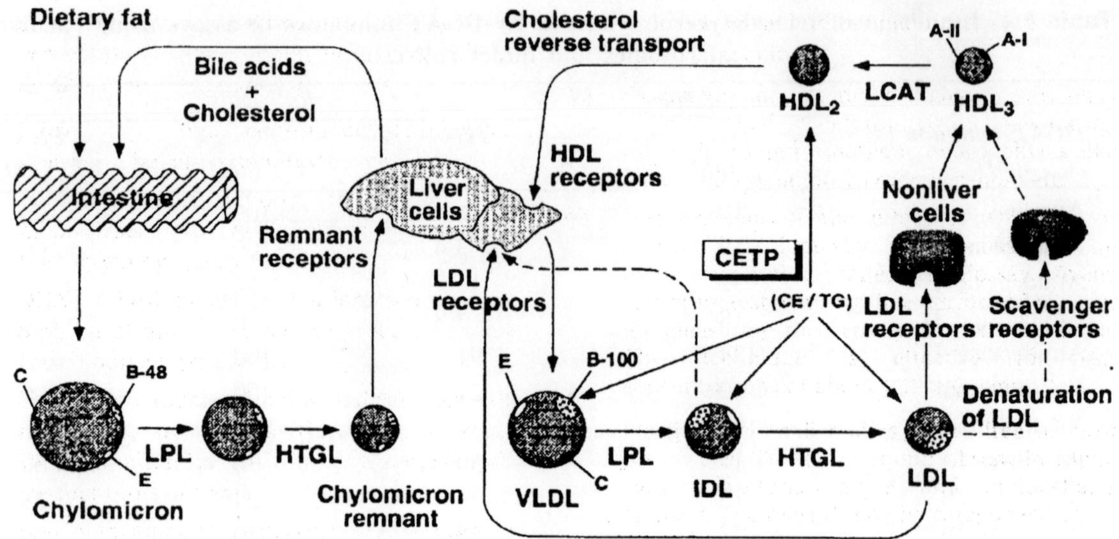

Fig. 7.10. Function of CETP, LPL (lipoprotein lipase) and HTGL (hepatic triglyceride lipase)

atherosclerosis; (5) antisense oligonucleotides and antibody against CETP inhibited the development of atherosclerosis in cholesterol-fed rabbits; and (6) antibody against CETP inhibited the development of atherosclerosis in cholesterol-fed rabbits. Therefore, inhibition of CETP is proposed as a novel target for anti-atherosclerotic drugs. Interestingly, the mechanism of CETP-mediated lipid transfer is still unclear. In fact, small molecules modulating the CETP activity have been searched for extensively for therapeutic and biochemical purposes.

Screening Methods

In vitro assay

Three methods have been reported for CETP assay. The rationale of each method is illustrated in Figure 7.11. Methods B and C are good for a high-throughput screening (HTS) format.

Method A

The rationale of method A is that HDL and LDL are separated by selective precipitation of LDL by dextran sulfate and Mg^{2+} after the reaction between LDL and reconstituted HDL containing radiolabeled CE by CETP. The method was originally described by Kato et al. The assay mixtures consist of reconstituted [^{14}C]CE-HDL as the donor for CE, LDL as the acceptor, 5,5′-dithiobis-2-nitrobenzoic acid, bovine serum albumin (BSA), partially purified CETP, and a test sample in Eppendorf tubes (1.5 ml). After a 30-min incubation at 37°C, the reaction is terminated by the addition of an LDL-precipitation solution. After standing for 20 min in an ice bath, the assay mixtures are centrifuged, and the supernatant solution containing [^{14}C]CE-HDL is analyzed for radioactivity. Furthermore, the [^{14}C]CE-LDL precipitate is also analyzed for radioactivity if necessary. Usually the blank and control transfer values are about 6% and 34% of initial [^{14}C]CE-HDL added under the assay conditions, respectively.

Method B

Bisgaier et al. reported a CETP assay using fluorescent cholesteryl 4,4-difluoro-5,7-dimethyl-4-bora-3a,4a-diaza-3-indacenedodecanoate (BODIPY-CE) in microemulsions. Microemulsions for donor/acceptor contain triolein, BODIPY-CE/cholesteryl oleate, and 1 -hexadecanoyl-2-[*cis*-9- octadecenoyl]-*sn*-glycero-3-phosphocholine. The assay mixtures consist of acceptor microemulsions, donor

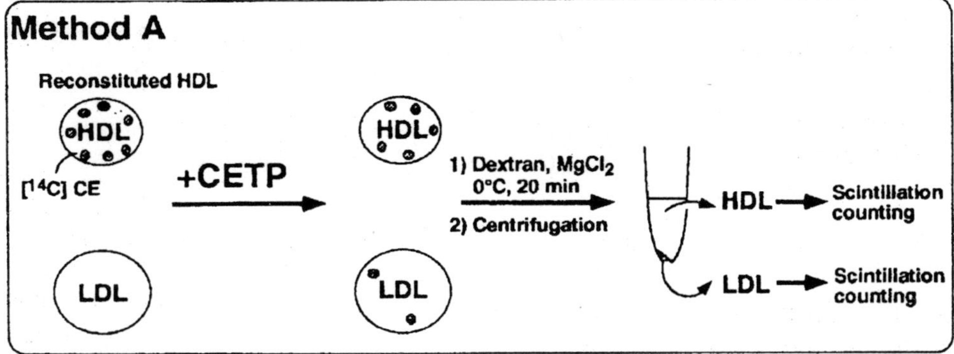

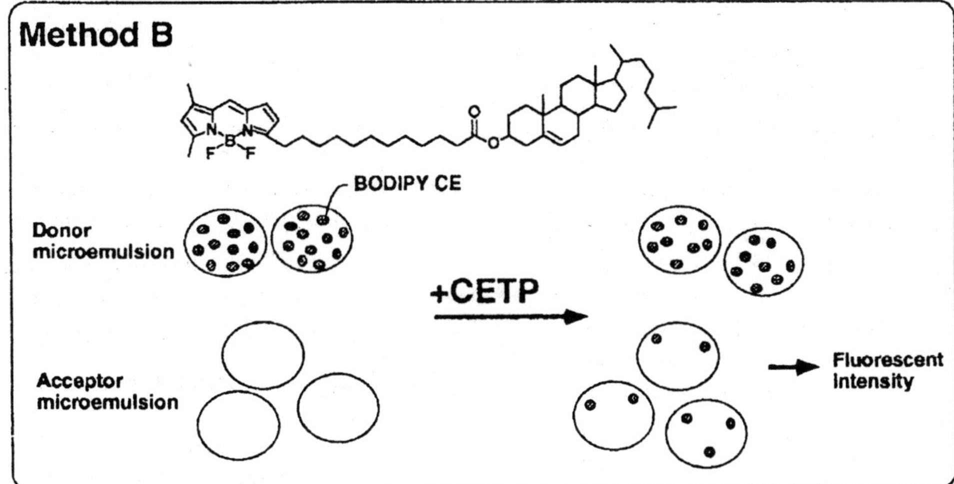

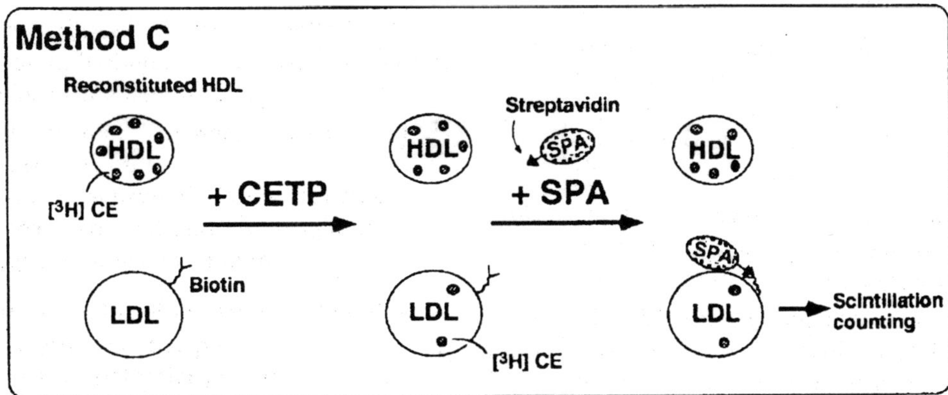

Fig. 7.11. Rotionales of three CETP assays.

microemulsions, and a test sample in each well of flat-bottom 96-well plates. After preincubation at 37°C for 10 min, the reaction is initiated by addition of CETP solution. The fluorescent intensity in each well of the plates is periodically (every 10 sec) detected at 37°C with a fluorescent 96-well plate reader equipped with 485- and 538-nm bandpass filters in the excitation and emission paths, respectively.

Method C

Most researchers have carried out CETP assay using a Scintillation Proximity Assay (SPA) kit. The reaction mixtures containing a test sample, [^{3}H]CE-HDL, and biotin-LDL, are thoroughly mixed. The reaction is initiated by the addition of CETP. After a 4-hr incubation at 37° C, the reaction is terminated by the addition of streptavidin SPA beads, and allowed to stand for 1 hr at room temperature. Finally, the transfer of [^{3}H]CE from [^{3}H]CE-HDL to LDL is measured by scintillation counter.

Ex vivo assay

Ex vivo tests for CETP inhibitors were reported using transgenic mice expressing human CETP and human apo A-I or hamsters. For example, a test sample dissolved in Cremophor EL solution (4 μl, final 10mg/kg) is administered to male mice (fasted overnight). Blood is taken at 4 and 24 hr after dosing, and is centrifuged immediately to obtain plasma. The plasma (25 μl) is used as a CETP source to determine the CETP activity by method A.

Inhibitors

Over 20,000 samples of microbial culture broths were subjected to our screening program for CETP inhibitors by method A. At first no BSA was added to the assay mixture, but many false-positive compounds such as fatty acids were isolated. To prevent this, the optimal concentration of BSA was tested and set up as 200 μM, resulting in a low hit rate in the primary screen. The serum albumin concentration in the assay is similar to that in human plasma. Finally, we discovered erabulenols from a fungal strain, and ferroverdins from an actinomycete strain, as novel CETP inhibitors.

Erabulenols A and B were isolated from the culture broths of fungal strain FO-5637, considered to belong to the genus *Penicillium*. Scleroderolide, previously reported as a fungal metabolite, was also isolated from culture broth. They have a tetracyclic ring, and erabulenols consist of a phenalenone skeleton and a trimethyltetrahydrofuran moiety. Very recently, three ferroverdins were isolated as very potent CETP inhibitors from the culture broth of *Streptomyces* sp. WK-5344. Ferroverdin A was known as a green pigment, but ferroverdins B and C were new compounds. They are a complex of one iron ion and three ligands with structures of*para*-vinylphenyl-nitrosohydroxybenzoate derivatives.

Novel compounds of synthetic or natural origin were reported to inhibit CETP activity. PD 140195, cholesterol derivatives of U-617 and U-95594, and an isoflavan CGS 25159 are synthetic inhibitors. Recently, synthetic pyridine derivatives, and bis-(2-aminophenyl) disulfides and 2-aminophenyl thio derivatives were disclosed. Wiedendiols and suberitenones were isolated from marine sponges, and U-106305 was isolated as a novel CETP inhibitor from a *Streptomyces* sp. A peptide from hog plasma was also reported to inhibit the activity. Additionally, known compounds such as strongylin A, puupehenone, chloropuupehenone, aureol, and avarol were reported to show CETP inhibitory activity. They were all previously isolated from marine sponges and are structurally similar to wiedendiols. We also observed that known fungal metabolites, sclerotiorin originally isolated as a yellow pigment, and L681512 compounds isolated as elastase inhibitors inhibit CETP activity.

Although it is difficult to compare their inhibitory activity due to the different assay methods, chloropuupehenone and ferroverdin B show very potent CETP inhibition, with nanomolar IC_{50} values. Some compounds gave quite different IC_{50} values depending on the assay conditions. For example, the IC_{50} value of sclerotiorin is 19 μM when assayed in the absence of BSA, and 67 μM in the presence of BSA. Therefore, the addition of a high concentration of serum albumin or whole plasma to the assay mixture is recommended to exclude a nonspecific-binding type of inhibitor. Accordingly, the CETP inhibitory activity of certain compounds should be reevaluated in the presence of serum albumin or plasma. In this sense, the highly potent CETP inhibition by ferroverdins B and C even in the presence of BSA is promising and further *ex vivo* and *in vivo* evaluation of the compounds is warranted.

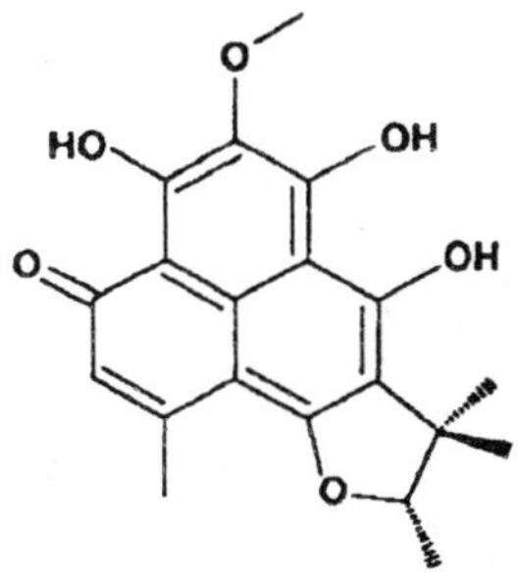

Erabulenol A

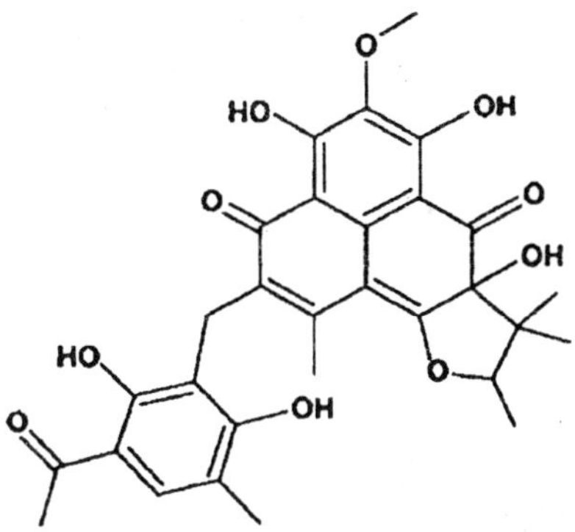

Erabulenol B

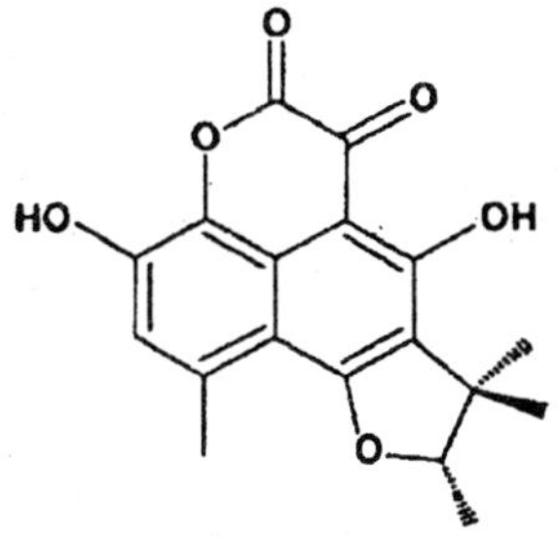

Sclerodereolide

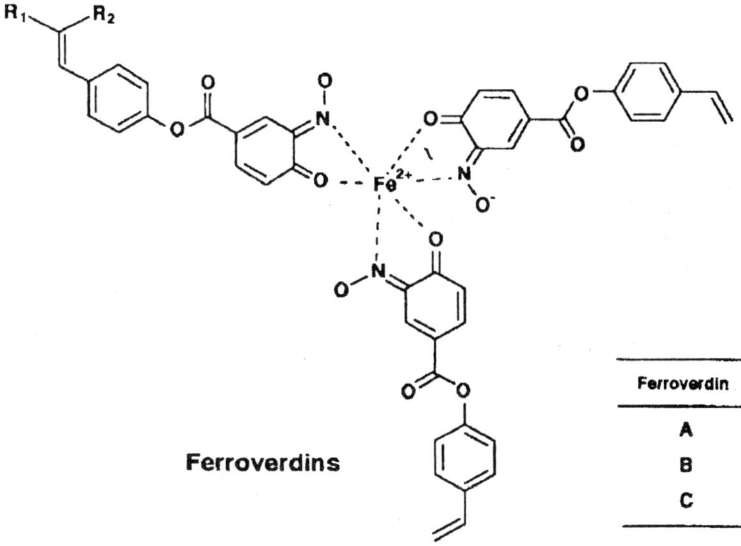

Ferroverdins

Ferroverdin	R_1	R_2
A	H	H
B	OH	H
C	H	COOH

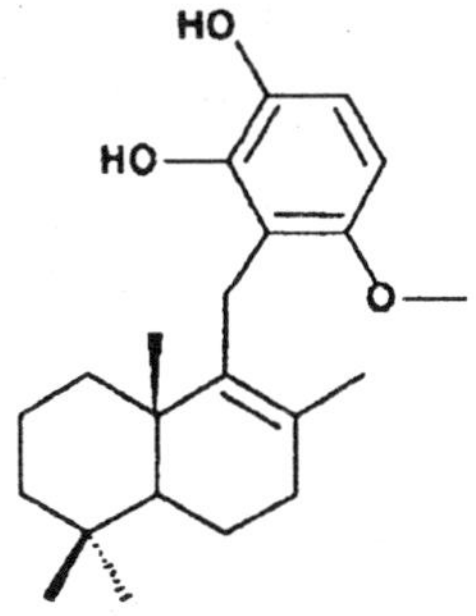

Wiedendiol-A

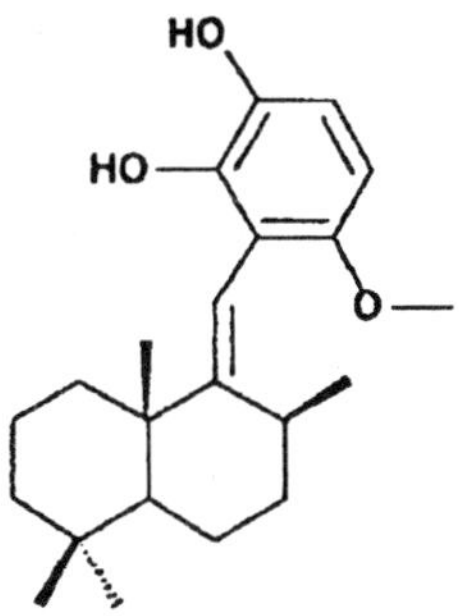

Wiedendiol-B

(A)

Fig. 7.12. Structures of CETP inhibitors of natural (A) and synthetic (B) origin.

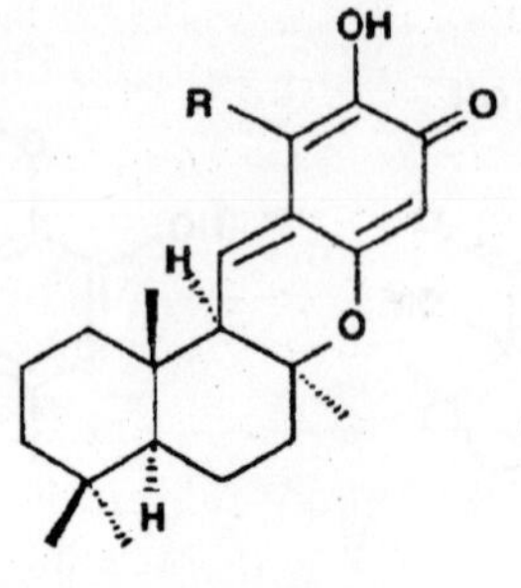

Chloropuupehenone Cl

Puupehenone H

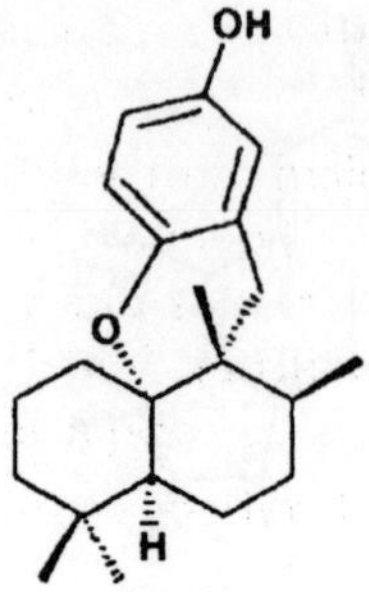

Aureol

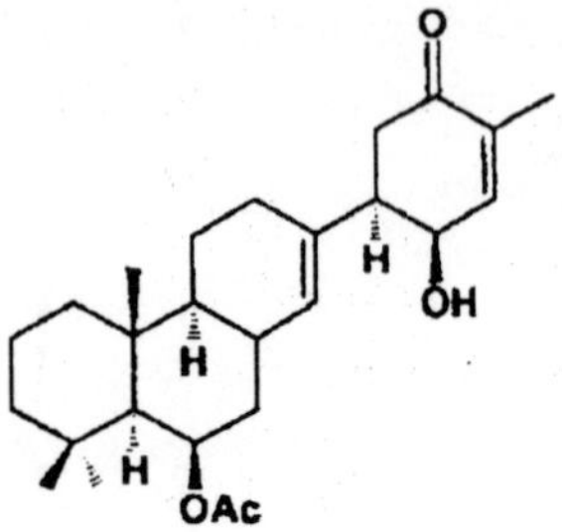

Suberitenone A

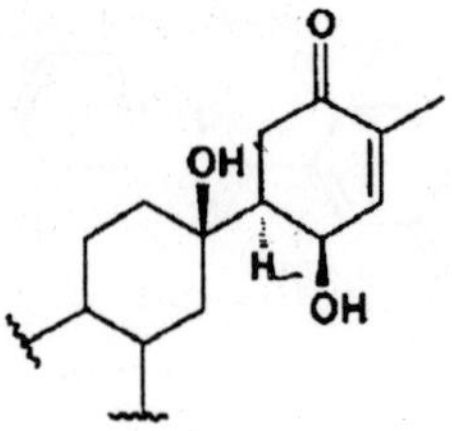

Suberitenone B

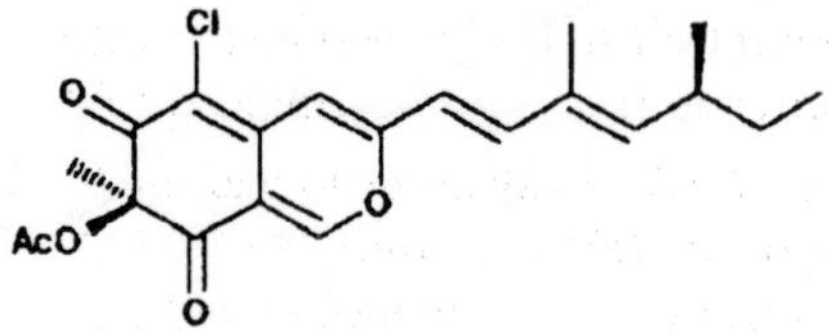

Sclerotiorin

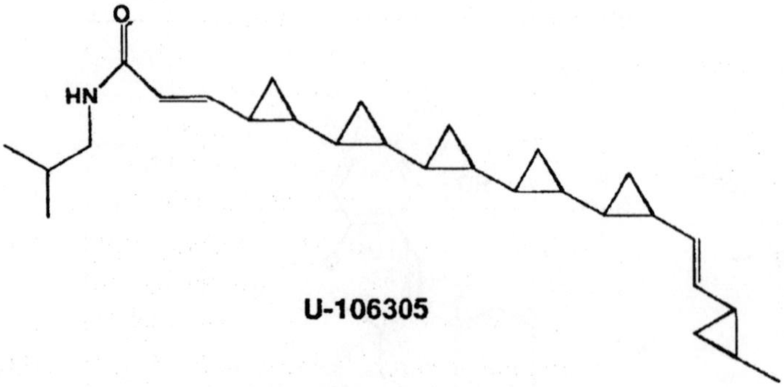

U-106305

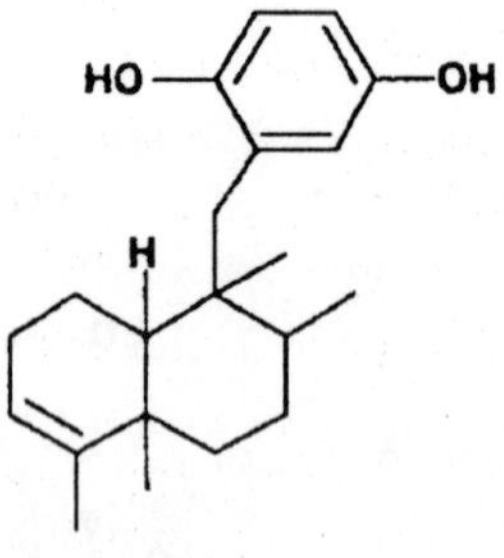

Avarol

Fig. 7.12. Continued.

Data have been presented for the *ex vivo* and *in vivo* evaluation of CETP inhibitors. *Ex vivo* efficacy was shown using hamsters for CGS 25159 (oral administration at 10 mg/kg) and using transgenic mice for sclerotiorin and L681512 (oral administration at 10 mg/kg). Furthermore, analysis of plasma lipoproteins from CGS 25159-treated (10 and 30 mg/kg, p.o.) hypercholesterolemic hamsters showed *in vivo* efficacy with an increase in HDL cholesterol.

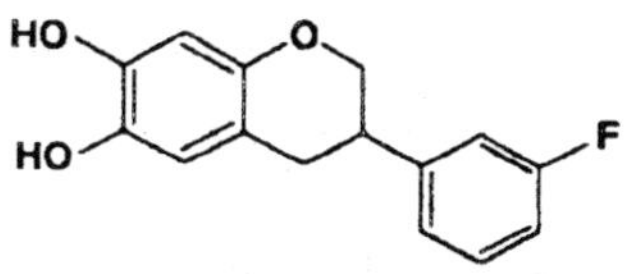

CGS 25159

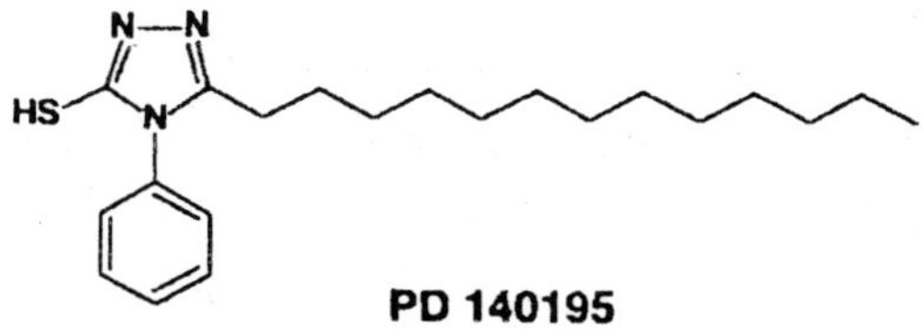

PD 140195

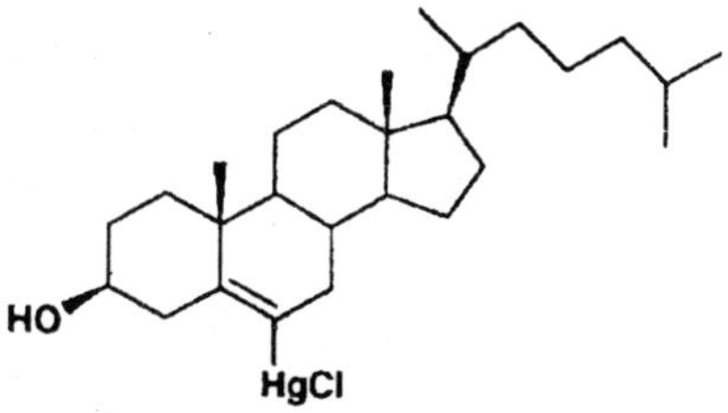

(B) U-617

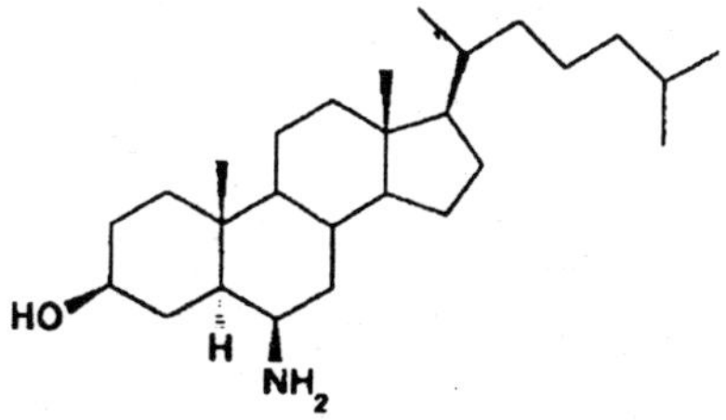

U-95594

Fig. 7.12. Continued.

Table 7.5. CETP inhibitors

Compound	*Origin*	*Assay method*	IC_{50} *(μM)*
Aureol	Sponge	C	22
Avarol	Sponge	C	25
Chloropuupehenone	Sponge	C	0.30
CGS25 159	Synthetic	A	10
Erabulenol A	Fungus	A	48
Erabulenol B	Fungus	A	58
Ferroverdin A	Actinomycete	A	21
Ferroverdin B	Actinomycete	A	0.62
Ferroverdin C	Actinomycete	A	2.2
L-681,512-1 ~ -4	Fungus	A	1.6 ~ 2.5
PD 140195	Synthetic	B/B(+BSA)	2.0/50
Puupehenone	Sponge	C	6.0
Sclerotiorin	Fungus	A (–BSA)	19
Scleroderolide	Fungus	A	95
Suberitenone A	Sponge	C	
Suberitenone B	Sponge	C	10
U-106305	Actinomycete	B	25
U-617	Synthetic	B	
U-95594	Synthetic	B	
Wiedendiol A	Sponge	C	5.0
Wiedendiol B	Sponge	C	5.0

Application of Inhibitors for the Biochemical Study of CETP

Since sclerotiorin, a member of the azaphilone family, was found to inhibit CETP activity, the effect of azaphilones on CETP activity was tested. A structure-specific CETP inhibition by azaphilones was shown. Electrophilic ketone(s) and/or enone(s) at both the C-6 and C-8 positions of the isochromane-like ring are necessary for eliciting CETP inhibitory activity. Several experiments strongly suggested that the drug inhibits CETP irreversibly. Sclerotiorin was reported to react with a primary amine such as ammonia and methylamine to yield sclerotioramine and *N*-methylsclerotioramine, respectively. Similarly, sclerotiorin reacts with α- and ε-amino residues of lysine to form the sclerotiorin adducts in our model reaction, which seems to explain the structure-specific CETP inhibition by azaphilones. Therefore, it is plausible that the drug modifies primary amines such as lysine or the *N*-terminal amino acid in the CETP molecule covalently. The amino acid sequence of human CETP revealed 25 lysine residues in the molecule, some of which are responsible for CETP activity. Furthermore, the *N*-terminal cysteine of both human and rabbit plasma CETP was modified by *para*-chloromercuriphenylsulfonate, resulting in inhibition of TG transfer activity. Therefore, covalent modification of such residues by sclerotiorin might impair the CETP activity.

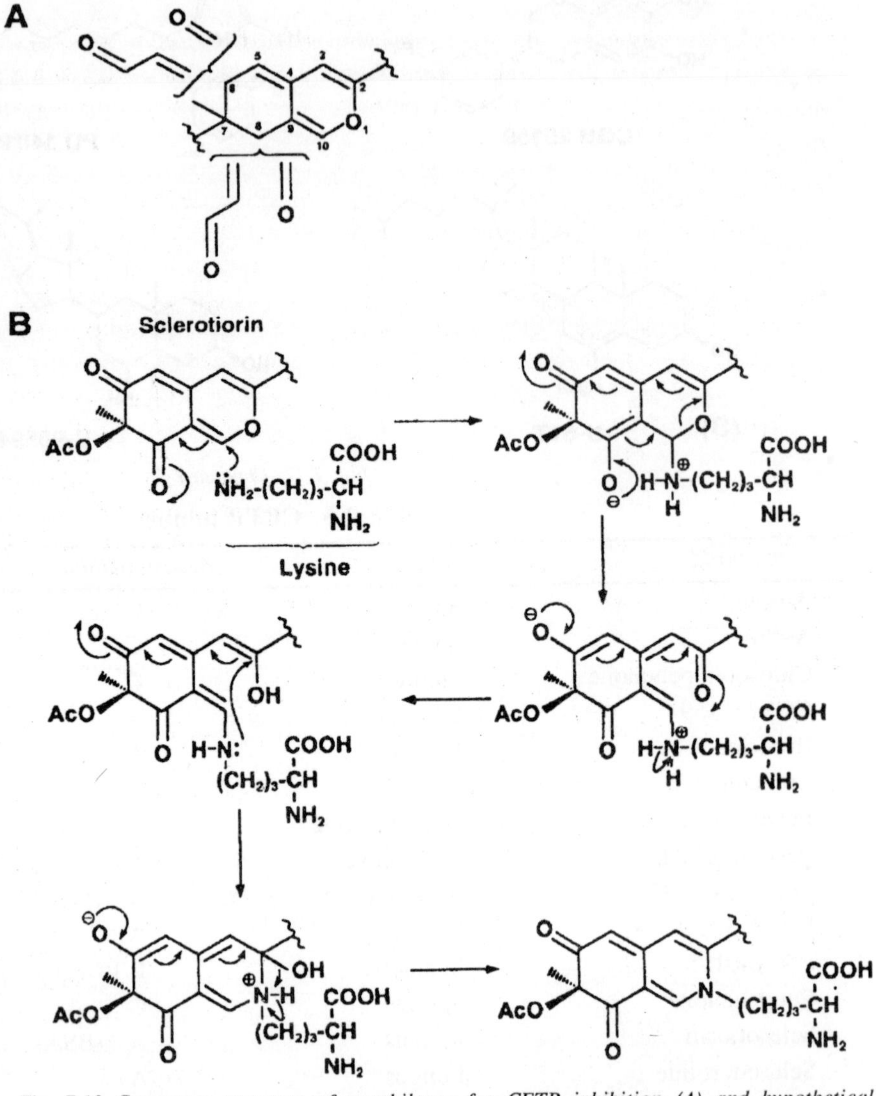

Fig. 7.13. Consensus structure of azaphilones for CETP inhibition (A) and hypothetical mechanism of reaction of sclerotiorin with ε-amino residue of lysine (B).

Swenson et al. observed the transfer of CE from vesicles to CETP by separating the vesicles and CETP through a gel-filtration column. Under similar conditions, 24% of [^{14}C]CE is transferred from [^{14}C]CE/PC vesicles to CETP. A thiol-modifying reagent, *para*-chloromercuriphenylsulfonate, inhibits this process, while sclerotiorin does not affect it essentially, but CETP lost the ability to transfer bound [^{14}C]CE to LDL. These findings indicate that the inhibitory mechanism of sclerotiorin is different from that of*para*-chloromercuri-phenylsulfonate. Previous studies showed that the binding of CETP to lipoproteins involves mainly ionic interactions, that is, negatively charged lipoproteins and positively charged CETP. Jiang et al. demonstrated, in fact, that point mutagenesis of positively charged amino acids including protonated ^{233}Lys within the conserved region of CETP reduced the HDL binding and CETP activities markedly. Therefore, it is plausible that sclerotiorin can modify such important lysine residues especially on the surface of the molecule to form a covalent bond as predicted from the model reaction.

The biological properties of sclerotiorin have not been studied in detail. We have investigated the effects of the drug on several enzymatic and biochemical reactions such as acyl-CoA:cholesterol acyltransferase, DGAT, phospholipase A2, PAF acetyl hydrolase, and gp 120-CD4 binding activities. Sclerotiorin did not show any inhibitory effects on the reactions at 100 μM except on type II phospholipase A2 (IC_{50} 1.5 μM). If our model of the reaction mechanism is valid, several lysine residues in the protein molecules might be modified by sclerotiorin. However, most enzymes appear to maintain their activity even after such modification, while CETP and type II phospholipase A2 lost their activity, suggesting differences in functional importance of lysine residues among proteins. Therefore, sclerotiorin is a useful tool with which to investigate whether lysine residues in proteins play a critical role in their biological functions. The binding site(s) of sclerotiorin on CETP remains to be defined.

Screening for Inhibitors of Macrophage-derived foam Cell Formation

From recent advanced research on ACAT genes, two isozymes, ACAT-1 and -2, are known to be present and to play different roles in the body. ACAT-1 is ubiquitous and expressed most in sebaceous gland, steroidogenic tissues, and macrophages, while ACAT-2 is expressed in the liver and intestine. The findings indicate that ACAT-1 contributes deeply to macrophage-derived foam cell formation in atherosclerosis and that ACAT-2 is responsible for absorption of dietary cholesterol from the intestine and lipoprotein production in the liver. A number of ACAT inhibitors including synthetic and natural inhibitors were reported. Researchers carried out assays using rat liver microsomes as the enzyme source in most cases, and inhibitors were evaluated in an animal model by measuring cholesterol absorption from intestines. The course of experiments is now recognized as an assay for the ACAT-2 isozyme.

We are interested in ACAT-1 inhibitors, which are expected to affect macrophages directly. In the early stages of atherosclerogenesis, macrophages penetrate the intima, efficiently take up modified LDL, store cholesterol and fatty acids as a form of neutral lipids such as CE and TG in the cytosolic lipid droplets, and are converted into foam cells, leading to the development of atherosclerosis in the arterial wall. We established an assay system of lipid droplet formation using intact mouse macrophages and searched for microbial inhibitors of the formation in macrophages. Once a compound is discovered, the inhibition site should be defined.

Screening Method

Nishikawa et al. reported that when mouse peritoneal macrophages are cultured in the presence of negatively charged liposomes, they take up the liposomes via the scavenger receptors and metabolize their components such as phospholipids and cholesterol to form lipid droplets containing neutral lipids in the cytosol. On the basis of their observation, we have developed cell-based assays by microscopic observation of oil red O-stained lipid droplets (morphological assay) and by measurement of [^{14}C]neutral lipids (CE and TG) synthesized from [^{14}C]oleic acid (biochemical assay). When macrophages are cultured in the presence of liposomes, a number of lipid droplets are observed in the cytosols in the morphological assay. For the primary screen, culture broths were selected that caused a reduction of the size and/or the number of lipid droplets without cytotoxic effect on macrophages. Then, the inhibition was confirmed in the biochemical assay. In control experiments with liposomes, the incorporation of [^{14}C]oleic acid into CE, TG, and PL is about 23%, 20%, and 10% of the total radioactivity added, respectively.

Effects of Known Lipid Metabolism Inhibitors on the Assays

First, effects of known inhibitors of lipid metabolism on the lipid droplet formation and the neutral lipid synthesis in macrophages were examined. Cerulenin (fatty acid synthase inhibitor), compactin (HMG-CoA reductase inhibitor), and hymeglusin (HMG-CoA synthase inhibitor) showed no effects, indicating that *de novo* biosynthesis of fatty acid and cholesterol is not involved in the process of lipid droplet formation. Pregnenolone (inhibitor of cellular cholesterol transport) and CL-283,546 (ACAT inhibitor) inhibited [^{14}C]CE synthesis specifically, with IC_{50} values of 5.0 and 0.03 8 μM, respectively. The inhibitors decreased cytosolic lipid droplets only partially even at the highest doses, which caused almost complete inhibition of [^{14}C]CE synthesis. In contrast, triacsin C (inhibitor of long-chain acyl-CoA synthetase) inhibited both [^{14}C]CE and [^{14}C]TG syntheses, with similar IC_{50} values of 0.19 and 0.10 μM, respectively. Furthermore, the triacsin C dose-dependent inhibition of lipid droplet formation was almost complete at 0.59 μM, a concentration that showed about 90% inhibition of [^{14}C]CE and [^{14}C]TG syntheses. These results show that inhibition of acyl-CoA synthetase by triacsin C causes a decrease in the cellular levels of acyl-CoA, the common substrate for CE and TG syntheses, leading to inhibition of the synthesis of neutral lipids and eventually to the complete disappearance of cytosolic lipid droplets in the macrophages. These findings imply that TG synthesis as well as CE synthesis is responsible for lipid droplet formation in mouse macrophages.

Inhibitors

Over 10,000 samples of microbial culture broths were subjected to the screening program in the morphological assay. We discovered beauveriolides and pheno-chalasins from fungal culture broths as novel inhibitors of lipid droplet formation in macrophages. Two structurally related cyclodepsipeptides, beauveriolide I and a novel compound named beauveriolide III, were isolated from the culture broth of *Beauveria* sp. FO-6979. Beauveriolides I and III caused a reduction in the number and size of cytosolic lipid droplets in macrophages at 10 μM without any cytotoxic effect on macrophages. They inhibited [^{14}C]CE synthesis specifically, with IC_{50} values of 0.8 and 0.4 μM, respectively. Studies on

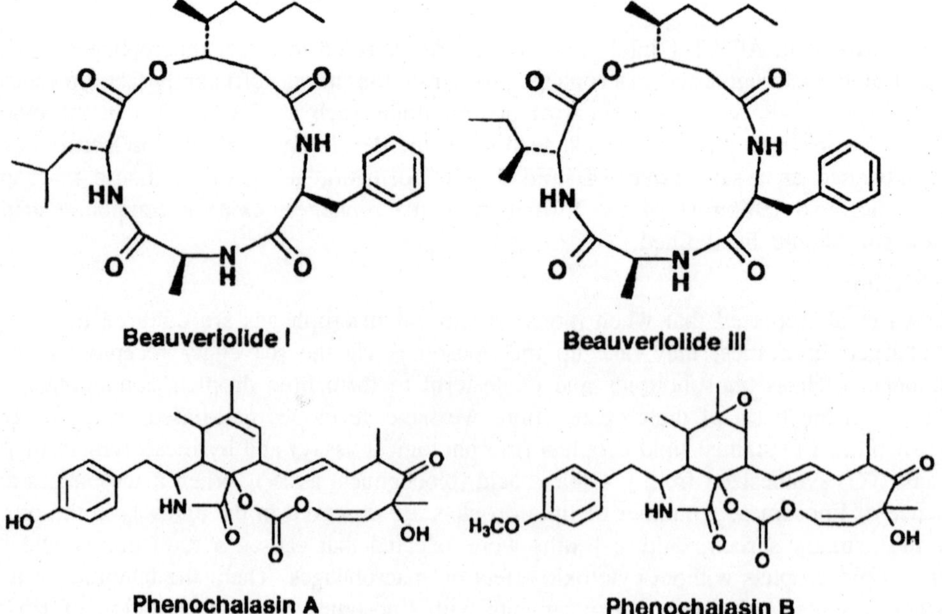

Fig. 7.14. Structures of inhibitors of lipid droplet formation in macrophages.

the mode of action revealed that they inhibit ACAT activity in microsomes prepared from both mouse macrophages and mouse liver, suggesting that beauveriolides inhibit ACAT-1 and -2 to similar extents. Among cyclodepsipeptides tested, beauveriolides I and III are the only ACAT inhibitors effective in morphological and bio-chemical assays using intact macrophages. We are planning to test beauveriolides in an *in vivo* model of atherosclerosis using LDL receptor-deficient mice.

Recently, phenochalasins A and B, belonging to the cytochalasan family, were isolated from the fungal culture broth of *Phomopsis* sp. FT-0211. Phenochalasin A has a unique phenol residue. Therefore, the effects of phenochalasins A and B and cytochalasin D on lipid droplet formation in macrophages were tested in morphological and biochemical assays. Phenochalasin A inhibits the formation in a dose-dependent manner at 0.5–20 μM without any toxic effect on macrophages. Cytochalasin D also inhibits lipid droplet formation but only in a narrow range of concentrations (0.5–1.5 μM), and with cytotoxic effects at higher concentrations ($>$2.0 μM). Phenochalasin B has a toxic effect on macrophages at concentrations tested (0.2–20 μM). From the biochemical assay, phenochalasin A and cytochalasin D inhibit CE synthesis specifically, with IC_{50} values of 0.64 and 2.4 μM, respectively, while phenochalasin B inhibits both CE and TG syntheses. Thus, these members of the cytochalasan family have different effects on lipid droplet formation in macrophages. Tabas et al. reported that cytochalasin D inhibits lipid droplet formation by specifically blocking CE synthesis in mouse macrophages, indicating that actin cytoskeleton is responsible for CE synthesis. However, our experiments suggested that phenochalasin A does not inhibit actin cytoskeleton, but the mechanism of action remains to be defined. Anyway, phenochalasin A is the best inhibitor of lipid droplet formation in macrophages among 10 cytochalasans tested.

From this screening work, it is expected that novel microbial products which affect the ACAT-1, TG synthetic pathway or unknown sites responsible for macrophage-derived foam cell formation will be discovered, leading to a new type of anti-atherosclerotic agent and providing a novel target for pharmaceutical intervention.

Future of Screening

Recent advances in biotechnology and molecular biology have provided researchers with a new strategy and methodology for drug discovery screens. Mammalian cells or microorganisms are easily manipulated to express or disrupt target genes, and swap similar genes, and such artificial organisms or expressed enzymes are introduced to automatic robotic or high-throughput screening systems.

Enzymes involved in biosynthetic or metabolic pathways have been targets in the development of new drugs. Squalene epoxidase in the sterol biosynthetic pathway, for example, is important not only as a promising target for cholesterol- lowering agents as described first, but also as a potential target for antifungal drugs. A screening system for squalene epoxidase inhibitors was constructed by using artificial microorganisms. Allylamine derivatives such as terbinafine and tolnaftate were originally synthesized as antifungal agents inhibiting fungal (or yeast) squalene epoxidase. Later, Banyu researchers found a new allylamine, NB-598, to be a potent inhibitor of mammalian squalene epoxidase, with the important implication that mammalian and fungal squalene epoxidases show different sensitivity to certain drugs. Meanwhile, the genes encoding squalene epoxidase were cloned from yeast, fungus and rat. Sakakibara et al. succeeded in cloning the rat squalene epoxidase gene by utilizing these inhibitors. They introduced the rat gene to yeast (*Schizosaccharomyces pombe* JY266) to construct a transformant *S. pombe* RSE, which possesses squalene epoxidases of both yeast and mammalian origins. The wild JY266 and transformant RSE strains have been utilized for screening for specific inhibitors of yeast or mammalian squalene epoxidase. Growth of the wild strain is inhibited almost completely by terbinafine even at 0.2 μg/ml and dose-dependently by tolnaftate (0.2–2.0 μg/ml), but growth is not inhibited by NB-598 (2.0 μg/ml). Conversely, the growth of the transformant in the presence of terbinafine or

Strain JY266

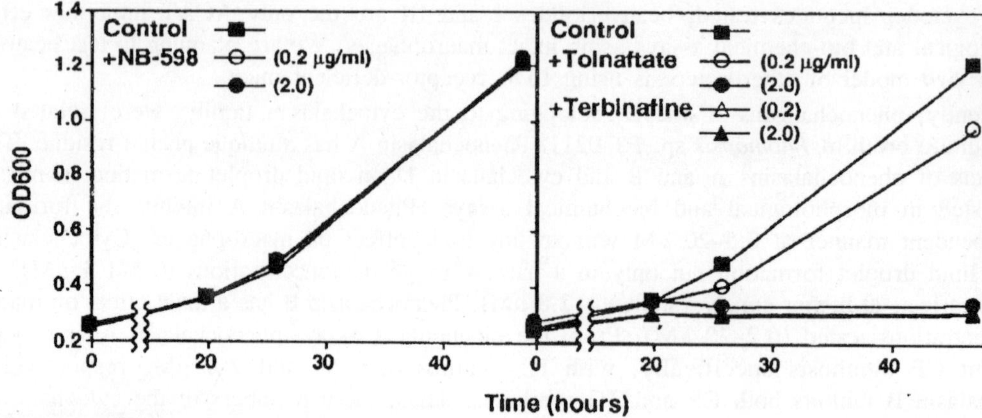

Strain RSE

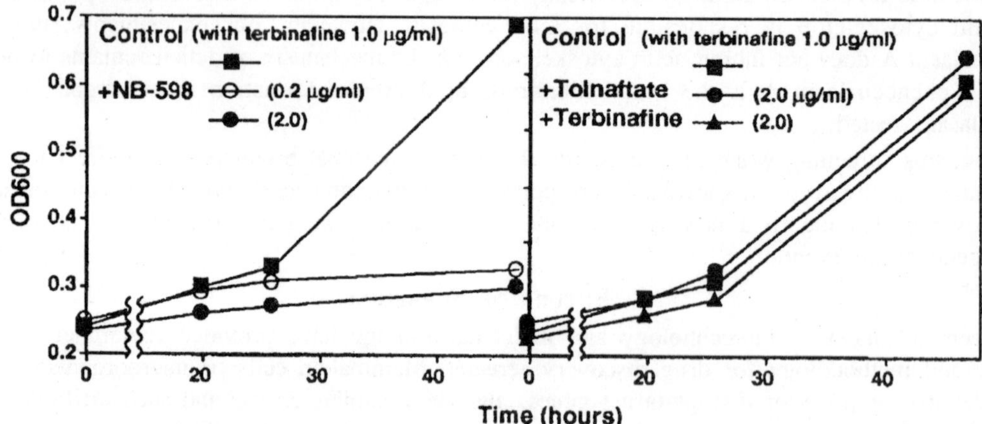

Fig. 7.15. Selective growth inhibition of S. pombe JY266 and RSE strains by terbinafine and tolnaftate and by NB-598.

tolnaftate (1.0 µg/ml) to block yeast squalene epoxidase is inhibited by NB-598 at 0.2 µg/ml, but not by a further addition of terbinafine nor tolnaftate at 2.0 µg/ ml. Ideally, a yeast strain swapping the yeast squalene epoxidase gene for the rat one is better than the transformant RES as a test organism for the screening because terbinafine is not needed for the assay. This strategy of using intact artificial organisms and manipulating desired genes is expected to spread in the near future. For example, even though host and pathogenic organisms possess the same enzymes, but with different characteristics like squalene epoxidase, this strategy will be useful in screening for specific inhibitors of the target enzymes.

Target enzymes expressed biotechnologically are also introduced to HTS systems. Merck researchers reported a new approach to drug screening by combinatorial enzymology. They have engineered a cell-free bacterial cell wall biosynthetic pathway to assay simultaneously six of the enzymes in the biosynthetic sequence. More than 40 compounds including penicillin and other beta-lactams and glycopeptides are used as antibiotics, but most of them inhibit the enzymes responsible for the last few steps in the cell-wall biosynthetic pathway. They aimed at the murein biosynthetic enzymes (MurA through MurF) involved in the earlier steps in this pathway as valid and promising targets for drug discovery. Since the pathway enzymes have evolved conserved binding motifs to bind structurally related pathway metabolites, an inhibitor that recognizes homologous binding motifs will likely bind to more than one enzyme in the pathway. They expect that modest inhibition of several enzymes will reduce flux through the pathway more effectively than potent inhibition of a single enzyme, and further that the frequency of target-mediated resistance to such a compound would be negligible. This approach can be applied to any therapeutically relevant metabolic pathway.

A number of projects on genome sequencing including that of human and pathogenic organisms are in progress worldwide. The achievements promise to be of great benefit to drug discovery. In 1998, the genome sequencing of *Mycobacterium tuberculosis* was completed. It was believed that tuberculosis caused by *M. tuberculosis* would eventually be eliminated, but the microorganism has proved to be very resilient and the disease continues to be a public health threat. *M. tuberculosis* has unique cell wall lipids called mycolic acids. These extremely long fatty acids form a broad family of more than 500 closely related structures and comprise about 30% of the dry weight of *M. tuberculosis*. Recently, Barry and co-workers identified an enzyme in mycolic acid biosynthesis that is targeted by isoniazid, the most widely used antituberculosis drug. Moreover, the complete genome sequence predicts that the microorganism produces about 250 distinct enzymes involved in fatty acid metabolism, while there are only 50 for *E. coli*. These findings imply that the enzymes are promising targets for new antituberculosis drugs.

New enzymes for drug discovery have been identified through biosynthetic studies on microbial metabolites. It has been long accepted that isopentenyl di-phosphate, an intermediate of sterols and terpenoids, is synthesized only through the mevalonate pathway. However, it has been shown that a mevalonate-independent (nonmevalonate) pathway of isopentenyl diphosphate biosynthesis is present

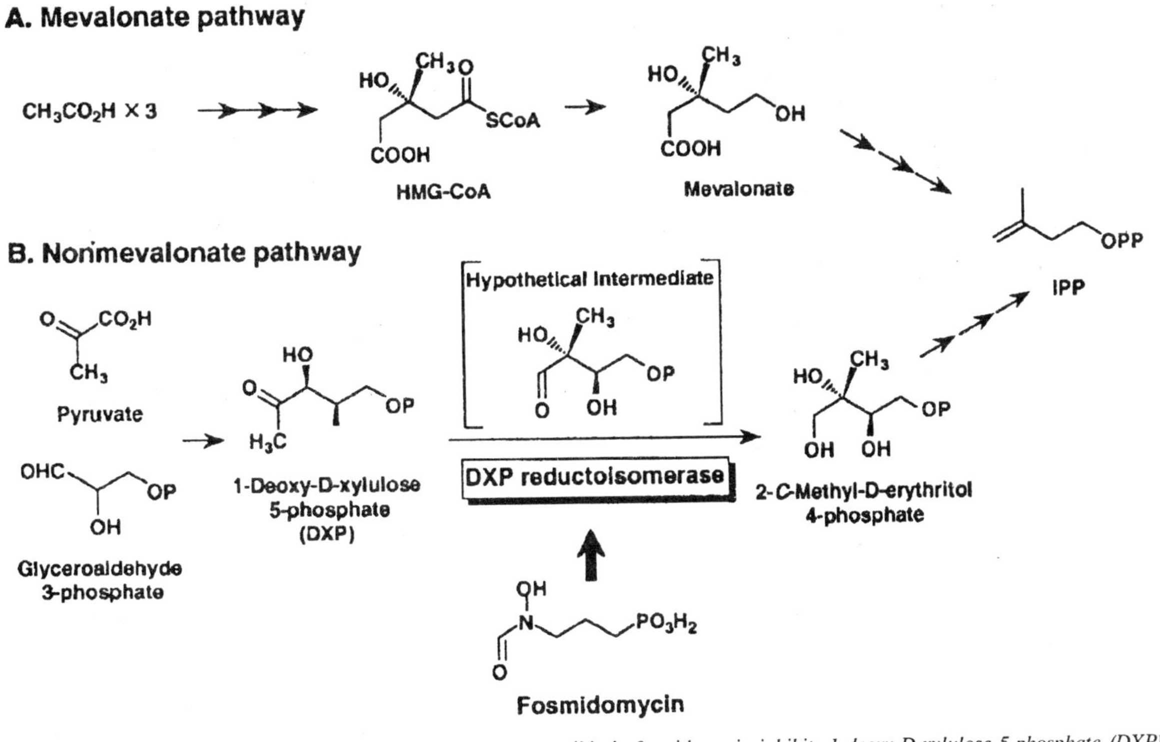

Fig. 7.16. Mevalonate pathway and nonmevalonate pathway. Antibiotic fosmidomycin inhibits 1-deoxy-D-xylulose 5-phosphate (DXP) reductoisomerase.

and essential for some bacteria, algae, plants, and malaria. Recent studies revealed that the initial step of this pathway is the formation of 1-deoxy-D-xylulose 5-phosphate (DXP) by condensation of pyruvate and glyceraldehyde 3-phosphate and the second step is the intramolecular rearrangement of DXP to 2-*C*-methyl-D-erythritol 4-phosphate via hypothetical intermediate 2-*C*-methylerythrose 4-phosphate. Seto and co-workers succeeded in the cloning and overexpression of the gene encoding the second reaction (DXP reductoisomerase), and established an assay system, leading to the finding that a known antibiotic fosmidomycin is a potent and specific inhibitor of DXP reductoisomerase. Moreover, *Plasmodium falciparum* strains possess the nonmevalonate pathway, and fosmidomycin was shown to be active against the malarial enzyme and to inhibit the *in vitro* growth of multidrug-resistant *P. falciparum* strains. Thus, enzymes involved in this nonmevalonate pathway are effective targets for new antibacterial and antimalarial drugs.

8

ANALYTICAL METHODS

The word chiroptical is descriptive of the techniques that use optical detection devices that are selective toward optically active (chiral) materials and/or molecules. They are used for structural investigation and analytical determination. There are three chiroptical techniques:

1. Polarimetry, which deals with the angular rotation of plane polarized light, usually at a single wavelength.
2. Optical rotatory dispersion (ORD), in which the angular rotation of the plane polarized light is measured as a function of the wavelength.
3. Circular dichroism (CD), in which the angular rotation is measured as a function of wavelength, but the light is circularly polarized.

Absorption of light energy is not essential to either polarimetry or ORD. It is, however, an integral part of the CD phenomenon making this method the most selective detector for chiral substrates.

THEORY

Theories of optical activity are described in detail in a number of studies. The physical phenomenon was first observed during experimental investigations of the transmission of solar radiation through Iceland spar, a natural form of CaCO3, by the French astronomer Arago. One year later, Biot was the first to demonstrate that solutions of certain organic compounds also rotate a beam of incident polarized light. Biot and Fresnel, working independently, reported that the rotatory power of a substance increases as the wavelength is decreased, the phenomenon now called ORD. By 1846, Haidinger had reported differences in the measured absorptions of left and right circularly polarized light, which is the origin of CD. The first experimental interpretation of the physical basis for optical activity was provided by Pasteur, who observed the hemihedrism of tartrate crystals, which was visually manifest by tetrahedral facets oriented either right or left with respect to the main crystal surfaces for two crystalline forms. His observation that a linearly polarized beam of light was rotated in opposite angular directions by aqueous solutions prepared from the separated crystal forms demonstrated the first direct connection between macroscopic and microscopic, or molecular, asymmetry.

The first theoretical model of optical activity was proposed by Drude in 1896. It postulates that charged particles (i.e., electrons), if present in a dissymmetric environment, are constrained to move in a helical path. Optical activity was a physical consequence of the interaction between electromagnetic radiation and the helical electronic field. Early theoretical attempts to combine molecular geometric models, such as the tetrahedral carbon atom, with the physical model of Drude were based on the use of coupled oscillators and molecular polarizabilities to explain optical activity. All subsequent quantum mechanical approaches were, and still are, based on perturbation theory. Most theoretical treatments are really semiclassical because quantum theories require so many simplifications and assumptions that their practical applications are limited to the point that there is still no comprehensive theory that allows for the predetermination of the sign and magnitude of molecular optical activity.

A chiral substance is defined by the International Union of Pure and Applied Chemistry (IUPAC) as one that interacts differently with left and right circularly polarized light. Two types of molecular optical activity are recognized: inherent dissymmetry characterized by large rotational strengths and inherently symmetrical, but asymmetrically perturbed, molecules for which rotational strengths are less by a factor of a thousand or so.

The first group is characterized by the absence of a plane of symmetry in the molecule, e.g., hexahelicine. The latter type requires the existence of a chromophore in close proximity to an asymmetric center, such as a carbonyl group adjacent to an asymmetric carbon atom.

Polarimetry

Unpolarized light is thought to consist of an infinite number of time-dependent electric and magnetic fields that vibrate in phase and at right angles to each other in planes that are orthogonal to the axis of propagation. Only the electric vector is considered in theoretical discussions of optical activity. Linearly polarized light is represented by only one of these planes and is given by the vector sum of two in-phase components of equal intensity that are circularly polarized in opposite directional senses. The components actually propagate in a helical manner with time; however, the polarization projection on the plane, which is orthogonal to the axis of propagation, is circular, thus, the acquired description of light as circularly polarized.

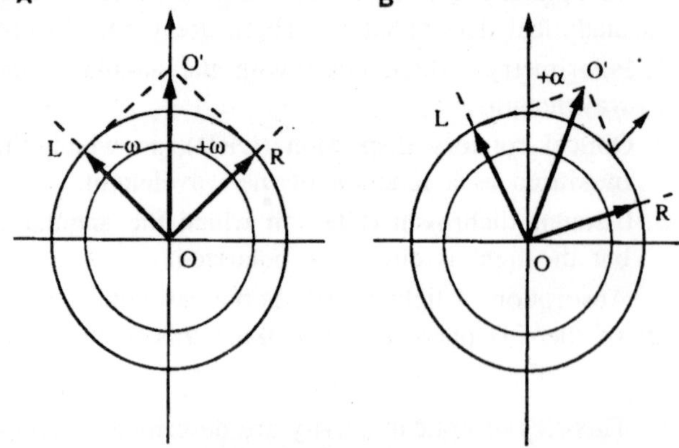

Fig. 8.1. The incident linearly polarized light OO′ is composed of left and right linearly polarized rotating components OL and OR of equal length.

As linearly polarized light is transmitted through an achiral medium, a single refractive index η is seen by both circularly polarized components, and their rates of propagation are equal. The result is that the vector sum is always a linearly polarized beam oriented along the direction of the incident beam, OO'. In contrast, because of the distinctly different interactions that occur between the two helical electromagnetic fields and the helical electronic motion in a chiral medium, two different refractive indices, η_L and η_R, are presented to the coherent beam (birefringence). There being two refractive indices, the left and right components propagate out of phase. On summing the vectors for the transmitted beam, represented for instance by the diagonal of a parallelogram for which OL and OR are adjacent sites, the polarization is still linear; however, a net rotation from the incident direction by an angle equal to α will have occurred. Rotational strengths are equal and opposite for optically active molecular or mirror-image pairs (enantiomers) of equal purity.

The magnitude of the optical rotation α (in degrees) is directly proportional to the refractive index difference and to the sample pathlength d, indicative of the fact that rotation is an extensive property, as shown in Eq. (1):

$$\alpha = (\pi d/\lambda)(\eta_L - \eta_R)(1800/\pi)$$
$$= (1800d/\lambda)(\eta_L - \eta_R) \quad \ldots(1)$$

and inversely proportional to the wavelength, in keeping with the observed increase in rotatory power with decreasing wavelength. The quantity $(1800/\pi)$ is included to convert radians to degrees. The magnitude of the birefringence $(\eta_L - \eta_R)$ that produces an angle of rotation equal to 1.0° at the Na–D line (590 nm), for a sample with a 10-cm pathlength, is only 3.2×10^{-8}. Because refractive indices are typically approximately 1.0, it is obvious that the absolute size of the birefringence effect is extremely small.

To normalize rotational values when comparing solutions of different concentrations, the specific rotation $[\alpha] = \alpha/c'd$ was defined, where c' was expressed in g/cm^3. This unit is an improper choice for making comparisons among substances with different molar masses M, and therefore $[\alpha]$ was replaced by the molecular rotation term $[\Phi] = [\alpha]$, M/100. In the older literature $[\Phi]$ was expressed in degrees × cm^2/decimole. Division by 100 had no physical meaning whatsoever and was introduced only to keep numbers small. IUPAC has determined that the term molecular rotation is improper and recommended that it be replaced with the more accurately descriptive molar rotation.

Optical Rotatory Dispersion

Two types of ORD were first described in 1852 by Biot. In his earliest quantitative experiments on quartz, he demonstrated that the optical rotatory power α varies inversely with the square of the wavelength: $\alpha = \kappa/\lambda^2$. Measurements on a large number of chiral organic compounds, dissolved in solvents both chemically and optically inactive, showed that most of these appeared to obey this law. Originally referred to as the "orthodox" class, these compounds are now thought to produce a plain or normal ORD curve. The distinctive property of the plain curve is that it is always concave to the $\alpha = 0$-axis, regardless of whether the dispersion is positive or negative. A substantial number of organic molecules, however, were found that did not appear to obey this law but had enormously large rotational powers compared with plain curves, which were limited to relatively narrow ranges in the spectra. Biot referred to this smaller group as the "heretical" class because of their anomalous behavior. Tartaric acid was the seminal example. In an effort to more accurately distinguish between the two types, Lowry specified that for normal ORD behavior, the specific rotation α and its first and second derivatives with respect to wavelength must all maintain the same sign throughout the wavelength range over which the medium is transparent. In other words, it is a mathematical statement to the effect that there should be no zero, no maximum, and no reversal of sign for α as the spectrum is scanned, that is, the curve is always concave to the axis.

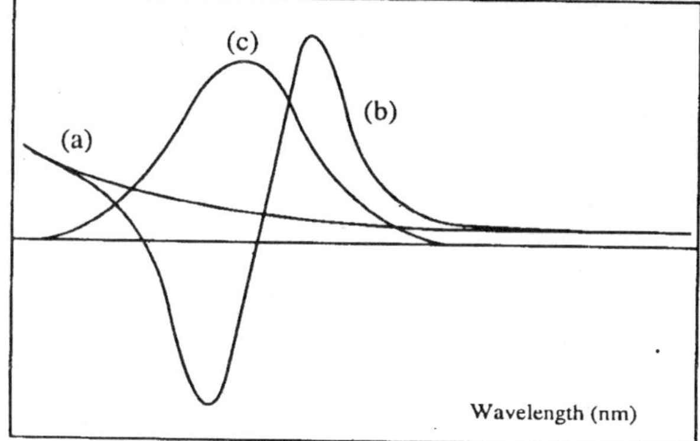

Fig. 8.2. Composite diagram of the three chiroptical dispersion spectra: (a) A positive plain ORD curve; (b) a positive anomalous ORD curve; (c) a positive CD curve for a single Cotton effect.

Among the first experimental discoveries regarding the origins of anomalous dispersion was the observation that the effect could be created by mixing pairs of natural products that generate plain ORD curves, provided they were of opposite signs and unequal rotatory strengths, for example, (l)-turpentine and (d)-camphor. This observation was to be of fundamental importance in the subsequent development of theories for anomalous dispersions. For solutions of tartaric acid, a single pure substance, the existence of an anomalous dispersion was more difficult to explain. It was first assumed that an equilibrium mixture of two molecular forms that generate plain curves of opposite signs must exist in solution. Eventually, however, the effect was correctly interpreted as being a consequence of the molecule having two asymmetric centers that give rise to the "required" unequal and opposite rotations.

The development of several mathematical models and interpretations followed, with the best interpretation being proposed by Drude in Eq. (2), where i = 1,2,3, ..., m:

$$\alpha = \Sigma_i \{k_i/\lambda^2 - \lambda_i^2 \qquad \ldots(2)$$

In modern terms, this is rewritten using molar rotational values by replacing α with $[\Phi]$ and k_i with A_i. Drude originally referred to λ_i as the "*characteristic vibrational*" wavelength, meaning that there were periods of vibration of the charged particles that, when close to the vibrational period of the incident light, would produce the anomalous effect. Again, in modern terms, these are identified with wavelengths of maximum absorbance in the electronic absorption spectra. Whenever $\lambda > \lambda_i$, that is, the wavelength of observation is outside the range of an absorption band, the Drude equation is reduced to the one-term Biot expression for a plain curve. As the value of λ approaches λ_i, α increases asymptotically, reaching infinity at $\lambda = \lambda_i$. Immediately past the maximum wavelength, α is numerically close to minus infinity, and as λ continues to decrease, the curve follows along an inverse asymptotic path towards zero.

The anomalous positive ORD curve is rounded at finite values for the maximum (peak) and minimum (trough) extremities. The crossover wavelength, where $\alpha = 0$, generally coincides with the wavelength of the maximum absorbance. An anomalous curve is always superimposed on a fundamental plain curve that is alluded to as the background rotation. Media confirmed to have just a single anomalous dispersion can be solved for λ_i. Historically, this procedure was used to predict the wavelength maximum for an incomplete absorbance band that could not be observed in its entirety because of instrumental limitations. This particular application of ORD is now obsolete.

An anomalous curve is referred to as a Cotton effect in honor of the French physicist Aime Cotton who, in 1892, was the first to point out that the absorption of light energy was the other physical property behind anomalous ORD and CD. Positive and negative anomalous dispersions are equally evident in practice. In ORD, the sign of a Cotton effect, by convention, is defined to be positive when the peak precedes the trough as the wavelength decreases and vice versa. A simple structural way of looking at the origins of ORD in a single molecule is to imagine that the fixed asymmetry of a saturated chiral group induces a degree of dissymmetry into an unsaturated and therefore symmetrical functional group or chromophore. In theory $\sigma - \sigma^*$ electronic excitations are possible for saturated molecules for which the theoretical limit of λ_i was determined to be ≈150 nm. Chromophores, on the other hand, absorb at much longer wavelengths in the easily accessible range of modern instrumentation. The closer 150 nm is approached, the harder it is to measure a spectrum. Whenever the induced dissymmetry is opposite in sign to the fixed asymmetry, anomalous dispersion is produced. The mutual

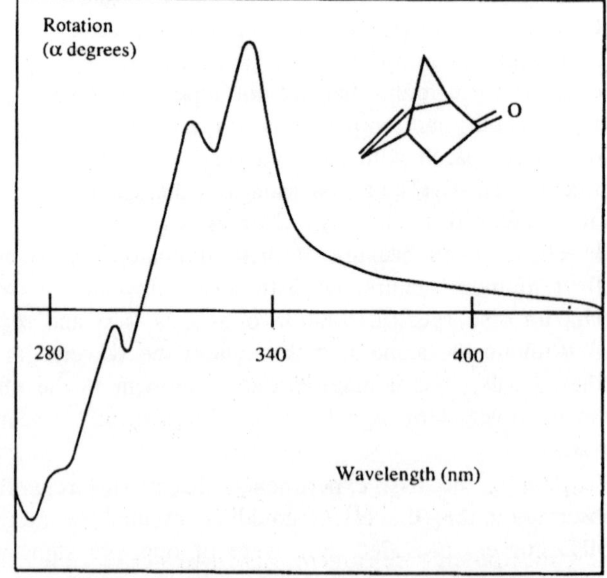

Fig. 8.3. The anomalous ORD spectrum consisting of several overlapping Cotton bands of the unsaturated rigid ketone, bicyclo(2,2,1)hept-5-enone, which shows how complex the spectrum can be, even for a single molecule.

proximity of the asymmetric center and the chromophore is a necessary prerequisite to CD induction. Dissymmetry is the preferred description for the induced chirality because the chromophore might well have a high degree of axial symmetry. How this perturbation might occur has never been satisfactorily explained.

In reality, the occurrence of a complete curve in the electronic spectrum is rare. Complete dispersions are more likely to be observed in the vibrational spectral range because of the increased spectral resolution. However, even there, dispersions are too often complicated by extensive band overlap. The same is true for electronic spectra where hidden absorption bands coupled vibronic excitations and interferences from bands associated with other chiral chromophores contribute to producing anomalous ORD curves that are so complex they have little utility in quantitative analytical applications.

Circular Dichroism

Because absorption is a prerequisite to CD activity, the phenomenon is limited to only those wavelength ranges that encompass an absorption band in any part of the electromagnetic spectrum. Outside the range of absorption, the CD signal is zero, which is the first important advantage CD has over ORD as an analytical detector. It should be emphasized, however, that the absence of a band is not evidence of the lack of chirality in the substrate.

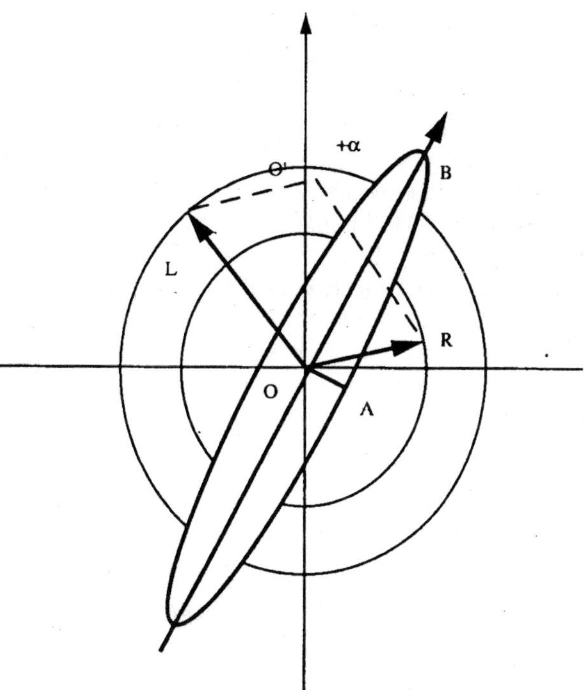

Fig. 8.4. Production of elliptically polarized light in CD. The direction of polarization of the incident beam is OO′.

At the time that Cotton was correctly interpreting the physical origins of anomalous ORD behavior, he proposed that there is also a difference between the absolute absorbances of the two circular polarized beams by a chiral medium (dichroism) and that the magnitude of the dichroism is proportional to the absorbance difference. Convention has dictated that the difference is always written as the absorbance of the left rotating beam minus the absorbance of the right, $\Delta A = A_L - A_R \neq O$. Using the Beer–Lambert law to convert A to molar units, the dichroism expression can be rewritten as $\Delta\varepsilon = \varepsilon_L - \varepsilon_R$, where ε has the units of L/mol cm. The wavelength of the maximum CD coincides with the crossover wavelength of the ORD dispersion. Shorter lengths for the vectors OL and OR are used to convey the fact that absorption has occurred. The absorbance difference at a given wavelength is then represented by unequal vector lengths OL ≠ OR. The resultant of OL and OR, given by the instantaneous diagonal vector OO′ of the parallelogram OLO′R, no longer oscillates in a single plane, but traces out the perimeter of an ellipse as OL and OR rotate around an angle 2π. The transmitted beam is rotated by the angle α from the original plane of polarization (owing to birefringence) and is elliptically polarized owing to dichroism.

The eccentricity of the elliptically polarized light is characterized by the term ellipticity Ψ equal to the arc- tangent of the ratio of the minor to the major axis of the ellipse. Because the ratio $(\Delta_\varepsilon/\varepsilon)$ necessary to produce an observable CD signal is as small as 1 part in 10^7, the ellipticity is approximated almost exactly by the expression $\Psi = \pi(\varepsilon_L - \varepsilon_R)/\lambda$, which is entirely analogous to Fresnel's equation that relates birefringence to α and points up the common origins of anomalous ORD and CD. In keeping with the older definitions of terms that are part of polarimetry, there are definitions for specific ellipticity $[\Psi] = \Psi.c'.d$, and molecular ellipticity $[\Theta] = [\Psi]$ M/100, where M is the molar mass. With appropriate substitutions, the molecular ellipticity can be expressed in terms of e, namely $[\Theta] = 3300(\varepsilon_L - \varepsilon_R) = 3300\ \Delta\varepsilon$. The numerical constant is the result of all the physical conversion factors. The survival of these arcane units is a consequence of the wealth of informational data already in the literature. The disclosure that CD is no more than a modified absorbance technique should ultimately motivate investigators to adopt the term molar ellipticity, Θ_M, in the CD analog of the Beer–Lambert law, that is, $y = \Psi = \Theta Mcd$.

Anomalous ORD and CD both originate from light absorption by a chiral species and as such contain the same information. A mathematical equation, the Kronig-Kramers transform, relates one to the other over the wavelength range of the absorption, namely, $[\Theta(\lambda)] = -2/\pi\ [\Theta(\lambda')](\lambda'^2/\lambda^2 - \lambda'^2)d\lambda'$. When the appropriate substitutions are made, the equation relating ORD to CD reduces to $\Theta = 40.28\Delta\varepsilon$.

Because all the rules that apply to absorbance detection apply equally well to CD, it is convenient to think of CD as a modified form of absorption spectrophotometry. Spectra are temperature- and pH-dependent; non-linear correlations of signal versus concentration are commonplace and are produced for the same reasons, such as chemical equilibria, polychromatic radiation, stray light, etc. Fluorescence emission CD (FDCD) spectroscopy is observed whenever an analyte meets all three of the structural prerequisites simultaneously, either intrinsically or extrinsically. Therefore, anyone with experience in absorption and emission spectrophotometries can easily become acquainted with the experimental capabilities of CD. Similarities end there, however, and the differences are what make CD detection unique, especially the enhanced selectivity that arises from the fact that CD bands can be positive or negative in sign. Electronic absorption bands are generally broad and lack the kind of resolution associated with the infrared range. In contrast to visible-UV absorptions, however, exciton coupling can divide CD bands into two sub-bands of opposite sign and unequal intensity separated by a characteristic crossover wavelength where the signal is zero, resulting in narrower bands than those given by absorption. Circular dichroism is used most often for the analysis of bulk samples and has seen limited use in liquid chromatography and capillary electrophoresis.

CD activity can be induced into molecules that are either chiral or achiral and is generally referred to as extrinsic CD. For chiral species, intrinsic and extrinsic CD effects are additive. Compared with intrinsic CD, the extent of extrinsic or induced chiroptical effects is small. One way to induce activity is to apply a static magnetic field whose strength is on the order of 10–20 k Gauss. Magnetically induced CD (MCD) was originally described by Verdet and correctly interpreted by Faraday in what has become known as the Faraday effect. A magnetic field of sufficient strength splits the degeneracy of the electronic ground and/or excited states (the Zeeman effect), resulting in absorbance differences between the two circularly polarized beams. The effect is entirely general and can be observed in every dielectric substance that transmits light. The magnitude of the effect depends on the relative orientations of the light path and the magnetic field strength and is at maximum when the fields are parallel. For a fixed geometry, the maximum signal is proportional to the sample pathlength and the analyte concentration. Poor sensitivities and even poorer selectivities associated with MORD and MCD make them unacceptable as analytical detectors.

A second way to induce chiroptical behavior is to associate a chiral center on one molecule with a chromophore on another by some aggregation or complexation reaction. If the chiral moiety is CD-inactive, only the resultant complex exhibits CD activity. The intensity of the induced CD signal is determined by two factors: the concentration of the complex that is formed and the magnitude of the induced *De* term. Magnitudes and selectivities of chemically induced CD are much greater than those of MCD and have correspondingly higher potential for analytical applications. Typically, the correlations of signal amplitudes with analyte concentrations are nonlinear.

Instrumentation

The basic instrumental needs for chiroptical methods are virtually the same as for other spectroscopic methods, namely, a stable unpolarized illuminating source of sufficient intensity, a wavelength-selection device, sample holder, and detector; polarizing elements are essential. Because the only parameter measured in polarimetry and ORD is rotation, the polarizing elements are common to both. A monochromatic source, such as an Na or Hg lamp, is all that is required for polarimetry. Deuterium or halogen lamps are of sufficient intensity for ORD, but highly intense (150–450W) Xe arc lamps are needed for CD.

Polarizing elements are transparent rhombs constructed by joining together two triangular prisms cut from a single crystal of calcite or quartz. The junction between the two parts may be just air or a light-weight balsam cement. The purpose of the junction is to physically separate the ordinary and extraordinary rays of the linearly polarized light beam, allowing only one ray to pass while the other is selectively reflected in a direction at a right angle to the first. Often, the reflected ray is fully absorbed to eliminate any interference with the transmitted ray. An excellent historic account of the assembly of the parts into working polarimeters is given by Lowry.

In polarimetry and ORD, the sample is placed between the first polarizing element (the polarizer), which remains fixed, and the second element (the analyzer), which can be rotated about the axis of propagation. Maximum intensity of the transmitted light is observed when the principal axis of the polarizer and analyzer are colinear and exactly parallel. The intensity is zero when they are crossed; that is, when the principal axes are orthogonal to each other. The most accurate way to determine the rotation angle α is to set the polarizer and analyzer in the crossed position using an achiral substrate and to measure the extent to which the analyzer has to be turned to restore the optical null position when the achiral sample is replaced by a chiral substrate.

Optical rotations are temperature-dependent. For the most accurate work, sample cells must be thermostatted. Solution concentrations are typically above 0.2 M for polarimetric detection, and path lengths range from 1.0 to 100 mm; volumes vary from 0.1 to 50 ml. Because rotations increase in magnitude with decreasing wavelength, the best sensitivities using conventional light sources are achieved in the UV. Accuracies are reported to be on the order of $\pm 0.2\%$ for rotations $> 1.0^0$. Only the most sophisticated high-sensitivity polarimeters meet the requirements for chromatographic detection. With a stable laser system as the illuminating source, rotations as small as 10^{-10} to 10^{-11} radians can be measured fairly accurately. High sensitivities are critically important in chromatography because concentrations of eluted components are very low, being limited by the retention capacity of the column materials, and because path lengths, viewed across the eluant exit tubes, are very short.

The first commercial ORD spectropolarimeters appeared in the 1950s but are no longer available. The ORD capability is typically offered as an add-on to a CD spectropolarimeter.

At present, technical difficulties associated with scanning chiroptical methods prevent the use of diode-array detection, and therefore wavelength is selected in CD with a scanning double monochromator set-up. The block diagram for CD differs from ORD instrumentation by the addition of an electrooptic modulator, placed immediately after the linear polarizer, to generate the phase-separated left and right circularly polarized component beams that are the origins of the elliptically polarized light beam. The physical parameter that was measured in the first CD instruments was the ellipticity of the transmitted beam. Greater accuracy and greatly improved sensitivities are achieved if the absorbance difference is measured, which is the procedure preferred by every contemporary CD instrument manufacturer.

Because of significant losses of radiant power on polarization and transmission through the double monochromator system needed to keep stray light to an absolute minimum, the light sources for CD detection must be intense. As a consequence, instrument compartments are purged with nitrogen to remove ozone that might be produced by the high-intensity radiation of oxygen. The detector is a photomultiplier tube. Wavelength ranges on commercial instruments extend from 180 to 850 nm. Instruments for the vibrational spectroscopy range are still only custom built. The ellipticity, or $\Delta\varepsilon$, scale should be calibrated daily against selected standards. Scale calibration is wavelength-dependent, and whenever the range of study is very broad, the use of more than one standard is recommended. Those most commonly used are androsterone, pantoylactone, (+)-camphor-10-sulfonic acid, and ammonium camphor-10-sulfonate for the near-UV, and alkaline nickel(II) tartrate in the visible.

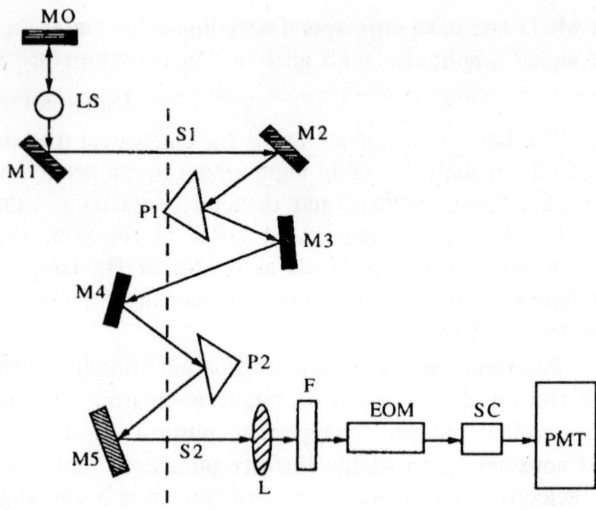

Fig. 8.5. Block diagram for a commercial double-monochromator CD spectropolarimeter.

With absorbance differences on the order of only 1 part in 10^7 for CD activity, the ratio of transmitted intensities for the left and right circularly polarized beams (I_L/I_R) is essentially one because the errors in $\Delta\varepsilon$ would be very large if I_L and I_R are measured directly.

$$\Delta\varepsilon = (\varepsilon_L - \varepsilon_R) = [(1/c\cdot d)\log(I_L I_R)] \qquad \ldots(3)$$

The problem is overcome instrumentally by measuring the intensities I_L and I_R separately, at a frequency of 5 kHz. This has the effect of producing an AC voltage proportional to the CD signal, riding on top of a steady-state DC component proportional to the total absorbance at each wavelength. The independence of IL and IR from the steady-state DC voltage indicates that the size of a CD signal is not dependent on the absolute magnitude of the absorption, and relatively strong CD signals can be obtained from overall weak absorbers. Although an absorbance difference is measured in CD detection, the total absorbance by the substrate and matrix is still a limiting feature because it can affect the intensities of the transmitted beams to be measured. Excessive amplification of very weak signals increases the noise level and adversely affects the quality of the CD signal.

The principal electronic excitations in the accessible UV range that lead to absorption by organic molecules are the $\pi - \pi^*$ transitions associated with the aromatic ring and the $n - \pi^*$ transitions of carbonyl functional groups. Excitations associated with $\pi - \pi^*$ transitions have a high probability, and absorbances are highly intense. To preserve the signal quality, solutions must be very dilute and/or path lengths must be short, which is the second advantage that CD has over polarimetry and ORD. The photomultiplier (PMT) measures the total transmitted intensity and is incapable of discriminating between chiral and achiral species. Besides affecting the signal/noise ratio, excessive absorptions reduce the linear dynamic range of the detector. At the low concentration end, the determining factor is the very small size of the CD signal, and the upper limit is determined by the total absorption. Ranges are often much narrower than they normally are using absorption detection.

Current CD instruments commercially available for analytical applications are limited to the electronic excitation range of the electromagnetic spectrum. The more sophisticated of these have the added capability of pulling an eluate from a chromatographic separation off-line into a microcell attachment where, instead of limiting detection to just one wavelength, a partial CD spectrum can be measured. Volumes can be as small as 10 nL. Instrumentation for the measurement of vibrational CD (VCD) and Raman optical activity (ROA) are still custom-built, although the prospects for their commercial development in the not too distant future are bright. A major disadvantage is, of course, that the emission intensities of tunable IR sources are generally weak.

An intriguing recent development in CD detection is its extension to the wavelength range of soft X-Rays using a synchrotron source. Although this might never become a routine analytical method, it has been speculated that from CD measurements made in this range, it will at last be possible to indisputably determine the absolute conformation of a chiral molecule of any size in solution. This would make it superior to NMR detection, which is limited to small molecules and single-crystal X-ray structure analyses, in which, for the want of other methods, structures are usually assumed to be the same in solution.

Analyte Selection

In deciding whether analytes are CD-active, it is not always a simple matter to inspect a molecular formula and be certain that the chromophore and the chiral center are mutually located in a manner that produces activity. Even if the molecular structure suggests that a chirally perturbed chromophore is present, the substance might only be available as an achiral racemic mixture and therefore is not detected by CD. Optimum wavelength ranges for CD detection are those where the absorption is minimum and the CD signal maximum. Absorptions for $n - \pi^*$ and $\pi - \pi^*$ transitions are generally weaker at wavelengths longer than 230 nm, where they appear as shoulders on the edges of the intense bands that reach a maximum at shorter wavelengths. Frequently, CD bands in the range of 230–340 nm are intense enough to allow quantitative analysis, e.g., for testosterone and dihydrotestosterone.

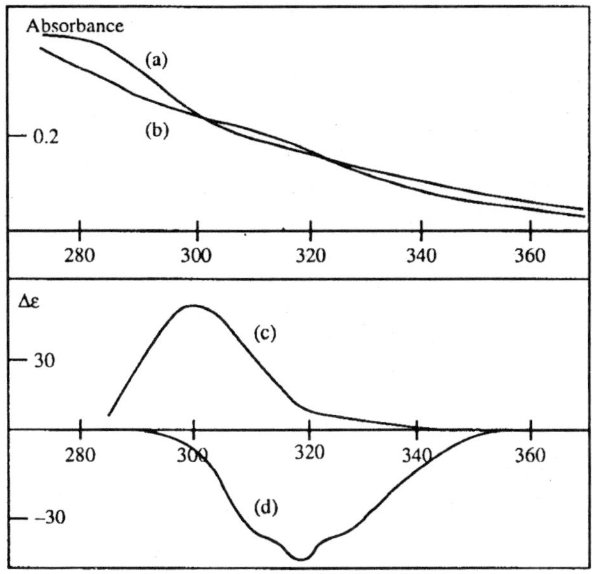

Fig. 8.6. Demonstration of the strong similarity between the absorbance spectra for (a) dihydrotestosterone and (b) testosterone in methylene chloride in contrast to their CD spectra (c) and (d), respectively.

Electronic excitation energies are shifted to longer wavelengths as the extent of molecular conjugation increases. The molecular symmetry that accompanies the structural planarity created by conjugation might reduce the number of potential achiral centers and the chances of observing intrinsic CD activity, for example, in organic dye molecules. Strong absorptions by dyes, however, are exploited by associating them with a chiral molecule to induce an extrinsic CD activity in the longer wavelength range, where passive absorption by the matrix is less of an interference. Other absorbers of this capability are colored chiral metal complexes that have the special advantage that their absorbances are generally of much lower intensity than those of organic dyes.

Similarities between CD and absorbance methods are also found between CD and fluorescence and CD and circularly polarized luminescence (CPL). Three prerequisites are needed to produce FDCD and CPL activities. Intense emission signals normally associated with fluorescence are attractive because limits of detection are lowered considerably. FDCD finds more uses as a chromatographic detection device. A CD signal is usually induced by some kind of molecular complexation reaction. Association can be with a simple molecule or with an aggregate of molecules, such as chiral micelles, which are known to be fluorescence enhancers. In cases of color induction combined with fluorescence induction, FDCD can lead to even higher levels of selectivity among analytes that have been derivatized by the same color reagent. Selectivity enhancement is a result of a number of circumstances. For example, not all of the sub-bands in the absorption or fluorescence spectrum of the derivative are necessarily CD-active; because only the chromophore next to the chiral center must fluoresce for CD activity, all other fluorescence that centers on the analyte, or in the matrix, will not interfere with the FDCD signal, and if a chiral center is lost in the derivatization process, that molecule will be removed from the list of interferences.

Chiroptical Detection in Chromatography

Only polarimetry and CD find practical use as chromatographic detectors. Important parameters to consider in modifying chiroptical detectors for use in chromatography are the very small sample volumes involved, which today can be handled with relative ease, and the very short time intervals that separate consecutive peaks, which has not been, and probably never will be, totally resolved. Peak overlap remains a significant problem. In molar terms, limits of detection are not particularly impressive, for example, micromolar levels, but in volumes as little as 1.0 μl, the limits of detection are actually at the nano- to picomole level and sometimes lower. Engineering priorities are to develop the technology to focus the beam on such small targets while maintaining the high level of radiance needed for chiroptic detection. CW lasers are an obvious place to start, but source noise and instability are problems to contend with. By exploiting the added radiance of pulsed lasers, limits of detection can be stretched to even lower levels. Laser sources, however, are limited in the number of their output wavelengths. Dye lasers offer the best, albeit still very narrow, ranges (approximately 60 nm). Current CD instruments, in which the source is laser illumination, really do operate at just a single wavelength, depriving the detector of its ability to identify an analyte. Options for multichannel LC–CD detection do exist. Stopped-flow accessories for commercial instruments are available that allow part of an eluted fraction to be taken off-line into a microcell placed in the regular sample compartment where data are measured in the normal way. The method still requires rapid scanning capabilities. Repeated injections and multiple scans can be averaged to improve the quality of the signal. A major deterrent to the progress in the early development of HPLC–CD detection was the lack of a dedicated instrument at a reasonable cost, the only option being a fully equipped CD instrument.

In 1998, Jasco International Co. introduced the first dedicated commercial polarimetric detector, the OR-990, and the first dedicated CD cum absorbance detector, the CD-1595, for HPLC. The CD detector operates in the 220-420 nm range, with a 20 nm bandwidth. The illuminating source is a 150W Hg–Xe lamp. Injections are typically in the microgram range. Minimum detectable amounts are on the 0.1 -ng scale. The sensitivity of the CD detector is typically 200 times higher than that of the OR-990 detector but of a factor of four lower than the absorbance detector of the CD-1959. The latter is the limiting factor in the combination of CD with absorbance detection when applied to enantiomeric purity measurements. This last assay has taken on considerable new meaning with the obsessive focus on measuring the enantiomeric purities of chiral drugs in the biotechnology and pharmaceutical industries.

Eventually these devices may turn out to be the starting point for the development of CD diode-array detectors. Adjusting the scanning speed for on-line, wide-spectrum CD measurements is a formidable problem. A major reason for the problem is the incongruity between the time it takes to accumulate CD data, even for just one spectral "pass" using the very best currently available diode array technology, and the typical dispersion time between chromatographic peaks. The situation may very well change as faster electronic detection devices become available.

If all the components of a sample loaded on an HPLC column are baseline-separated, any conventional detector will work, unless the object of the separation is to determine or confirm the stereochemical conformation of an enantiomer. In achiral systems, (solvent and/or stationary phase) enantiomers have identical retention times and are not separable. The problem has a solution if two detectors are used in series, e.g., CD and absorbance. Because the enantiomers elute together, the absorbance detector measures the sum of their concentrations, and the CD detector measures the difference *D*A. Solving the simultaneous equations gives the concentrations for both enantiomers.

Historically, the experimental limitations of this procedure give totally meaningless results when enantiomeric ratios are greater than 95: 5, or within 5% of being racemic. Concepts that have evolved as potential solutions to these experimental limitations making them capable of improving on the accuracies of enantiomeric purity determinations are the g-factor and principal component analysis (PCA) treatments of eluted band intensities as a function of time. These are especially useful in cases in which bands are asymmetrical, which is frequent. The g-factor is defined as the ratio of the CD intensity to the absorbance intensity $\Delta A/A$. One attribute of this factor is that for an enantiomerically pure material, the g-ratio does not change with concentration. Should a change in the g-factor occur during the elution of a band, it is clear evidence for an enantiomeric impurity. Ideal traces documenting the total resolution of bands for two pure enantiomers in a racemic mixture would consist of two horizontal lines with constant g-values of equal and opposite signs. Over the time interval between the elutions, the traces are separated by signals that are excessively noisy. This occurs because calculated g-factors in the ranges in which no CD-active species is being eluted correspond to zero divided by zero. With PCA, the number of components that are coeluted can be derived by reduction of a matrix of signal intensities versus concentrations versus time data for a series of solutions with prepared compositions.

Ostensibly, the better alternative is to separate the enantiomers on a chiral HPLC system, typically done by reacting both enantiomers of a racemic mixture with a third chiral species. The chiral derivativizing agent is an integral part of either the mobile phase or the stationary phase. The products are two diastereoisomer derivatives with different retention times. The same principle was used in classic experiments in which, for example, (–)brucine was added to separate enantiomers by fractional crystallization. It is still the only viable option to discriminate among enantiomeric forms by NMR. The numerous problems associated with chiral chromatographic methods are familiar:

1. The number of chiral derivatizing agents that are 100% enantiomerically pure is extremely small.
2. Differences in retention times are very small if the material has several chiral centers.
3. In practice, chiral solvents can be used as mobile phases only once.
4. Even if derivatization is accomplished, baseline separation is not guaranteed.
5. Racemization of the analyte may occur on the column during elution.

The protocol for separating a partial racemic mixture calls for the chromatographic conditions to be modified in such a way that the minor component elutes first and is not lost in the trailing edge of the band for the major component. Errors encountered in the determination of enantiomeric excesses when they are in the range of 98–100%, or close to unique protocol is required for every chiral analyte assayed by chiral-HPLC, requiring considerable development time and constant review of the procedure.

Direct Chiroptical Detection

In this context, direct means separation of the substrate, except solvent extraction, is not a part of the analytical work up. Only CD has the necessary selectivity to function as a direct detector. Chiral molecules that do not absorb (e.g., most simple sugars) do not interfere. Achiral molecules that absorb interfere to the extent that their absorption lowers the signal/noise ratio and the limits of detection.

Naturally occurring pigments and coloring agents added to pharmaceuticals are among the worst interferences. Overlapping bands from multiple CD-active analytes are also a concern, although there is less of a tendency for this to happen with CD compared with absorption because bands are generally narrower and often have opposite signs. Curve-fitting algorithms might be used to resolve overlapping bands, but these kinds of solutions often lead to ambiguous results. More and more attention will be given to pattern- recognition strategies that involve data analyses that use chemometric methods such as principal component analyses and artificial neural networking.

Molar ellipticities in the preferred wavelength range of 230 to 340-nm for underivatized analyses typically differ by only a factor of two or three. By comparison, linear dynamic ranges are much greater than this, and the limiting property in discriminating among CD signals is the analyte concentration rather than the rotational strength of the chiral chromophore. Limits of direct CD measurements made on bulk samples using direct transmission detection are similar to those for absorbance, approximately 100 nM for a 1.0-cm pathlength.

Reference CD Spectra

There are no comprehensive data files for CD spectra for standard reference materials (SRM) that compare with the exhaustive libraries which have been compiled for absorbance data in the electronic and vibrational spectroscopy ranges. Analysts are required to create their own CD spectral files using SRM prepared by the usual purveyors of fine chemicals. A significant problem with an SRM is that although it might meet the industry specifications for chemical purity, its enantiomeric purity is open to question. The few cases in which absolute enantiomeric purity might be assured involve natural products whose syntheses are under total enzymatic control. To prove 100% enantiomeric purity is beyond current capabilities. The problem is compounded even more with the risk that the material might racemize after its extraction from its natural environment. Therefore, it is not possible to assume absolute enantiomeric purity with firm conviction.

The superficial observation that CD spectra for enantiomers are exact mirror images of each other is only true if the two SRM used to calibrate the CD have equivalent enantiomeric purities. And even if the spectra are exact images, the evidence is not irrefutable proof that both SRM are 100% enantiomerically pure. Added complications arise when an analyte molecule has two asymmetric centers for which there are a total of four optical isomers (R,R; R,S; S,R; and S,S). Together they constitute two pairs of diastereoisomers for which there are two pairs of "equivalent" CD spectra. It is conceivable then that the wrong analyte could be identified and assayed. The practical solution of these disconcerting uncertainties is to run regular checks on there producibility of the spectrum for a chemically pure SRM that has been "defined" to be enantiomerically pure. This is done by adding spectral data for every new issue of an SRM, supplied from different product lots by different manufacturers, to an ever- increasing data pool and periodically updating the statistically averaged spectrum as the reference spectrum. The inability to get standards of absolute enantiomeric purities takes on an even greater practical significance when attempts are made to assay enantiomeric excesses or enantiomeric purities in mixtures of isomers that may have been produced synthetically.

Applications

The ubiquity of the aromatic ring and carbonyl chromophores in the molecular structure of natural products means that the number of potential analyses is enormously large. Djerrasi pointed out the analytical potential of chiroptical methods as long ago as 1960, but even now, the number of investigations is small, which is explained in part by the enormity of the field of separation sciences. Most analysts would argue that the obsession with separation is because problems with interferences are minimized. On the other hand, for many of these processes, their potential was illustrated using carefully chosen synthetic laboratory mixtures, most of which were so simple they did not even begin to address the complexities that are encountered in the analysis of real samples.

The emphases of this section reflect the author's own special interests in using CD detection to directly determine chiral substrates. The majority of the systems described are drug substances. Direct analytical applications over the last 20 or so years have clearly demonstrated that a priori expectations of serious interference problems are ill-founded. Analytical sensitivities similar to those for absorbance spectrophotometry are readily accessible, and a high degree of analytical selectivity is obtained because of that very same property that makes ORD and CD such useful structural tools, namely, the sensitivity of a chromophore to its chiral environment. Substrates are organized into three groups:

1. Those with chiral chromophores that absorb in the near-UV.
2. Those that are either chiral or achiral but do not absorb and are derivatized to absorb in the visible.
3. Those that are achiral and absorb and have optical activity induced by interaction with a chiral host.

Chiral Chromophores that Absorb in the Near-UV

The major analytes in this category are the alicyclic compounds (alkaloids and terpenes); heterocyclic compounds (barbiturates, benzodiazapams, indole alkaloids, quinolines, nucleic acids, and nucleotides); aminoacids and peptides; oligopeptides; and proteins (globular, nucleo-, and lipo-); saccharides and polysaccharides; and condensation products of saccharides with all the other analytes, e.g., glucuronides and glycoproteins. Thus far, most analyses have been done on solid and solution forms of the drug substances. A few illustrations are reported in which CD was used in the direct analysis of biological extracts.

Morphine Alkaloids

The first series of compounds assayed directly by CD detection were the morphine alkaloids. They were supported in aqueous solutions, in a chiral cholesteric liquid crystal solvent, and mixed in pellet form with solid KBr. Contrary to expectations, the homogeneous aqueous solution medium gave the best selectivity among 10 related opiates and the most quantitative results. The pH-dependence of phenol substituted analogs, which in some instances caused the sign of the CD signal to invert, enhanced the selectivity. Heroin was assayed both directly and as the morphine hydrolysate. Direct multicomponent analyses were made for prepared mixtures of morphine, codeine, thebaine, noscapine, and opium extracts.

Aromatic Amines

The strong structural similarities and the proliferation of enantiomeric forms in the phenethylamine and catecholamine series are major reasons for the considerable difficulties encountered in their analyses. Absorbance bands in the 250- to 320-nm range are identified with the aromatic ring and are non-discriminatory. Chiroptical detection methods have a slight edge over absorbance and a large advantage over electrochemical detection because of the birefringence factor. An ORD detection assay was developed to analyze mixtures of ephedrine and pseudoephedrine. An unprecedented advantage was found in the determinations of amphetamine and methamphetamine in cases in which achiral excipients such as lidocaine, procaine, and benzocaine had been added to deliberately confuse the assay by absorbance detection. These additives have absorbance spectra and retention times in achiral liquid chromatography that are too similar to the analytes.

Antibiotics

All the tetracyclines have intense visible CD spectra, with some degree of discrimination among them possible. The β-lactam antibiotics have very similar near-UV absorbance spectra, making some kind of separation the method of choice for their determination. Discrimination between the penicillin and cephalothin groups by CD detection, however, turned out to be an elementary exercise when mixtures of Pen-V and cephalothin were simultaneously determined with equal imprecisions in prepared laboratory mixtures. In contrast, discriminations among individual members of either β-lactam group is a very difficult prospect that will, in all likelihood, require a prior chemical derivatization. An ORD study reported the discrimination between the neomycin B and C amino- glycoside antibiotics. However, the strong similarities between the absorbance and CD spectra for the polymixin and bacitracin antibiotics make their discriminations by direct assay impractical unless there is first a derivatization step.

Alkaloids

Other alkaloids assayed with varying degrees of success include the quinine–quinidine, cinchonine–cinchonidine, digoxin–digitoxin, L-hyoscyamine–atropine, and pilocarpine–isopilocarpine diastereoisomeric forms. Being diastereoisomers, these have different chromatographic retention times, yet their assays are confused when compositions of the enantiomeric mixtures change. Prepared binary mixtures of the first two pairs of diastereoisomers were easily quantified using direct CD detection. Observed signals for the digoxins and pilocarpines, on the other hand, are so weak that the best possible analysis was qualitative identification. The CD spectra for the colchicine, strychnine, brucine, and tubocurarine alkaloids, all potent poisons, have been characterized in strong aqueous acids. No reports of their being assayed by chiroptical methods have appeared.

Vitamins

In the area of vitamin analyses, CD spectra have been characterized for the water-soluble vitamins B2 and C. When they occur together, their distinction by direct measurement is an elementary procedure. Both were successfully assayed in the extracts of pharmaceutical preparation, as was B12. Analysis of the fat-soluble D2 and D3 vitamins (ergocalciferol and cholecalciferol) has not been equally successful. Vitamin D extracted from natural sources has a single conformational stereochemistry that is one of several isomers produced in synthetic preparations. To certify that the natural form is present in a synthetic product, where it can be accurately assayed in the presence of the other isomers, is a formidable analytical task. Whether direct CD detection can satisfactorily solve it is currently unknown. A prior non-selective derivatization reaction might be required on all isomers. The A and E vitamins are achiral and not subject to chiroptical detection unless first derivatized by reaction with a chiral host.

Steroids

The seminal work on steroid analyses using chiroptical detection was done by Djerrasi by the determination of hecogenin acetate in the presence of tigonenin acetate. Every steroid is chiral and therefore amenable to polarimetric detection after chromatographic separation. Chromophores are fairly uncommon, and analysis by ORD or CD is therefore less suitable. The only unsaturation in the cholesterol molecule, for example, is the isolated Δ^5-double bond, which has an absorbance maximum at 205 nm. Unsaturation coupled with chirality provides some selectivity, as ably demonstrated by the work of Potapov for analogs of progesterone Even simpler than that is the direct discrimination between the ketosteroids testosterone and dihydrotestosterone, which have opposite signs in methylene chloride solution.

Gergely promoted the development of ORD methods for the Δ^4-3-Ketosteroids and the 17-Keto- and 17-Ethynyl derivatives. The 17-Keto derivative is often present as an impurity in the manufacture of 1 7-Ethynyl-substituted steroids and is easily quantitated by mathematically fitting the spectrum for the mixture using weighted spectra for the components or by measuring the spectra in two solvents. In the second option, data at two wavelengths are used to prepare simultaneous equations that are solved for the concentrations of both components. The latter was used to quantitate mixtures of corticosteroids and Δ^4-3-Ketosteroids. For the most accurate results, however, chemometrics methods are recommended with full spectral data.

Carbohydrates

Natural Products in Plant Extracts Although included in this subsection, the only carbohydrates that meet the condition of absorbing in the near-UV are the keto-, amido-, and carboxylate-substituted sugars. Fully saturated sugars absorb only at wavelengths less than 200 nm and in general have incompletely developed spectra, with many not reaching a maximum signal. In the near-UV, excellent analytical data have been obtained for the in situ determination of D-fructose in honey and of the N-acetyl content of chitosan in crustacean shells. Simple sugars commonly exist in the form of equilibrium mixtures of open-chain and cyclic anomers, in which equilibrium must be established and the temperature controlled for the most accurate and reproducible measurements. Aldoses are typically determined by high-performance liquid chromatography (HPLC) using absorbance detection at approximately 300 nm. Polarimetry can be, and has been, used whenever information on the enantiomeric forms of the eluants is needed. Kuo and Yeung combined both these detectors for the analysis of several saccharides in laboratory mixtures. An advantage is that the focus is narrowed to cover only chiral absorbers, which simplifies the analytical identification of the eluates. Of the systems in which HPLC with CD detection was used, the most common are the simplest ketoses, D-fructose, D-tagatose, D-sorbose, turanose, D-ribose, and vitamin C.

Aminoacids, Peptides, and Proteins

Most of the findings related to CD detection of steroids and carbohydrates apply equally well to these analyses. Without derivatization, only aminoacids with aromatic side-chain substituents are CD-active in the near-UV. Signals are generally weak, and enantiomeric purity measurements using polarimetry detection are not quantitative. Peptides and proteins have stronger rotatory powers with obvious potential for clinical analyses. Nevertheless, the major exploitations of these data are toward elucidating secondary and tertiary structural information in aqueous media. With respect to analytical applications, there is a larger role for these macromolecules as auxiliary or host substrates in determining low-molecular-weight substances that bind to the hosts in stereo-controlled ways, such as warfarin to human serum albumin for which FDCD is the preferred detector. The ubiquitous involvement of these materials in chirality induction for the purposes of assaying small molecules, determining enantiomeric purities, quality control, and quantitative structure-activity relationships (QSAR) is reviewed later in this article. The detector that is common to all these applications is CD.

Natural Products in Plant Extracts

A special example of the analytical selectivity of CD is its ability to directly assay natural products in plant extracts. Because there are no reference standards for plant materials, an assay is deemed to be successful if the results lie within the expected compositional ranges for that material. Analyses are not fully quantitative. Direct assays have been described for tetrahydrocannabinol and cannabidiol in marihuana extracts; S-Nicotine in leaf extracts from tobacco and tobacco products; Pen-V extracted from a crude fermentation broth; vitamin C from a variety of whole fruits, fruit juices, and whole vegetables; reserpine alkaloids from Rauwolfia; pyrethroid insecticide s; and amaryllidacea alkaloids; atropine from digitalis; and humulone from hops. Obviously, the most serious interferences would be from the absorbance by the plant pigments and light-scattering from suspended materials. The CD assays offer the advantage that the pigments are not fully extracted into the selected solvents, leaving the near-UV virtually transparent to absorption.

Exceptions to this last observation are encountered when the colored materials happen to be present in the same phase where, because of their excessive absorbances, the signal-to-noise ratio is decreased.

This kind of complication was successfully handled in direct analytical assays devised for lysergic acid diamide (LSD) and phencyclidine (PCP) in illicit drugs spiked with intensely colored dyes; for L-cocaine, morphine, and methadone in the pharmaceutical product commonly referred to as Brompton's cocktails; and for D-pseudoephedrine in children's Sudafed.

Substrates Made CD-Active by Color Induction

From what has been learned from the near-UV studies, the selectivity and the sensitivity of CD detection are greatly enhanced if the CD-active absorption bands are shifted from the wavelength range where the matrix absorbances are highest. With a few exceptions, the range of least interference is the visible. Wavelengths arr shifted by using selective color or fluorescence derivatization reactions on chiral analytes as they exist in the matrix.

Color derivatizations can be broadly divided between reversible and irreversible reactions. Reversible reactions typically involve some kind of complex formation equilibrium. The color originates on the host and is imparted to the analyte on the formation of the complex. The combination of chirality and absorbance that produces CD activity is limited to only the complex. Any absorbance by uncomplexed host or any residual chirality on the uncomplexed analyte is not detected and are therefore not interfering. Because these are equilibrium reactions, the correlation between the experimental elliptically and the analyte concentration is non-linear. An elegant and simple illustration of the capabilities of this kind of procedure is the determination of cholesterol in human gallstones in which association between the chiral cholesterol and colored bilirubin produced the CD-active complex. Analogous reactions could be exploited for other naturally occurring pigments. Other colored host molecules with obvious potential as reversible derivatizing agents are organic dyes and metal complexes of the first-row transition metals. Dyes, of course, are inherently strong absorbers, whereas transition metal complexes are not; however, the CD signals for the complexes are of similar intensities. Dyes are used as prosthetic binding groups in the CD analysis of peptides, proteins, and oligo- and polysaccharides, although more often, the object of the study is to discover stereochemical information about macromolecular structures in solution and at binding sites. Their applications as hosts for the chemical analysis of simple molecules, oligopeptides, and nucleic acids using CD detection will ultimately follow.

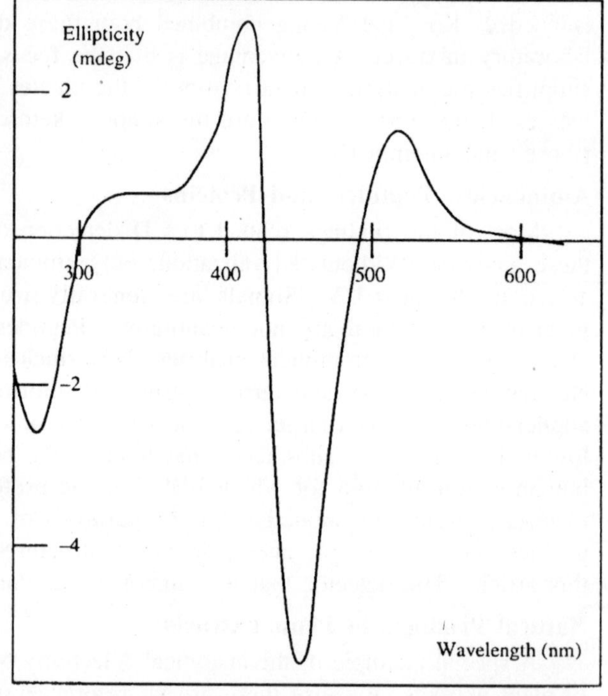

Fig. 8.7. Extrinsic (induced) CD spectrum for the complex formed between cholesterol and bilirubin in chloroform solution.

An example of a colored metal complex as an analytical prosthetic reagent is alkaline Cu(II)-tartrate, which is used routinely for the determination of total-plasma protein. Detection is by absorbance. If racemic tartrate is replaced by the L-enantiomer, the analytical reagent itself is CD-active. Exchanges of analyte ligands with the L-tartrate induce significant changes from the CD spectrum of the host complex—changes that can be used not only for structural information about interactions occurring between the ligands in the first coordination sphere, but also as an analytical method selective toward the incoming ligand. The assay is a take-off from the analytical discrimination between neomycin B and neomycin C using ORD detection. The discrimination power of CD detection allied with the ligand exchange reaction on copper-L-tartrate was demonstrated for the amikacin, gentamycin, kanamycin, neomycin, and streptomycin antibiotics. The same host complex used to measure enantiomeric excesses or ratios in difficult-to-measure compositional ranges is addressed below.

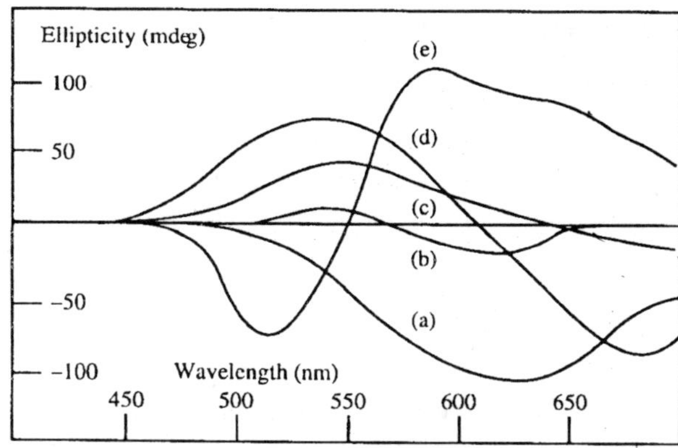

Fig. 8.8. CD spectra for (a) the chiral Cu(II)-L-tartrate metal complex and for mixed complexes of this host with equimolar amounts of (b) kanamycin, (c) amilacin, (d) gentamycin, and (e) streptomycin.

The choice of an irreversible color-induction reaction requires more ingenuity and greater care in execution. If the extended molecular unsaturation required to produce the color is too exhaustive, the chiral centers could be systematically eliminated, and must be avoided. Reaction conditions are much more unfavorable. Reagents are generally toxic and corrosive, and reaction conditions are anhydrous, e.g., the measurement of plasma cholesterol using a modified Chugaev reagent.

Substrates Made CD-Active by Chirality Induction

Although the heading implies that the analyte is achiral, it does not have to be. Greater analytical selectivity can be engendered by specific mutual influences of intrinsic and extrinsic chirality properties. Chirality induction reactions are generally reversible. Many are used extensively in chiral liquid chromatography. Developments presented here are the changes toward chiroptical detection and the applications of direct spectral measurements. Optimal conditions are achieved when chirality resides only on the derivatizing agent, and the chromophore is limited to the analyte. On reaction, the CD activity is exclusive to the molecular complex. Potential interferences from host and guest are inconsequential. The best hosts are linear and cyclic forms of oligo- and polysaccharides, such as the oligomaltoses and the cyclodextrins, which absorb only in the far-UV. Oligomaltoses are more soluble but less selective than are cyclodextrins. Virtually any material that has been used as a stationary phase in chiral chromatography is a candidate for direct homogeneous association reactions, and many others will ultimately appear, e.g., cryptands, vesicles, micelles, peptides, proteins, enzymes, antibodies, and nucleic acids.

Complexation is an equilibrium process. It is recommended that the host molecule be kept in large compositional excess over the analyte, thereby maximizing the mass-action effect and complexing as much of the analyte as possible. The larger the formation constant, the straighter the correlation line between the experimental elliptically ΔA and the analyte concentration. The β- and γ-cyclodextrins were used in exploratory investigations as analytical reagents and to determine achiral forms of barbiturates, phenethylamines, benzodiazepin-2-ones, and phencyclidine and its analogs. Initial assays were done on prepared laboratory mixtures, but successful assays were also reported for secobarbital in seconal suppositories, meperidine in demerol dispensary products, and diazepam and flurazepam in pharmaceutical preparations.

The CD spectra for chiral complexes, formed by chirality induction on organic dyes by oligomaltoses and oligocelluloses, were used to elucidate the rotational direction of the helical structures of the hosts in aqueous media. CD spectra of chiral derivatives formed by the association of aromatic residues, such as 9-Anthroate and p-Hydroxycinnamate with analogous oligosaccharides, were used to probe the local stereo- chemistry of the ring linkages and conformational arrangements of adjacent groups in acyclic polyols.

Protein hosts, whose absorbance and CD spectra are dominated by intense signals in the far-UV range (190–230 nm) are appropriate choices for introducing chirality into any molecule that absorbs at longer wavelengths, e.g., associative complexations of proteins, enzymes, and/or oligopeptides with warfarin; bilirubin and its analogs; and a few dye molecules. Beside the generation of analytical data, structural modifications at the active sites can be monitored over two spectral ranges: the far-UV, where the active group is the peptide bond, and the near-UV, where the absorber is the guest molecule. In addition, CD ought to be seriously considered as an alternative detector for immunoassays because the experimental selectivity might overcome some of the limitations associated with polyclonal antibodies.

Determination of Enantiomeric Excess in Partial Racemic Mixtures

For all types of chemical analysis, the quality of the results ultimately relates to the chemical purity of the best available SRM. For naturally chiral substances, there is the additional more serious concern over what constitutes absolute enantiomeric purity. Not even mass spectroscopy, which provides assurance that a substance is chemically pure, can be used to report absolute enantiomeric purities. To actually report an enantiomeric purity higher than 99% is truly beyond the capability of current analytical methodology. As noted previously, the fact is that results are measured relative to an enantiopurity defined to be 100%. Chemical purities aside, the measurement of enantiomeric purity and enantiomeric excess is technically the same, the difference being the extent of racemization. There are only two experimental options, either enantiomeric separations or multivariate spectroscopic analyses, that involve either two distinct detectors or multiple-wavelength detection for a single detector, as noted above. The newly described derivatization reactions fulfill the second option.

If the chosen derivatization reaction is chirality induction, a simple two-step process is to measure the CD spectrum for the underivatized partial racemic mixture, followed by a measure of the net spectrum after the addition of the derivatizing agent to the mixture. Fundamentally, the reaction is the simple competitive instantaneous complexation of the enantiomers with, for example, β-cyclodextrin, in which two diastereoisomers are formed. These might have different formation constants, or different induced spectra, or both. Regardless, the result is a change in the original CD spectrum. The two unknown enantiomeric concentrations are calculated by solving the simultaneous equations that describe the additivity of the two enantiomers in the case of the original solution and the two diastereoisomers in the case of the derivatized solution. The method was used with limited success in the measurement of enantiomeric distribution for prepared non-racemic mixtures of R- and S-Nicotine. The poor results could in part be attributed to the spectral changes being very small.

More accurate results were achieved by exchanging both the enantiomers in prepared non-racemic mixtures of ephedrines and pseudoephedrines with the coordinated L-tartrate ligand of the Cu(II)-L-tartrate host complex dissolved in 0.10 M aqueous base. The first CD spectrum is that for the parent complex and the second for the mixed ligand complexes, where only one of the two bonded L-tartrate ligands on Cu(II) is exchanged by either the (+)- or the (–)-ephedrine or pseudoephedrine enantiomers. The total signal is the sum of three terms, the CD signal from the decreased concentration of the parent complex, plus the CD signal from the 1:1 complex of Cu(II) with one L-tartrate and the (+) enantiomer, plus the CD signal from the 1:1 complex of Cu(II) with one L-tartrate and the (–) enantiomer. With careful control of the reaction conditions, the detection limit for the enantiomeric purity was on the order of ±2%. In fact, changes in the CD signal on complexation was so large that almost equivalent results were more easily obtained using polarimetric measurements at only four wavelengths.

CD Detection/Ligand Exchange for Assays of Peptides, Oligopeptides, and Proteins

With literally thousands of potential new drug substances in the combinatorial chemistry pipeline and the expanding emphasis on chiral drugs, the development of low-cost, routine quality-control procedures is becoming a priority in pharmaceutics and biotechnology. Ligand-exchange derivatization, coupled to CD detection, has the potential to do that for peptides, oligopeptides, and proteins.

Regulatory agencies have already set the standards for quality control (QC) for chiral drug substances. If it is a company's decision to market a chiral drug as a single enantiomer (the eutomer), the submission for regulatory approval must also include the equivalent chirality information for the other, non-therapeutic enantiomeric form (the distomer). An accurate determination of the enantiomeric purity of both forms is essential. Furthermore, chemical racemization will alter the eutomer to distomer ratio with time, diminishing the therapeutic property of the eutomer. Another very significant factor in QC, therefore, is to be able to accurately measure the rate of change of enantiomeric purity and decide when the meaningful therapeutic value of the eutomer has expired. By replacing the L-tartrate ligand of the Cu(II)- derivatizing agent described above with D-histidine, a very selective host complex for ligand exchange was created. Much of the analytical selectivity accomplished by full spectrum visible-range CD detection is attributable to the specifics of the ligand–ligand interactions that ostensibly occur within the first coordination sphere of the complex. The extent of the selectivity that is accomplished for peptides and proteins is extraordinarily high.

It was also determined that the CD spectral changes are extremely sensitive to changes in the amino acid sequence among residues that are far removed from the binding sites. A case in point is the individualized CD spectral changes for the exchange of D-histidine with human, human LysPro, porcine, and bovine insulin forms, all of which are 51 amino acid residue proteins. It is a known fact that proteins bind to Cu(II) ion in aqueous base by first substitution via the N-atom at the amine terminus. Chelation is completed by second and third substitutions into the metal first coordination sphere through the N-atoms of the first and second peptide functional groups. Because all four insulins have identical initial sequences, the observed CD spectral changes on ligand exchange are caused by some other structural variations. The only differences in the insulin residue sequences occur either at or adjacent to the acid terminus of the B-chain. Human insulin differs from human LysPro by the simple exchange of lysine and proline residues at positions B-28 and B-29. Porcine and human insulins differ by one residue, alanine for threonine, at position B-30. The only explanation that accounts for this is that the metal ion is enclosed by an extensive, flexible, chiral, three-dimensional architecture and that subtle differences in the conformational properties of the enclosure bring different residues into the realm of the ligand to metal ion electronic transitions. With the D-histidine kept in very large excess over the insulin analytes, there is a good quantitative linear correlation of the CD signal with concentration. What many researchers may have failed to realize in drug modeling is that when two chiral molecules interact, the stereochemical conformations of both change, and these changes may be just as significant in the mechanism of drug action as the absolute conformations of the participants themselves.

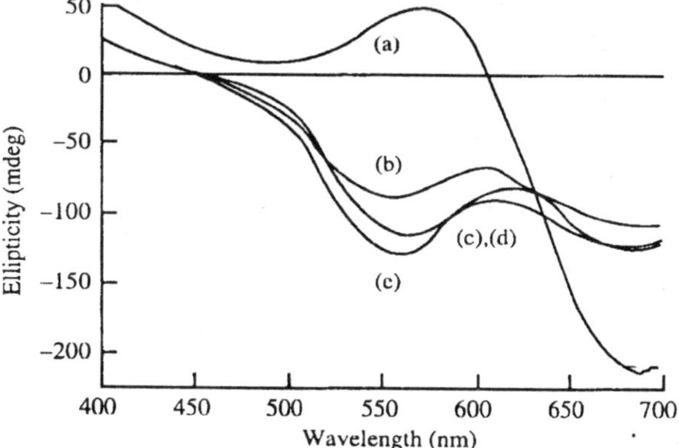

Fig. 8.9. CD spectra for (a) the Cu(II)-D-histidine host complex and for the mixed ligand complexes with (b) bovine insulin, (c) human insulin, (d) porcine insulin, and (e) human LysPro insulin.

In other tests of the ligand exchange/CD detection assay procedure, it was demonstrated that 51 of a total of 53 di- and tripeptides could be uniquely identified by the character of the changes in the CD spectra for the mixed Cu(II)-peptide-D-histidine complexes. A series of 19 neuropeptides was the focus of another investigation. Neuropeptides are invariably chiral molecules and, because of the peptide bond, are CD-active. Once again, all but two of the analogs were individually distinguishable by the CD spectra for the mixed ligand complexes. For the two exceptions, ICI 174,864 and PLO17, the terminal amine group is substituted and, as such, it is not competitive with D-histidine in binding to the Cu(II) ion. In other words, substitution did not occur. To determine whether the CD spectra had characteristic properties that could be associated with the structure of first coordination spheres of the metal complexes, a Y-correlation matrix of the CD data was subjected to principal component analysis (PCA). All of the spectra can be accounted for mathematically by only four factors. The spectral data for each neuropeptide analyte can be graphically represented by a single point in an X–Y plot of the first two principal components, PC1 and PC2.

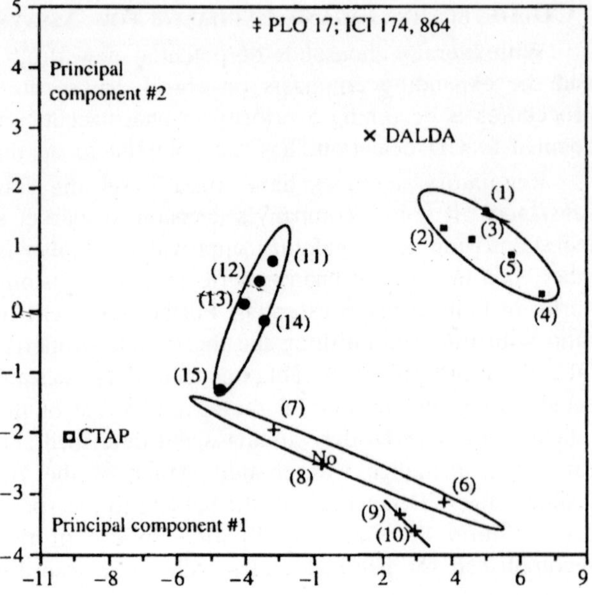

Fig. 8.10. Cluster plot of the first and second principal components derived by PCA from spectral data.

When the points are subjected to a hierarchical clustering algorithm, the neuropeptides are observed to aggregate according to their preferences for the δ, μ, or κ protein receptors. This calibration model has the potential to become a prototypical- predictive in vitro model for correlating CD spectroscopic data with quantitative structure-activity relationships (QSAR) and, on further substantiation, may become a viable procedure for new drug forms.

Despite the fact that the system is a mixed equilibrium reaction, in quantitative terms, a strong linear correlation exists between PC1 and analyte concentrations. A recurring chiral property in many of the neuropeptides is the presence of at least one D-enantiomeric residue, e.g., natural and designer enkephalins such as DALDA, DAGO, and DPDPE. Locating the position of the D-form in a sequence is a challenging endeavor that is being systematically studied on two series of model penta- and hexapeptides.

The role of D-enantiomeric forms in biotechnology drug substances is a very real interest and more especially in view of the recent recognition of the existence of D-serine, which functions as neurotransmitter in mammalian brain tissue. The D-enantiomer is synthesized in the brain from the natural L-form catalyzed by serine racemase. The intent of this article was to demonstrate, based on a wealth of relatively new experimental data, that there is sufficient analytical selectivity and sensitivity to accept polarimetry and CD as viable and easy-to-use analytical detection methods. In contrast to other detectors, they provide the capability of making direct analytical assays after a sample work-up that is a simple solvent extraction and of measuring enantiomeric purities in the ranges specified by the FDA for the process and quality control for new chiral drug substances. In the future, broader applications will be developed, especially as the current analytical emphasis turns toward nucleic acid protein interactions and the CD properties of intact single cells.

Immunoassays for Macromolecules

Current guidance documents for the assessment of analytes and their metabolites in biological fluids are focused primarily on the quantification of small molecules using chromatographic and mass spectrometry platforms. Specific recommendations coming out of these guidances fall short in the immunoassay realm. The antibody binding of analytes directly from biological fluids confers a practicality and specificity unique to these assays. These assays are typically nonlinear and experience specific issues associated with the protein matrix, e.g., the presence of endogenous materials, to name just one. Until the authorities propose a guideline targeted at best practices in developing and validating ligand binding assays (antibody-based immunoassays) to support pharmacokinetics/toxicokinetics (PK/TK), the following recommendations, based on the paper generated by a 10-member panel from Biotech, Pharma, and CROs.

Assay development and implementation are dynamic processes. The life-cycle steps of development, validation, and in-study assay monitoring can be reassessed throughout the process as the analyst benefits from the experience of extended use, adds stability data, or updates current precision and accuracy data. During early immunoassay development, it is important to assess the "intended use" of the assay. When the intended use is to support pharmacokinetics in either nonclinical PK/TK or clinical bioequivalence (BE) studies, developing a validatable assay is of utmost importance. A well-thought-out validation plan and fully documented assay methods and results that support the validation are crucial. To withstand the scrutiny of the authorities, and to guarantee the optimal method is applied to your drug development process, the following parameters should be assessed critically, validated to specific criteria, and fully documented.

Assessment Parameters

The goal of the development phase for immunoassays is to establish a method that can consistently produce a reliable result culminating in a validation plan with established target acceptance criteria for accuracy and precision. The following recommended parameters are assessed critically during early development, evaluated in late development, and finally, confirmed during validation.

Reference Material

Inherent to macromolecules is the associated variability (i.e., glycosylation and deamidation) of the material from different preparations. Therefore, it is not usually feasible to obtain a "reference standard" for a macromolecule drug for use in bioanalysis. Typically, what is obtained is a well-characterized product. Therefore, it is important to clearly state the source of the material and to refer to any documentation describing characteristics of that material. Whenever possible, the standards, the validation samples, and quality control (QC) samples should be prepared from separate vials of the same source material. In the case of lyophilized material, it is preferred to reconstitute two separate vials to prepare standards and QCs. In circumstances of limited availability of reference material (e.g., drug interaction studies where the pure standard is not available except from a limited source of commercial kits), standards and QC samples can be prepared from single aliquots after checking the comparability between lots or other commercial sources. In any circumstance, the lot numbers, batch numbers, and supporting documentation should be carefully monitored. This is a critical parameter that should be evaluated during method transfers and cross-validation studies.

Assay Format/Reagent Selection

Assay formats more recently have been defined as much by the platform (ELISA, RIA, Bioveris, Luminex) as by the type of immunoassay (direct or indirect binding, sandwich, competition or inhibition). Considering several different formats before selecting one is optimal, if time allows, because there are pros and cons to each format. Solid phase formats include glass, treated plastics, and coated plates (e.g., streptavidin). As antibody binding to the coated surface is highly dependent on pH, buffer content, salt concentration, detergents, nonspecific carrier protein, temperature, and shaking, any relevant conditions should be tested during the development of an immunoassay. When solid phase formats prove difficult, solution phase binding, for instance using coated beads, can result in a practical and sensitive assay. The antibody or pair of antibodies selected for the assay format is the primary critical reagent for an immunoassay because it will ultimately define the specificity and sensitivity of the assay. Therefore, whenever possible, as many antibodies or pairs should be tested hand-in-hand with the selection of the assay format before moving into further development. This may include whole or fragmented monoclonals, polyclonals, and combinations as the assay format demands. The time it takes to develop and purify unique reagent antibodies demands that this start as early in the drug development process as possible.

Other critical reagents are those that impact the sensitivity, ruggedness, and consistency of the assay and especially include the detection system. It is a recommendation that a list of critical reagents and criteria for their acceptance be identified before initiating sample analysis. These must also be sourced, characterized, documented, and stored under conditions defined by stability investigation. When in-house reagents make up any part of the immunoassay, it is important to define and document the source, preparation, expiration, storage conditions, and acceptance criteria for their use to ensure a reliable result. Once the final conditions are established, it is important to understand the assay's accuracy and precision capabilities because target criteria should be set for both before entering into validation. It is also good practice during validation to "stress the system" in a manner representing a true sample analysis run. Therefore, if the "batch" size is expected to be unusually large, a comparable batch, run during validation, should demonstrate that it could achieve the same acceptance criteria. It is particularly useful to evaluate the variability of QCs on every plate to predict the outcome expected during sample analysis. The established/validated format should be used during sample analysis. Changes to the format must be revalidated to the extent that a consistent format is confirmed. The acceptability of changes to critical reagents should be documented before placing them into the sample analysis assays.

Specificity and Selectivity

One challenge of interpreting results derived from immunoassays is understanding exactly what the assay is detecting. Fundamental to this is knowing to what the antibody binds, that is, determining the antibody's specificity. A related parameter, selectivity, refers to the assay's ability to solely measure the target analyte in the presence of other protein constituents in the sample, some in very high concentrations. Typically, experiments designed to determine the antibody's specificity involve assessing their cross-reactivity with similar compounds. When feasible, it is suggested that the sample matrix is spiked with physio-chemically similar compounds or variants of the target analyte.

Selectivity is the easier of the two parameters to assess experimentally. After the assay format is relatively fixed, multiple lots (at least 10 normals and 10 of the intended patient population in the case of clinical samples) of the sample matrix should be spiked near the lower limit of quantification and the recovery of the analyte should be calculated. The percent recovery of spike (expressed as relative error or %RE) is calculated as: 100× (observed mean conc − nominal concentration)/nominal concentration. This will aid in finally selecting a lower limit of quantification, before initiating assay validation. An additional experiment to understand selectivity involves spiking both the diluent and the matrix with standard curve calibrators to detect matrix effects at all concentrations across the range of calibration.

Interfering substances, especially in patient populations, that require some evaluation may include prescription and over-the-counter medication, herbal medications, dietary substances, and even the presence of antidrug antibodies and associated immune complexes. During sample analysis, new matrix conditions may develop that would require further investigation and could include hemolysis, lipemia, rheumatoid factor, and so on. Both specificity and selectivity experiments, if performed during the late development phase, after the assay format and critical reagents are fixed, may be cited in the validation report. Otherwise the experiments can be performed during validation. In both cases, the *a priori* acceptance criteria should be applied and acceptable recovery should be realized in at least 80% of the samples. Additionally, as lots of critical reagents are replenished, these types of assessments must reconfirm their acceptability.

Sample Collection Process/Matrix/Sample Preparation/Minimum Required Dilution

As mentioned, the ability of the antibody to bind to its target is the basis for assay sensitivity; therefore, maintaining the integrity of the analyte is vital. Frequently overlooked, the selection of sample matrix type and process for collection are crucial elements in bioanalysis. Rigorous investigation should go into the stability of the sample as it is collected, the anti-coagulant requirements, protease inhibitors, and other possible additives, and it should include the postprocessing storage. Furthermore, a process must be defined that provides for sample tracking "from cradle to grave" documenting the chain of custody, the sample ID, and the time spent at each location and temperature through analysis. After analysis, the archival and destruction process should be identified.

For practical reasons, the matrix of choice for immunoassays is typically serum. The plate washers or automated systems used during sample analysis easily clog when plasma is used, which then has the potential to impact the validity of the result. However, protein analytes, including cytokines that are identified as labile and prone to degradation in serum, would preferentially be collected in plasma. When collecting citrated plasma, it is wise to clearly identify the salt form of citrate (Na, K, Li) so that it is transparent what the comparable matrix should be for QC preparation.

Whenever possible, the matrix expected in the samples should be used in the preparation of the standard calibrators and QCs. Individual donors (found acceptable when assayed as blank and spiked) are pooled to produce the standard curve and QC matrix; then aliquots are spiked to produce the standard curve and QCs. Some matrices are difficult to obtain. To accommodate this, as long as the QCs prepared in the intended matrix demonstrate the accuracy and precision expected, non-matrix standard curve calibrators are acceptable.

QC accuracy assessments can be challenging when the therapeutic drug shares an endogenous protein. In this case, the endogenous protein concentration can either be added to or subtracted from the final value. Before establishing the calculations, the necessary experiments must be performed, and the consistency of the endogenous value contribution must be documented.

In cases where the endogenous interferents do not generate a linear signal, then a minimum required dilution (MRD) may be applied. A MRD is the dilution of a matrix that finally permits an accurate and precise measurement of analyte. Although the diluting sample reduces the sensitivity of the assay, it may be required to develop and validate an accurate and precise method.

Standard Calibrators and Standard Curves

As described in the Guidance for the Industry, May 2001, the "calibration curve is the relationship between instrument response and known concentrations of the analyte" in the matrix of interest. In immunoassays, the affinity and avidity of the antibody(ies) used to develop the standard curve are fundamental to the range because they define the sensitivity of the assay. The antibody (or pairs) once selected should be used throughout validation and sample analysis. During the development phase, it is a good idea to use many more calibrators and replicates evenly across the range to thoroughly describe the concentration-response relationship and to investigate the "best fit." Thereafter, select at least six to eight calibrators, over the entire range of the curve before the start of validation. Once validation begins, the standard curve calibrators should not be adjusted. Spiked standard curve points may be used outside the quantification range of the curve to help fit the curve, but they are not used in the assessment. "Best-fit" can be evaluated in a straightforward manner by fitting several regression methods to the data generated during the development phase. The relative error of the back-calculated standard calibrators should be calculated. As expected, the regression that consistently generates the most accurate and precise data is selected for confirmation in the validation phase. Usually a four- or five-parameter logistic with/without weighting describes the s-shaped immunoassay curve optimally; however, the smoothed spline has also been used with success with some platforms. It is important to critically assess whether the curves fall consistently above or below the expected concentration. This "trending" can invalidate a regression model.

Precision/Accuracy: Role of QCs

One function of the QC sample (or validation samples as they are sometimes called when used during the validation phase) is to mimic the study sample. Therefore, the therapeutic drug is spiked into a neat sample matrix, and not into a diluted or otherwise modified matrix. The QCs should be stored preferably along with the samples in the same freezer or at least in a comparable freezer. Documentation of freezer conditions will be critical to provide evidence that the conditions of samples and QCs are similar. A second function of the QC sample is to measure the degree to which the assay is under control as determined by the assessment of accuracy and precision in multiple runs. Accuracy is described as the % relative error (%RE) or the amount the assayed value deviates from the nominal value. The precision is described as the % coefficient of variation (%CV) by dividing the standard deviation by the mean value recovered value.

During development, preliminary assessments are conducted to predict not only the QC concentration values to be used but also the target acceptance criteria. In this case, it is prudent to include more QC levels than will finally be used during validation. For instance, three levels prepared at the LLOQ will likely provide a clear indication of which QC is acceptable and where the assay cannot support the target acceptance. The same can be performed for the ULOQ. At least three levels between the two asymptotes are necessary because these will be used during sample analysis. For the validation process, five QC levels should be selected for testing, based on the accurate and precise readout: the final LLOQ to be confirmed; the LQC; less than three times the LLOQ; the MQC, placed about the middle of the curve; and the HQC, placed no more than 75% below the ULOQ and the ULOQ.

During validation, the five QCs should be tested in a minimum of six runs, at least in duplicate. It is not acceptable to discard any runs during this testing. The inter- and intrabatch precision and accuracy from all runs performed should be reported. It is generally expected that the precision and accuracy acceptance be at least 20–25% of the target range with a Total Error not exceeding 30%.

During sample analysis, only the LQC, MQC, and HQC defined during validation need to be run in duplicate with every assay. The precision and accuracy should conform to that established during validation. Typically, run acceptance criteria also require that at least one QC at each concentration level is acceptable, and that four out of the six QCs assayed must be acceptable. It is recommended that method acceptance criteria that are consistent with the validation be used during sample analysis.

Range of Quantification

It is important to understand that the LLOQ and ULOQ have been selected because they define the true, accepted limits of the standard curve. Standard curve points below or above the LLOQ and ULOQ, respectively, are considered extrapolated and cannot be used to report sample concentrations. The LLOQ and the ULOQ validation samples and not the standard curve samples spiked into neat matrix define the standard curve range of quantification.

With certain toxicokinetic studies or therapeutic drugs dosed in high concentrations, the expected concentration in the sample may be well outside the quantification range as defined by the ULOQ. These samples must be diluted into the accepted range of the standard curve to determine an initial concentration and then multiplied by the dilution factor to determine the final concentration of the analyte in the sample. Although it is preferable to dilute the sample in matrix, in many cases, the process is performed in a buffer diluent.

Sample Stability (Bench Top, 4°C, –70°C)

The underlying reason that samples are tracked from "cradle to grave" is to document the integrity of the sample. Stability testing under all conditions to which a set of samples in a study is exposed supports the statement of integrity. Therefore, such testing of QC samples in matrix comprises evaluating stability during sample collection and processing: –20°C or –70°C long-term storage to cover the time from when the sample is processed to its final analysis, bench top under conditions similar to analysis, resident time in laboratory refrigerators and freezers, and freeze-thaw to cover the expected or possible cycles. Another consideration is to test the stability of the analyte in intermediate stock solutions if stored for later analysis. The samples should be thawed under the same conditions used to thaw study samples. Similarly, refreeze the samples for a length of time that would ensure complete freezing, usually 12–24 hours. Samples should be assayed using a freshly prepared standard curve, and acceptable QCs should be used to monitor assay performance. The stability samples should meet the criteria for acceptance as defined for in the validation plan.

Dilutional Linearity and Parallelism

Dilutional linearity is the ability of a QC sample spiked at a high concentration (at least as high as the expected C_{max} in a study) to be acceptably diluted into the range of the standard curve so that the initial concentration determined off the regression and multiplied by the dilution factor produces a final concentration with an accuracy and precision expected for that assay. Usually, serial dilutions are employed to ensure that at least two to three fall on the acceptable range of the curve so that linearity can be demonstrated. When a study design produces samples that require a dilution greater than that established, it is advisable to employ an equivalent dilutional QC that is run in the assay. To evaluate the "hook effect," dilute a very high QC (100- to 1000-fold greater than the ULOQ) so that the expected concentration read off the regression reads above the ULOQ. Parallelism is determined in a manner similar to dilutional linearity but with incurred samples. This is usually not possible until after the initiation of a study. When incurred samples are available, one strategy is to pool the C_{max} samples to create parallelism QCs. Serially dilute the sample so that at least two to three fall on the acceptable range of the curve to demonstrate linearity.

Robustness and Ruggedness

Robustness and ruggedness experiments are used to demonstrate how reproducible a method is when conditions vary. An assay method protocol defines the exact steps to be followed to ensure an accurate and precise result. Unfortunately, slight-to-large deviations occur in the everyday process, which may or may not impact the result. Assay conditions like incubation temperature or exposure to light define the robustness of the assay, whereas changes to the routine, for instance, multiple analysts or different instruments, define the ruggedness. The actual batch size for a routine sample analysis run is frequently overlooked but is often an impactful ruggedness measurement that should be assessed.

Run Acceptance Criteria

Because validation QCs are used to assess the overall accuracy and precision of the method during the validation phase, no runs initiated for validation may be eliminated due to QC failure. Therefore, the acceptance criteria for the standard curves are used to accept each assay. At the conclusion of the validation, run acceptance criteria for QCs to be used in-study are summarized and run acceptance criteria are established based on this data. During sample analysis, the standard curve should be evaluated for acceptance before evaluating the QCs. Once the curve has been accepted, then the performance of the QCs should be evaluated. The acceptance criteria established during the precision and accuracy (4–6–20 rule) should be followed as described.

Partial Validation, Method Transfer, and Cross-validation

Method validations can be classified into three broad categories, full, partial, and cross. A full validation is done for any new methods and involves method development, prestudy, and in-study validation. It is essential that a full validation be conducted for changes in species (e.g., rat to mouse), change in matrix within a species (e.g., rat serum to rat urine). However, a partial validation is sufficient when a minor change is made to an already fully validated method as described below.

Partial Validation

A partial validation is conducted when minor changes to a method are made. These may include method transfer, changes to anticoagulant (e.g., EDTA, heparin, citrate), changes in the reagents used in the method (especially pivotal reagents such as the primary antibody or secondary antibody), sample processing changes (e.g., how fast a clot needs to be spun, collection vessels, and storage condition), changes to sample volume (e.g., if the volume of sample is changed from 100 to 200 μL per well), extension of the concentration range, selectivity issues (e.g., different disease population and concomitant medication), conversion of a manual to an automated method, qualification of an analyst, and so on. Partial validations can range from a single intra-assay accuracy and precision run to a nearly full validation. Although sample-processing changes may only require one run, several runs would typically be expected for changes to lots of reagents. Transferring an analytical method may require substantially more experimentation. Typically, for partial validations, three accuracy and precision runs are conducted and the inter- assay accuracy and precision criteria are compared against the original validated assay. If these criteria are met, the change to the method will be accepted and the proper documentation should be made to the method or method standard operating procedure (SOP). Other validation parameters have to be compared depending on the situation where these experiments are conducted to scientifically justify the change; e.g., if the method is to be used with a diseased population different to the original intended use of this method, then additional selectivity experiments must be conducted to evaluate the matrix effect.

Method Transfer

Method transfer is the situation in which the method is fully validated in one laboratory (sending laboratory) and transferred to another laboratory (receiving laboratory) and requires at least a partial validation. The parameters to evaluate during this partial validation are accuracy and precision of the method, selectivity, bench- top stability, and so on. In addition to the required documentation (e.g., method description, validation report, and certificate of analysis), the sending laboratory should provide information on those factors that may affect the ruggedness of the assay (e.g., identifying pivotal reagents and material). The method transfer process can be conducted in a multiphase manner, a transfer phase in which the sending laboratory participates in the transfer of the method at the receiving laboratory; the feasibility evaluation phase, in which the receiving laboratory runs the assay independently; the validation phase, which could be the phase where the partial validation is conducted; and finally a qualification phase in which both the sending and the receiving laboratory assays blinded samples. The method transfers require a plan or protocol that defines the process (e.g., experiments to be conducted) and the acceptance criteria. It is not uncommon for the sending laboratory to send personnel to physically demonstrate and train the personnel at the receiving laboratory.

Once the transferred method is validated at the receiving laboratory, an ideal scenario is to have both the sending and the receiving laboratories analyze blinded, 30 spiked samples covering the standard curve range, and 30 pooled incurred samples. The two sets of data may be compared by using a predefined statistical equivalence test. Alternatively, the differences between the two sets of data may be compared using an agreed to range of acceptability. Any acceptance criteria must be set *a priori* and documented in a plan or protocol before executing this phase of the method transfer process.

Cross-Validation

Cross-validation is conducted when two validated bioanalytical methods are used within the same study or submission, for example, ELISA assay to Biacore and ELISA to a liquid chromatography/mass spectrometry. It is recommended that test samples (spiked and/or pooled incurred samples) be used to cross-validate the bioanalytical methods. Data should be evaluated using an appropriate predefined acceptance criteria or statistical method. It should be cautioned that many times the methods that are being cross-validated may not have the same range of quantification. In these situations, it is necessary to prepare spiked samples within the range that are common to both methods for comparison.

Total Error versus 4-6-20 Rules

Total Error

The total error of a measurement takes into account both the systematic error (bias) and the random error components. Any measurement that is made during an experiment consists of both of these error parameters, and it is not possible to separate these two. Therefore, it is scientifically correct to use the total error criteria to assess the acceptability of a quality control result during a run.

As described in this chapter, prestudy validation runs are accepted based on the standard-curve acceptance criteria. No run acceptance criteria are applicable for prestudy validation sample assessments; i.e., no run can be rejected due to poor validation sample performance during accuracy and precision evaluation, and all data from the prestudy validation runs are reported without exceptions. In some cases, there may be assignable cause (e.g., technical issues) for removal of a validation sample data point before the calculation of the cumulative mean. Exclusion is applied at the end of the validation study period and must be documented as described in the documentation section.

For each in-study run, the standard curve must satisfy criteria described in the standard-curve section; however, run acceptance is based primarily on the performance of the QC samples. When using total error for ligand binding assays of macromolecules, the run acceptance criteria recommended in the precision and accuracy section requires that at least four of six (67%) QC results must be within 30% of their nominal values, with at least 50% of the values for each QC level satisfying the 30% limit. The recommended 4–6–30 rule imposes limits simultaneously on the allowable random error (imprecision) and systematic error (mean bias). If the application of an assay requires a QC target acceptance limit different than the 30% deviation from the nominal value, then prestudy acceptance criteria for precision and accuracy should be adjusted so that the limit for the sum of the interbatch imprecision and absolute mean RE is equal to the revised QC acceptance limit.

Documentation

It is critical to document the information generated during the development of a method in a laboratory notebook or other acceptable format. Iformation on the following assessments should be generated during assay development: critical assay reagent selection and stability, assay format selection (antibody[ies], diluents, plates, detection system, etc.), standard-curve model selection, matrix selection, specificity of the reagents, sample preparation, preliminary stability, and a preliminary assessment of assay robustness. At the end of the development portion of the assay life cycle, a draft method or an assay worksheet should be generated to be referred to during the prestudy validation.

A validation plan should be written before the initiation of the prestudy validation experiments. Alternatively, reference to an appropriate SOP can be made to ensure that a documented outline exists for the experiments required for prestudy validation. This plan can be a stand-alone document or can be contained in a laboratory notebook or some comparable format. The documentation should include a description of the intended use of the method under consideration and a summary of the performance parameters to be validated that should include, but may not be limited to, standard curve, precision and accuracy, range of quantification, specificity and selectivity, stability, dilutional linearity, robustness, batch size, and run acceptance criteria. The plan should include a summary of the proposed experiments and the target acceptance criteria for each performance parameter studied.

After completion of the validation experiments, a comprehensive report should be written. The format of the report may be dictated by internal policies of the laboratory; however, such reports should summarize the assay performance data and deviations from the method SOP or validation plan and any other relevant information related to the conditions under which the assay can be used without infringing the acceptance criteria.

Cumulative standard curve and QC data tables containing appropriate statistical parameters should be generated and included with the study sample values in the final study report. Unlike the prestudy validation, failed runs are not included in these tables. Additional information to be included in the final report is a description of deviations that occurred during the study, a table of the samples that underwent repeat analysis and the reasons, and a table with details on all failed runs.

The primary focus in the analytical considerations of immunoassays for macromolecules should be in the development phase. By thoroughly defining each component of the immunoassay in the first phase of the assay life cycle, the resulting validation plan should be concise and the validation process should be straightforward. Several facets of the assay defined in the late development stage, such as specificity and dilutional linearity, can appropriately be included in the final validation report.

A typical validation will include at least six precision and accuracy assays to define the consistency of the assay. Within those assays, several parameters can be defined, including early stability, specificity, selectivity, and range of quantification. No assay run should be eliminated except for a true and documented analyst's error.

The validation QC samples define the range of the assay, and no values below the LLOQ or above the ULOQ may be reported. Within the six validation assay

runs, the validation samples are used to define the cumulative precision and accuracy. During validation, no validation sample may be eliminated to show the true profile of the assay.

During sample analysis before assessing the QC samples for acceptance, the standard curve must be deemed appropriate by predetermined criteria. Only after the curve is accepted may the assessment of QC samples continue. QC sample results determine whether the assay run is valid. Acceptance criteria can be based on 4-6-20 rule or on Total Error and should be predicated on the criteria used in both the development and the prestudy validation phase. Overall, the immunoassay is a highly sensitive assay that can be used to quantify protein and peptide drugs in a biological matrix, often routinely in the μg/mL range.

9

Advanced Aseptic Processing

Blow-Fill-Seal (BFS) technology was developed in the early 1960s and was initially used for filling many liquid product categories, such as non-sterile medical devices, foods, and cosmetics. The technology has now developed to an extent that BFS systems are used today throughout the world to successfully aseptically produce sterile pharmaceutical products, such as respiratory solutions, ophthalmics, and wound care products. BFS is an advanced aseptic processing technique within which plastic containers are formed by means of molded extruded polymer granules that are filled and sealed in one continuous process. This differs from conventional aseptic processing where container formation, preparation, sterilization, and container filling and closure are all separate processes. Due to the level of automation of the entire process, very little human intervention is necessary during manufacture as compared to traditional aseptic filling. This is considered an advanced aseptic filling process. It is therefore possible to achieve very high levels of sterility confidence with a properly configured BFS machine designed to fill aseptically.

Outline of the BFS Process

The pharmaceutical BFS process combines the formation of plastic containers by blow/vacuum molding extruded pharmaceutical grade polymers, with an aseptic solution filling system.

Polymer granules are continuously fed to a machine hopper through an adiabatic screw extruder. Within the extruder the polymer is subjected to high temperature (generally greater than 160°C) and pressure (up to 350 bar) and becomes molten. It is then extruded through a die and pin set to form an open-ended tube of molten polymer known as a parison. The parison is supported by sterile air (parison support air) that is fed into the center of the parison through a sterilizing grade air filter fed with oil free compressed air. The parison is held in position by a parison clamp, which on some machines also serves to seal the bottom of the parison. A mold set in two halves then moves over to the parison and closes around it. Molding is facilitated by vacuum slots in the mold. The molded plastic is severed from the continuously extruding parison by a hot knife, and is then shuttled within the mold set to the filling position.

The filling mandrels are comprised of a set of filling tips that are held within a protective air shower; this is a small area within the filling machine that is typically fed with sterile filtered air. When the molds are beneath the air shower, the filling tips are lowered into the neck of the partially formed container and the containers are filled. The mandrels then return to the protective air shower, and the containers are sealed by a second mold set (head mold), which forms the neck and closure of the BFS containers. The entire cycle takes only a few seconds and therefore, results in minimal exposure of the open container to the surrounding clean room/air shower environment. The mold then opens and the filled containers surrounded by excess polymer are released. Excess plastic is then removed (typically this is done on-line by means of a mold specific cropping tool).

Liquid product is fed to the BFS machine from a holding tank or vessel. The product pathway is sterilized in place prior to receiving product, and product is sterilized by means of in-line sterilizing grade filters. Usually more than one stage of sterile filtration is on the product pathway.

Filling Environment

Aseptic BFS machines are housed within classified clean areas of a minimum specification of class M5.5 for 0.5 μm particles and greater (or equivalent), at rest. The new generation of BFS machines also is capable of operating with significantly decreased particle levels. The localized filling environment, or "air shower," is of a higher classification, which meets the specification of class M3.5 for 0.5 μm particles and greater.

Total particle levels should meet the required specifications and be measured, with the machine at rest, at defined intervals by means of a laser particle counter (or other suitable instrument) to demonstrate continued compliance.

Levels of viable contamination, however, are of importance in operation. Microbiological monitoring for viable contaminants should be carried out to coincide with routine manufacture with normal levels of dynamic activity. As with traditional aseptic filling, viable contamination within the clean area should be controlled by means of an effective routine cleaning and disinfecting program and the adoption of appropriate clean room behaviors and practices by trained personnel. BFS technology has the advantage of being able to operate without continuous personnel presence within the clean area. However, operators will need to enter the area to start up the machinery and to attend to the machine as necessary to make routine adjustments. It is a requirement within the European forum that clean room garments worn to enter the class M5.5 (FS209E) clean room be of a standard appropriate for a higher (M3.5) classification clean room.

A routine microbiological environmental monitoring program should be established and documented based on historical and operational data to demonstrate continued compliance with specifications, as well as to monitor trends. A typical monitoring regime within the clean room would include quantitative air and surface monitoring. Semiquantitative air monitoring by the use of settle plates also is useful in supplying data associated with a longer period of time in operation (up to 4 h exposure). Recommended limits for viable contaminants in clean rooms are quoted in various guidelines, including the current United States Pharmacopoeia (USP) and directive 91/356/EEC. Alert and Action levels should be clearly defined based upon both operational data and published recommendations.

Consideration should also be given to monitoring the localized filling zone (air shower). Although access to this area will be prohibited (and also extremely dangerous) during operation, some monitoring for viable and non-viable contaminants may be possible at rest (e.g., at the end of a product batch). It may also be feasible to install a remote means of obtaining samples during operation.

Means of BFS Container Contamination from the Environment

As previously stated, for aseptic BFS, container filling occurs in a localized air shower provided with sterile filtered air. However, there is a short period of time between container formation and filling when the open container is transferred from the parison formation position to the filling position, and when the open container is exposed to the clean room environment. Therefore, it may be possible for contaminants from the room environment to enter the container during this shuttling period.

Air used to form the parison (parison support air) is typically sterile filtered air. If this is not the case, non-sterile air may be able to enter the parison during parison formation. It was demonstrated during a simple practical experiment that broth filled units (totaling over 44,000) manufactured over several days in a highly contaminated environment remained sterile. The environment was contaminated by means of high levels of personnel activity in order to generate contaminants in keeping with those generated under normal conditions.

During a more controlled study carried out within an environment artificially contaminated with high levels of individual nebulized spores of *Bacillus subtilis*, a level of contamination within the environment was achieved that led to the contamination of broth filled units. The results were extrapolated to suggest a contamination rate of 1 unit in 4×10^6, with a surrounding environmental contamination of 1 cfu/m^3.

Routes of air-borne contamination into BFS containers were investigated during a study using Sulfur hexafluoride (SF_6) tracer gas. During this experiment, the tracer gas was released at a known concentration into a clean room that housed an aseptic BFS machine. Levels of the tracer gas were then measured within subsequently filled BFS units. The study concluded that the container was effectively protected by the localized air shower. Although not necessarily representative of deposition of microbial contaminants, there also was conclusive evidence of some room air within the BFS containers. The control of environmental contamination within the clean room is therefore important.

Extensive process simulation (broth fill) results for BFS effectively demonstrate that high levels of sterility confidence can be obtained with a properly configured and validated machine. However, in order to maintain high levels of sterility assurance, it is important that levels of microbial contamination are controlled within the filling environment.

Contamination from Product Components

As with traditional aseptic filling, in order to comply with pharmaceutical good manufacturing practices (GMP), it is important to minimize contamination at all stages of manufacture. Raw materials should be of a high quality and tested for microbial contamination. Water used for product manufacture should be of low bioburden and high purity (preferably water for injection quality, although this requirement is dependent upon the nature of the product being manufactured).

A program of bioburden testing for each product batch at various stages of manufacture should be established and documented. This will be dependent upon the manufacturing process, but as a minimum should include bioburden analysis of bulk solutions prior to any sterile filtration. The maximum life of the bulk solution in a non-sterile environment (generally within a mixing tank) should be limited to prevent increase in bioburden beyond an acceptable level. Bioburden testing at this stage should be carried out on samples taken at the end of the holding period to give "worst case" data.

BFS technology often results in considerable machine down time, especially as associated with activities such as Clean In Place (CIP) and Steam In Place (SIP), in order to prepare a machine for manufacture. Initial machine adjustments will then be necessary in order for integral and cosmetically acceptable units of the correct fill volume to be consistently produced. It, therefore, can be advantageous to fill larger product batches once this is achieved. In order to facilitate this with respect to maintaining a low bioburden throughout all stages of liquid processing, it is a common practice to have a sterilized storage vessel into which bulk product is filtered through a sterilizing grade filter. This sterilized bulk solution can then be used to feed the filling machine without escalation of microbial levels. Further stages of sterile filtration are required on the filling machine closer to the point of fill. A facility for sampling products during the course of the filling stage prior to further filtration can be incorporated. This will give data to confirm the low/zero bioburden of the product prior to the final stages of filtration, during the course of a longer batch.

The BFS container is produced from high-grade virgin polymer granules. Studies have investigated the lethality of the extrusion process with respect to container sterilization, the most recent of which is discussed in the validation section. Bioburden testing of polymer granules can be carried out in order to establish base line data. Virgin polymer granules, if handled and stored correctly, should be of very low bioburden.

Equipment—Interventions and Maintenance

In order to produce sterile pharmaceutical products with a high degree of sterility confidence, it is of key importance that the equipment be operated by experienced and trained personnel with a full understanding of both the technology and aseptic processing. Operator intervention during machine operation is limited due to the nature of the technology; however, BFS machines are complex and some operator activity will be required from time to time during normal manufacture. Clearly documented rules are imperative in order to clarify which activities are prohibited during batch manufacture and which are permitted. For example, if a fault occurs that requires immediate corrective action involving the sterile product pathway, or within the direct vicinity of the filling zone, these would typically be prohibited activities that would lead to termination of the product batch. Activities such as parison and fill volume adjustments are part of the normal operation of the machinery and are permitted. A proceduralized means of documenting these activities should exist, however routine they may be.

Interventions should be categorized according to their potential for affecting the product being manufactured, and only those with no risk to product sterility should be permitted during operations.

As with all machinery, BFS machines must be properly maintained in order to maintain effective operation with the minimum of operator activity. A documented preventative maintenance program should be in place and specify appropriate frequencies for all machine components and associated systems and services. Maintenance activities should ensure that moving parts are sufficiently (but not overly) lubricated, and that excess lubricants are removed at regular intervals to maintain the cleanliness of the machine. Abrasion among moving parts, particularly hoses and flexible pipe work, can be a problem with BFS machines and can cause undesirable particle generation and leaks that lead to unplanned maintenance and downtime. Moving parts should be inspected at regular intervals to avoid abrasion and to check for wear and tear. Regular seal changes with reconciliation of new/old seals should also be included.

Coolant systems are an integral part of container formation and serve to cool the molds and, if applicable, the parison clamp assembly. Coolant, although not in direct contact with product pathways, is in close proximity to the containers, and maintenance should be carried out to prevent coolant leakage. Coolant systems are prone to microbiological contamination and should be routinely treated to keep the bioburden under control. Coolant systems should be regularly sampled and tested for bioburden to ensure continuous compliance to a predefined specification.

Validation of BFS Systems

BFS machinery and associated equipment for aseptic manufacture should be constructed in such a way that the product pathways are of hygienic design with hygienic valves and minimal joints to facilitate cleaning and sterilizing in place.

Clean in Place (CIP)

As for all machinery involved in aseptic manufacture, CIP is necessary for all equipment that has product contact. This would typically include a bulk mixing tank, transfer lines, and the BFS machine itself, and may also include a holding vessel with associated transfer lines. CIP validation should be carried out to establish routine CIP practices that will clean the manufacturing equipment so that no contamination of subsequent products manufactured that would alter the safety, identity, quality, or purity of the drug beyond the predetermined requirements can occur. CIP procedures should be established by cleaning validation following the manufacture of worst case products (i.e., those that are most difficult to remove down to acceptable levels due to their solubility or activity). Means of measuring CIP efficacy include analysis of swabs taken directly from product contact machine parts and analysis of rinse waters. When establishing areas for swabbing, the specific equipment design needs to be taken into account, and those areas that are potentially most problematic should be selected for analysis (e.g., filter housings or areas that may cause product hold-up).

Steam in Place (SIP)

Aseptic BFS machines are subject to SIP sterilization following standard CIP cycles. SIP cycles are routinely measured by thermocouples located in fixed positions along the product pathway. Validation of SIP cycles should be carried out to demonstrate that consistent sterilization temperatures are achieved throughout the equipment in order to prove that the system can be effectively sterilized. Validation should also identify suitable positions for routine use, or justify the fixed probe positions already in place. SIP validation is generally carried out using additional thermocouples and should include the use of Biological Indicators (appropriate for moist heat sterilization). Test locations should include areas that may be prone to air or condensation entrapment. An accurate engineering line drawing of the system in order to aid identification of suitable test locations and to document test locations selected should be available.

Qualification of Aseptic Filling

The standard and most appropriate method for the qualification of aseptic filling is by means of a broth fill (or media fill). Using this method, units of liquid microbiological growth media (usually a full strength general-purpose media, such as Tryptone Soy Broth), are filled and incubated. Following an appropriate incubation period, the units are inspected for contamination. In this way, an indication of the level of contamination during the filling process can be evaluated.

There is no appropriate defined sterility confidence level that can be translated directly into acceptance criteria for broth fill contamination for BFS processes. The most commonly recognized acceptance criteria is a sterility assurance level (SAL) of 10^{-3}, although it is accepted that modern aseptic filling techniques such as BFS can achieve a higher SAL and that this should be reflected by broth fill results and acceptance criteria for this recognized advanced technology.

Broth fills should be a major part of the operational qualification of a new BFS machine to demonstrate aseptic processing capability prior to product manufacture (typically three successful consecutive broth fills are required) and should be carried out at defined intervals thereafter.

Broth fills should be carried out under conditions that are representative of those during normal operation. If there is to be a deviation from routine processes, it should only be in the direction of presenting a greater, rather than a lesser, challenge to the process. Due to the level of automation of BFS technology, it is extremely difficult to take "extra care" in order to reduce the chance of container contamination during a broth fill; therefore, results are not as operator- dependent as other less automated aseptic manufacturing processes.

New facilities should contain some background environmental monitoring data. It is important that environmental monitoring data be obtained during the course of broth fill batches to demonstrate a normal level of environmental contamination—the validity of broth fill results carried out in an environment having consistently lower contamination levels than those obtained during routine batch manufacture could be questioned.

Batch manufacture, storage, and transfer should be carried out in accordance with routine procedures and with the same operators. The machine should be cleaned and sterilized as normal, although if an overkill cycle is used routinely for sterilization, a partial sterilization (although still meeting standard sterilization parameters) may be chosen as "worst case."

Broth filled BFS units should generally meet all of the necessary product acceptance criteria, such as fill volume, wall thickness, container integrity, and cosmetic acceptability. The necessary operator activity at the start of a product batch is arguably more intrusive than at any other stage of manufacture. Product units routinely produced at the very start of a batch will usually be discarded due to fill volume, cosmetic, or other deficiencies as the machine set-up is adjusted. However, during a broth fill, it is a good practice to retain and incubate all start-up units (except any leaking units) to demonstrate that start-up activities have not affected product sterility. Such units should be segregated from the subsequent units that meet the acceptance criteria and labeled accordingly.

In addition, it can be useful to retain and incubate reject units filled during the course of a broth fill batch (again, excluding leaking units) for additional information. Again, these should be segregated from acceptable units and labeled accordingly. Although such units would be rejected during normal production, microbial contamination found in such units can be indicative of a problem that requires attention.

During the course of a broth fill, operator activity will be necessary as with routine manufacture. However, additional activities can be carried out to cover all permissible activities in order to provide evidence that product sterility is not affected. Such interventions should be planned and documented with the batch documentation.

Frequency and size of broth fills must be clearly defined. Size of fill is usually based upon the statistical probability of detecting an acceptably low incidence of microbial contamination. Tables have been published to this effect, but the BFS operator must decide both the size and frequency of broth fills based upon their specific facility, routine product batch sizes, and operation. For high-speed BFS machines, filling routine product batches in excess of 100,000 units, relatively large broth fill batches, in comparison with traditional aseptic filling lines, are both feasible and appropriate.

The internal surfaces of broth filled units should be fully wetted to ensure capture of any contaminants within the broth. This is commonly achieved by agitation or inversion of the units either prior to or during the incubation period.

Incubation time and temperature should be such that macroscopic microbial growth of a wide range of common isolates will be detected. This should be routinely demonstrated by including positive control units inoculated with a low level of compendial microorganisms. It is desirable to perform additional testing to demonstrate that the incubation time and temperature selected will promote the growth of isolates obtained from machine operating environments. The Pharmaceutical BFS Operators Association recommends incubation of 14 days at 25–32°C.

Some of the media fills carried out were full production batch volumes with hundreds of thousands of units filled in a single batch. In addition to the figures within the table, a run of over 1,500,000 units was recorded with the detection of a single contaminated unit.

It is clearly impractical to carry out very high numbers of broth filled units on a routine basis, but if unpreserved products are manufactured, and if practicable, it is good practice to fill broth directly following product batches with no further machine flushing or sterilization.

Given the high performance demonstrated during media fills, acceptance criteria should be based upon what can be realistically achieved. During broth fills of a standard size, any incidence of contamination among the units filled should lead to an investigation. In the absence of a cause, even with very low levels of contamination, consideration should be given to machine recommissioning.

Machine recommissioning should also be carried out if modifications to a filling machine have been made that may have an effect on process capability (e.g., changes to the sterile product pathway or air shower).

BFS Containers

The BFS container is formed as an integral part of the process from medical grade virgin polymer granules. A recent study investigated the lethality of the extrusion process when challenged with a high bioburden of spores. The spores of the test organism Bacillus subtilis var. niger were selected as they are known to be resistant to dry heat; the same strain was selected as the organism of choice for Biological Indicators used in dry heat sterilization processes. A series of broth fills were carried out using polymer batches inoculated with various levels of spores between 2×10^1 and 2×10^5 spores per gram. The broth filled units were then incubated in line with the company's routine broth fill procedure (25–32°C for 14 days). Spore contamination of units was observed with batches of polymer inoculated with high spore levels. The experiment demonstrated a relationship between polymer contamination and product contamination that was dependent upon both the level of contamination in the polymer and the resistance of the contaminant (in terms of D-value) to dry heat sterilization. The study also demonstrated inactivation of the spores on the granules with strong evidence of lethality associated with the extrusion process.

Routine bioburden testing of virgin pharmaceutical grade polymer granules tends to give very low or zero counts per gram of polymer tested, with contaminants generally much more heat labile than *Bacillus subtilis* spores. The study detailed was also carried out using a BFS machine adjusted to extrude at the lower end of the operating temperature range for extrusion. Therefore, it can be concluded that the extrusion process renders the contaminants unavailable, with sufficient bioburden reduction/ inactivation for it to be appropriate for aseptic formation of BFS containers. This is further endorsed by routine broth fill data.

The closures of BFS containers are formed within the automated process by the head mold set which closes around the top of the severed section of parison following filling. The integrity of the container and closure is generally tested by a manual or automated method of leak detection performed outside of the filling environment following removal of excess plastic (deflashing) from the filled product units.

In order to minimize the number of leaking units produced, it is important that mold sets are correctly aligned. Very slight misalignment of molds may potentially lead to the production of units with very slight leaks that may be difficult to detect by routine methods. Therefore, correct molding is of key importance and usually can be checked easily by careful and experienced visual examination of units.

Container integrity testing can be carried out very effectively by a bacterial challenge test. Using this method, sterile broth filled units are submerged for a period of time (e.g., 24 hours) within a buffered solution that contains a high level bacterial challenge. (There are no regulations or guidelines that specify which organism to use, but it would seem logical to use a factory isolate or a relatively small organism such as a *Pseudomonas* spp.) Units are then removed, incubated, and checked for growth of the challenge organism. An absence of growth shows an integral unit and closure. This method is extremely sensitive and although this is not a test that is practical to perform on a routine basis, it can be a useful tool for infrequent use.

Filtration

Hydrophilic and hydrophobic sterilization grade filters are used throughout the BFS process for the sterilization of product and air, respectively. Filters should be purchased from an approved supplier and should be certified as meeting the regulatory requirements for sterilizing grade filters. By definition this means that the filter will have full bacterial retention when subjected to an aqueous challenge of *Brevundimonas diminuta* at a minimum concentration of 1×10^7 cfu/cm^2 of filter surface area.

Hydrophobic filters do not come into direct product contact and, therefore, the standard bacterial retention test alone generally is sufficient validation. However, as hydrophilic filters are in direct product contact, additional validation will be necessary for each product type in order to demonstrate that the filters selected for product sterilization do not alter the safety, identity, strength, quality, or purity of the drug product. Qualification of hydrophilic filters will also be necessary in order to demonstrate that the specific product type, in conjunction with a bacterial challenge, does not affect the efficacy of the filter. Validation of filters by means of bacterial retention tests requires specialist equipment and is often arranged between the filter manufacturer and the BFS operator.

Aseptic pharmaceutical BFS technology for the manufacture of sterile liquid products demonstrates high levels of sterility assurance when correctly operated and configured. The technology is continually improving as more expertise is developed. However, an understanding of the means of potential container contamination and the implementation of systems operating to minimize these means is important in order to maintain the high standards achievable with this technology.

10

Product Analysis

All pharmaceutical finished products undergo rigorous QC testing in order to confirm their conformance to predetermined specifications. Potency testing is of obvious importance, ensuring that the drug will be efficacious when administered to the patient. A prominent aspect of safety testing entails analysis of product for the presence of various potential contaminants.

The range and complexity of analytical testing undertaken for recombinant biopharmaceuticals far outweighs that undertaken with regard to 'traditional' pharmaceuticals manufactured by organic synthesis. Not only are proteins (or additional biopharmaceuticals such as nucleic acids) much larger and more structurally complex than traditional low molecular mass drugs, their production in biological systems renders the range of potential contaminants far broader. Recent advances in analytical techniques render practical the routine analysis of complex biopharmaceutical products. An overview of the range of finished-product tests of recombinant protein biopharmaceuticals is outlined below. Explanation of the theoretical basis underpinning these analytical methodologies is not undertaken, as this would considerably broaden the scope of the text.

Table 10.1 The range and medical significance of potential impurities present in biopharmaceutical products destined for parenteral administration

Impurity	*Medical consequence*
Microorganisms	Potential establishment of a severe microbial infection – septicaemia
Viral particles	Potential establishment of a severe viral infection
Pyrogenic substances	Fever response that, in serious cases, culminates in death
DNA	Significance is unclear – could bring about an immunological response
Contaminating proteins	Immunological reactions. Potential adverse effects if the contaminant exhibits an unwanted biological activity

Protein-Based Contaminants

Most of the chromatographic steps undertaken during downstream processing are specifically included to separate the protein of interest from additional contaminant proteins. This task is not an insubstantial one, particularly if the recombinant protein is expressed intracellularly.

In addition to protein impurities emanating directly from the source material, other proteins may be introduced during upstream or downstream processing. For example, animal cell culture media are typically supplemented with bovine serum/foetal calf serum (2–25 per cent), or with a defined cocktail of various regulatory proteins required to maintain and stimulate growth of these cells. Downstream processing of intracellular microbial proteins often requires the addition of endonuleases to the cell homogenate to degrade the large quantity of DNA liberated upon cellular disruption. (DNA promotes increased solution viscosity, rendering processing difficult. Viscosity, being a function of the DNA's molecular mass, is reduced upon nuclease treatment.)

Minor amounts of protein could also potentially enter the product stream from additional sources, e.g. protein shed from production personnel. Implementation of good manufacturing practice (GMP), however, should minimize contamination from such sources.

The clinical significance of protein-based impurities relates to (a) their potential biological activities and (b) their antigenicity. Whereas some contaminants may display no undesirable biological activity, others may exhibit activities deleterious to either the product itself (e.g. proteases that could modify/ degrade the product) or the recipient patient (e.g. the presence of contaminating toxins).

Their inherent immunogenicity also renders likely and immunological reaction against protein-based impurities upon product administration to the recipient patient. This is particularly true in the case of products produced in microbial or other recombinant systems (i.e. most biopharmaceuticals). Although the product itself is likely to be non-immunogenic (usually being coded for by a human gene), contaminant proteins will be endogenous to the host cell, and hence foreign to the human body. Administration of the product can elicit an immune response against the contaminant. This is particularly likely if a requirement exists for ongoing, repeat product administration (e.g. administration of recombinant insulin). Immunological activation of this type could also potentially (and more seriously) have a sensitizing effect on the recipient against the actual protein product.

In addition to distinct gene products, modified forms of the protein of interest are also considered impurities, rendering desirable their removal from the product stream. Although some such modified forms may be innocuous, others may not. Modified product '*impurities*' may compromise the product in a number of ways, e.g.:

1. Biologically inactive forms of the product will reduce overall product potency;
2. Some modified product forms remain biologically active, but exhibit modified pharmacokinetic characteristics (i.e. timing and duration of drug action);
3. Modified product forms may be immunogenic.

Removal of Altered Forms of the Protein of Interest from the Product Stream

Modification of any protein will generally alter some aspect of its physicochemical characteristics. This facilitates removal of the modified form by standard chromatographic techniques during downstream processing. Most downstream procedures for protein-based biopharmaceuticals include both gel-filtration and ion-exchange steps. Aggregated forms of the product will be effectively removed by gel filtration (because they now exhibit a molecular mass greater by several orders of magnitude than the native product). This technique will also remove extensively proteolysed forms of the product. Glycoprotein variants whose carbohydrate moieties have been extensively degraded will also likely be removed by gel-filtration (or ion-exchange) chromatography. Deamidation and oxidation will generate product variants with altered surface charge characteristics, often rendering their removal by ion exchange relatively straightforward. Incorrect disulfide bond formation, partial denaturation and limited proteolysis can also alter the shape and surface charge of proteins, facilitating their removal from the product by ion exchange or other techniques, such as hydrophobic interaction chromatography.

The range of chromatographic techniques now available, along with improvements in the resolution achievable using such techniques, renders possible the routine production of protein biopharmaceuticals which are in excess of 97–99 per cent pure. This level of purity represents the typical industry standard with regard to biopharmaceutical production.

A number of different techniques may be used to characterize protein-based biopharmaceutical products, and to detect any protein-based impurities that may be present in that product. Analysis for non-protein-based contaminant is described in subsequent sections.

Product Potency

Any biopharmaceutical must obviously conform to final product potency specifications. Such specifications are usually expressed in terms of 'units of activity' per vial of product (or per therapeutic dose, or per milligram of product). A number of different approaches may be undertaken to determine product potency. Each exhibits certain advantages and disadvantages.

Bioassays represent the most relevant potency-determining assay, as they directly assess the biological activity of the biopharmaceutical. Bioassay involves applying a known quantity of the substance to be assayed to a biological system that responds in some way to this applied stimulus. The response is measured quantitatively, allowing an activity value to be assigned to the substance being assayed.

All bioassays are comparative in nature, requiring parallel assay of a 'standard' preparation against which the sample will be compared. Internationally accepted standard preparations of most biopharmaceuticals are available from organizations such as the World Health Organization (WHO) or the United States Pharmacopeia. An example of a straightforward bioassay is the traditional assay method for antibiotics. This usually entailed measuring the zone of inhibition of microbial growth around an antibiotic-containing disc, placed on an agar plate seeded with the test microbe. Bioassays for modern biopharmaceuticals are generally more complex. The biological system used can be whole animals, specific organs or tissue types, or individual mammalian cells in culture.

Bioassays of related substances can be quite similar in design. Specific growth factors, for example, stimulate the accelerated growth of specific animal cell lines. Relevant bioassays can be undertaken by incubation of the growth-factor-containing sample with a culture of the relevant sensitive cells and radiolabelled nucleotide precursors. After an appropriate time period, the level of radioactivity incorporated into the DNA of the cells is measured. This is a measure of the bioactivity of the growth factor. The most popular bioassay of EPO involves a mouse-based bioassay (EPO stimulates red blood cell production, making it useful in the treatment of certain forms of anaemia; Chapter 10). Basically, the EPO-containing sample is administered to mice along with radioactive iron (^{57}Fe). Subsequent measurement of the rate of incorporation of radioactivity into proliferating red blood cells is undertaken. (The greater the stimulation of red blood cell proliferation, the more iron taken up for haemoglobin synthesis.)

One of the most popular bioassay for interferons is termed the 'cytopathic effect inhibition assay'. This assay is based upon the ability of many interferons to render animal cells resistant to viral attack. It entails incubation of the interferon preparation with cells sensitive to destruction by a specific virus. That virus is then subsequently added, and the percentage of cells that survive thereafter is proportional to the levels of interferon present in the assay sample. Viable cells can assimilate certain dyes, such as neutral red. Addition of the dye followed by spectrophotometric quantitation of the amount of dye assimilated can thus be used to quantitate percentage cell survival. This type of assay can be scaled down to run in a single well of a microtitre plate. This facilitates automated assay of large numbers of samples with relative ease. Although bioassays directly assess product potency (i.e. activity), they suffer from a number of drawbacks, including:

1. *Lack of precision*. The complex nature of any biological system, be it an entire animal or individual cell, often results in the responses observed being influenced by factors such as metabolic status of individual cells, or (in the case of whole animals) subclinical infections, stress levels induced by human handling, etc.

2. *Time*. Most bioassays take days, and in some cases week, to run. This can render routine bioassays difficult, and impractical to undertake as a quick QC potency test during downstream processing.
3. *Cost*. Most bioassay systems, in particular those involving whole animals, are extremely expensive to undertake.

Because of such difficulties alternative assays have been investigated, and sometimes are used in conjunction with, or instead of, bioassays. The most popular alternative assay system is the immunoassay.

Immunoassays employ monoclonal or polyclonal antibody preparations to detect and quantify the product. The specificity of antibody–antigen interaction ensures good assay precision. The use of conjugated radiolabels (RIA) or enzymes (EIA) to allow detection of antigen–antibody binding renders such assays very sensitive. Furthermore, when compared with a bioassay, immunoassays are rapid (undertaken in minutes to hours), inexpensive, and straight-forward to undertake. The obvious disadvantage of immunoassays is that immunological reactivity cannot be guaranteed to correlate directly to biological activity. Relatively minor modifications of the protein product, although having a profound influence on its biological activity, may have little or no influence on its ability to bind antibody. For such reasons, although immunoassays may provide a convenient means of tracking product during downstream processing, performing a bioassay on at the very least the final product is usually necessary to prove that potency falls within specification.

Determination of Protein Concentration

Quantification of total protein in the final product represents another standard analysis undertaken by QC. A number of different protein assays may be potentially employed.

Table 10.2. Common assay methods used to quantitate proteins. The principle upon which each method is based is also listed

Method	*Principle*
Absorbance at 280 nm (A_{280}; UV method)	The side chain of selected amino acids (particularly tyrosine and tryptophan) absorbs UV at 280 nm
Absorbance at 205 nm (far-UV method)	Peptide bonds absorb UV at 190–220 nm
Biuret method	Binding of copper ions to peptide bond nitrogen under alkaline conditions generates a purple colour
Lowry method	Lowry method uses a combination of the Biuret copper-based reagent and the 'Folin–Ciocalteau' reagent, which contains phosphomolybdic-phosphotungstic acid. Reagents react with protein, yielding a blue colour that displays an absorbance maximum at 750 nm
Bradford method	Bradford reagent contains the dye Coomassie blue G-250 in an acidic solution. The dye binds to protein, yielding a blue colour that absorbs maximally at 595 nm
Bicinchonic acid method	Copper-containing reagent that, when reduced by protein, reacts with bicinchonic acid yielding a complex that displays an absorbance maximum at 562 nm
Peterson method	Essentially involves initial precipitation of protein out of solution by addition of trichloroacetic acid. The protein precipitate is redissolved in NaOH and the Lowry method of protein determination is then performed
Silver-binding method	Interaction of silver with protein – very sensitive method

Detection and quantification of protein by measuring absorbency at 280 nm is perhaps the simplest such method. This approach is based on the fact that the side chains of the amino acids tyrosine and tryptophan absorb at this wavelength. The method is popular, as it is fast, easy to perform and is non-destructive to the sample. However, it is a relatively insensitive technique, and identical concentrations of different proteins will yield different absorbance values if their content of tyrosine and tryptophan vary to any significant extent. Hence, this method is rarely used to determine the protein concentration of the final product, but it is routinely used during downstream processing to detect protein elution off chromatographic columns, and hence track the purification process.

Measuring protein absorbance at lower wavelengths (205 nm) increases the sensitivity of the assay considerably. Also, as it is the peptide bonds that are absorbing at this wavelength, the assay is subject to much less variation due to the amino acid composition of the protein.

The most common methods used to determine protein concentration are the dye-binding procedure using Coomassie brilliant blue, and the bicinchonic-acid-based procedure. Various dyes are known to bind quantitatively to proteins, resulting in an alteration of the characteristic absorption spectrum of the dye. Coomassie brilliant blue G-250, for example, becomes protonated when dissolved in phosphoric acid, and has an absorbance maximum at 450 nm. Binding of the dye to a protein (via ionic interactions) results in a shift in the dye's absorbance spectrum, with a new major peak (at 595 nm) being observed. Quantification of proteins in this case can thus be undertaken by measuring absorbance at 595 nm. The method is sensitive, easy and rapid to undertake. Also, it exhibits little quantitative variation between different proteins.

Protein determination procedures using bicinchonic acid were developed by Pierce Chemicals, who hold a patent on the product. The procedure entails the use of a copper-based reagent containing bicinchonic acid. Upon incubation with a protein sample, the copper is reduced. In the reduced state it reacts with bicinchonic acid, yielding a purple colour that absorbs maximally at 562 nm.

Silver also binds to proteins, an observation that forms the basis of an extremely sensitive method of protein detection. This technique is used extensively to detect proteins in electrophoretic gels, as discussed in the next section.

Detection of Protein-based Product Impurities

SDS polyacrylamide gel electrophoresis (SDS-PAGE) represents the most commonly used analytical technique in the assessment of final product purity. This technique is well established and easy to perform. It provides high-resolution separation of polypeptides on the basis of their molecular mass. Bands containing as little as 100 ng of protein can be visualized by staining the gel with dyes such as Coomassie blue. Subsequent gel analysis by scanning laser densitometry allows quantitative determination of the protein content of each band (thus allowing quantification of protein impurities in the product).

The use of silver-based stains increases the detection sensitivity up to 100 fold, with individual bands containing as little as 1ng of protein usually staining well. However, because silver binds to protein non-stoichiometrically, quantitative studies using densitometry cannot be undertaken.

SDS-PAGE is normally run under reducing conditions. Addition of a reducing agent such as β-mercaptoethanol or dithiothreitol (DTT) disrupts interchain (and intrachain) disulfide linkages. Individual polypeptides held together via disulfide linkages in oligomeric proteins will thus separate from each other on the basis of their molecular mass.

The presence of bands additional to those equating to the protein product generally represent protein contaminants. Such contaminants may be unrelated to the product or may be variants of the product itself (e.g. differentially glycosylated variants, proteolytic fragment, etc.). Further characterization may include western blot analysis. This involves eluting the protein bands from the electrophoretic gel onto a nitrocellulose filter. The filter can then be probed using antibodies raised against the product. Binding of the antibody to the '*contaminant*' bands suggests that they are variants of the product.

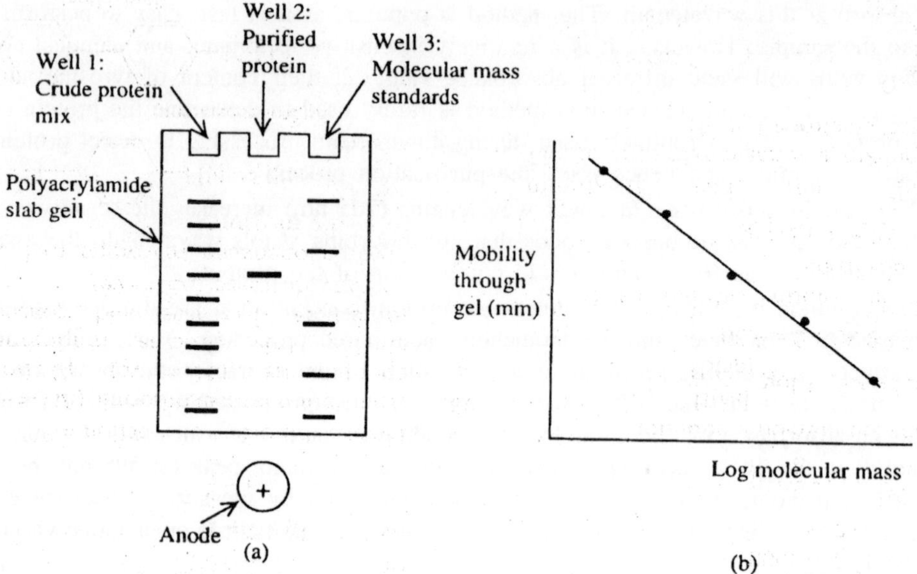

Fig. 10.1. Separation of proteins by SDS-PAGE.

One concern relating to SDS -PAGE-based purity analysis is that contaminants of the same molecular mass as the product will go undetected as they will co-migrate with it. Two-dimensional electrophoretic analysis would overcome this eventuality in most instances. Two-dimensional electrophoresis is normally run so that proteins are separated from each other on the basis of a different molecular property in each dimension. The most commonly utilized method entails separation of proteins by isoelectric focusing in the first dimension, with separation in the second dimension being undertaken in the presence of SDS, thus promoting band separation on the basis of protein size. Modified electrophoresis equipment that renders two- dimensional electrophoretic separation routine is freely available. Application of biopharmaceutical finished products to such systems allows rigorous analysis of purity.

Isoelectric focusing entails setting up a pH gradient along the length of an electrophoretic ġel. Applied proteins will migrate under the influence of an electric field until they reach a point in the gel at which the pH equals the protein's isoelectric point pI (the pH at which the protein exhibits no overall net charge; only species with a net charge will move under the in- fluence of an electric field). Isoelectric focusing thus separates proteins on the basis of charge characteristics. This technique is also utilized in the biopharmaceutical industry to determine product homogeneity. Homogeneity is best indicated by the appearance in the gel of a single protein band, exhibiting the predicted pI value. Interpretation of the meaning of multiple bands, however, is less straightforward, particularly if the protein is glycosylated (the bands can also be stained for the presence of carbohydrates). Glycoproteins varying slightly in their carbohydrate content will vary in their sialic acid content and, hence, exhibit slightly different pI values. In such instances, isoelectric focusing analysis seeks to establish batch-to-batch consistency in terms of the banding pattern observed. Isoelectric focusing also finds application in analysing the stability of biopharmaceuticals over the course of their shelf life. Repeat analysis of samples over time will detect deamidation or other degradative processes that alter protein charge characteristics.

Capillary Electrophoresis

Capillary electrophoresis systems are also likely to play an increasingly prominent analytical role in the QC laboratory. As with other forms of electrophoresis, separation is based upon different rates of protein migration upon application of an electric field. As its name suggests, in the case of capillary electrophoresis, this separation occurs within a capillary tube. Typically, the capillary will have a diameter of 20–50 μm and be up to a 1 m long (it is normally coiled to facilitate ease of use and storage). The dimensions of this system yield greatly increased surface area:volume ratio (compared with slab gels), hence greatly increasing the efficiency of heat dissipation from the system. This, in turn, allows operation at a higher current density, thus speeding up the rate of migration through the capillary. Sample analysis can be undertaken in 15–30 min, and on-line detection at the end of the column allows automatic detection and quantification of eluting bands.

The speed, sensitivity, high degree of automation and ability to quantitate protein bands directly render this system ideal for biopharmaceutical analysis.

High-performance Liquid Chromatography

HPLC occupies a central analytical role in assessing the purity of low molecular mass pharmaceutical substances. It also plays an increasingly important role in analysis of macromolecules, such as proteins. Most of the chromatographic strategies used to separate proteins under 'low pressure' (e.g. gel filtration, ion exchange, etc.) can be adapted to operate under high pressure. Reverse-phase-, size-exclusion- and, to a lesser extent, ion-exchange-based HPLC chromatography systems are now used in the analysis of a range of biopharmaceutical preparations. On-line detectors (usually a UV monitor set at 220 or 280 nm) allows automated detection and quantification of eluting bands. HPLC is characterized by a number of features that render it an attractive analytical tool. These include:

1. Excellent fractionation speeds (often just minutes per sample);
2. Superior peak resolution
3. High degree of automation (including data analysis);
4. Ready commercial availability of various sophisticated systems.

Reverse-phase HPLC (RP-HPLC) separates proteins on the basis of differences in their surface hydophobicity. The stationary phase in the HPLC column normally consists of silica or a polymeric support to which hydrophobic arms (usually alkyl chains, such as butyl, octyl or octadecyl groups) have been attached. Reverse-phase systems have proven themselves to be a particularly powerful analytical technique, capable of separating very similar molecules displaying only minor differences in hydrophobicity. In some instances a single amino acid substitution or the removal of a single amino acid from the end of a polypeptide chain can be detected by RP-HPLC. In most instances, modifications such as deamidation will also cause peak shifts. Such systems, therefore, may be used to detect impurities, be they related or unrelated to the protein product. RP-HPLC finds extensive application in, for example, the analysis of insulin preparations. Modified forms, or insulin polymers, are easily distinguishable from native insulin on reverse-phase columns.

Although RP-HPLC has proven its analytical usefulness, its routine application to analysis of specific protein preparations should be undertaken only after extensive validation studies. HPLC in general can have a denaturing influence on many proteins (especially larger, complex proteins). Reverse-phase systems can be particularly harsh, as interaction with the highly hydrophobic stationary phase can induce irreversible protein denaturation. Denaturation would result in the generation of artifactual peaks on the chromatogram. Size-exclusion HPLC (SE-HPLC) separates proteins on the basis of size and shape. As most soluble proteins are globular (i.e. roughly spherical in shape), separation is essentially achieved on the basis of molecular mass in most instances. Commonly used SE-HPLC stationary phases include silica-based supports and cross-linked agarose of defined pore size. Size-exclusion systems are most often used to analyse product for the presence of dimers or higher molecular mass aggregates of itself, as well as proteolysed product variants.

Calibration with standards allows accurate determination of the molecular mass of the product itself, as well as any impurities. Batch-to-batch variation can also be assessed by comparison of chromatograms from different product runs. Ion-exchange chromatography (both cation and anion) can also be undertaken in HPLC format. Though not as extensively employed as reverse-phase or size-exclusion systems, ion-exchange-based systems are of use in analysing for impurities unrelated to the product, as well as detecting and quantifying deamidated forms.

Mass Spectrometry

Recent advances in the field of mass spectrometry now extend the applicability of this method to the analysis of macromolecules such as proteins. Using electrospray mass spectrometry, it is now possible to determine the molecular mass of many proteins to within an accuracy of ± 0.01 per cent. A protein variant missing a single amino acid residue can easily be distinguished from the native protein in many instances. Although this is a very powerful technique, analysis of the results obtained can sometimes be less than straightforward. Glycoproteins, for example, yield extremely complex spectra (due to their natural heterogeneity), making the significance of the findings hard to interpret.

Immunological Approaches to Detection of Contaminants

Most recombinant biopharmaceuticals are produced in microbial or mammalian cell lines. Thus, although the product is derived from a human gene, all product-unrelated contaminants will be derived from the producer organism. These non-self proteins are likely to be highly immunogenic in humans, rendering their removal from the product stream especially important. Immunoassays may be conveniently used to detect and quantify non-product-related impurities in the final preparation (immunoassays generally may not be used to determine levels of product-related impurities, as antibodies raised against such impurities would almost certainly cross-react with the product itself).

The strategy usually employed to develop such immunoassays is termed the 'blank run approach'. This entails constructing a host cell identical in all respects to the natural producer cell, except that it lacks the gene coding for the desired product. This blank producer cell is then subjected to upstream processing procedures identical to those undertaken with the normal producer cell. Cellular extracts are subsequently subjected to the normal product purification process, but only to a stage immediately prior to the final purification steps. This produces an array of proteins that could co- purify with the final product. These proteins (of which there may be up to 200 as determined by two-dimensional electrophoretic analysis) are used to immunize horses, goats or other suitable animals. Therefore, polyclonal antibody preparations capable of binding specifically to these proteins are produced. Purification of the antibodies allows their incorporation in radioimmunoassay or enzyme-based immunoassay systems, which may subsequently be used to probe the product. Such multi-antigen assay systems will detect the sum total of host-cell-derived impurities present in the product. Immunoassays identifying a single potential contaminant can also be developed.

Immunoassays have found widespread application in detecting and quantifying product impurities. These assays are extremely specific and very sensitive, often detecting target antigen down to parts per million levels. Many immunoassays are available commercially, and companies exist that will rapidly develop tailor-made immunoassay systems for biopharmaceutical analysis.

Application of the analytical techniques discussed thus far focuses upon detection of proteinaceous impurities. A variety of additional tests are undertaken that focus upon the active substance itself. These tests aim to confirm that the presumed active substance observed by electrophoresis, HPLC, etc. is indeed the active substance, and that its primary sequence (and, to a lesser extent, higher orders of structure) conform to licensed product specification. Tests performed to verify the product identity include amino acid analysis, peptide mapping, N-terminal sequencing and spectrophotometric analyses.

Amino Acid Analysis

Amino acid analysis remains a characterization technique undertaken in many laboratories, in particular if the product is a peptide or small polypeptide (molecular mass ≤10 kDa). The strategy is simple. Determine the range and quantity of amino acids present in the product and compare the results obtained with the expected (theoretical) values. The results should be comparable.

The peptide/polypeptide product is usually hydrolysed by incubation with 6 mol l^{-1} HCl at elevated temperatures (110°C), under vacuum, for extended periods (12–24 h). The constituent amino acids are separated from each other by ion-exchange chromatography and identified by comparison with standard amino acid preparations. Reaction with ninhydrin allows subsequent quantification of each amino acid present.

Although this technique is relatively straightforward and automated amino acid analysers are commercially available, it is subject to a number of disadvantages that limits its usefulness in biopharmaceutical analysis. These include:

1. Hydrolysis conditions can destroy/modify certain amino acid residues, in particular tryptophan, but also serine, threonine and tyrosine;
2. The method is semi-quantitative rather than quantitative;
3. Sensitivity is at best moderate; low-level contaminants may go undetected (i.e. not significantly alter the amino acid profile obtained), particularly if the product is a high molecular mass protein.

These disadvantages, along with the availability of alternative characterization methodologies, limit application of this technique in biopharmaceutical analysis.

Peptide Mapping

A major concern relating to biopharmaceuticals produced in high-expression recombinant systems is the potential occurrence of point mutations in the product's gene, leading to an altered primary structure (i.e. amino acid sequence). Errors in gene transcription or translation could also have similar consequences. The only procedure guaranteed to detect such alterations is full sequencing of a sample of each batch of the protein, which is a considerable technical challenge. Although partial protein sequencing is normally undertaken, the approach most commonly used to detect alterations in amino acid sequence is peptide (fingerprint) mapping.

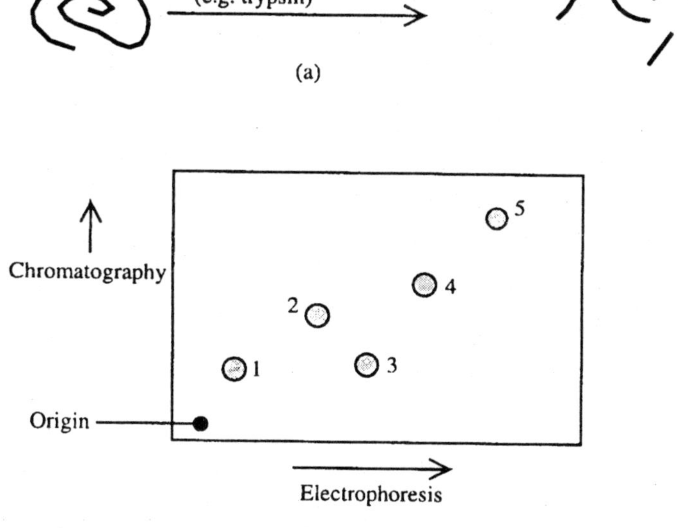

Fig. 10.2. Generation of a peptide map.

Peptide mapping entails exposure of the protein product to a reagent that promotes hydrolysis of peptide bonds at specific points along the protein backbone. This generates a series of peptide fragments. These fragments can be separated from each other by a variety of techniques, including one- or two-dimensional electrophoresis, and RP-HPLC in particular. A standardized sample of the protein product when subjected to this procedure will yield a characteristic peptide fingerprint, or map, with which the peptide maps obtained with each batch of product can subsequently be compared. If the peptides generated are relatively short, then a change in a single amino acid residue is likely to alter the peptide's physicochemical properties sufficiently to alter its position within the peptide map. In this way, single (or multiple) amino acid substitutions, deletions, insertions or modifications can usually be detected. This technique plays an important role in monitoring batch-to-batch consistency of the product, and also obviously can confirm the identity of the actual product. The choice of reagent used to fragment the protein is critical to the success of this approach. If a reagent generates only a few very large peptides, a single amino acid alteration in one such peptide will be more difficult to detect than if it occurred in a much smaller peptide fragment. On the other hand, generation of a large number of very short peptides can be counterproductive, as it may prove difficult to resolve all the peptides from each other by subsequent chromatography. Generation of peptide fragments containing an average of 7–14 amino acids is most desirable.

The most commonly utilized chemical cleavage agent is cyanogen bromide (it cleaves the peptide bond on the carboxyl side of methionine residues). V8 protease, produced by certain staphylococci, along with trypsin are two of the more commonly used proteolytic-based fragmentation agents. Knowledge of the full amino acid sequence of the protein usually renders possible pre-determination of the most suitable fragmentation agent for any protein. The amino acid sequence of hGH, for example, harbours 20 potential trypsin cleavage sites. Under some circumstances it may be possible to use a combination of fragmentation agents to generate peptides of optimal length.

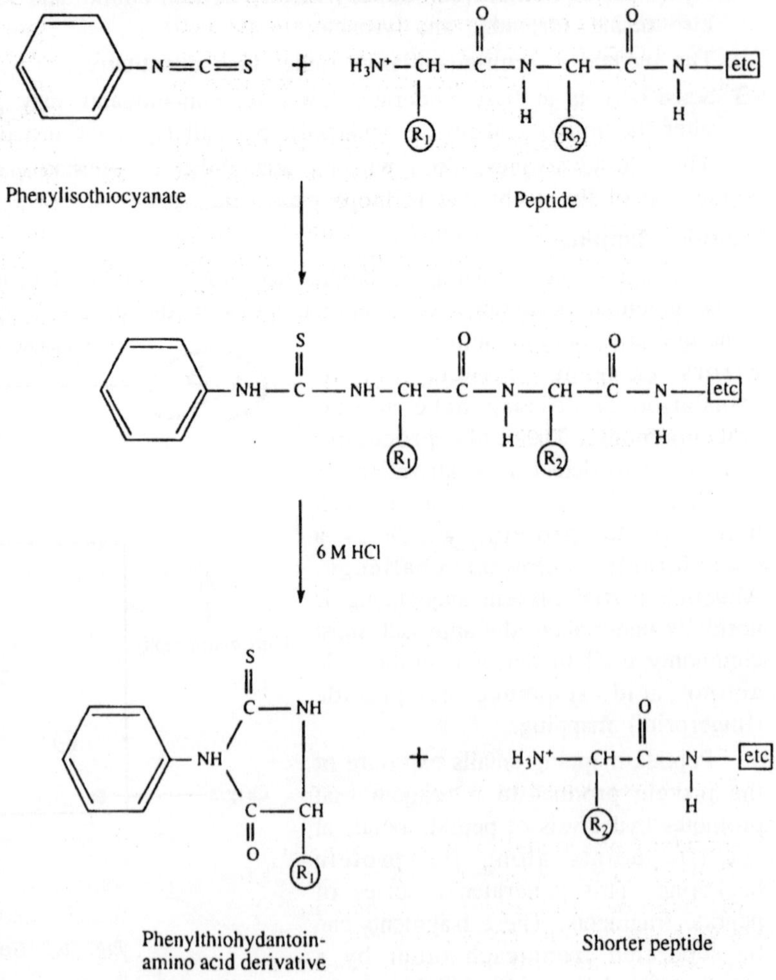

N-terminal Sequencing

N-terminal sequencing of the first 20–30 amino acid residues of the protein product has become a popular quality control test for finished biopharmaceutical products. The technique is useful, as it:

1. Positively identifies the protein;
2. Confirms (or otherwise) the accuracy of the amino acid sequence of at least the N-terminus of the protein;
3. Readily identifies the presence of modified forms of the product in which one or more amino acids are missing from the N-terminus.

Phenylisothiocyanate + Peptide

6 M HCl

Phenylthiohydantoin-amino acid derivative + Shorter peptide

Fig. 10.3. The Edman degradation method, by which the sequence of a peptide/polypeptide may be elucidated.

N-terminal sequencing is normally undertaken by Edman degradation. Although this technique was developed in the 1950s, advances in analytical methodologies now facilitate fast and automated determination of up to the first 100 amino acids from the N-terminus of most proteins, and usually requires a sample size of less than 1 μmol to do so. Analogous techniques facilitating sequencing from a polypeptide's C-terminus remain to be satisfactorily developed. The enzyme carboxypeptidase C sequentially removes amino acids from the C-terminus, but often only removes the first few such amino acids. Furthermore, the rate at which it hydrolyses bonds can vary, depending on what amino acids have contributed to bond formation. Chemical approaches based on principles similar to the Edman procedure have been attempted. However, poor yields of derivatized product and the occurrence of side reactions have prevented widespread acceptance of this method.

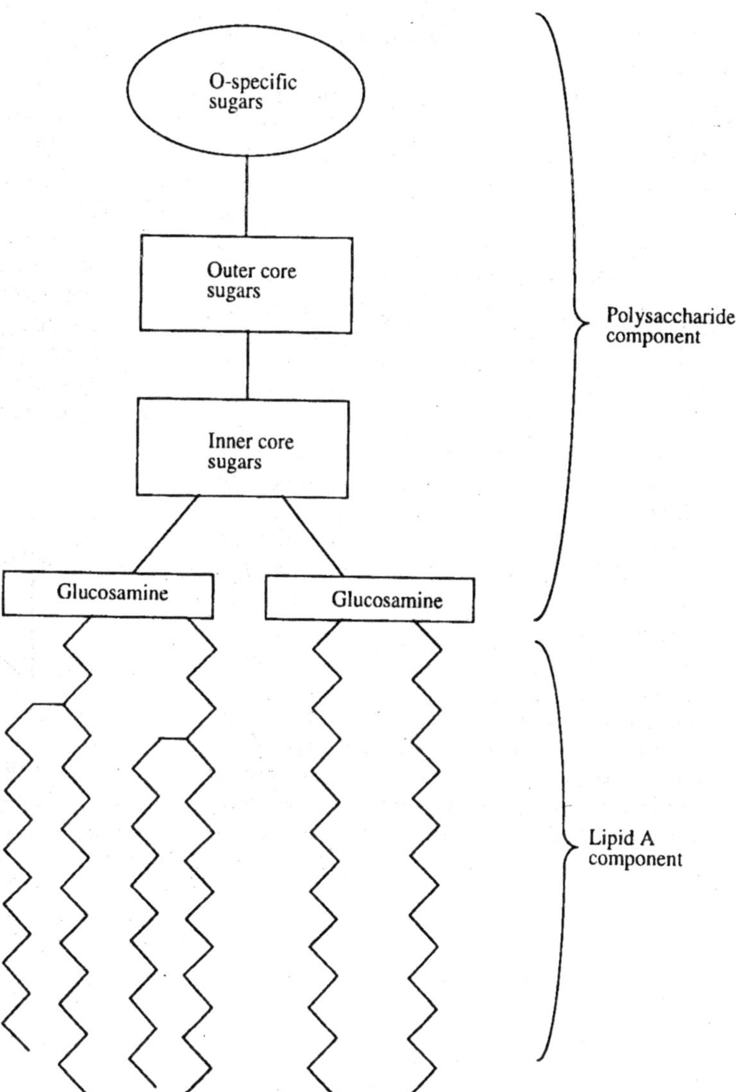

Fig. 10.4. Structure of a generalized LPS molecule.

Analysis of Secondary and Tertiary Structure

Analyses such as peptide mapping, N-terminal sequencing or amino acid analysis yield information relating to a polypeptide's primary structure, i.e. its amino acid sequence. Such tests yield no information relating to higher-order structures (i.e. secondary and tertiary structure of polypeptides, along with quaternary structure of multi-subunit proteins). Although a protein's three-dimensional conformation may be studied in great detail by X-ray crystallography or NMR spectroscopy, routine application of such techniques to biopharmaceutical manufacture is impractical, both from a technical and an economic standpoint. Limited analysis of protein secondary and tertiary structure can, however, be more easily undertaken using spectroscopic methods, particularly far-UV circular dichroism. More recently proton-NMR has also been applied to studying higher orders of protein structure.

Endotoxin and other Pyrogenic Contaminants

Pyrogens are substances that, when they enter the blood stream, influence hypothalamic regulation of body temperature, usually resulting in fever. Medical control of pyrogen-induced fever proves very difficult, and in severe cases results in patient death. Pyrogens represent a diverse group of substances, including various chemicals, particulate matter and endotoxin (LPS), a molecule derived from the outer membrane of Gram-negative bacteria. Such Gram-negative organisms harbour 3–4 million LPS molecules on their surface, representing in the region of 75 per cent of their outer membrane surface area. Gram-negative bacteria clinically significant in human medicine include *E. coli*, *Haemophilus influenzae*, *Salmonella enterica*, *Klebsiella pneumoniae*, *Bordetella pertussis*, *Pseudomonas aeruginosa*, *Chylamydia psittaci* and *Legionella pneumophila*.

In many instances the influence of pyrogens on body temperature is indirect. For example, entry of endotoxin into the bloodstream stimulates the production of IL-1 by macrophages. It is the IL-1 that directly initiates the fever response (hence its alternative name, '*endogenous pyrogen*').

Although entry of any pyrogenic substance into the bloodstream can have serious medical consequences, endotoxin receives most attention because of its ubiquitous nature. Therefore, it is the pyrogen most likely to contaminate parenteral (bio)pharmaceutical products. Effective implementation of GMP minimizes the likelihood of product contamination by pyrogens. For example, GMP dictates that chemical reagents used in the manufacture of process buffers be extremely pure. Such raw materials, therefore, are unlikely to contain chemical contaminants displaying pyrogenic activity. Furthermore, GMP encourages filtration of virtually all parenteral products through a 0.45 or 0.22 μm filter at points during processing and prior to filling in final product containers (even if the product can subsequently be sterilized by autoclaving). Filtration ensures removal of all particulate matter from the product. In addition, most final product containers are rendered particle free immediately prior to filling by an automatic pre-rinse using WFI. As an additional safeguard, the final product will usually be subject to a particulate matter test by QC before final product release. The simplest format for such a test could involve visual inspection of vial contents, although specific particle detecting and counting equipment is more routinely used.

Contamination of the final product with endotoxin is more difficult to control because:

1. Many recombinant biopharmaceuticals are produced in Gram-negative bacterial systems; thus, the product source is also a source of endotoxin.
2. Despite rigorous implementation of GMP, most biopharmaceutical preparations will be contaminated with low levels of Gram-negative bacteria at some stage of manufacture. These bacteria shed endotoxin into the product stream, which is not removed during subsequent bacterial filtration steps. This is one of many reasons why GMP dictates that the level of bioburden in the product stream should be minimized at all stages of manufacture.
3. The heat stability exhibited by endotoxin means that autoclaving of process equipment will not destroy endotoxin present on such equipment.
4. Adverse medical reactions caused by endotoxin are witnessed in humans at dosage rates as low as 0.5 ng per kilogram body weight.

Endotoxin, the Molecule

As its name suggests, LPS consists of a complex polysaccharide component linked to a lipid (lipid A) moiety. The polysaccharide moiety is generally composed of 50 or more monosaccharide units linked by glycosidic bonds. Sugar moieties often found in LPS include glucose, glucosamine, mannose and galactose, as well as more extensive structures such as L-glycero-mannoheptose. The polysaccharide component of LPS may be divided into several structural domains. The inner (core) domains vary relatively little between LPS molecules isolated from different Gram-negative bacteria. The outer (O-specific) domain is usually bacterial-strain specific. Most of the LPS biological activity (pyrogenicity) is associated with its lipid A moiety. This usually consists of six or more fatty acids attached directly to sugars such as glucosamine. Again, as is the case in relation to the carbohydrate component, lipid A moieties of LPS isolated from different bacteria can vary somewhat. The structure of *E coli*'s lipid A has been studied in the greatest detail; its exact structure has been elucidated and it can be chemically synthesized.

Pyrogen Detection

Pyrogens may be detected in parenteral preparations (or other substances) by a number of methods. Two such methods are widely employed in the pharmaceutical industry.

Historically, the rabbit pyrogen test constituted the most widely used method. This entails parenteral administration of the product to a group of healthy rabbits, with subsequent monitoring of rabbit temperature using rectal probes. Increased rabbit temperature above a certain point suggests the presence of pyrogenic substances. The basic rabbit method, as outlined in the European Pharmacopoeia, entails initial administration of the product to three rabbits. The product is considered to have passed the test if the total (summed) increase of the temperature of all three animals is less than 1.15°C. If the total increase recorded is greater than 2.65°C then the product has failed. However, if the response observed falls between these two limits the result is considered inconclusive, and the test must be repeated using a further batch of animals.

This test is popular because it detects a wide spectrum of pyrogenic substances. However, it is also subject to a number of disadvantages, including:

1. It is expensive (there is a requirement for animals, animal facilities and animal technicians);
2. Excitation/poor handling of the rabbits can affect the results obtained, usually prompting a false positive result;
3. Subclinical infection/poor overall animal health can also lead to false positive results;
4. Use of different rabbit colonies/breeds can yield variable results.

Another issue of relevance is that certain biopharmaceuticals (e.g. cytokines such as 1L-1 and TNF) themselves induce a natural pyrogenic response. This rules out use of the rabbit- based assay for detection of exogenous pyrogens in such products. Such difficulties have led to the increased use of an *in vitro* assay; the *Limulus* ameobocyte lysate (LAL) test. This is based upon endotoxin-stimulated coagulation of amoebocyte lysate obtained from horseshoe crabs. This test is now the most widely used assay for the detection of endotoxins in biopharmaceutical and other pharmaceutical preparations.

Development of the LAL assay was based upon the observation that the presence of Gram- negative bacteria in the vascular system of the American horseshoe crab, *Limulus polyphemus*, resulted in the clotting of its blood. Tests on fractionated blood showed that the factor responsible for coagulation resided within the crab's circulating blood cells, i.e. the amoebocytes. Further research revealed that the bacterial agent responsible of initiation of clot formation was endotoxin.

The endotoxin molecule activates a coagulation cascade quite similar in design to the mammalian blood coagulation cascade. Activation of the cascade also requires the presence of divalent cations such as calcium or magnesium. The final steps of this pathway entail the proteolytic cleavage of the polypeptide coagulogen, forming coagulin, and a smaller peptide fragment. Coagulin molecules then interact non-covalently, forming a 'clot' or 'gel'.

The LAL-based assay for endotoxin became commercially available in the 1970s. The LAL reagent is prepared by extraction of blood from the horseshoe crab, followed by isolation of its amoebocytes by centrifugation. After a washing step, the amoebocytes are lysed and the lysate dispensed into pyrogen-free vials. The assay is normally performed by making a series of 1:2 dilutions of the test sample using (pyrogen-free) WFI(and pyrogen-free test tubes). A reference standard endotoxin preparation is treated similarly. LAL reagent is added to all tubes, incubated for 1 h, and these tubes are then inverted

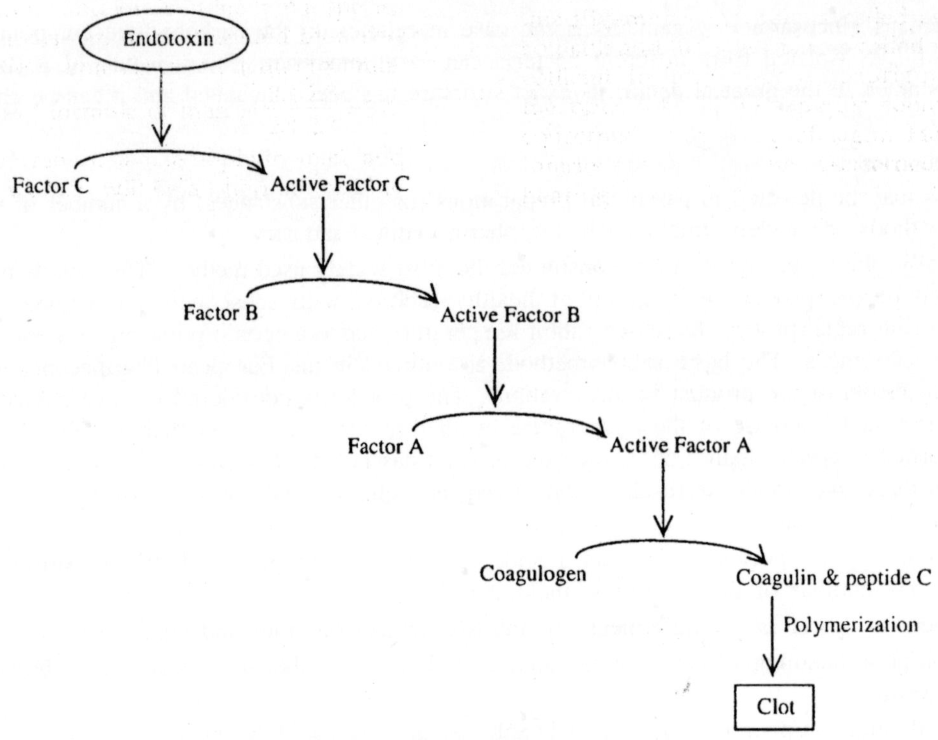

Fig. 10.5. Activation of clot formation by endotoxin.

to test for gel (i.e. clot) formation, which would indicate presence of endotoxin. More recently, a colorimetric-based LAL procedure has been devised. This entails addition to the LAL reagent of a short peptide, susceptible to hydrolysis by the LAL clotting enzyme. This synthetic peptide contains a chromogenic tag (usually *para*-nitroaniline, pNA) which is released free into solution by the clotting enzyme. This allows spectrophotometric analysis of the test sample, facilitating more accurate end-point determination. The LAL system displays several advantages when compared with the rabbit test, most notably:

1. Sensitivity – endotoxin levels as low as a few picograms per millilitre of sample assayed will be detected;
2. Cost – the assay is far less expensive than the rabbit assay;
3. Speed – depending upon the format used, the LAL assay may be conducted within 15–60 min.

Its major disadvantage is its selectivity: it only detects endotoxin-based pyrogens. In practice, however, endotoxin represents the pyrogen that is by far the most likely to be present in pharmaceutical products. The LAL method is used extensively within the industry. It is used not only to detect endotoxin in finished parenteral preparations, but also in WFI and in biological fluids, such as serum or cerebrospinal fluid. Before the LAL assay is routinely used to detect/quantify endotoxin in any product, its effective functioning in the presence of that product must be demonstrated by validation studies. Such studies are required to prove that the product (or, more likely, excipients present in the product) do not interfere with the rate/extent of clot formation (i.e. are neither inhibitors nor activators of the LAL-based enzymes). LAL enzyme inhibition could facilitate false-negative results upon sample assay. Validation studies entail, for example, observing the effect of spiking endotoxin-negative product with know quantities of endotoxin, or spiking endotoxin with varying quantities of product, before assay with the LAL reagents. All ancillary reagents used in the LAL assay system (e.g. WFI, test tubes, pipette tips for liquid transfer, etc.) must obviously be endotoxin free. Such items can be rendered endotoxin free by heat. Its heat-stable nature, however, renders very vigorous heating necessary in order to destroy contaminant endotoxin. A single autoclave cycle is insufficient, with total destruction requiring three consecutive autoclave cycles. Dry heat may also be used (180°C for 3 h or 240°C for 1 h).

GMP requires that, where practicable, process equipment coming into direct contact with the biopharmaceutical product stream should be rendered endotoxin free (depyrogenated) before use. Autoclaving, steam or dry heat can effectively be used on many process vessels, pipework, etc., which are usually manufactured from stainless steel or other heat-resistant material. Such an approach is not routinely practicable in the case of some items of process equipment, such as chromatographic systems. Fortunately, endotoxin is sensitive to strongly alkaline conditions; thus, routine cleaning in place of chromatographic systems using 1 mol l^{-1} NaOH represents an effective depyrogenation step. Gentler approaches, such as exhaustive rinsing with WFI (until an LAL test shows the eluate to be endotoxin free), can also be surprisingly effective. It is generally unnecessary to introduce specific measures aimed at endotoxin removal from the product during downstream processing. Endotoxin present in the earlier stages of production is often effectively removed from the product during chromatographic fractionation. The endotoxin molecule's highly negative charge often facilitates its effective removal from the product stream by ion-exchange chromatography. Gel-filtration chromatography also serves to remove endotoxin from the product. Although individual LPS molecules exhibit an average molecular mass of less than 20 kDa, these molecules aggregate in aqueous environments and generate supramolecular structures of molecular mass 100–1000 kDa.

The molecular mass of most biopharmaceuticals is considerably less than 100 kDa. The proteins would thus elute from gel-filtration columns much later than contaminating endotoxin aggregates. Should the biopharmaceutical exhibit a molecular mass approaching or exceeding 100 kDa, then effective separation can still be achieved by inclusion of a chelating agent such as EDTA in the running buffer. This promotes depolymerization of the endotoxin aggregates into monomeric (20 kDa) form. Additional techniques capable of separating biomolecules on the basis of molecular mass (e.g. ultrafiltration) may also be used to remove endotoxin from the product stream.

DNA

The clinical significance of DNA-based contaminants in biopharmaceutical products remains unclear. The concerns relating to the presence of DNA in modern biopharmaceuticals focus primarily upon the presence of active oncogenes in the genome of several producer cell types (e.g. monoclonal antibody production in hybridoma cell lines). Parenteral administration of DNA contaminants containing active oncogenes to patients is considered undesirable. The concern is that uptake and expression of such DNA in human cells could occur. There is some evidence to suggest that naked DNA can be assimilated by some cells at least, under certain conditions. Guidelines to date state that an acceptable level of residual DNA in recombinant products is of the order of 10 pg per therapeutic dose.

DNA hybridization studies (e.g. the '*dot blot*' assay) utilizing radiolabelled DNA probes allows detection of DNA contaminants in the product, to levels in the nanogram range. The process begins with isolation of the contaminating DNA from the product. This can be achieved, for example, by phenol and chloroform extraction and ethanol precipitation. The isolated DNA is then applied as a spot (i.e. a 'dot') onto nitrocellulose filter paper, with subsequent baking of the filter at 80°C under vacuum. This promotes (a) DNA denaturation, yielding single strands, and (b) binding of the DNA to the filter. A sample of total DNA derived from the cells in which the product is produced is then radiolabelled with ^{32}P using the process of nick translation. It is heated to 90°C (promotes denaturation, forming single strands) and incubated with the baked filter for several hours at 40°C. Lowering the temperature allows reannealing of single strands via complementary base-pairing to occur. Labelled DNA will reanneal with any complementary DNA strands immobilized on the filter. After the filter is washed (to remove non-specifically bound radiolabelled probe) it is subjected to autoradiography, which allows detection of any bound probe.

Quantification of the DNA isolated from the product involves concurrent inclusion in the dot blot assay of a set of spots, containing known quantities of DNA, and being derived from the producer cell. After autoradiography, the intensity of the test spot is compared with the standards. In many instances there is little need to incorporate specific DNA removal steps during downstream processing. Endogenous nucleases liberated upon cellular homogenization come into direct contact with cellular DNA, resulting in its degradation. Commercial DNase's are sometimes added to crude homogenate to reduce DNA-associated product viscosity. Most chromatographic steps are also effective in separating DNA from the product stream. Ion-exchange chromatography is particularly effective, as DNA exhibits a large overall negative charge (due to the phosphate constituent of its nucleotide backbone).

Microbial and Viral Contaminants

Finished-product biopharmaceuticals, along with other pharmaceuticals intended for parenteral administration, must be sterile (the one exception being live bacterial vaccines). The presence of microorganisms in the final product is unacceptable for a number of reasons:

1. Parenteral administration of contaminated product would likely lead to the establishment of a severe infection in the recipient patient.
2. Microorganisms may be capable of metabolizing the product itself, thus reducing its potency. This is particularly true of protein-based biopharmaceuticals, as most microbes produce an array of extracellular proteases.
3. Microbial-derived substances secreted into the product could adversely affect the recipient's health. Examples include endotoxin secreted from Gram-negative bacteria, or microbial proteins that would stimulate an immune response.

Terminal sterilization by autoclaving guarantees product sterility. Heat sterilization, however, is not a viable option in the case of biopharmaceuticals. Sterilization of biopharmaceuticals by filtration, followed by aseptic filling into a sterile final-product container, inherently carries a greater risk of product contamination. Finished-product sterility testing of such preparations thus represents one of the most critical product tests undertaken by QC. Specific guidelines relating to sterility testing of finished products are given in international pharmacopoeias.

Biopharmaceutical products are also subjected to screening for the presence of viral particles prior to final product release. Although viruses could be introduced, for example, via infected personnel during downstream processing, proper implementation of GMP minimizes such risk. Any viral particles found in the finished product are most likely derived from raw material sources. Examples could include HIV or hepatitis viruses present in blood used in the manufacture of blood products. Such raw materials must be screened before processing for the presence of likely viral contaminants.

A variety of murine (mouse) and other mammalian cell lines have become popular host systems for the production of recombinant human biopharmaceuticals. Moreover, most monoclonal antibodies used for therapeutic purposes are produced by murine-derived hybridoma cells. These cell lines are sensitive to infection by various viral particles. Producer cell lines are screened during product development studies to ensure freedom from a variety of pathogenic advantageous agents, including various species of bacteria, fungi, yeast, mycoplasma, protozoa, parasites, viruses and prions. Suitable microbiological precautions must subsequently be undertaken to prevent producer cell banks from becoming contaminated with such pathogens. Removal of viruses from the product stream can be achieved in a number of ways. The physicochemical properties of viral particles differ greatly from most proteins, ensuring that effective fractionation is automatically achieved by most chromatographic techniques. Gel-filtration chromatography, for example, effectively separates viral particles from most proteins on the basis of differences in size.

In addition to chromatographic separation, downstream processing steps may be undertaken that are specifically aimed at removal or inactivation of viral particles potentially present in the product stream. Significantly, many are 'blanket' procedures, equally capable of removing known or potentially likely viral contaminants and any uncharacterized/undetected viruses. Filtration through a 0.22 μm filter effectively removes microbial agents from the product stream, but fails to remove most viral types. Repeat filtration through a 0.1 μm filter is more effective in this regard. Alternatively, incorporation of an ultrafiltration step (preferably at the terminal stages of downstream processing) also proves effective. Incorporation of downstream processing steps known to inactivate a wide variety of viral types provides further assurance that the final product is unlikely to harbour active virus. Heating and irradiation are amongst the two most popular such approaches. Heating the product to between 40 and 60°C for several hours inactivates a broad range of viruses. Many biopharmaceuticals can be heated to such temperatures without being denatured themselves. Such an approach has been used extensively to inactivate blood-borne viruses in blood products. Exposure of product to controlled levels of UV radiation can also be quite effective, while having no adverse effect on the product itself.

Viral Assays

A range of assay techniques may be used to detect and quantify viral contaminants in both raw materials and finished-biopharmaceutical products. No generic assay exists that is capable of detecting all viral types potentially present in a given sample. Viral assays currently available will detect only a specific virus, or at best a family of closely related viruses. The strategy adopted, therefore, usually entails screening product for viral particles known to be capable of infecting the biopharmaceutical source material. Such assays will not normally detect newly evolved viral strains, or uncharacterized/unknown viral contaminants. This fact underlines the importance of including at least one step in downstream processing that is likely to inactivate or remove viruses indiscriminately from the product. This acts as a safety net. Current viral assays fall into one of three categories:

- Immunoassays;
- Assays based on viral DNA probes;
- Bioassays.

Generation of antibodies that can recognize and bind to specific viruses is straightforward. A sample of live or attenuated virus, or a purified component of the viral caspid, can be injected into animals to stimulate polyclonal antibody production (or to facilitate monoclonal antibody production by hybridoma technology). Harvested antibodies are then employed to develop specific immunoassays that can be used to screen test samples routinely for the presence of that specific virus. Immunoassays capable of detecting a wide range of viruses are available commercially. The sensitivity, ease, speed and relative inexpensiveness of these assays render them particularly attractive. An alternative assay format entails the use of virus-specific DNA probes. These can be used to screen the biopharmaceutical product for the presence of viral DNA. The assay strategy is similar to the dot blot assays used to detect host-cell-derived DNA contaminants, as discussed earlier. Viral bioassays of various different formats have also been developed. One format entails incubation of the final product with cell lines sensitive to a range of viruses. The cells are subsequently monitored for cytopathic effects or other obvious signs of viral infection. A range of mouse-, rabbit- or hamster-antibody production tests may also be undertaken. These bioassays entail administration of the product to a test animal. Any viral agents present will elicit production of antiviral antibodies in that animal. Serum samples (withdrawn from the animal approximately 4 weeks after product administration) are screened for the presence of antibodies recognizing a range of viral antigens. This can be achieved by enzyme immunoassay, in which immobilized antigen is used to screen for the virus-specific antibodies. These assay systems are extremely sensitive, as minute quantities of viral antigen will elicit strong antibody production A single serum sample can also be screened for antibodies specific to a wide range of viral particles. Time and expense factors, however, militate against this particular assay format.

Miscellaneous Contaminants

In addition to those already discussed, biopharmaceutical products may harbour other contaminants, some of which may be intentionally added to the product stream during the initial stages of downstream processing. Examples could include buffer components, precipitants (ethanol or other solvents, salts, etc.), proteolytic inhibitors, glycerol, anti-foam agents, etc. In addition to these, other contaminants may enter the product during downstream processing in a less controlled way. Examples could include metal ions leached from product-holding tanks/pipework, or breakdown products leaking from chromatographic media. The final product containers must also be chosen carefully. They must be chemically inert and be of suitable quality to eliminate the possibility of leaching of any substance from the container during product storage. For this reason, high-quality glass vials are often used.

In some instances it may be necessary to demonstrate that all traces of specific contaminants have been removed prior to final product filling. This would be true, for example, of many proteolytic inhibitors added during the initial stages of downstream processing to prevent proteolysis by endogenous proteases. Some such inhibitors may be inherently toxic, and many could (inappropriately) inhibit endogenous proteases of the recipient patient.

Demonstration of absence from the product of breakdown products from chromatographic columns may be necessary in certain instances. This is particularly true with regard to some affinity chromatography columns. Various chemical-coupling methods may be used to attach affinity ligands to the chromatographic support material. Some such procedures entail the use of toxic reagents, which, if not entirely removed after coupling, could leach into the product. In some cases ligands can also subsequently leach from the columns, particularly after sustained usage or overvigorous sanitation procedures. Improvements in the chemical stability of modern chromatographic media, however, have reduced such difficulties, and most manufacturers have carried out extensive validation studies regarding the stability of their product.

Sophisticated analytical methodologies facilitate detection of vanishingly low levels of many contaminants in biopharmaceutical preparations. The possibility exists, however, that uncharacterized contaminants may persist, remaining undetected in the final product. As an additional safety measure, finished products are often subjected to 'abnormal toxicity' or '*general safety*' tests. Standardized protocols for such tests are outlined in various international pharmacopoeias. These normally entail parenteral administration of the product to at least five healthy mice. The animals are placed under observation for 48 h and should exhibit no ill effects (other than expected symptoms). The death or illness of one or more animals signals a requirement for further investigation, usually using a larger number of animals. Such toxicity testing represents a safety net, designed to expose any unexpected activities in the product that could compromise the health of the recipient.

Validation Studies

Validation can be defined as 'the act of proving that any procedure, process, equipment, material, activity or system leads to the expected results'. Routine and adequate validation studies form a core principle of GMP as applied to (bio)pharmaceutical manufacture, as such studies help assure the overall safety of the finished product. All validation procedures must be carefully designed and fully documented in written format. The results of all validation studies undertaken must also be documented, and retained in the plant files. As part of their routine inspection of manufacturing facilities, regulatory personnel will usually inspect a sample of these records, to ensure conformance to GMP.

Validation studies encompass all aspects of (bio)pharmaceutical manufacture. All new items of equipment must be validated before being routinely used. Initial validation studies should be comprehensive, with follow-up validation studies being undertaken at appropriate time intervals (e.g. daily, weekly or monthly). It is considered judicious to validate older items of equipment with increased frequency. Such studies can forewarn the manufacturer of impending equipment failure. Some validatory studies are straightforward, e.g. validation of weighing equipment simply entails weighing of standardized weights. Autoclaves may be validated by placing external temperature probes at various points in the autoclave chamber during a routine autoclave run. Validation studies should confirm that all areas within the chamber reach the required temperature for the required time.

Periodic validation of clean room air (HEPA) filters is also an essential part of GMP. After their installation, HEPA filters are subjected to a leak test. Particle counters are also used to validate cleanroom conditions. A particle counter is a vacuum-cleaner-like machine capable of sucking air from its surroundings at constant velocity and passing it through a counting chamber. The number of particles per cubic metre of air tested can easily be determined. Furthermore, passage of the air through a 0.2 μm filter housed in the counter will trap all airborne microorganisms. By placing the filter on the surface of a nutrient-agar-containing Petri dish, trapped microorganisms will grow as colonies, allowing determination of the microbial load per cubic metre of air.

In addition to equipment, many processes/procedures undertaken during pharmaceutical manufacture are also subject to periodic validation studies. Validation of biopharmaceutical aseptic filling procedures is amongst the most critical. The aim is to prove that the aseptic procedures devised are capable of delivering a sterile finished product, as intended.

Aseptic filling validation entails substituting a batch of final product with nutrient broth. The broth is subject to sterile filtration and aseptic processing. After sealing the final product containers, they are incubated at 3 0–37 °C, which encourages growth of any contaminant microorganisms. (Growth can be easily monitored by subsequently measuring the absorbance at 600 nm.) Absence of growth validates the aseptic procedures developed.

Contaminant-clearance validation studies are of special significance in biopharmaceutical manufacture. Downstream processing must be capable of removing contaminants such as viruses, DNA and endotoxin from the product steam. Contaminant-clearance validation studies normally entail spiking the raw material (from which the product is to be purified) with a known level of the chosen contaminant and subjecting the contaminated material to the complete downstream processing protocol. This allows determination of the level of clearance of the contaminant achieved after each purification step, and the contaminant reduction factor for the overall process.

Viral clearance studies, for example, are typically undertaken by spiking the raw material with a mixture of at least three different viral species, preferably ones that represent likely product contaminants, and for which straightforward assay systems are available. Loading levels of up to 1×10^{10} viral particles are commonly used. The cumulative viral removal/inactivation observed should render the likelihood of a single viral particle remaining in a single therapeutic dose of product being greater that one in a million. A similar strategy is adopted when undertaking DNA clearance studies. The starting material is spiked with radiolabelled DNA and then subjected to downstream processing. The level of residual DNA remaining in the product stream after each step can easily be determined by monitoring for radioactivity. The quantity of DNA used to spike the product should ideally be somewhat in excess of the levels of DNA normally associated with the product prior to its purification. However, spiking of the product with a vast excess of DNA is counterproductive, in that it may render subsequent downstream processing unrepresentative of standard production runs.

For more comprehensive validation studies, the molecular mass profile of the DNA spike should roughly approximate to the molecular mass range of endogenous contaminant DNA in the crude product. Obviously, the true DNA clearance rate attained by downstream processing procedures (e.g. gel filtration) will depend to some extent on the molecular mass characteristics of the contaminant DNA. Other manufacturing procedures requiring validation include cleaning, decontamination and sanitation (CDS) procedures developed for specific items of equipment/processing areas. Of particular importance is the ability of such procedures to remove bioburden. This may be assessed by monitoring levels of microbial contamination before and after application of CDS protocols to the equipment item in question.

11

Biocatalysts for Organic Chemistry

Cross-linked enzyme crystals, one of the most exciting new developments in biocatalysis to come along since people first began to use enzymes to do chemistry, are biocatalysts that the average organic chemist can use as easily as many other standard chemical reagents. Indeed, this new form of enzyme has the potential to transform biocatalysis from an esoteric specialization into the widely practiced synthetic technique it deserves to be. First, the development of cross-linked enzyme crystals (CLCs) will be discussed from a historical perspective. Next, a summary of the properties of enzymes in this form compared to soluble and immobilized enzymes will be presented. Finally, a review of recent applications of CLCs to show how they are bringing biocatalysis into the mainstream of organic synthesis, particularly with respect to the pharmaceutical industry, will be given.

Throughout the bulk of this chapter, CLC will be used as an abbreviation for cross-linked enzyme crystal. Occasionally, the abbreviation CLEC will also be used to indicate cross-linked enzyme crystal. This acronym is a registered trademark of Altus Biologics, Inc. and will be used in discussing work done with various cross-linked enzyme crystals which are commercially available from Altus. Finally, the notation CPC will be used to denote cross-linked protein crystal.

Table 11.1. Commercially available cross-linked enzyme crystals

Product	*Synthetic utility*
ChiroCLEC-BL (Subtilisin protease)	Resolution of amino acids, amines, and amino acid analogs
ChiroCLEC-CR (*Candida rugosa* lipase)	Resolution of alcohols, acids and esters
ChiroCLEC-EC (Penicillin acylase)	Resolution of amino acids and amines; protection/deprotection
ChiroCLEC-PC (*Burkholderia cepacia* lipase)	Resolution of acids, esters, and alcohols
PeptiCLEC-BL (Subtilisin protease)	Coupling of a-amino acid esters to amines, amino acid, or or peptides
PeptiCLEC-TR (Thermolysin protease)	Coupling of a-amino acids to amines, amino acids, or peptides
SynthaCLEC-PA (Penicillin acylase)	Antibiotic synthesis

History

The first reported preparation of cross-linked enzyme crystals was by Quiocho and Richards in 1964. They prepared crystals of carboxypeptidase-A and cross-linked them with glutaraldehyde. The material they prepared retained only about 5% of the activity of the soluble enzyme and showed a measurable increase in mechanical stability. The authors quite correctly predicted that "cross-linked enzyme crystals, particularly ones of small size where the diffusion problem is not serious, may be useful as reagents which can be removed by sedimentation and filtration." Two years later the same authors reported a more detailed study of the enzymic behavior of CLCs of carboxypeptidase-A. In this study they reported that only the lysine residues in the protein were modified by the glutaraldehyde cross-linking. The CLCs were packed in a column for a flow-through assay and maintained activity after many uses over a period of 3 months.

Little was done in the area of cross-linked enzyme crystals over the next 10 years. In 1977, the kinetic properties of CLCs of the protease subtilisin were reported by Tuchsen and Ottesen. They reported that cross-linked enzyme crystals of subtilisin were highly effective catalysts with increased thermal stability and increased stability toward acid compared to the soluble enzyme. They further reported that the CLCs of subtilisin showed essentially no autodigestion at 30°C. Like Quiocho and Richards before them, Tuchsen and Ottesen found that only the lysine residues of the enzyme were affected by the glutaraldehyde treatment.

Another gap of almost 10 years occurred before work in the area of CLCs picked up again. In 1985, a group at the Louis Pasteur University in Strasbourg, France, prepared cross-linked crystals of horse liver alcohol dehydrogenase. The activity of the enzyme in CLC form was maintained and the coenzyme was found to be firmly bound to the crystals. The cross-linked crystals could be used as redox catalysts with no addition of coenzyme. The authors also reported the increased stability of CLCs toward organic solvents.

Up to this time CLCs had been prepared largely for academic interest and showed significant stability but generally only very low activity when compared to the soluble enzymes from which they were derived. Cross-linked enzyme crystals were transformed from a mildly interesting, esoteric area of academic research into a viable commercial technology when Navia and St. Clair reported for the first time the development of cross-linked enzyme crystals (CLECs) which combined high activity with the high stability already associated with CLCs. The use of cross-linked enzyme crystals in biocatalysis finally started to become more common in 1992–1993 when Altus Biologics was formed to commercialize the technology developed by Navia and co-workers. Altus has obtained very broad patent coverage for its technology. Today many different enzymes are available in the cross-linked crystal format exclusively from Altus Biologics under the ChiroCLEC, PeptiCLEC, and SynthaCLEC brand names.

Properties

Having briefly outlined the historical development of cross-linked enzyme crystals, a discussion of their properties as compared to soluble and immobilized enzymes is in order.

Structure

First and foremost, cross-linked enzyme crystals are crystals. Within the crystal lattice the concentration of protein approaches the theoretical limit. This is important to the process development chemist, who would much rather use a small quantity of a very active catalyst in a reactor than fill it with an immobilized enzyme. Typically an immobilized enzyme contains only 1–10% by weight enzyme, with the remaining carrier material simply occupying valuable reactor space. The crystallinity is absolutely required to achieve the stability exhibited by CLCs. Cross-linked soluble thermolysin and cross-linked precipitate of thermolysin are no more stable than the soluble enzyme. Crystals of proteins (and enzymes) are not solid structures. They typically contain 30–65%, by volume, open channels, which are usually filled with solvent. In the case of cross- linked crystals of thermolysin, the diameter of those channels is about 25 Å. Cross-linked enzyme crystals and cross-linked protein crystals (CPCs) are micro- porous materials with pore surface areas between 500 and 2000 m^2/mg. This is the same range as for inorganic zeolites. CLCs, however, have pore diameters in the range of 3–8 nm, as compared to 0.2–1.0 nm for normal inorganic zeolites. Indeed, CLCs can be thought of as bioorganic zeolites. The macroporous nature of CLCs enables small molecules to penetrate easily into the crystals. Diffusion is not rate limiting, as long as microcrystals (10–100 μm) of enzymes are used to catalyze chemical reactions.

While it has been well established that glutaraldehyde reacts with the side-chain amino groups of lysine residues, the exact nature of the bonds formed is unclear. The stability exhibited to acid appears to eliminate simple imine formation as the mechanism. Aqueous glutaraldehyde forms a mixture of oligomers of various lengths and structures. It is thought that an enzyme crystal which is treated with such a mixture is able to self-select the best cross-linking agents from the mixture for its unique set of side-chain functionalities and their arrangement in space.

Purity

Commercially available, soluble enzyme preparations are generally very crude mixtures containing from less than 1% to about 10% active enzyme. The remaining materials present in these mixtures commonly include buffer salts, cell debris from the fermentation process, and even other enzymes, which may or may not have beneficial activities. Pure soluble enzymes tend to be prohibitively expensive due to the often complex chromatography used to achieve the purification, and frequently prove to be less stable in the purified state. Crystallization is an inexpensive, standard purification technique in organic chemistry. Cross- linked enzyme crystals are therefore, by definition, highly purified forms of enzymes. In contrast to crude enzyme preparations, the high purity of CLCs has several benefits when they are used to conduct chemistry. The most obvious benefit is that the chemist is putting fewer impurities into the reaction to begin with, so he or she can expect a cleaner reaction product and easier workup when the reaction is complete.

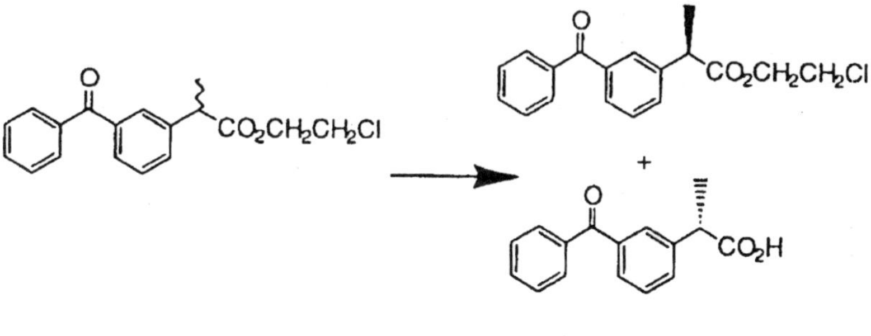

$CO_2CH_2CH_2Cl$ → $CO_2CH_2CH_2Cl$ + CO_2H

S-ketoprofen

Fig. 11.1. Resolution of racemic ketoprofen by enzyme catalyzed ester hydrolysis.

Another major benefit of the purity of CLCs relates to the fact that many commercially available enzyme products actually contain more than one enzyme, and these contaminating enzymes can often lead to undesired side reactions. In the case of a resolution this can mean the difference between success and failure. For example, in the resolution of racemic ketoprofen by ester hydrolysis, the enantioselectivity using crude *Candida rugosa* lipase is poor ($E = 5$). The E value represents the ratio of the specificity constants of the enzyme for the two enantiomers of the substrate and allows one to compare directly the selectivity of different enzymes in a reaction. In contrast, using the purified CLC form of the enzyme gives an $E = 66$, which makes it a viable method for obtaining pure S-ketoprofen.

Stability

Probably the most striking and valuable characteristic of cross-linked enzyme crystals is the remarkable stability they exhibit in comparison to soluble and immobilized enzymes. They can withstand exposure to organic solvents, high temperatures, mechanical stress such as shear, extremes of pH, and even exposure to proteases.

Organic Solvent Stability

Many of the compounds the organic chemist works with in the pharmaceutical industry are not very soluble in water. Enzymes are generally rapidly denatured in the presence of water-miscible organic solvents. Consequently, enzyme-catalyzed reactions which are typically water based have historically been viewed as a technique which was irrelevant to the organic chemist. The remarkable stability of cross-linked enzyme crystals has changed everything.

It is difficult to overstate the significance of the organic solvent stability of CLCs. This stability allows the organic chemist to use enzymes in a much broader set of reaction conditions than was ever possible before. Since it is now possible to use enzymes with the standard type of conditions under which they normally work, chemists are much more likely to try a biocatalytic step when developing a new synthetic scheme. Thus CLCs are the biocatalysts of choice for the organic chemist, and their commercial availability is spearheading an increase in the use of enzymes in the pharmaceutical industry.

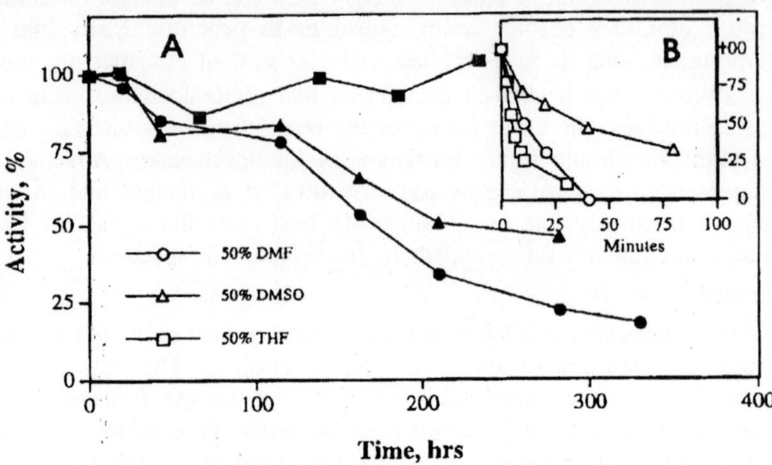

Fig. 11.2. Stability of (A) CRL-CLEC and (B) commercial CRL in the presence of water-miscible organic solvents.

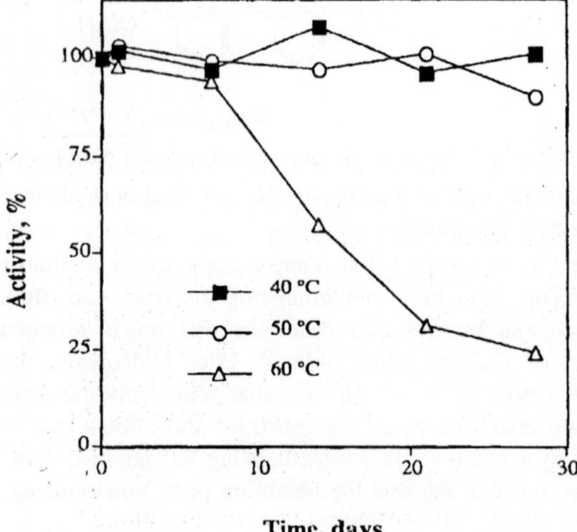

Fig. 11.3. Stability of thermolysin CLEC at elevated temperatures. In comparison, the half-life of soluble thermolysin is only 10 hr at 50°C.

Thermal stability

Soluble enzymes are typically easily inactivated by heat. It does not require much energy to disrupt the hydrogen bonds and other weak forces which hold an enzyme in its active conformation. Like the organic solvent stability, the thermal stability of CLCs can be two to three orders of magnitude greater than that of the soluble protein. When an enzyme forms a crystal, a very large number of stabilizing contacts are formed between individual enzyme molecules. Energy must be put into the system in order to disrupt these new contacts. On top of that, additional energy is required to break the covalent cross-links before the CLC begins to dissolve and then denature. CLCs therefore are much more stable than the same enzyme in solution.

The increased thermal stability offers several major benefits to the organic chemist using CLCs as catalysts. First, no special storage conditions are required for CLCs. Unlike soluble and immobilized forms, which must be shipped and stored cold, CLCs are stable for years at room temperature. Second, since enzyme catalyzed reactions are generally slower in organic solvents and with non-natural substrates, the ability to run such reactions at higher temperatures to increase the rate is a significant benefit to the chemist.

Mechanical stability

Testing has shown that CLEC catalysts are stable for long periods of time under standard fine chemical production conditions such as agitation, pumping, and filtration. As a process is scaled up from the bench, through pilot scale and production, there is an increase in the mechanical shear and pressure to which the catalyst is exposed to. CLCs of thermolysin and *Candida rugosa* lipase under high or moderate shear mixing showed little or no loss in average particle size. Extended agitation of an aqueous CLEC suspension at high mixing speeds using a flat turbine (high shear) and an A310 propeller blade (moderate shear) showed virtually no particle breakage. Under the more drastic treatment of continuous pumping using a high-shear centrifugal pump for 24 hr, particle fracturing for ChiroCLEC-CR was seen only at the highest speed. CLEC particles are mechanically stable under the highest shear conditions seen in fluid transfer and agitation.

Stability to proteolysis

Enzymes in the cross-linked crystal form are essentially impervious to degradation by exogenous proteases and from autolysis, in the case of CLCs of proteases themselves. This stability makes the enzyme-catalyzed preparation of peptides and peptide mimics truly practical. Further, one could conceive of using multiple enzymes in "one-pot" reaction systems mimicking natural biosynthetic cascades. Indeed, the application of this concept has been reported for a mixture of lipoamide dehydrogenase and lactate dehydrogenase.

General Applications

The primary focus of this section will be the use of cross-linked enzyme crystals as catalysts of chemical reactions and particularly those reactions of relevance to the pharmaceutical industry. Before beginning this discussion, however, a brief look at the use of CLCs in chromatography is given, since this application also has possible uses in the pharmaceutical industry.

Chromatography

Cross-linked enzyme crystals and cross-linked protein crystals can be thought of as bioorganic zeolites. In addition, CLCs and CPCs are chiral in nature and in the case of cross-linked enzyme crystals also contain special binding sites. It has recently been shown that CLCs and CPCs can be packed in high-performance liquid chromatography (HPLC) columns and used as unique stationary phases. These "*bioorganic zeolite*" columns are able to perform separations via size exclusion, adsorption, and chiral discrimination. The materials showed excellent stability over 500 runs cycling between water and 50% acetonitrile. This application of CLCs may become much more important in the future if large-scale chromatography becomes more widely accepted and utilized in the manufacture of pharmaceutical active ingredients and intermediates.

Biocatalysis

The major application of cross-linked enzyme crystals in the pharmaceutical and fine chemicals industry is in biocatalysis or the use of CLCs to catalyze various chemical reactions. In this section we will review recent applications, grouped by reaction type.

Resolutions

Resolutions of racemic mixtures are by far the most frequent applications of biocatalysts in the pharmaceutical industry. Repic et al., of the process research and development group at Novartis,

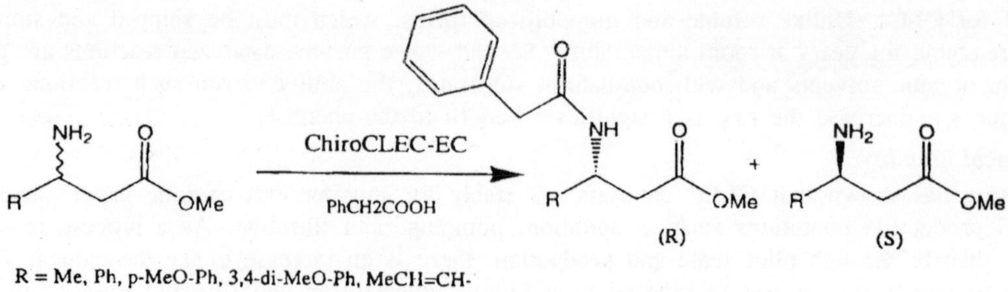

R = Me, Ph, p-MeO-Ph, 3,4-di-MeO-Ph, MeCH=CH-

Fig. 11.4. Resolution of β-amino esters via selective acylation.

recently published work to develop a method for the resolution of racemic β-amino acid esters, an important class of intermediates for the preparation of peptidomimetics. The Novartis group used Chiro-CLEC-EC in 2% aqueous toluene to selectively acylate several different β-amino esters. The authors were able to isolate the desired isomer of the amino esters in >95% ee in a simple one-step reaction and described it as a method which could be amenable for large-scale preparation.

The bicyclic aminoalcohol, 3-quinuclidinol, is an important synthon for the preparation of cholinergic receptor ligands, anesthetics, and drugs for the treatment of Alzheimer's disease and asthma. P. Bossard at Lonza AG developed and patented an enantioselective acylation of racemic 3-quinuclidinol using ChiroCLEC-BL, the CLC form of subtilisin. The reaction was run in 2-methyl-3-butanol with vinyl butyrate used as the acylating agent. The pure (*R*) enantiomer was obtained in 68% yield and 96.2% ee after crystallization.

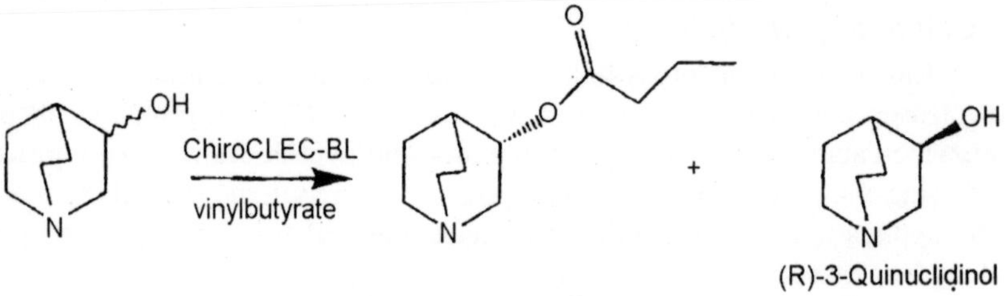

(R)-3-Quinuclidinol

Fig. 11.5. Resolution of (R,S)-3-quinuclidinol via selective acylation.

The natural products epothilone A and B are structurally different from taxol but have similar anticancer activity. Significantly, they have been reported to be much more active against cell lines exhibiting multiple-drug resistance. Taylor and co-workers at the University of Notre Dame have recently published an elegant, formal total synthesis of epothilone A. In this work, the authors used the CLC form of *Burkholderia cepacia* (formerly *Pseudomonas cepacia*) lipase (ChiroCLEC-PC) to resolve a key alcohol intermediate by selective acylation with vinyl acetate in *t*-butyl methyl ether. The enantioselectivity was >20:1 at 47% conversion and efficiently provided gram quantities of the desired (*R*) alcohol. Since the unreacted (*S*) alcohol can easily be epimerized by a simple oxidation–reduction sequence and the catalyst reused without significant loss in activity, the method is ideally suited for scale-up.

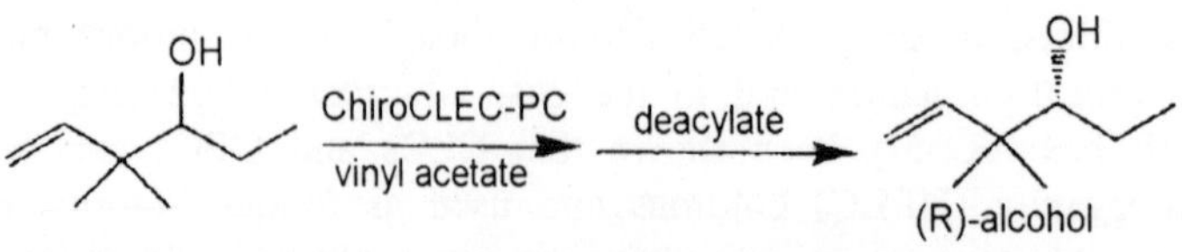

(R)-alcohol

Fig. 11.6. Resolution of key alcohol intermediate for epothilone A and B.

Researchers at the biotech company EntreMed, Inc., have recently prepared and tested 2-phthalimidino-glutaric acid analogs of thalidomide and found them to be potent inhibitors of tumor metastasis. The key to the success of their synthesis was a resolution via enantioselective ester hydrolysis catalyzed by ChiroCLEC-BL, the CLC form of the protease subtilisin. The authors were able to isolate both enantiomers of the desired product with good optical purity (95% ee).

Peptide synthesis

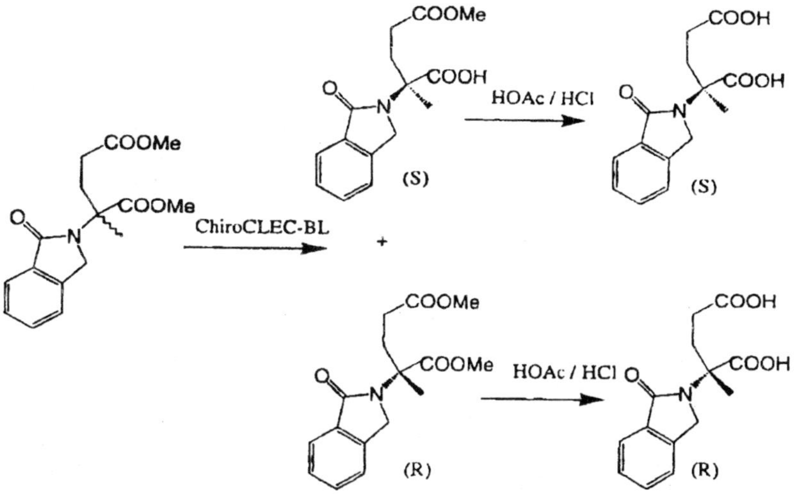

Peptide synthesis is an extremely important area of chemistry for the pharmaceutical industry, and like any specialized area of chemistry, has its own set of unique problems associated with it. Racemization and purification of final products are two of the most difficult problems in this area. The use of enzymes has been explored as a possible answer to these problems since 1938. However, proteases needed to catalyze peptide synthesis are subject to rapid autolysis under the conditions needed to affect peptide coupling, so this has generally not been a practical approach until cross-linked enzyme crystals of proteases became available. The synthetic utility of protease-CLCs was demonstrated by the thermolysin CLC (PeptiCLEC-TR)-catalyzed preparation of the aspartame precursor Z-Asp-Phe-OMe. The product was obtained in good yield (95%) and the reaction was repeated over 19 cycles in pure ethyl acetate at 55°C with no loss in enzyme activity.

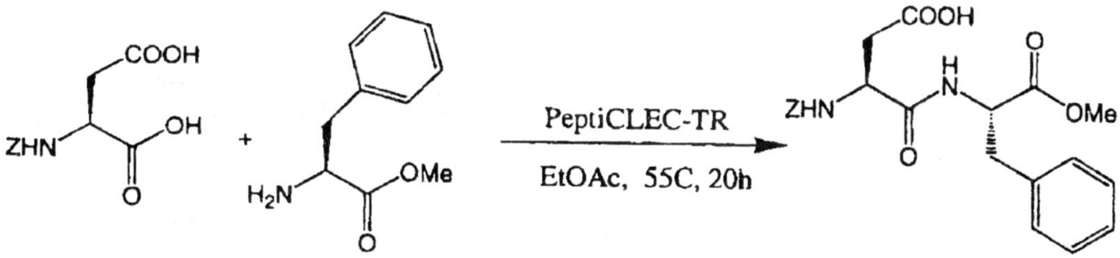

Fig. 11.7. Synthesis of 2-phthalimidino-glutaric acid analogs.

Fig. 11.8. Synthesis of aspartame precursor.

Biologically active peptides are generally metabolized very quickly by the body and often present bioavailability problems. Pharmaceutical companies circumvent these problems by designing peptide mimics which might contain non- natural amino acids and/or functional isosteres. The synthetic potential for using cross-linked enzyme crystals to prepare peptidomimetics was demonstrated in recent work by Margolin et al. A variety of chiral alkylamide derivatives of amino acids and peptides were prepared by CLC-catalyzed (PeptiCLEC-BL) coupling reactions. The power in this approach is that racemic carboxy and/or amine components can be stereoselectively coupled to give the desired (*S,S*) products and thereby eliminate several steps from the process. In the coming years, we will no doubt see many new peptidomimetic drugs come to market which are produced via CLC-catalyzed coupling reactions.

Regioselective reactions

Regioselective reactions in systems which contain multiple functional groups are an area ideally suited for biocatalysis. Linhardt and co-workers at the University of Iowa's Division of Medicinal and Natural Products Chemistry recently published the synthesis of a series of 1′-O-acyl sucrose derivatives. Using Chiro-CLEC-BL (the CLC of subtilisin) and vinyl esters of the acylating agent in pyridine as

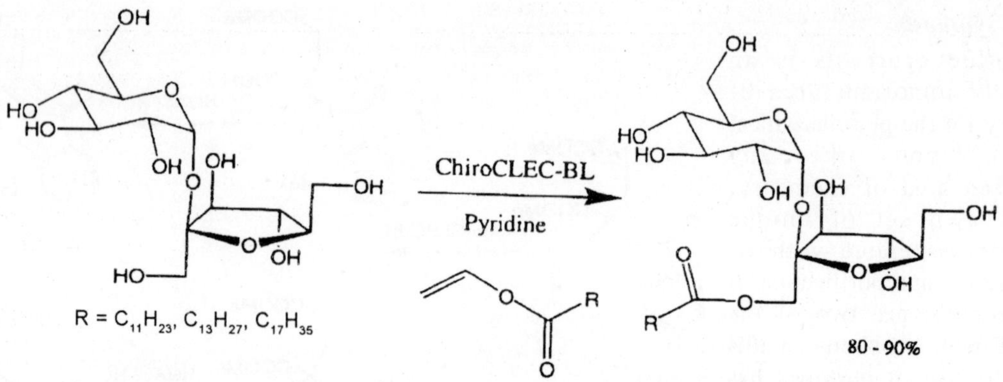

Fig. 11.9. Regioselective acylation using ChiroCLEC-BL.

solvent, the authors prepared 1′-O-lauryl sucrose, 1′-O-myristyl sucrose, and 1′-O-stearyl sucrose in 80–90% yield. Their method represents a "green" alternative to the tin chemistry previously used.

Carbon–carbon bond-forming reactions

Carbon–carbon bond-forming reactions are some of the most important transformations in organic chemistry. Sobolov et al. reported that CLCs of fructose 1,6-diphosphate aldolase from rabbit muscle are much more stable than the soluble enzyme. The synthetic potential of these CLCs was demonstrated by the preparation of a series of compounds.

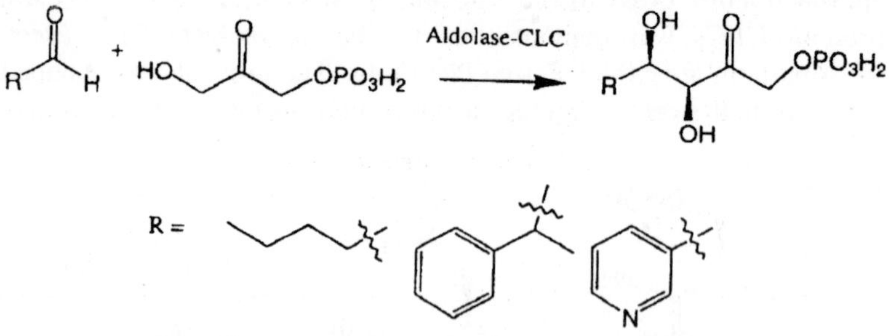

Fig. 11.10. Aldolase-CLC-catalyzed C-C bond formation.

Reductions

Reduction of achiral precursors is often used to produce chiral products. The advantage of this approach is that the theoretical yield of product is 100% compared to the 50% theoretical maximum for the resolution of racemates. Cross-linked crystals of lactate dehydrogenase have been used to prepare L-lactic acid from pyruvic acid in an electrolytic cell. The LDH CLCs maintained constant activity over 25 days and were much less sensitive to pH than the soluble enzyme. Horse liver alcohol dehydrogenase has been crystallized and cross-linked with the cofactor bound to the enzyme and the resulting CLCs used to reduce a number of ketones to chiral alcohols. The CLCs exhibited activity similar to the soluble enzyme and were more stable toward heat and the presence of alcohols. The cofactor remained tightly bound to the CLC and could be regenerated in situ with a high turnover number.

Haring and Schreier have modified the active site of subtilisin cross-linked enzyme crystals by introducing selenium into it and thereby converting the enzyme into a peroxidase. The rigid CLC matrix allowed them to chemically modify subtilisin without loss of the tertiary structure. The kinetic resolution of racemic 2-hydroxy-1-phenylethyl hydroperoxide was demonstrated using the semisynthetic CLC. The reaction time was 25–30 min with an ee of 97%. The authors demonstrated the stability of these semisynthetic CLCs by cycling their enzyme 10 times.

INDUSTRIAL APPLICATIONS

The true value of cross-linked enzyme crystals is that this technology minimizes many if not all of the problems which have limited the industrial use of enzymes to date. Issues of stability, purity, and cost are all addressed favorably by cross-linked enzyme crystal technology. The first large-scale commercial application of cross-linked enzyme crystals was the use of glucose isomerase CLCs to produce high-fructose corn syrup. While this is not a pharmaceutical or a biotechnological application, it is included here because it serves to demonstrate the economic viability of the technology in a very cost-sensitive business. In this application the CLCs were attached to the surface of a polystyrene-cellulose-titanium oxide composite carrier in a ratio of 9:1 carrier:enzyme. The catalyst had a half-life of 150 days at 57°C, and 12–18 tons of dry sugar product could be produced per kilogram of enzyme.

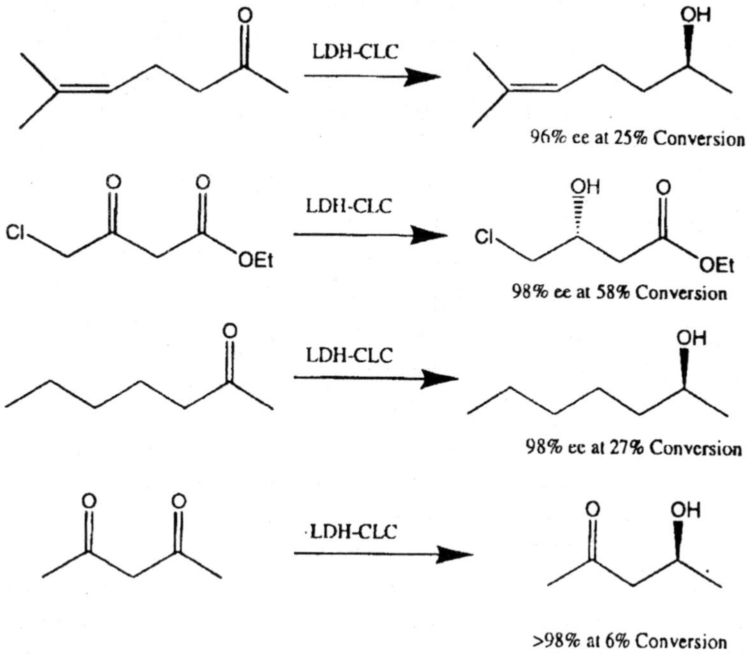

LDH-CLC

96% ee at 25% Conversion

LDH-CLC

98% ee at 58% Conversion

LDH-CLC

98% ee at 27% Conversion

LDH-CLC

>98% at 6% Conversion

Fig. 11.11. Reduction of ketones with LDH-CLC.

A group at Industrial Research Limited in New Zealand recently reported the results of a study to determine if a cross-linked enzyme crystal-catalyzed resolution can compete with alternative chiral technologies in the pharmaceutical and chemical process industries. The group used the enantioselective hydrolysis of α-phenylethyl acetate catalyzed by ChiroCLEC-PC as a model system. Based on their results with 270 kg of racemate, they evaluated the economics of running the process at the 600-kg batch scale and concluded that "this process is economically feasible".

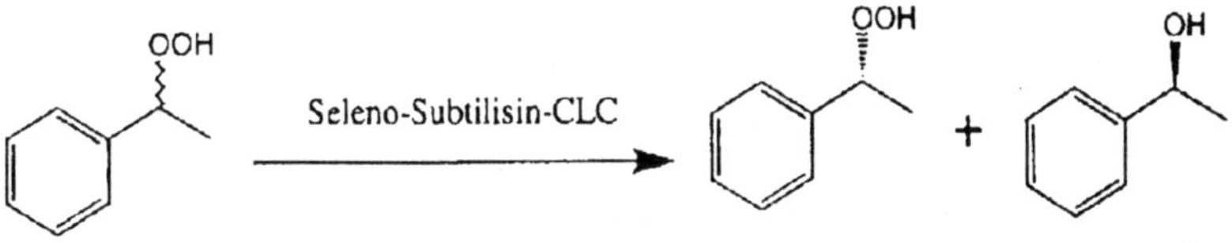

Seleno-Subtilisin-CLC

Fig. 11.12. Resolution using semisynthetic seleno-subtilism CLC.

As discussed earlier in the chapter, the use of CLCs did not begin to take off until Altus Biologics was formed and commercialized the technology in 1993. Since it takes several years for a new drug to be developed and commercialized and many do not make it all the way to the market, there are few examples in the public domain of recent drug introductions which are produced using a CLC step. The syntheses of Chiroscience's single-isomer MMPIs (matrix metalloprotease inhibitors) D1927 and D2163 were elegantly achieved via the use of PeptiCLEC-TR. In these cases the key molecular structure and a final element of asymmetry were introduced via a PeptiCLEC-TR-mediated amide bond formation.

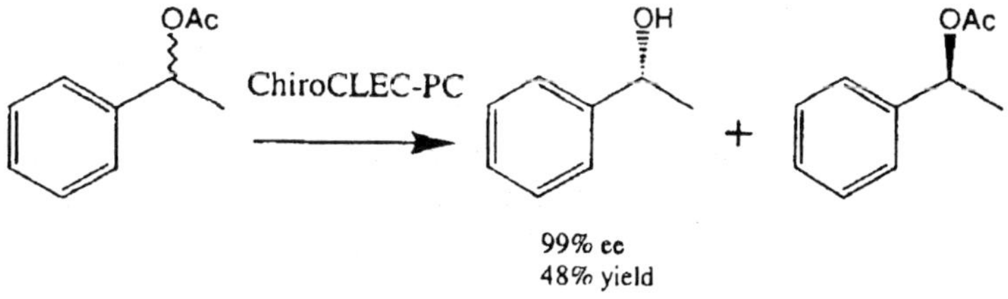

In the very important therapeutic class of antibiotics, both 6-APA (6-aminopenicillinic acid) and 7-ADCA (7-aminodeacetoxycephalosporanic

ChiroCLEC-PC

99% ee
48% yield

Fig. 11.13. Resolution of racemic α-phenylethyl acetate via ChiroCLEC-PC.

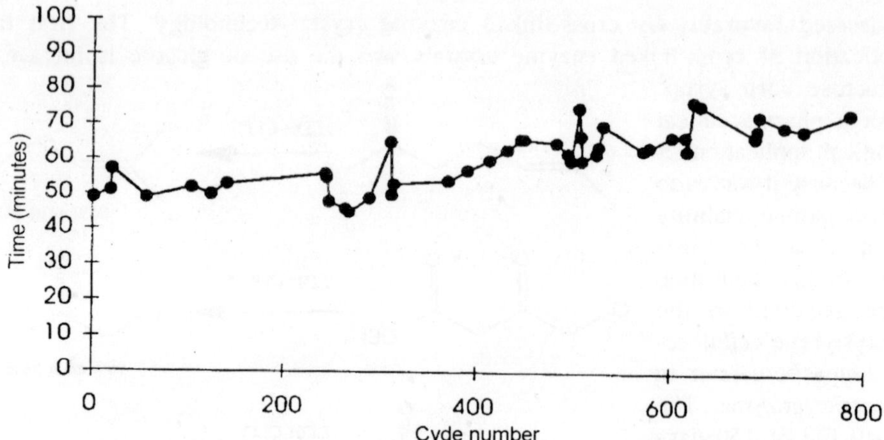

Fig. 11.14. Repetitive batch hydrolysis of penicillin-G to 6-aminopenicillanic acid.

acid) are being produced today on multi-ton scale using the cross-linked crystal form of penicillin-G amidase. The stability of enzymes in the cross-linked crystal form is again clearly demonstrated by the multicycle piloting reaction run for the hydrolysis of penicillin-G. Like all "new technologies," cross-linked enzyme crystals were not developed overnight. Almost 30 years separate the first report of cross-linked enzyme crystals from the introduction of truly useful, commercially available CLEC products.

The tremendous advantages of purity, stability, and ultimately economy of using enzymes in CLC form have only very recently been discovered by the organic chemist and in fact is still an ongoing process. As the examples in this chapter illustrate, a wide variety of synthetic targets, especially in the pharmaceutical area, are being successfully prepared using cross-linked enzyme crystals. Further, processes for large-scale manufacturing employing CLC steps have been developed and successfully employed. It is a certainty that many of the exciting new therapeutic agents which will reach the market in the coming years will be manufactured by processes which include the use of cross-linked enzyme crystals.

12

Activity of Ketone Reductases

While Baker's yeast (*Saccharomyces cerevisiae*) was domesticated over 4000 years ago for bread and beverage production, it was not until the early part of the twentieth century that its potential for asymmetric ketone reductions was appreciated. Since then, baker's yeast, which is inexpensive, simple to handle, nonpathogenic, and reduces a wide range of ketones, has become an important reagent for organic synthesis. Such applications of baker's yeast reductions have been reviewed extensively, and these can provide important precedent for deciding whether baker's yeast is likely to accept a novel substrate as well as guidance in predicting the major product. Some of these reviews also comment on the efforts to isolate and characterize enzymes catalyzing asymmetric ketone reductions from baker's yeast; however, there appears to have been no systematic attempt to link the recently completed genome sequence of *S. cerevisiae* to enzymes with synthetic utility, and this is the focus of the present review. The goal of this chapter is to uncover all yeast genes that might participate in the reduction of exogenous ketones, which is the first step toward rational improvements in cofactor and enzyme levels by recombinant DNA techniques, an approach that is still in its infancy.

Source of Reducing Equivalents

The ability of baker's yeast to reduce exogenously added ketones is closely related to the fermentation process that converts carbohydrates such as glucose or starch to ethanol and carbon dioxide via glycolysis and the subsequent decarboxylation and reduction of pyruvate. Efficient ethanol and carbon dioxide production directly influences the efficiencies of both bread making and brewing, and *S. cerevisiae* has been subjected to intense selective pressure over the preceding four millennia to optimize carbohydrate assimilation. During fermentation, the metabolic goal is to convert all available carbohydrate to ethanol, a process that does not require oxygen. Glycolysis depletes the cytoplasmic pool of NAD^+, as this cofactor is used to oxidize glyceraldehyde-3-phosphate to 1,3-*bis*-phosphoglycerate. The NADH-dependent reduction of acetaldehyde yielding ethanol is a major route to regenerating the NAD needed for additional carbohydrate assimilation. On the other hand, any pyruvate decarboxylated to acetyl-coenzyme A (acetyl-CoA) in preparation for oxidative phosphorylation results in an excess of NADH in the cytoplasm. This is believed to be the major source of NADH available to reduce exogenously added ketones by the subset of enzymes that accept this cofactor.

The pentose phosphate pathway is the other major route by which glucose is assimilated by baker's yeast, and this pathway yields excess reducing equivalents in the form of NADPH. The fate of the ribulose 5-phosphate depends on the cellular requirements for pentose sugars, but it can be converted by a series of equilibria into intermediates in glycolysis (glyceraldehyde 3-phosphate and fructose 6-phosphate). The possibility that the pentose phosphate pathway can operate as a cycle has been debated

1/2 Glucose → Glyceraldehyde-3-phosphate → (NAD^+ → NADH) → 1,3-*bis*-Phosphoglycerate → (ADP → ATP) → 3-Phosphoglycerate → Pyruvate → ($2\ CO_2$) → CH_3CHO Acetaldehyde → (NADH → NAD^+) → CH_3CH_2OH Ethanol

Pyruvate → (CoASH, NAD^+ → CO_2, NADH) → Acetyl-CoA

Starting point for Krebs Cycle and oxidative phosphorylation

for some time, although the consensus is that this situation is not normally encountered in sugar-grown baker's yeast. The two oxidative steps at the beginning of the pentose phosphate pathway are believed to be the major source of NADPH required for endogenous biosynthetic pathways when baker's yeast is grown on sugars. When ethanol is used as the carbon source, acetaldehyde dehydrogenase (which catalyzes the $NADP^+$-dependent oxidation of acetaldehyde to acetate) is likely to be the major source of NADPH. This cofactor is required by the majority of yeast reductases that accept exogenous ketones.

Glucose → (ATP → ADP) → Glucose-6-phosphate → ($NADP^+$ → NADPH) → 6-Phosphogluconolactone → ($NADP^+$ → NADPH, CO_2) → Ribulose-5-phosphate → Glyceraldehyde-3-phosphate, Fructose-6-phosphate

To facilitate synthetically useful ketone reductions, the quantities of reduced nicotinamides must be kept relatively high. It is experimentally difficult to measure the levels of cellular NADH and NADPH in situ, and optimization of this key parameter is therefore generally performed by trial and error using the rate of ketone reduction as the dependent variable. The nature of the carbon source, the supply of oxygen, and other growing conditions affect the levels of reducing equivalents, and variation of these experimental parameters can therefore improve the performance of baker's yeast-mediated ketone reductions. For NADH, controlling the partitioning of pyruvate between ethanol and glycerol production (which consumes NADH) and oxidative phosphorylation (which does not regenerate cytoplasmic NAD^+) has the greatest influence on the supply of NADH available for reducing exogenous ketones. For NADPH, the level of carbon flux through the pentose phosphate pathway versus that through glycolysis has the greatest impact on the quantity of cytoplasmic NADPH. The factor(s) controlling these fluxes are not well understood in *S. cerevisiae*. In addition, it appears that the cytoplasmic NADH and NADPH pools are independent in baker's yeast, since this organism lacks both a cytoplasmic pyridine nucleotide transhydrogenase [which interconverts reduced and oxidized NAD(H) and NADP(H)] and NAD(H) kinase activities. This point is important, since many reductases are specific for either NADH or NADPH. Furthermore, Kielland-Brandt and co-workers recently demonstrated that expressing a membrane- bound bacterial transhydrogenase in *S. cerevisiae* resulted in a net transfer of reducing equivalents from NADPH to NADH. While this shift may be useful in certain applications, most previously characterized yeast enzymes that accept synthetically important ketones are specific for NADPH.

Multiple Baker's Yeast Reductases and Streoselectivity in Whole Cell-mediated Reductions

Baker's yeast is able to reduce a broad variety of ketones because of the presence of a large complement of reductase enzymes. In nearly all cases, the physiological substrate(s) for these enzymes are not known; instead they have been purified on the basis of activity toward a specific ketone. For this reason, it is important to keep in mind that descriptions such as "important" and "major" contributors to ketone reductions are meaningful only in the context of specific substrates. These practices have also led to ad-hoc naming of yeast reductases that often derive from the order of elution from specific chromatographic columns or reflect the nature of the assay substrate used during the purification, which often leads to confusion when trying to compare results from different laboratories. In many cases, different groups have purified reductases with similar but nonidentical physical properties and it is not clear whether these differences are yeast strain-related or whether the enzymes are distinct. For all of these reasons, the number and properties of ketone reductases produced by baker's yeast is still ambiguous. All of the ketone and keto-ester reductases purified from baker's yeast as of 1998, along with their physical properties, have been tabulated recently by Straathof. An important goal for future studies in this area will be the linking of this biochemical information to the corresponding yeast genes using the complete genome sequence of *S. cerevisiae*.

The presence of multiple reductases with overlapping substrate specificities but differing stereoselectivities often leads to mixtures of alcohol products when whole yeast cells are used for ketone reductions. Several ingenious methods have been devised to overcome these problems. These include changing the substrate structure or concentration, altering the carbon source, performing reactions in organic solvents or two-phase systems, immobilization of the yeast cells, or adding inhibitors or sulfur compounds to the reductions. All of these strategies are aimed at decreasing the catalytic activities of competing enzymes while leaving that of the target enzyme

largely undisturbed. The major difficulty with all of these approaches is that they are empirical and their effects on the reductions of novel substrates are not easily predictable. On the other hand, recombinant DNA technology provides a potentially powerful route to improving the stereoselectivities of yeast reductions rationally. This possibility had been recognized earlier, although it has only been explored systematically in recent years. In this approach, desirable enzymes are overexpressed while competing reductases are eliminated by knocking out the corresponding genes. The major advantage of this metabolic engineering strategy over previous methods is that the enzyme whose level is manipulated is known unambiguously. Knocking out individual reductase genes also provides a simple means to determine whether a given enzyme contributes significantly to biotransformations of individual substrates. This approach will become even simpler once construction of a complete library of single-gene knockout strains is completed within the next few years.

General Approach to Identifying Yeast Genes Encoding Potential Ketone Reductases

Using rational metabolic engineering to tailor the stereoselectivity of yeast-mediated reductions is feasible only when all of the relevant genes are known and the relationships between enzyme and acceptable substrates are defined. We are far from this ideal. For a few reductase proteins, amino acid sequence data has linked biochemical data with the corresponding gene conclusively. In other cases, reductases have been isolated from yeast cells and their substrate specificities have been defined to a greater or lesser extent, but the absence of amino acid sequence data has precluded matching to the appropriate gene. Given the ability of baker's yeast cells to reduce a seemingly endless variety of ketones, it seems unlikely that all of the yeast ketone reductases have been isolated, and our efforts to identify all genes encoding potential reductases gives a total number of candidates—49—that is much larger than the number of purified reductases.

The availability of the genome sequence allowed us to approach the problem of identifying all potential ketone reductases by detecting yeast proteins with sequence similarity to known reductases, whether from baker's yeast or other species. In some cases, sequence identities of more than 50% were shared with known reductase proteins, making the identification of a putative yeast reductase protein unambiguous. In other cases, the level of sequence identity was much lower (25–35%). In these cases, the yeast protein sequences were grouped according to membership in previously recognized superfamilies—short-chain alcohol dehydrogenases/reductases, medium-chain alcohol dehydrogenases, etc.—to allow an informed choice as to their potential as authentic reductase enzymes. Accordingly, these yeast protein sequences were aligned with one another and with a superfamily representative whose catalytic activity and three-dimensional structure had been established (except for short-chain alcohol dehydrogenases, where no related crystal structure is available). Those yeast proteins that conserved residues known to be critical for catalysis and whose sequence insertions and/or deletions could be reasonably accommodated by the known protein structure were accepted as potential yeast ketone reductases. We have not attempted to model the yeast reductase proteins using the known X-ray crystal structures, although this may be useful in certain cases. Despite a good deal of effort, it is not yet possible to predict reliably the substrate or stereoselectivity of yeast reductases on the basis of computer modeling alone.

One caveat with the genetic approach to identifying yeast reductases is the possibility that their expression may be restricted to specific situations or they may be pseudo-genes that are not expressed under any growth conditions. Gene chip technology offers one approach to addressing these issues by making a genome-wide snapshot of mRNA levels available. While levels of transcription are not always correlated with protein levels, such measurements provide at least some guidance. Clearly, those potential reductases transcribed at reasonable levels are candidates worthy of further investigation. The catalytic efficiency of reductases also plays an important role in determining whether a given candidate is "important" for a given substrate, particularly at low substrate concentrations.

Lactate Dehydrogenases

Baker's yeast contains at least four lactate dehydrogenases, three of which are located in the mitochondrion and one in the cytoplasm. Electron flow in the mitochondrial enzymes is linked to cytochromes rather than nicotinamides. Their apparent physiological function is the reversible interconversion of pyruvate and lactate, and it is not clear whether any of these four enzymes accept ketones other than pyruvate, which would limit their importance in organic synthesis.

Alcohol Dehydrogenases

Selection for efficient conversion of carbohydrates to ethanol and carbon dioxide has shaped baker's yeast over the past four millennia. One manifestation is the high levels of glycolytic enzymes in the yeast cytoplasm (ca. 30% of total protein). Another is a high level of catalytic activities for the conversion of pyruvate to ethanol by the action of pyruvate decarboxylase and alcohol dehydrogenases. Pyruvate decarboxylation is essentially irreversible under physiological conditions, and it is critical that the cells avoid high concentrations of acetaldehyde given its propensity to react spontaneously with a variety of cellular nucleophiles. It is therefore not surprising that several redundant genes encoding related alcohol dehydrogenases are present in the yeast genome.

Five of the yeast alcohol dehydrogenases (encoded by the SFA1, ADH1, ADH2, ADH3, and ADH5 genes) appear to be Zn(II)-dependent enzymes that share a high degree of sequence similarity with mammalian alcohol dehydrogenases. The alcohol dehydrogenase encoded by the ADH4 gene is an iron-dependent enzyme that is a member of a different family. A multiple sequence alignment of the five Zn(II)-dependent enzymes with horse liver alcohol dehydrogenase (HLADH) revealed a number of conserved residues, several of which are known to be critical for structure and function of the horse liver enzyme. Horse liver alcohol dehydrogenase contains two Zn(II) ions, a "structural Zn(II)" ligated by Cys97, Cys1 00, Cys103, and Cys111, and a "catalytic Zn(II)" ligated by Cys46, His67, and Cys174. The conservation of all seven residues that serve as ligands for the two Zn(II) ions is one important indication that all five yeast genes encode bonafide alcohol dehydrogenases.

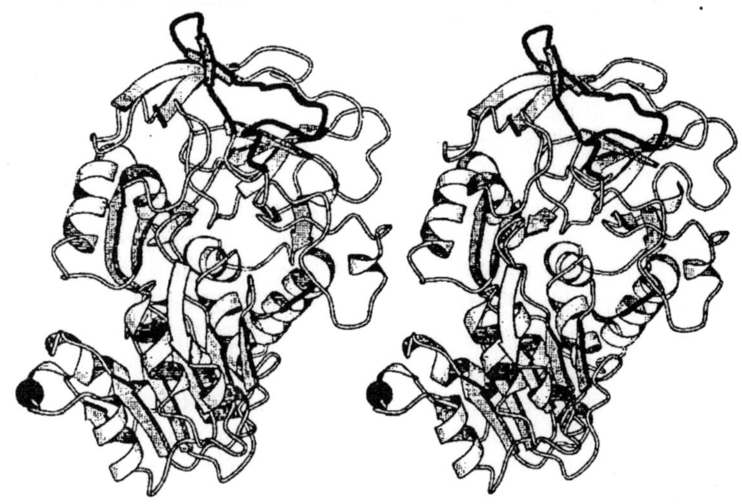

Fig. 12.1. Stereoview of the HLADH structure showing positions of insertions and deletions in similar yeast protein sequences.

The sequences of these five yeast proteins are also congruent with the experimental three-dimensional structure of the horse liver enzyme, implying that these will have the same overall fold. The length of the Sfal protein (Sfalp) is virtually the same as that of the horse liver enzyme except for a three-amino acid insertion after Asp245 (HLADH numbering), which is located in a surface loop between a β-strand and an α-helix near the entrance to the active site. The proteins encoded by the ADH1, ADH2, ADH3, and ADH5 genes also share a 22-amino acid deletion compared to the HLADH sequence. This region is part of a surface loop in HLADH relatively far from the active site.

The contribution of these alcohol dehydrogenases to reductions of exogenous ketones is unclear. While mammalian alcohol dehydrogenases accept a variety of ketones and aldehydes, yeast alcohol dehydrogenase I has a relatively narrow substrate specificity that is restricted largely to simple ketones. Whether the substrate specificities of enzymes encoded by the ADH2, ADH3, ADH5, and SFA1 genes are similarly restricted awaits experimental investigation, although this seems likely given their high degree of sequence similarity.

Medium-Chain Alcohol Dehydrogenases

The *S. cerevisiae* genome also contains a number of other genes related to the above-mentioned alcohol dehydrogenases, and their sequences place all of these proteins in the medium chain alcohol dehydrogenase superfamily. Oxidoreductases in this superfamily are generally metal ion-dependent and composed of two domains, a catalytic domain (composed of the N-terminal and C-terminal regions) and a central cofactor-binding domain that contains a Rossman fold. The closest relative of the six putative baker's yeast proteins whose three-dimensional structure is known is human χχ alcohol dehydrogenase. The number of critical residues shared with this enzyme and the locations of sequence insertions and deletions relative to secondary structure elements of the human enzyme suggests that all six of these putative yeast proteins are bonafide dehydrogenases, although their substrates and physiological roles are unknown at this time.

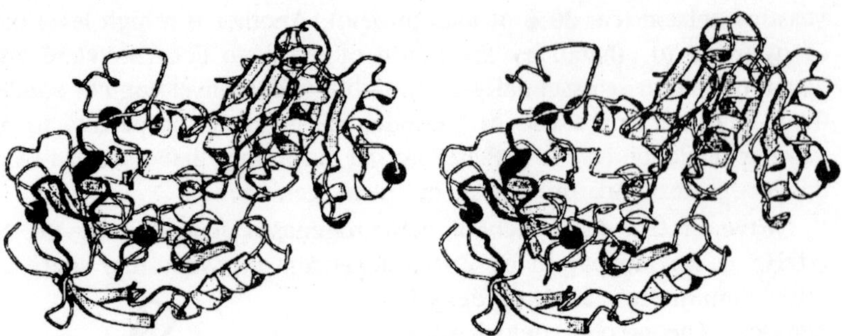

Fig. 12.2. Stereoview of the χχ alcohol dehydrogenase structure showing positions of insertions and deletions in similar yeast protein sequences.

The six putative yeast reductases share several key residues that are also conserved in a global sequence alignment of medium-chain alcohol dehydrogenases constructed by Person and co-workers. A subset of this superfamily employ an essential metal ion and all six putative yeast enzymes conserve both the Cys46 and His67 residues (χχ alcohol dehydrogenase numbering) that ligate the catalytic Zn(II). The residue that acts as the third ligand to the catalytic Zn(II) (Cys 174, χχ alcohol dehydrogenase numbering) is not conserved between all of the yeast proteins and the human enzyme, however. Both the proteins encoded by the YMR318c and YCR105w genes feature a cysteine at this position; however, this position is occupied by a glutamate in those encoded by the YAL060w, SOR1, and YLR070c genes. Interestingly, the residue at this position in the YAL061wp (glutamine) has limited ability to bind Zn(II), suggesting that the metal ion coordination may be different in this case. Virtually all of superfamily members possess the G–X–G–X–X–G motif characteristic of the Rossman fold, and this is true of the six putative yeast reductases as well. In addition, the complete conservation of several glycine residues in the C-terminal region implies that the overall fold of the χχ alcohol dehydrogenase may be preserved in the putative yeast proteins.

Human χχ alcohol dehydrogenase is also known as formaldehyde dehydrogenase since it oxidizes the spontaneous formaldehyde-glutathione adduct to a thioester that is subsequently hydrolyzed to regenerate reduced glutathione and formate by a separate hydrolase. This sequence may be a detoxification pathway for formaldehyde. Several features of the six putative yeast protein sequences argue that while they are likely to possess alcohol dehydrogenase activity, their substrate specificities may be quite different. Residues known to be important in substrate binding in χχ alcohol dehydrogenase (e.g., Asp57 and Arg115) are not conserved between the human enzyme and the six putative yeast proteins. The yeast open reading frames also contain a variety of insertions and deletions that are likely to affect the substrate-binding pocket. Of the six, the proteins encoded by the YMR318c and YCR105w genes are most closely related to human χχ alcohol dehydrogenase. The major difference is a large deletion between residues Lys113 and Cys132 (χχ alcohol dehydrogenase numbering), which form a loop in the human enzyme that makes up part of the substrate-binding pocket. In addition to this deletion, the sequences of putative yeast proteins encoded by the YAL061w and YAL060w genes also differ from the χχ alcohol dehydrogenase by a 14-amino acid insertion after residue Pro95. This insertion—which occurs in a surface loop in χχ alcohol dehydrogenase—would change the substrate-binding site substantially.

The final member of the yeast medium-chain alcohol dehydrogenase super- family, encoded by the ZTA1 gene, differs in several key aspects from the six putative yeast reductases. Most important, this enzyme lacks the residues that ligate the catalytic Zn(II) ion, in common with other crystallin homologs. Related metal-free proteins are capable of reducing quinones; however, the catalytic activity and substrate specificity of the protein encoded by ZTA1 is currently unknown.

Short-Chain Alcohol Dehydrogenases

The short-chain alcohol dehydrogenases constitute a second superfamily whose members are widely distributed across all three phylogenetic kingdoms. Sequence analysis of the yeast genome revealed a large number of potential proteins that would be part of this superfamily, and we have recently demonstrated that at least one of these is a key player in stereoselective reductions of β-keto esters (*vide infra*) and it is likely that closely related proteins may also participate in similar reductions. Short-chain alcohol dehydrogenases are metal- independent enzymes that can be distinguished by a conserved Y–X–X–X–K motif. Unfortunately, no crystal structure of a dehydrogenase with high sequence similarity to yeast short-chain alcohol dehydrogenases is currently available, so it is not possible to interpret sequence differences in this context. Because the number of potential short-chain alcohol dehydrogenases is quite large, the discussion has been divided into three subsections (potential β-keto ester reductases, distantly related short-chain dehydrogenases and aryl alcohol dehydrogenases).

Potential β-keto ester reductases

Yeast-mediated reductions of β-keto esters have been the most-utilized biotransformation involving this organism. Several groups have purified yeast enzymes that accept β-keto esters; however, the corresponding gene had not been identified for any β-keto ester reductase member of the short-chain alcohol dehydrogenase superfamily. α-Acetoxyketone reductase reduces a variety of β-keto esters to L-alcohols with very high enantio- and diastereoselectivity. Based on amino acid sequence data, it was suggested that this enzyme corresponded to the YJR105w open reading frame. We have shown subsequently that this assignment was incorrect.

To identify the correct yeast gene, we purified α-acetoxyketone reductase according to Shieh and determined the amino acid sequences of Lys-C fragments (since the N-terminus was blocked). Data obtained from three separate fragments corresponded precisely to the protein encoded by *S. cerevisiae* GRE2 gene, which has sequence similarity to plant dihydroflavinol and cinnamoyl-CoA reductases (both known members of the short-chain alcohol dehydrogenase superfamily). The Gre2p sequence was used as a probe in Basic Local Alignment Sequence Tool (BLAST) analysis of the *S. cerevisiae* genome, and three closely related putative proteins were identified.

The nature of residues conserved between the putative open reading frames and the Gre2p and plant cinnamoyl-CoA reductase argues strongly that the proteins encoded by the YDR541c, YGL157w, and YGL039w genes are all likely to be functional reductases. That all sequences share that consensus Y–X–X–X–K motif places them securely in the short-chain dehydrogenase superfamily. Moreover, their conservation of residues that are also identical between plant dihydroflavinol and cinnamoyl-CoA reductases from different species suggests that their catalytic activities have been identified correctly. On the other hand, whether the substrate specificities of these putative proteins overlap with that of a-acetoxyketone reductase is unknown.

Other short-chain alcohol dehydrogenases

Using a variety of known short-chain alcohol dehydrogenases as probes for BLAST searching of the yeast genome revealed an additional eight putative proteins that are more distantly related. All eight share the Y–X–X–X–K motif as well as a glycine-rich motif near the N-termini that may represent an NAD(P)H-binding site. In the absence of an X-ray crystal structure of a related dehydrogenase, it is not possible to determine whether the pattern of insertions and deletions would be compatible with a known architecture. The assignment of this group of proteins as potential reductases is tenuous at best.

Aryl alcohol dehydrogenases

The *S. cerevisiae* genome encodes four very closely related proteins with high sequence similarity to known aryl alcohol dehydrogenases. These enzymes are characterized by the Y–X–X–X–K motif and are members of the short-chain dehydrogenase family. In addition, two other proteins (encoded by YFL057c and AAD15) correspond to the C-terminal half of the longer sequences. It is particulârly interesting that four of the six open reading frames can be derived from alternate start codons in the AAD14 protein sequence. The reason for this apparent genetic redundancy is not known, nor is the physiological role of these proteins. Whether these enzymes participate in reductions of exogenous ketones is also not known.

Aldose Reductase Family

Enzymes of the aldo-keto reductase superfamily are also widely distributed within the phylogenetic kingdoms. In baker's yeast, these enzymes may play a role in protection against osmotic stress by producing sugar-derived polyols. On the other hand, at least one of these enzymes (encoded by the YPR1 gene) also plays a major role in the stereoselective reduction of exogenous β-keto esters. We have shown recently that manipulating the level of the YPR1 protein by recombinant DNA techniques results in useful stereochemical changes in whole-cell-mediated reductions, conclusively linking this gene to the aldoketo reductase isolated by both Sih and Nakamura. Using the Ypr1p and related aldo-keto reductase sequences as probes for BLAST searches of the *S. cerevisiae* genome uncovered five additional putative proteins that were closely related to one another and to human aldose reductase, whose X-ray crystal structure has been determined. It is very likely that these additional five proteins are also ketone reductases, and they may be participants in reductions of β-keto esters. Support for this notion is also provided by the demonstration that the YBR149w open reading frame corresponds to a reductase purified by Nakamura and co-workers on the basis of its ability to reduce a variety of α-carbonyl compounds. The structure and function of another member of this family, yeast xylose reductase, has been reviewed recently.

A number of key residues are conserved completely between human aldose reductase and the six yeast protein sequences. A catalytic mechanism in which Tyr48, Lys77, and His110 play key roles was proposed for human aldose reductase by Gabbay and co-workers on the basis of its X-ray crystal structure. In this mechanism, Tyr48 acts as a general acid to protonate the nascent alcohol during carbonyl reduction, and this proton transfer is facilitated by interaction with the side chain of Lys77. The side chain of Hisl 10 was proposed to influence the stereochemistry of reduction by positioning the substrate correctly. All three of these residues are conserved among all six yeast open reading frames. In addition, other amino acids conserved between the human and yeast sequences match relatively well with residues conserved between mammalian aldose reductases, further suggesting that the yeast sequences are functional reductase enzymes.

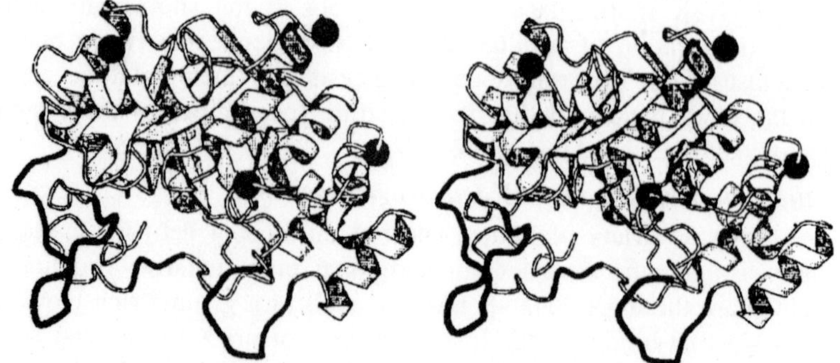

Fig. 12.3. Stereoview of human aldose reductase showing positions of insertions and deletions in similar yeast protein sequences.

The locations of sequence insertions and deletions present in the yeast sequences are congruent with the three-dimensional structure of human aldose reductase. Most occur between secondary structure elements, as would be expected for proteins with the same overall fold but differences in surface-exposed loops. The major difference between the human enzyme and those encoded by YPR1, GCY1, and ARA1 is an eight-amino acid deletion between residues Arg217 and Ser226, which forms a loop at the entrance to the active site. In addition to this deletion, the sequences of the Yjr096w and Ydl124w proteins also have a large deletion (22 and 16 amino acids, respectively) between residues Lys119 and Leu138 (human enzyme numbering). This region corresponds to a large surface-exposed loop in human aldose reductase, which in principle could be deleted without requiring major changes in the protein architecture.

Taken together, the evidence strongly suggests that all six of the yeast al- dose reductase superfamily members are catalytically active. Further explorations of these proteins are likely to yield correlations with previously isolated yeast reductases.

D-Hydroxyacid Dehydrogenase Family

Members of the D-hydroxyacid dehydrogenase family catalyze the stereoselective reduction of small α-keto acids such as hydroxypyruvate, pyruvate, etc. Enantiomerically pure α-hydroxy acids are valuable synthetic intermediates, and a variety of ingenious approaches to these compounds have been described. Sequence similarity searching of the *S. cerevisiae* genome revealed five open reading frames that were similar to members of the D-hydroxyacid dehydrogenase family, although one (YPL275w) appeared to lack the N-terminal domain common to this superfamily and may be nonfunctional, at least for this type of reduction. A multiple sequence alignment of the five yeast open reading frames with the sequence of *Hyphomicrobium methylovorum* D-glycerate dehydrogenase revealed that several key residues were conserved and the pattern of sequence insertions and deletions might be reasonably accommodated by the known structure of D-glycerate dehydrogenase. Based on these observations, it appears likely that the five open reading frames encode active reductases; however, it is not clear whether the α-keto ester reductases isolated previously from baker's yeast correspond to one or more of these open reading frames.

An alignment of nine authentic D-hydroxyacid dehydrogenases from a variety of sources revealed several conserved residues, and many of these were also shared by the five yeast open reading frame sequences. From the crystal structure of D-glycerate dehydrogenase, three residues were suggested to play key roles in catalysis: Arg240, Glu269, and His287. Both the arginine and histidine residues are conserved in all five yeast open reading frames. A glutamate is present in three of the yeast sequences at the position corresponding to Glu269; however, the remaining two proteins have a glutamine at this position. Such a substitution has also been observed in *Pseudomonas* sp. 101 formate dehydrogenase. In the proposed catalytic mechanism, Glu269 is proposed to hydrogen bond with the conserved histidine (His287), thereby raising its pK_a and facilitating its role in protonating the nascent alcohol. Interestingly, the authors note that the side chain of Asp264 may also participate in catalysis, and this residue is conserved in all five yeast open reading frames. The side chain of Arg240 is proposed to interact with the carboxylate of bound substrate and thereby ensure productive substrate binding, and this residue is also present in all five yeast sequences.

The structure of D-glycerate dehydrogenase consists of two domains, an N-terminal catalytic domain and a C-terminal cofactor-binding domain with a typical Rossman fold topology. Insertions in the yeast open reading frame sequences relative to that of D-glycerate dehydrogenase are the major difference in overall primary structure. These occur mainly in the catalytic domain and are largely confined to loops between secondary structure elements, suggesting that these would be accommodated by the D-glycerate dehydrogenase architecture.

Fatty Acid Synthase

Baker's yeast appears to contain only a single pair of genes encoding the subunits of fatty acid synthase (FAS1 and FAS2). This complex reduces a β-keto thioester intermediate stereoselectively to the corresponding D-alcohol during each elongation cycle and also accepts a variety of other β-keto esters as substrates, although it requires an unsubstituted α-position. We have recently shown that the fatty acid synthase complex also reduces an α-keto-β-lactam. While the reduction product did not have the stereochemistry required for the Taxol side chain, the result suggested that fatty acid synthase has a broader substrate tolerance than might have been anticipated.

Fatty acid biosynthesis occurs in the cytoplasm, whereas degradation is localized to the mitochondrion. No other *S. cerevisiae* open reading frame sequences appear to share high sequence similarity with the FAS2 protein. The only other yeast enzyme that catalyzes a similar reaction is 3-oxoacyl-(acyl-carrier-protein) reductase, the product of the OAR1 gene. This is a mitochondrial enzyme that likely functions in the oxidative direction. Moreover, the OAR1 protein possesses the Y–X–X–X–K motif typical of short-chain alcohol dehydrogenases, a motif that is absent from fatty acid synthase.

Gene-Protein Relationships

A major motivation in collecting the information was to facilitate matching biochemical information for yeast reductases with the corresponding gene. Classical genetics has revealed the connection between gene and protein in several cases including yeast alcohol dehydrogenases and fatty acid synthase. In cases where even a fragment of amino acid sequence data from a purified reductase is available, the gene assignment is unequivocal. This method was used to show that the GRE2 gene encodes α-acetoxyketone reductase, YPR1 encodes yeast aldo-keto reductase, GRE3 encodes xylose reductase, ARA1 encodes D-arabinose dehydrogenase, and YBR149w encodes another member of the aldo-keto reductase superfamily. The major disadvantage of this approach is the time and effort required to isolate each protein and determine its amino acid sequence.

Amino acid sequence comparisons with known reductases will continue to play a major role in identifying enzymes in baker's yeast and other species. Several groups have identified key sequence patterns in different reductase superfamilies that allow one to determine whether a protein sequence is consistent with a role in carbonyl reductions.

Matching physical properties of purified enzymes to those predicted by computer analysis of yeast open reading frames offers a second approach to matching protein with gene. Molecular weight can be measured easily by gel electrophoresis, and such data are routinely included in all papers in which a yeast reductase has been isolated. Unfortunately, the resolution of this technique is limited to accuracies of ±5%, which is not sufficient to distinguish between related proteins. For example, the six members of the aldo-keto reductase family identified in the *S. cerevisiae* genome are predicted to have an average molecular weight of 35,443 Da, with a standard deviation of 1943 Da (5.5%). A similar situation holds for other families, reveals that the vast majority of potential yeast reductases have predicted molecular weights between 30 and 40 kDa. The isoelectric point for purified yeast reductases would be valuable corroborating evidence in assigning the appropriate gene and these values differ significantly, even for proteins in the same superfamily. Unfortunately, such data have not been reported for any of the reductases reported to date.

The behavior of knockout mutants can provide another method to connect a reductase enzyme with the appropriate gene. Clearly, individual deletions of most of these genes are not lethal, indicating that the proteins are involved in nonessential pathways or there are redundant enzymes. Deletion of open reading frame Ybr1 59w, however, was lethal. The sequence of this enzyme indicated distant relationship to short-chain alcohol dehydrogenases. Whether this will be a general observation must await completion of the systematic gene deletion project.

In the short term, the most productive method for identifying yeast reductases will involve testing deletion strains for an inability to reduce ketones that are accepted by the parent strain. This search can be focused on the most likely candidates if a homologous enzyme from another species with similar stereo-selectivity has been identified. Ideally, a single knockout mutation would abrogate the reduction of a given ketone. On the other hand, if more than one yeast enzyme is responsible for product formation, gene knockouts may instead alter the stereo-selectivity of whole-cell reductions. In fact, such a result provides some of the strongest evidence that incomplete stereoselectivity is the result of multiple enzymes rather than a single reductase with incomplete discrimination. The advantage of this approach is that it is rapid and requires little biochemical or genetic expertise, since all the strains are (or shortly will be) commercially available. One disadvantage of this strategy is that it identifies only those gene products that participate in reducing the specific substrate under investigation. In addition, it will be difficult to identify contributing enzymes if two or more have the same stereoselectivity for a given substrate or if knocking out one gene affects the levels of other enzymes. While knocking out one participant might be expected to reduce the rate of reduction, this analysis can be complicated by changes in overall growth rate as a result of the mutation.

The increased regulatory demands for optically pure drugs and agrochemicals coupled with pressures to minimize the environmental impacts of chemical processes makes enzyme-mediated processes logical alternatives. The need for chiral ketone reductions often arises in synthetic schemes, and baker's yeast has proven particularly adept at such transformations, even on industrial scales. The low cost and experimental simplicity associated with reductions by intact yeast cells provides a strong motivation to employ this organism, particularly because the use of whole yeast cells removes the need to purify enzymes or supply nicotinamide cofactors. Unfortunately, the large number of ketone reductases produced by baker's yeast can lead to side products, and efforts to optimize yeast reductions are therefore focused on minimizing these undesired reactions. The availability of genome sequence information, coupled with knowledge of which genes are likely to encode desirable and competing reductase enzymes, should allow for a rational approach to strain improvement by recombinant DNA techniques.

13

ENGINEERING *STREPTOMYCES AVERMITILIS*

Streptomycetes are gram-positive, filamentous soil bacteria that have two characteristic features: (1) a complex life cycle that includes mycelial differentiation and sporulation, and (2) the ability to produce a variety of secondary metabolites with therapeutic value. The application of chemical mutagenesis and mutasynthesis have provided important technical tools in the development of industrial cultures for the production of antibiotics and other therapeutic compounds. More recently, the application of recombinant DNA technology in *Streptomyces* spp. has offered the possibility of manipulating the expression of specific genes and the design of new mutants with enhanced ability to produce natural and novel secondary metabolites. Due to the fact that each Streptomycetes soil isolate usually presents distinct characteristics in terms of growth properties, media requirements, genome instability, transformation capability, and recombination proficiency, a significant effort is frequently needed to adapt recombinant DNA techniques to each strain of interest. When successfully developed, genetic engineering strategies can be used to improve the growth characteristics of particular cultures in industrial fermentation, to increase antibiotic production, and to produce novel antibiotic structures.

An extremely desirable but challenging objective is the ability to carry out molecular genetic manipulations within high-titer strains already used for the commercial production of secondary metabolites, significantly reducing timelines and effort required to develop novel therapeutic agents, compared to classical process development from environmental isolates. In this chapter, we shall describe how we have applied these approaches to the development of novel avermectins. *Streptomyces avermitilis* produces eight closely related polyketide macro- cyclic lactones with potent activity against both ecto- and endoparasites. Following the discovery of avermectins in 1979, they have been developed to commercialization and have enjoyed outstanding success in parasite control in the fields of animal health care, agriculture, and human infections. Avermectins were originally isolated as agents which could kill nematodes. It was soon realized that these compounds had a broad spectrum of activity, not only against essentially all roundworms found in the mammalian corpus, including the gastrointestinal tract, lung, heart, and eye, but also against ectoparasites such as mites, biting flies, and ticks. The mode of action of avermectins, and the closely related milbemycins, is believed to be the irreversible opening of chloride channels in muscle membranes. These chloride channels were initially believed to be associated with γ-aminobutyric acid (GABA) receptors, but more recent data have implicated glutamine-gated chloride channels, a mechanism which would account for the efficacy of the compounds against both roundworms and arthropods.

In nematodes, it has been proposed that avermectins block the activities associated with pharyngeal function, feeding, hydrostatic pressure regulation, and/or secretion, thereby causing paralysis of the parasite and facilitating its elimination from the host. In mammals, use of chloride channels as neurotransmitters is restricted to the central nervous system. As a consequence, the blood/brain barrier is believed to prevent the drug from reaching the glutamine-gated chloride channels and accounting for the excellent therapeutic index and safety profile of the avermectins. The combination of such potent activity against a wide variety of parasites and very safe performance in mammals has made avermectins the most successful antiparasitic product ever developed for animal health applications.

Chemical Structure of Avermectins and Biosynthesis

Eight naturally occurring, structurally related avermectins are produced by *Streptomyces avermitilis*. The avermectin polyketide structure is derived from seven acetate and five propionate residues, together with a single 2-methylbutyric acid or isobutyric acid residue which forms the *sec*-butyl or isopropyl group attached to the C25 of the spiroketal moiety. The avermectin aglycone is further modified by glycosylation at C13, with the attachment of two *O*-methylated oleandrose residues and *O*-methylation at C5. Thus, *S. avermitilis* produces all the eight different combinations of avermectin resulting from variability at the C5, C22,23, and C25 positions.

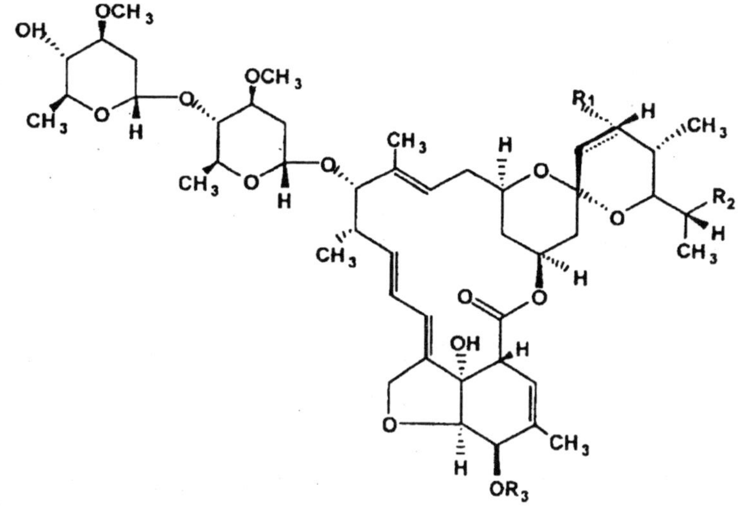

Fig. 13.1. Structure of the avermectin molecules.

The avermectin biosynthetic genes encompass a region of approximately 85 kb of the *S. avermitilis* genome which have been cloned and sequenced by us, by the Merck group, and by the Kitasato group. The DNA sequence of the avermectin biosynthetic region was recently published. The avermectin polyketide synthase (PKS) genes have a

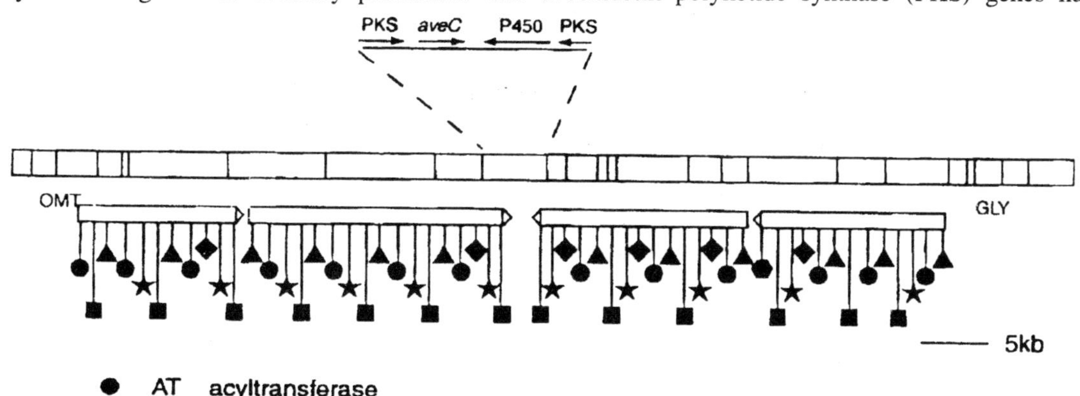

Fig. 13.2. Physical map of the avermectin biosynthetic gene cluster.

type I modular organization consisting of four large multifunctional open reading frames (ORFs) that encode a 12-module system. These PKS genes are required for the biosynthesis of the avermectin aglycone. Additional ORFs are located adjacent to the PKS genes and encode polypeptides involved in postpolyketide modifications. A set of 8 genes to make dTDP-oleandrose from glucose and attach it to the avermectin aglycone is located within an 11-kb *Pst*I fragment. The deduced gene products have homology to enzymes involved in the biosynthesis of other 6-deoxy sugars and are listed below using the nomenclature from Ikeda et al:

aveBI	glycosyl transferase (*dnmS*, *eryBV*, *eryCIII*)
aveBII	dTDP-glucose 4,6-dehydratase (*dnmM*, *ery gdh*)
aveBIII	α-D-glucose-1-phosphate thymidylyltransferase (*dnmL*)
aveBIV	dTDP-4-keto-6-deoxy-L-hexose 4-reductase (*dnmV*, *eryBIV*)
aveBV	dTDP-4-keto-6-deoxyhexose 3,5-epimerase (*dnmU*, *eryBVII*)
aveBVI	dTDP-4-keto-6-deoxy-L-hexose 2,3-dehydratase (*dnmT*, *eryBVI*)
aveB VII	dTDP-6-deoxy-L-hexose 3-*O*-methyltransferase (*eryBIII*)
aveB VIII	dTDP-4-keto-6-deoxy-L-hexose 2,3-reductase (*eryBII*)

Although the pathway of 6-deoxysugar biosynthesis in antibiotic-producing bacteria has not been established, recent work by Madduri et al. verifies the function predicted for *aveBIV* and homologs *dnmV* and *eryBIV*. In addition, these authors were able to modify a step in the biosynthesis of dTDP-L-daunosamine and produce the C-4 epimeric form of daunosamine by inactivating the normal *dnmV* gene in *Streptomyces peucetius* and replacing it with the heterologous *aveBIV* or *eryBIV* gene from *S. avermitilis* or *Saccharopolyspora erythraea*, respectively.

Analysis of the avermectin biosynthetic genes has presented the potential to engineer specific changes in the biosynthetic pathway. In the next three sections, the discussion will focus on the genetic basis for the biosynthesis of the eight natural avermectin components and discuss experiments to identify the genes involved in the differences detected at the C5, C22,23, and C25 positions. Later in the chapter, we will discuss how it is possible to manipulate the producing microorganism to direct the biosynthesis of novel avermectins. Finally, there will be a discussion of possible approaches applied to titer improvement.

The A and B Forms of Avermectins: The Role of the C5 *O*-Methyltransferase

Avermectins produced by *S. avermitilis* that have a hydroxyl group at C5 are the B components, and avermectins containing a methoxy group at C5 are the A components. The enzyme catalyzing the methylation of the hydroxyl group at C5 is a C5 *O*-methyltransferase (OMT). The corresponding gene (*aveD*) was identified within a 3.4-kb *Bam*HI fragment by complementing a *S. avermitilis* OMT-deficient mutant previously isolated by screening after random chemical mutagenesis. The gene encoding OMT maps near the left side of the avermectin biosynthetic gene cluster in the *S. avermitilis* genome. DNA sequence analysis of this chromosomal region by us and by Ikeda et al. revealed a potential open reading frame, and the predicted amino acid sequence of this ORF contains conserved domains found in other methyltransferases. Ikeda et al. determined that the *aveD* mutant K2034 had a single base-pair change which would lead to Thr23→Ile substitution. We examined an *aveD* mutant obtained during mutagenesis of *S. avermitilis* and determined that a single base-pair change resulted in Trp267→termination codon. The AveD protein from this mutant is missing the last 17 amino acids. In addition, disruption of the promoter region of *aveD* eliminated both C5 *O*-methylation activity and C5 keto reduction, presumably because *aveF* (which has a deduced gene product resembling a 3-ketoacyl-ACT/CoA reductase) and *aveD* are part of an operon.

The 1 and 2 Forms of Avermectins: The Role of the C22,23 Dehydratase

Avermectins produced by *S. avermitilis* that have a hydroxyl group at C23 are the 2 components, and avermectins containing double-bond carbons at C22,23 are the 1 components. Both 1 and 2 forms of avermectin are produced during fermentation. Pioneering studies to characterize the PKS system of the erythromycin biosynthetic gene cluster demonstrated that each biosynthetic step in the assembly of the polyketide chain has a separate active site. These steps are organized in sets, one set for each chain extension and (where appropriate) reduction cycle. The order of the structural genes in the biosynthetic gene cluster is related to the order in which the sets of activities act in the polyketide biosynthesis. Based on this model, the avermectin dehydratase (DH) domain in Module 2 should be responsible for the reduction at C22,23. To determine if this dehydratase functioned in the production of the 1 and 2 forms of avermectins, we investigated a region of the avermectin PKS which corresponds to the PKS module 2. A cosmid library of *S. avermitilis* was constructed and cosmid clones containing ketosynthase and dehydratase regions were identified by hybridization. A *Bam*HI restriction map was constructed by analysis of overlapping cosmids and hybridization. Sequence analysis identified a region of module 2 that contained >72% homology with the DH oligo probe and a putative conserved DH active site histidine.

A comparison of the deduced amino acid sequence of the module 2 DH from *S. avermitilis* with the conserved active site motif of other known DH shows that this *S. avermitilis* DH consensus sequence was altered from HxxxGxxxxP to HxxxGxxxxS. We designed an amino acid replacement strategy to change the serine (S) residue to a proline (P) residue (since all active DH domains that had been identified contain the conserved sequence HxxxGxxxxP). An *Xho*I restriction site was introduced in the corresponding DNA sequence to follow the gene replacement event. Chromosomal DNA isolated from transformants was analyzed by PCR and *Xho*I digestion to identify gene replacement events. Twenty-three isolates did not produce avermectins, and DNA sequence analysis of 5 avermectin nonproducing isolates confirmed the S-to-P change.

Since avermectin production seemed to require the presence of the serine residue in the conserved motif, we investigated gene replacement of a portion of the module 2 DH region with portions of DH region from module 7 or module 12. The DH domain for reduction at C4,C3 was identified, sequenced, and contained the motif HxxxGxxxxP. A gene replacement strategy was designed to exchange 51 amino acids from this region with 51 amino acids from module 2 DH. Two isolates that were confirmed by DNA sequence analysis to have undergone gene replacement produced avermectins at the normal B2:B1 ratio, suggesting that the conserved DH motif HxxxGxxxxP did not provide complete dehydratase activity to module 2 DH.

The DH domain (nonfunctional) for reduction at C13,C12 was identified, sequenced, and contained the motif YxxxGxxxxS. A gene replacement strategy was designed to exchange 38 amino acids from this region with 38 amino acids from module 2 DH. Three isolates that were confirmed by DNA sequence analysis to have undergone gene replacement produced avermectins at the normal B2:B1 ratio, suggesting that altering the putative C22,23 DH by replacing the active site H (histidine) with a Y (tyrosine) did not affect avermectin production. Previous experiments to alter the active-site histidine in the erythromycin module 4 DH or the fatty acid DH enzyme resulted in the elimination of erythromycin biosynthesis or the disruption of fatty acid biosynthesis.

The above results show that the dehydratase reaction that takes place at C22,23 in the fermentation to produce both 1 and 2 avermectins is probably not located in the PKS at the predicted module 2, since replacing a portion of this region with the inactive module 10 DH domain did not affect the amounts of 1 and 2 avermectins produced. Therefore, the identification and mapping of the gene encoding the C22,23 dehydratase remain to be elucidated.

The a and b Forms of Avermectins: C25 Substituents

As discussed earlier, the avermectin polyketide backbone is derived from seven acetate and five propionate extender units added to an α branched-chain fatty acid starter, which is either (*S*(+)-α-methylbutyric acid or isobutyric acid. The C25 position of naturally occurring avermectins has two possible substituents: a *sec*-butyl residue derived from the incorporation of *S*(+)-α-methylbutyryl-CoA ("a" avermectins), or an isopropyl residue derived from the incorporation of isobutyryl-CoA ("b" avermectins). These α branched-chain fatty acids, which act as starter units in the biosynthesis of the polyketide ring, are derived from the α branched-chain amino acids isoleucine and valine through a branched-chain amino acid transaminase reaction followed by a branched-chain α-keto acid dehydrogenase (BCDH) reaction.

Novel Avermectins Modified at the C25 Side Chain: Successful Application of Mutasynthesis

Bu'Lock et al. had shown initially that supplementation of *S. avermitilis* fermentations with a range of fatty acids resulted in their uptake and incorporation to generate novel avermectins modified at the C25 side chain of the molecule. This approach, described as precursor-directed biosynthesis, has been employed to produce many new antibiotics, but the co-expression of the parent molecule interferes with the detection and isolation of the novel analogs. To circumvent these difficulties, the elegant technique of "*mutational biosynthesis*" or "*mutasynthesis*" was developed. In this approach, a mutant of an organism, deficient in the production of an essential precursor for the secondary metabolite of choice, is isolated, and precursor-directed biosynthesis is then employed to generate only the novel analogs. In applying mutasynthesis to the production of novel avermectins, the elimination of branched-chain α-keto acid dehydrogenase (BCDH) was targeted. This multienzyme complex is responsible for supplying the 2-methylbutyryl- and isobutyryl-CoA "starter units" that initiate natural avermectin biosynthesis, and which are derived from branched-chain amino acid metabolism. However, it was unclear whether this approach would be feasible, for several reasons.

Thus, labeling studies had demonstrated that not only were the "*starter units*" incorporated intact at the C25 position initiating avermectin biosynthesis, but that they were also degraded by subsequent enzymes of branched- chain amino acid catabolism, and incorporated into the 8 "*propionate*" and 6 "*acetate*" units of the macrolide. Consequently, if branched-chain amino acid catabolism was a major source of avermectin' s "*propionate*" and "acetate" extender units, disruption of this pathway could compromise novel avermectin expression. In addition, 2-methylbutyryl- and isobutyryl-CoA (along with isovaleryl-CoA produced by the comparable metabolism of leucine) also initiate the biosynthesis of the long, branched-chain fatty acids that are the major cellular fatty acids present in *Streptomyces* and other bacterial genera including *Bacillus*. Previous studies had shown an obligate growth requirement for 2-methylbutyric, isobutyric, and isovaleric acids for *bkd*-deficient mutants of *B. subtilis*. Furthermore, the branched-chain α-keto acid dehydrogenase of *B. subtilis* had been shown to be responsible not only for the oxidative decarboxylation of branched-chain α-keto acids, but also for the oxidative decarboxylation of pyruvic acid. Labeling studies had shown that every carbon atom in avermectin can be derived from glucose; thus, concomitant inactivation of pyruvate dehydrogenase, a key enzyme of glucose metabolism, could also compromise novel avermectin co-expression.

bkd Mutants Isolated after Chemical Mutagenesis

Some *bkd* mutants of *S. avermitilis* were isolated using a radioactive screening approach. Unlike comparable mutants of *B. subtilis*, pyruvate dehydrogenase was not concomitantly inactivated, nor did the *S. avermitilis* mutants demonstrate an obligate requirement for 2-methylbutyric, isobutyric, and isovaleric acid supplementation. Analysis of these mutants confirmed the absence of long, branched-chain fatty acids, and indicated that the observed increase in the levels of the C16:1 unsaturated fatty acid ensures the required level of "*membrane fluidity*" normally provided by the C15 and C17 ante-iso-fatty acids resulting from initiation of fatty acid biosynthesis with 2-methylbutyric acid. Most important, the *bkd*-deficient mutants of *S. avermitilis* produced no avermectins in the absence of supplementation with fatty acids. However, natural avermectins were produced upon supplementation with isobutyric acid or (*S*)-2-methylbutyric acid, and novel avermectins with other fatty acids. Branched-chain α-keto acid dehydrogenase thus plays a pivotal and singular role in branched-chain precursor supply in *S. avermitilis*. In the absence of exogenous supplementation, *bkd*-deficient mutants can produce neither long, branched-chain fatty acids nor avermectins and, in addition, cannot grow on branched-chain amino acids as sole carbon source.

BKD Mutants Constructed by Recombinant DNA Technology

The BCDH complex is a multienzyme complex composed of four functional components: a branched-chain α-keto acid dehydrogenase and decarboxylase (E1 [αβ]), a dihydrolipoamide acyltransferase (E2), and a dihydrolipoamide dehydrogenase (E3). The BCDH complex catalyzes the oxidative decarboxylations of α-ketoisovalerate, α-keto-β-methylvalerate, and α-ketoisocaproate (the deamination products of the branched-chain amino acids valine, isoleucine, and leucine, respectively), releasing CO_2 and generating the corresponding acyl-CoA analogs and NADH. The genes encoding the components of the BCDH complex of *Pseudomonas putida* and the pyruvate dehydrogenase (PDH) and BCDH dual-purpose complex of *B. subtilis* and *Bacillus stearothermophilus* have been cloned and found to be clustered in the following sequence: gene encoding E1α, gene encoding E1β, gene encoding E2, and gene encoding E3. Recently, the genes for the branched-chain fatty acid-specific BCDH from *B. subtilis* were cloned and sequenced. This operon consisted of only the three genes encoding the E1α, E1β, and E2 components. Additionally, the sequences of several eukaryotic genes encoding either E1α or E1β BCDH subunits have been reported.

To understand further the importance of the BCDH-catalyzed reaction as a source of precursors for natural avermectin production and to manipulate the production of these antibiotics, we decided to clone and analyze the genes encoding the BCDH multienzyme complex from *S. avermitilis*. PCR primers were designed to encompass conserved regions of known *bkd* genes, and multiple sets of primers were used to amplify *S. avermitilis* genomic DNA. Two strong PCR products were detected and sequenced. Computer analysis suggested that the deduced amino acid sequences of the amplified PCR products were similar to several published E1-α subunits. Probes were generated from the PCR products and used to screen a cosmid library of *S. avermitilis* genomic DNA. The hybridizing regions were cloned and restriction maps were generated. First, we identified a cluster of genes encoding the E1α, E1β, and E2 components of a BCDH complex of *S. avermitilis*. These genes were designated *bkdA*, *bkdB*, and *bkdC* by analogy with the nomenclature introduced to describe similar genotypes of *P. putida*. When *bkdA* and *bkdB*, encoding the E1α and E1β BCDH subunits, were coexpressed in *Escherichia coli*, a functional E1(αβ) BCDH activity was detected. However, when the genomic copies of these genes were inactivated by gene disruption, no obvious phenotypic changes were observed, suggesting that these genes were silent or that their functions could be accomplished by other genes.

Soon after, we reported the cloning and characterization of a gene cluster encoding another BCDH in *S. avermitilis*, *bkdFGH*. These genes are located approximately 12 kb downstream of the *bkdABC* gene cluster. An *S. avermitilis bkd* mutant was then constructed by deletion of a genomic region comprising the 5′ end of *bkdF*. The mutant exhibited a typical *bkd* phenotype, lacking BCDH activity, and it was unable to make natural avermectins in a medium lacking both *S*(+)-α-methylbutyrate and isobutyrate. However, supplementation with *S*(+)-α-methylbutyrate restores production of the corresponding "a" avermectins, while supplementation with cyclohexanecarboxylic acid results in the formation of a novel cyclohexyl avermectin without the co-expression of the natural analogs.

These results confirmed that branched-chain amino acid catabolism via the BCDH reaction provides the fatty acid precursors for natural avermectin biosynthesis in *S. avermitilis*. In contrast, *B. subtilis* appears to possess two mechanisms for branched-chain precursor supply. The dual substrate pyruvate/branched-chain α-keto acid dehydrogenase (*aceA*) and an α-keto acid dehydrogenase (*bfmB*), which also has some ability to metabolize pyruvate, appears to be primarily involved in supplying the branched-chain initiators of long, branched-chain fatty acid biosynthesis. Two mutations are therefore required to generate the *bkd* phenotype in *B. subtilis*.

Mutasynthesis

The *bkd* mutants were subjected to an intensive effort to generate novel avermectins by mutasynthesis. More than 800 potential precursors were fed and more than 60 novel avermectins were obtained covering a wide range of functional groups. These include carbon–carbon double bonds, triple bonds, and S or O atoms in the form of ethers. Cyclic fatty acids are also incorporated along with benzoic acid, and thienoic and furoic acids. Alkyl or alkoxy substituents are accepted, but not polar substituents such as hydroxy or amino groups. In addition to these α-branched carboxylic acids, straight-chain acids such as acetic and propionic acid and β-branched acids such as isovaleric acid are also

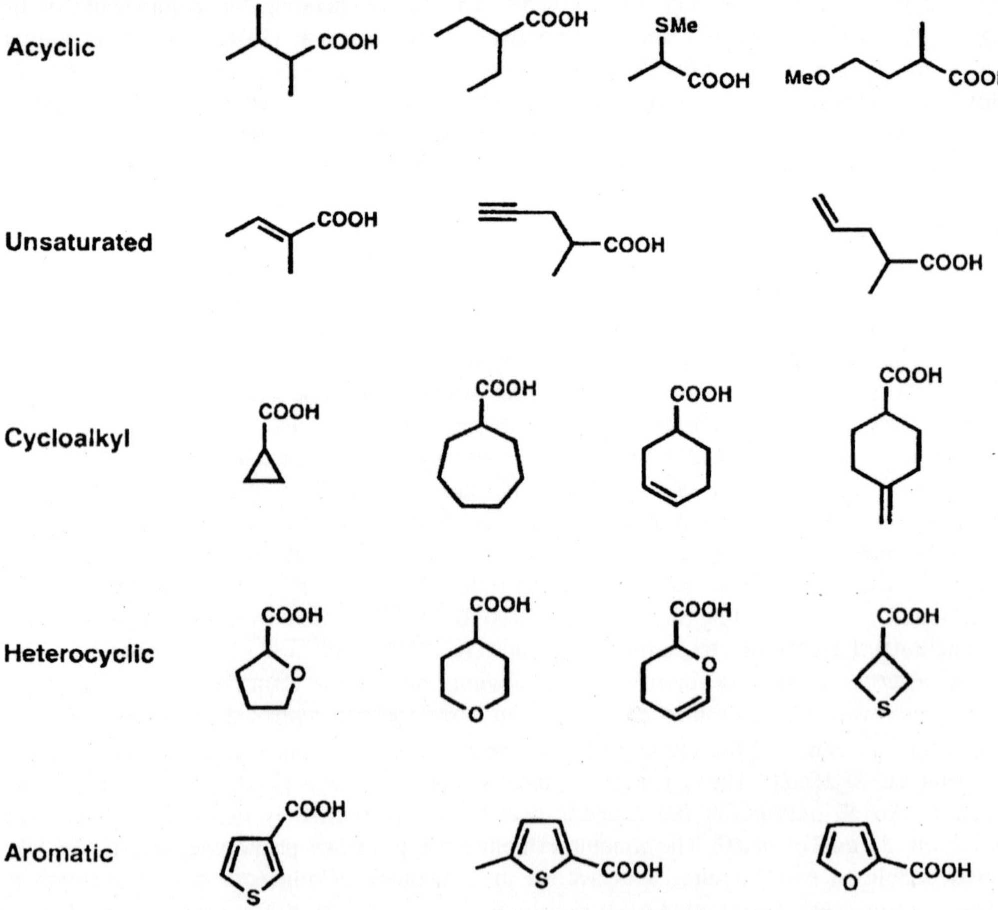

Acyclic

Unsaturated

Cycloalkyl

Heterocyclic

Aromatic

Fig. 13.3. Examples of carboxylic acids incorporated into novel avermectins.

incorporated. The amazing promiscuity of the loading domain of the avermectin PKS has been more recently exploited with its replacement into a wide range of polyketide synthases and triketide lactone model systems. The most intensely studied system, to date, involves the substitution of the avermectin loading domain into the erythromycin PKS. Thus, a wide range of novel erythromycins were produced when these chimeric constructs of *S. erythraea* were supplemented exogenously with fatty acids.

Novel Avermectin, Doramectin

The potency and spectrum of the novel avermectins was initially profiled *in vitro* using a range of nematode and arthropod parasites. Promising candidates were then tested *in vivo* using endoparasite (nematode-infected rats) and ectoparasite (rabbit ear mite) models. The best candidates were subsequently evaluated for efficacy, persistence, and desirable pharmacokinetics in cattle infected with three species of nematodes (*Dictyocaulus viviparus, Cooperia oncophera, Ostertagia ostertagi*). The results of these studies suggested that the novel cyclohexyl B1 avermectin, doramectin, obtained by the incorporation of cyclohexanecar-boxylic acid, appeared to offer advantages over Ivermectin, the existing article of commerce. Formulation evaluation studies showed that there was considerable scope for manipulating the pharmacokinetic profile of doramectin via the formulation vehicle. An oil-based vehicle of sesame oil:ethyl oleate (90: 10) was found to provide high therapeutic and persistent efficacy against a wide range of endo-and ectoparasites, with excellent injection-site toleration, and so doramectin was selected for development.

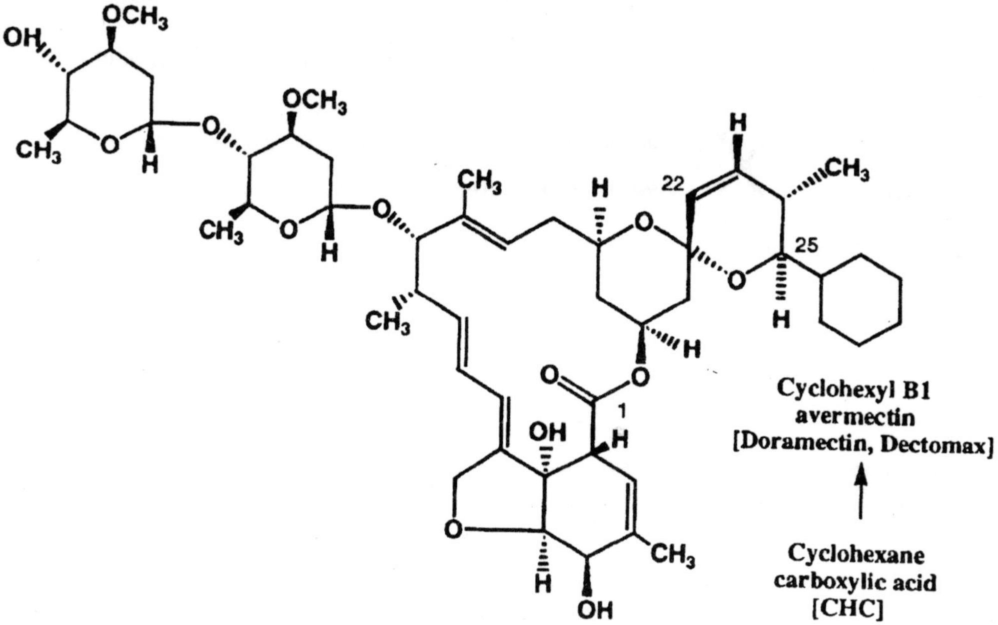

Cyclohexyl B1 avermectin [Doramectin, Dectomax]

Cyclohexane carboxylic acid [CHC]

Fig. 13.4. Structure of the doramectin molecule.

Titer Improvement: Manipulations of the Precursor Flow in the Production of Doramectin

As discussed above, when a *S. avermitilis bkd* mutant (lacking BCDH activity) is grown in a fermentation medium supplemented with the unnatural branched- chain fatty acid, cyclohexanecarboxylic acid (CHC), the novel CHC-derived avermectin, doramectin, is produced. Initial studies using radiolabeled CHC showed that the efficiency of incorporation of CHC into cyclohexyl-avermectins was low, accounting for less than 10% of the total precursor added. As CHC is one of the most expensive components of the doramectin fermentation, a more detailed analysis of the CHC flux was undertaken. Two pathways have previously been identified for the metabolism of CHC by microorganisms. The less common route (4-hydroxy pathway) involves the aromatization of CHC to protocatechuic acid via trans-4-OH-CHC, 4-keto-CHC, and *para*-hydroxybenzoic acid. The primary metabolic route (2-hydroxy pathway) is an initial β-oxidation of CHC to 2-OH-CHC, and thence to 2-keto-CHC and pimelic acid. The 4-hydroxy pathway utilizes P450 hydroxylases, while the 2-hydroxy pathway has been proposed to involve coenzyme-A-activated intermediates (*vide infra*). In addition to the catabolism of CHC, *B. subtilis* has been shown to incorporate exogenously supplied CHC to ω-cylohexane fatty acids. Such fatty acid biosynthesis would be anticipated to initiate from cyclohexyl-CoA, the presumptive starter unit for doramectin biosynthesis. A detailed analysis of products derived from 14C-labeled CHC showed the presence of key intermediates from the 2- and 4-hydroxy pathways, ω-cylohexane fatty acids, and cyclohexyl-avermectins, indicating that all presumed routes of CHC flux were operating in *S. avermitilis*.

In order to enhance CHC incorporation into doramectin, we initiated efforts to decrease CHC flux in other pathways. Since a strategy to alter CHC incorporation into lipids would be more difficult to achieve, our initial focus was on decreasing the oxidative catabolism of CHC. Although most of the metabolites of the 4-hydroxy pathway were present at too low a level for effective quantitation, ^{14}C-4-OH-CHC was readily detected by scanning radioautography after thin-layer chromatography. This offered an useful method of screening mutagenized cultures for blocked mutants, and such mutants were easily isolated using this screen.

The 2-hydroxy pathway is analogous to the latter stages of branched-chain amino acid catabolism and the β-oxidation of fatty acids which utilize coenzyme A derivatives. Branched-chain acyl-CoA

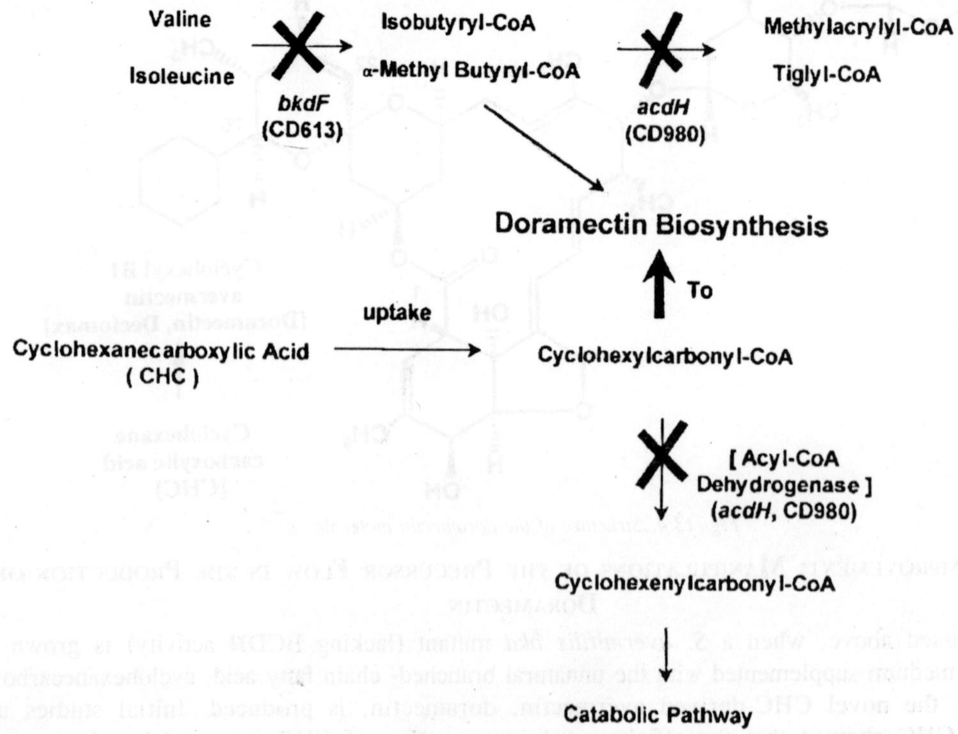

Fig. 13.5. Doramectin titer improvement through disruption of the acdH gene in S. avermitilis.

dehydrogenase acts at the third step of the branched-chain amino acid catabolic pathway, catalyzing the conversion of 2-methylbutyryl-CoA and isobutyryl-CoA into tiglyl-CoA and methacrylyl-CoA, respectively. We recently reported the cloning and nucleotide sequencing of *acdH*, a gene encoding an acyl-CoA dehydrogenase (AcdH), from *S. avermitilis*. AcdH protein expressed in *E. coli* showed a broad range of substrate specificity, oxidizing isobutyryl-CoA, *n*-butyryl-CoA, *n*-valeryl-CoA, isovaleryl-CoA, and cyclohexylcarbonyl-CoA, to their respective 2,3-unsaturated derivatives.

In addition, a *S. avermitilis acdH* mutant constructed by insertional inactivation of the *acdH* gene was unable to grow on solid minimal medium containing valine, isoleucine, or leucine as sole carbon sources and had a decreased ability to process isobutyryl-CoA via a methacrylyl-CoA intermediate to methylmalonyl-CoA. These results were consistent with the *acdH* gene encoding an acyl-CoA dehydrogenase with a broad substrate specificity that has a role in the catabolism of branched-chain amino acids in *S. avermitilis*.

We speculated that the *S. avermitilis* AcdH is also responsible for the catabolic conversion of the doramectin precursor cyclohexylcarbonyl-CoA into cyclohexenylcarbonyl CoA, in a similar way as the acyl CoA analogs of 2-methylbutyrate and isobutyrate are catabolized in the third step of the isoleucine and valine catabolic pathways, respectively. The ultimate objective of our work was to attain a doramectin titer improvement by optimizing the amount of intracellular cyclohexylcarbonyl-CoA available for doramectin production. To that end, the *acdH* gene was disrupted by gene replacement in a high-producer *S. avermitilis bkd* mutant. As a result of this manipulation a doramectin titer increase of approximately 20% was observed.

S. avermitilis and the biosynthesis of avermectins constitute an interesting example where traditional techniques such as chemical mutagenesis and protoplast fusion combined with recombinant DNA technology have been successfully applied in mutant isolation and strain improvement. In addition, this system offered the first opportunity to apply mutasynthesis to the production of better analogs, an application that had never before been exploited commercially. An intense doramectin development effort was therefore initiated with the *bkd*-deficient mutants of *S. avermitilis*. The first step in this process involved the isolation of mutants deficient in 5-*O*-methyltransferase activity to maximize levels

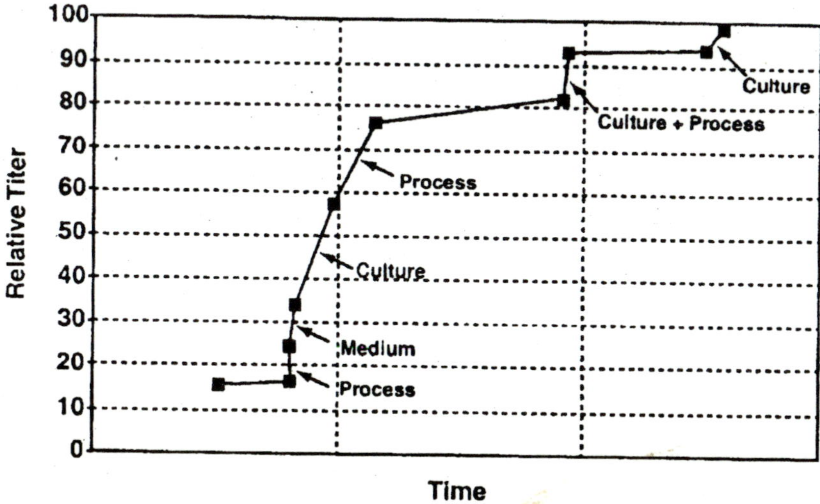

Fig. 13.6. Impact of culture and process on doramectin titer improvement.

of the more bioactive class B avermectins. Thereafter, a combination of strain improvement, employing random mutagenesis, directed enhancements through protoplast fusion approaches, genetic engineering of knockout strains, and process improvement efforts, involving optimization of medium and fermentation (batch feeding, control parameters, etc.), were pursued. In common with development efforts for most secondary metabolites, culture and process improvement contributed almost equally to potency enhancements. These efforts in concert with parallel development of an optimal recovery process have permitted commercially viable expression levels to be achieved, and doramectin has been launched in all major global markets under the trade name of Dectomax. Thus, doramectin represents the first commercially successful application of mutasynthesis plus a complex combination of strain design through genetic engineering, and fermentation and recovery process technologies.

14

CHROMATOGRAPHIC METHODS OF ANALYSIS

The word "*chromatography*" is derived from the Greek words "chroma" and "graphein," which mean "color" and "to write," respectively, or "*color writing*." The initial use of the term is attributed to Tswett, who separated colored bands of plant pigments on a chromatographic column that consisted of an adsorbant powder that was washed with a liquid solvent termed the mobile phase. Substitution of this liquid mobile phase by a gas constitutes the fundamentals of *gas chromatography* (GC), where the solute to be separated is vaporized and carried down the length of a tube that contains an immobile solid or liquid phase, i.e., the stationary phase. The gaseous mobile phase serves to move the solute vapors along the column at rates dependent on several factors, the most important of these being temperature.

GAS CHROMATOGRAPHY

The first reported use of a vapor as the mobile phase is attributed to Martin and Synge in 1941. They used the principles of partition chromatography, whereas James and Martin, in 1952, described the first application of this method, gas–liquid chromatography (GLC), for the analysis of fatty acids and amines. Gas adsorption chromatography (GSC), on the other hand, involves the use of a solid stationary phase and separation is based on an adsorptive mechanism. This technique was first described in 1947 in a doctoral thesis by Prior, under the supervision of Professor Cremer, and subsequently in their 1951 publication. It was not, however, until 1955–1956 that the first commercial gas chromatographs were built. Rapid progress in instrumentation and increased use of GC followed with the introduction of novel detectors, such as the flame ionization detector, development of the capillary column, and the introduction of temperature programming and microsyringes for sample injection.

Utility

The introduction of GC as an analytical technique has had a profound impact on both qualitative and quantitative analysis of organic compounds. Identification of compounds by GC can be accomplished by their retention times on the column as compared to known reference standards, by inference from sample treatment prior to chromatography, or by the concept of retention index. The latter method and tables of retention indices with associated conditions have been reported. Although qualitative data and analytical techniques for identification of compounds are well-established and relative retention data for over 600 substances also have been published, the main utility of GC undoubtedly lies in its powerful combination of separation and quantitative capabilities. Use in quantitative analysis involves the implementation of two techniques being performed concurrently, i.e., separation of components and subsequent quantitative measurement.

The use of GC was first included in the United States Pharmacopoeia (USP) in the sixteenth edition in 1960, and became an official method of the British Pharmacopoeia (BP) in 1968. GC has found widespread use in pharmaceutical analysis by virtue of its applications to purity and control analysis of raw materials, content and quality assessment of dosage forms (including product stability), and in the quantitative measurement of drugs in biological fluids. The latter application is important for therapeutic drug monitoring, pharmacokinetic studies, and bioavailability assessments. In fact, in a survey on GC use, a major application of this technique was in the field of pharmaceuticals.

When this article was first written several years ago, it appeared that the advent and establishment of high-performance liquid chromatography (HPLC) in pharmaceutical analysis had somewhat diminished with the utilization of GC. However, new regulatory requirements for drug approvals by the Federal Drug Administration (FDA) and other regulatory agencies around the world, more particularly with respect to the determination of organic volatile impurities (OVI's) as well as other impurities and related substances, has resulted in more extensive use being made of GC in modern compendia, such as the USP 24th edition and the 1999 edition of the BP. Perusal of the current USP indicates that many more GC applications have been introduced since the 22nd edition of the USP. New inclusions have been incorporated in the tables in this article. Similarly, the recent edition of the BP also includes numerous new applications.

GC remains the chromatographic method of choice for thermally stable volatile compounds and for drugs, which are difficult to measure by HPLC due to detector insufficiency and/or inadequate resolution by the HPLC technique. The use of capillary columns in GC makes the method particularly attractive for difficult multicomponent analysis since extremely high resolution can be readily attained.

Modus Operandi

As previously mentioned, GC is a two-phase system that consists primarily of a stationary (solid and/or liquid) and mobile (gas) phase. When a liquid stationary phase is used (GLC), the liquid is immobilized as a thin film supported on a finely divided, inert solid support usually consisting of siliceous earth, crushed firebrick, glass beads, or in some cases, the inner wall of a glass tube. In GSC, the stationary phase is an active adsorbent, such as alumina, silica gel, or carbon, which is tightly packed into a tube. Separation of components takes place in this tube (chromatographic column) following the introduction of sample at the tube inlet, which is subsequently swept through the column, partitioning or being dynamically adsorbed (or both) between the stationary and mobile phases during transit. The degree and speed of separation of components is governed by several factors, such as temperature, gas flow rate, and the physicochemical properties of the individual components being separated, as well as those of the stationary and to a lesser extent, mobile phase. Obviously, therefore, molecules with greater affinity for the stationary phase will spend more time either adsorbed to or partitioned within that phase and thus take longer to emerge from the column. On emerging at the outlet, each component passes into a detector system that produces a signal that can be related to the mass of the individual component being detected. This signal is usually amplified electronically and subsequently recorded on a chart-recorder, integrator, or captured by an online data system. The resulting response is in the form of a signal–time plot or chromatogram, and is subsequently evaluated for either qualitative or quantitative use.

Theoretical Principles and Rate Theory

A general account of chromatographic theory was presented in volume 2 of Encyclopedia of Pharmaceutical Technology. Therefore, the following discussion will focus specifically on GC theory. The separation of the component of a mixture depends upon the column performance (efficacy) and the relative retention capability of the stationary phase (selectivity). The former determines the width of the peaks relative to the length of time a component spends in the column, while the latter determines the relative position of each emerging component (resolution).

When the sample is introduced into the column, usually in the form of a zone of vapor, it takes the form of a narrow band. During transit through the column, various factors influence the width of this band, which is continuously increased due to various dispersion processes. These include diffusion of the solute, resistance to mass transfer between and within phases, and the influence of flow irregularities and perturbations. A simple concept, the "*theoretical plate*," carried over from distillation processes, has been used to compare columns and account for the degree of dispersion that influences bandwidth. A chromatographic column may be considered to consist of numerous theoretical plates where the distribution of sample components between the stationary and mobile phase occurs. Hence, a measure of the efficiency of a GC column may be obtained by calculating the number of theoretical plates, N, in the column from:

$$N = 16\left(\frac{t}{w}\right)^2 \quad \text{or} \quad N = 5.54\left(\frac{t^2}{w_{1/2}}\right) \qquad \ldots(1)$$

where t is the retention time of the substance, w is the width of the base of the peak obtained by extrapolation (tangential extension of the sides of the relevant peak) of the relevant peak to the baseline, and $w_{1/2}$ is the peak width at half height.

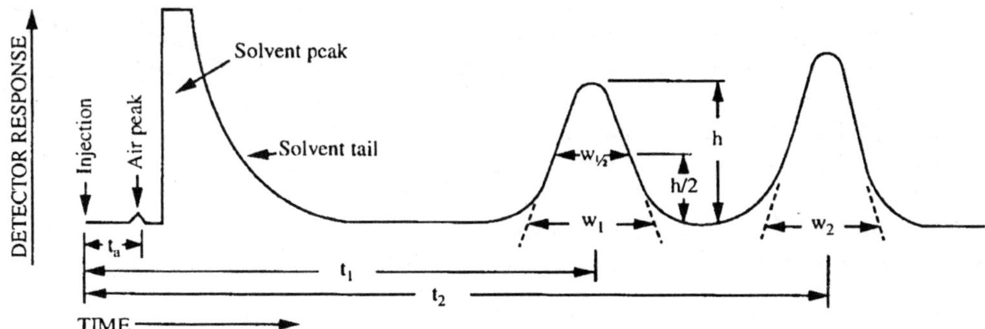

Fig. 14.1. Chromatographic separation of two substances.

The higher the value of N for a column, the more efficient it will be. Columns with high efficiency allow smaller samples to be injected into shorter columns at lower temperatures, which results in high resolution of components in less time.

Column performance under different conditions or the comparison of different columns may be assessed by considering the height equivalent of a theoretical plate (HETP). Thus, HETP = L/N where L is the length of the column. Van Deemter, Zuiderweg, and Klinkenberg derived an equation for dispersion in chromatography:

$$\text{HETP} = 2\lambda d_p + \frac{2\gamma D_g}{\mu} + \frac{8k'd_f^2}{\Pi^2(1+k')^2 D_l}\mu \qquad \ldots(2)$$

where λ is a constant related to the geometry of the column packing particles, d_p is the average diameter of the solid support particles, γ is a factor to correct for the "*tortuosity*" of the column's gas channels, D_g and D_l are solute diffusion coefficients in the gas and liquid phases respectively, d_f is the liquid film (stationary phase) thickness, k' is the partition coefficient of the solute, and μ is the linear gas velocity. Therefore, the Van Deemter equation expresses HETP as a function of the average mobile phase velocity μ and for a specific column, the equation has the general form:

$$\text{HETP} = A + \frac{B}{\mu} + C\mu \qquad \ldots(3)$$

where A is the eddy diffusion term that results from flow inequalities in the column packing, B is the molecular diffusion term (when divided by μ it reflects axial diffusion in the mobile phase), and C reflects resistance to mass transfer from the stationary phase. The linear gas velocity, μ may be obtained from:

$$\mu = \frac{\text{Length of column}}{\text{Retention time of an unretained component (e.g., air)}} \qquad \ldots(4)$$

The flow dependence of the three terms in the Van Deemter equation gives rise to a hyperbola when HETP is plotted against μ for a single component. The minimum is the flow rate at which the column will function at optimum efficiency. For maximum efficiency, these terms must be minimized, i.e., keep HETP as small as possible. Minimization of the A parameter is readily accomplished by using small uniform packing material particles in small diameter columns. Decreasing the particle diameter, d_p, lowers the HETP. However, below a certain particle size, flow of carrier gas through the column is restricted and results in pressure increases, which limits the reduction in particle size. Since λ is a measure of the column packing particle irregularities, the more uniform the size and shape of these particles, the smaller the value of λ.

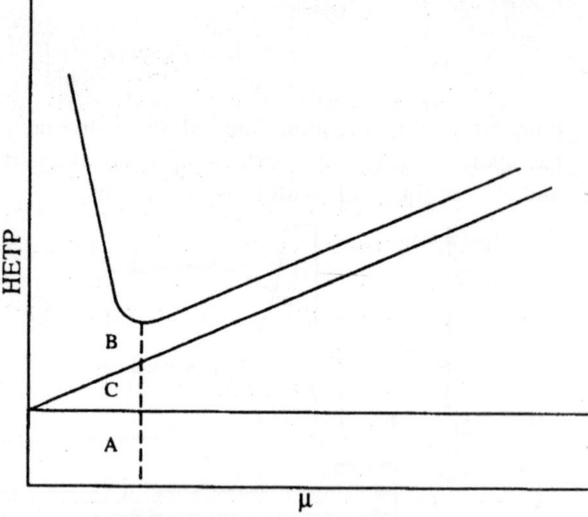

Fig. 14.2. Plot of HETP vs. flow velocity.

The B parameter relates to the diffusivity of the solute in the carrier gas. Increases in molecular diffusion will result in increases in band broadening, which may, however, be controlled to some extent by increasing the gas pressure. The use of a high-molecular-weight carrier gas will retard diffusivity and result in the best efficiency. However, detector function may be affected by the type of carrier gas used; hence, for the purposes of expediency, a compromise is often made by employing hydrogen or helium, which allows rapid analysis albeit with somewhat reduced efficiency. These aforementioned gases, which can rapidly diffuse into the stationary phase, are used at higher flow rates than nitrogen, another commonly used carrier gas.

The remaining parameter, C, is a measure of the mass transfer of the solute molecules from the stationary into the gas phase and depends upon several variables. These include the transfer of solute from liquid to gas and vice versa. Use of thin films of liquid phase will thus allow faster analysis at lower operating temperatures, although sample capacity will be reduced. Viscosity of the liquid stationary phase also affects mass transfer and therefore, should be kept as low as possible at the lowest possible temperature.

Golay and Giddings, respectively, described a modification of the rate theory for capillary columns (hollow tube with inner wall coated with liquid phase) and the random walk, non-equilibrium theory. The former derived an equation to describe the efficiency of an open tubular column, while the random walk theory describes chromatographic separation in terms of statistical moments. The non-equilibrium theory involves a rigorous mathematical treatment to account for incomplete equilibrium between the two phases. Selectivity is a function of the efficiency of the stationary phase with respect to its interactions with the solute vapor. Selection of an appropriate liquid stationary phase will even allow the separation of compounds that have the same vapor pressure. Separation is thus determined by the solubilities of the respective solutes in the stationary phase. Hence, the partition coefficient, k, is an extremely important parameter and is given by the following relationship:

$$k = \frac{\text{Concentration of solute in liquid phase}}{\text{Concentration of solute in gas phase}} \qquad \ldots(5)$$

The efficiency of a stationary phase for a particular separation is measured by α, the relative retention, which is the ratio of two adjusted retention times:

$$\alpha = \frac{t_2 - t_a}{t_1 - t_a} \qquad \ldots(6)$$

where t_2 is the retention time of one of the components, t_1 is the retention time of a second or reference component in the mixture determined on the same column using the same separation conditions, and t_a is the retention time for an unretained compound, such as air. It is thus seen that a reflects the ratio of the partition coefficients for two components being separated under identical conditions and is a useful parameter for the identification of compounds when one of the components is a reference standard material. In order to express how well two peaks are actually separated, a resolution term, R, may be determined, i.e.,

$$R = \frac{2(t_2 - t_1)}{W_2 + W_1} \qquad \ldots(7)$$

where t_2 and t_1 are the retention times of the two components, and W_2 and W_1 are the corresponding widths of the bases of the peaks. Resolution is a measure of both column and stationary phase efficiency and relates peak width and maximal separation. In order to obtain complete separation (baseline resolution) between two peaks, the value of R must be a minimum of 1.5.

System components/Equipment

Gases

While in principle any gas may be used in GC as the carrier, a prerequisite stipulates that the gas be inert with respect to both sample and stationary phase at the operating temperature. The carrier gas plays a critical role in the separation process and indeed, contributes to the efficiency of the system, as was shown in the Van Deemter equation where HETP depends on solute diffusivity in the gas phase. In practice, however, the importance of this role is relegated to a somewhat lower priority since the choice of carrier gas is usually dictated by the detector requirements. Helium is the gas of choice for use with the thermal conductivity detector (TCD), and allows greater sensitivity as compared to nitrogen. The electron capture detectors (ECD), on the other hand, are more efficient when nitrogen or argon–methane mixtures are used as carrier gas, while no noticeable difference in sensitivity is evident between nitrogen and helium when using the flame ionization detector (FID). Thermionic detectors (TD), such as the nitrogen–phosphorus detector (NPD) utilize nitrogen or helium as the carrier gas. Similarly, the photoionization detector (PID) uses oxygen-free nitrogen or helium, while nitrogen is used as carrier gas with the flame photometric detector (FPD). All gases used as carriers in GC should be of high purity. A report on carrier gas purity in GC has been comprehensively discussed by Perretta, and procedures for the preparation of "clean" gases were published previously. Traces of hydrocarbons can lower detector sensitivity (FID), trace amounts of water can desorb contaminants in the column, which leads to high background signals and/or "ghost peaks," while traces of oxygen can cause degradation of certain liquid phases, such as polyglycol and poly-amides, which results in changes of solute retention times. Moisture can be removed by placing cartridges that contain an appropriate molecular sieve fitted in-line between the gas cylinder and the instrument. These type of filters also serve to remove other small, trace level contaminants, such as low-molecular weight hydrocarbons, and may be regenerated by heating with a slow flow of nitrogen for a few hours. Oxygen traps also should be used to protect stationary phases from oxidative degradation.

Flow Control

The carrier gas is fed into the GC via a pressure regulator, while flow controllers are used to control the mass flow rate. Maintenance of an accurate and constant carrier gas flow rate is essential for solute elution reproducibility in both qualitative and quantitative analysis. Normally, gas flow rates will decrease due to an increase in gas viscosity and column back pressure, with an increase in temperature, especially during temperature programmed work. Differential flow controllers are thus essential to assure a constant mass flow rate independent of the resistance of the column. In addition, detectors usually require gas flow control, and this can be accomplished using pressure regulators operating against flow restrictors. Gas flow rates can be simply measured at the end of the column with a soap bubble flow meter or by using rotometers. While flow control was previously adjusted manually, various manufacturers now offer software and associated hardware to effect such changes.

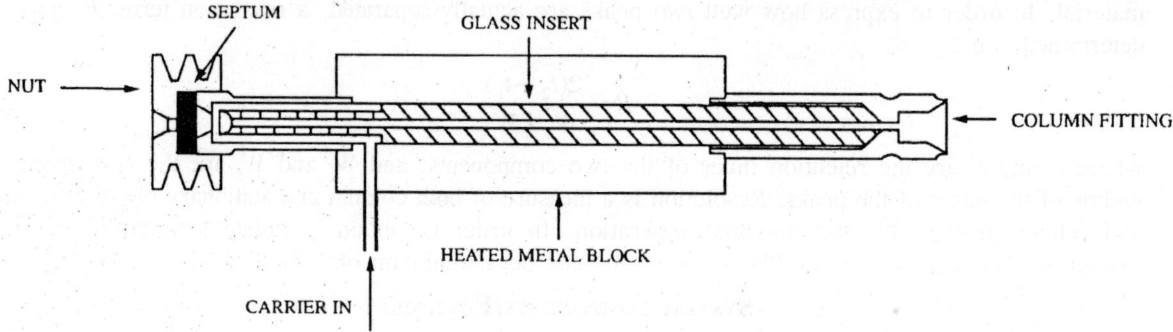

Fig. 14.3. Injection block.

Sample Inlets

Various sample inlet systems have been designed with a primary objective of facilitating satisfactory vaporization of samples and subsequent transfer to the column as a compact "plug" in the shortest possible time and in an accurate and reproducible manner. Additional considerations for efficient sample introduction include maintenance of constant carrier gas flow rate and temperature during sample injection. Considerable differences, however, exist between the manner of sample injection and the actual injecting system, depending on whether packed columns or capillary columns are used. Therefore, sample volume considerations must be taken into account; whereas 1–10 μl is usual for packed columns, several orders of magnitude less is used with capillary columns. Inlet systems for packed columns usually consist of a heated injection block with a minimum dead volume port (to reduce band spreading) which is sealed with a special rubber septum through which the injection syringe needle may be inserted. Compounds which are thermally sensitive and unstable when in contact with metal surfaces may be protected by using glass liners that minimize the sample contact time with the metal injection block.

The foregoing discussion relates to the flash vaporization sample introduction technique that involves injection of sample into a precolumn zone that is kept at a temperature of 30–50° C higher than that of the column. This facilitates instantaneous sample vaporization. Samples also may be introduced by on-column injection where the sample is injected directly into the head of the column, which results in better precision than flash vaporization. Inlet systems for packed columns can often be used with capillary columns as well. However, the much smaller injection volumes and slower gas flow rates used with capillary columns, especially small-bore open tubular capillaries (0.25 mm i.d.), require different sampling techniques.

Split injection

Early capillary inlets utilize an inlet splitter, which splits the sample into two unequal portions, the smaller of which goes into the column. The major function of the inlet splitter is not only to redirect the amount of sample placed on the column but also to permit rapid flushing of the injection chamber so that the sample in the column is followed by pure carrier gas, thereby avoiding sample dilution. The larger portion of sample is vented out of the system and the ratio of the two flows, the split ratio, typically ranges from 1:10 to 1:500. Since split injection is a flash vaporization technique, the possibility of sample discrimination exists. All sample components must be divided in the same ratio irrespective of differences in molecular weight, component concentration, polarity, injected volume, and inlet temperature for optimum reproducibility. Although the discriminatory effect can be minimized through the use of different inlet configurations, quantitative results by sample splitting are often not as good as by splitless and on-column techniques.

Splitless injection

Splitless injection utilizes a "*solvent effect*' and allows a relatively large amount of dilute sample (1–5 μl) to be injected. The sample is vaporized and then carried onto the column on which it must be reconcentrated prior to analysis. This is essential in order to prevent band broadening. In order to prevent column overloading, the amounts of components being separated should be less than 50 ng. The large excess of solvent used to prepare the sample is backflushed 30–60 s after injection in order to minimize the occurrence of a long solvent tail, which can obscure any early eluting peaks. There are two mechanisms for reconcentrating the solutes at the head of the column. Grob and Grob utilized the "*solvent effect*," whereby the solvent acts as a barrier to the sample components, which facilitates their condensation and concentration at the head of the column. This is due to the fact that when the sample components encounter a liquid phase mixed with retained solvent, the front of the sample plug undergoes stronger retention than the rear of the plug. In order to minimize column deterioration that can result from solvent overloading, a solvent in which the liquid phase is not readily soluble should be used. Both dichloromethane and hexane have been widely used and care should be taken to see that the initial column temperature is 10–30°C below the boiling point of the solvent selected.

Another method of reconcentrating the components at the head of the column is to keep the column temperature low enough to condense the solutes (cold trapping). A general guideline for the use of this pre- column concentration technique is that compounds with boiling points 100°C higher than the column temperature will be cold trapped. Therefore, splitless injection should be used when component concentrations are too low for detection by split injection (<0.1% sample) or when only a very limited amount of sample is available.

On-column injection

When dealing with thermolabile compounds, vaporization of the sample can result in degradation during this process. Schomburg et al. described an on-column injection technique whereby the sample never encounters temperatures higher than the column temperature. This method also has been shown to be extremely useful for the separation of compounds that have low volatility and samples that have a wide boiling range. Using very fine long fused silica needles attached to a microsyringe and inserted into the capillary column bore, on-column systems have been described. The fine needles are too fragile for normal septum piercing, hence other methods have been devised in which a septum-free valved inlet is used. Inlet modifications that incorporated air-cooling of the column inlet were later designed to overcome vaporization in the needle that resulted from the slow injections necessary to achieve a narrow band of injected sample.

Automatic injection

The injection process has been automated, thus facilitating batch processing of large numbers of samples that are completely unattended. Various automatic injector systems are commercially available for use with both packed and capillary columns. These are mainly based on the use of syringe injection and pneumatically operated under microprocessor control. Injector loops are largely used for the introduction of gases into the column, while manual injection continues to be extensively used. In the latter instance, the operator's injection technique can dramatically influence the quality of the analysis. A skilled operator may achieve precisions of the order of ±1% with manual syringes by careful debubbling of the syringe, and using sample sizes at least 50% of the syringe capacity to minimize needle hold up and setting errors, as well as using a very reproducible injection technique. However, the advent of automatic samplers considerably enhances injection precision and accuracy. In addition, the tedious process of carefully cleaning and flushing the syringe between samples to avoid cross-contamination during manual injections is readily accomplished automatically.

Oven and Temperature Controls

The column is usually suspended in an insulated thermostatically controlled air oven through which the air is very rapidly circulated by means of fans or pumps. This allows accurate temperature control to within 0.1°C and minimizes thermal gradients. Provision is also made for the temperature to be rapidly increased and for the equally rapid cooling required with temperature-programmed work.

Injection port temperatures for packed columns include thermostatically controlled heating. These parts should be hot enough to rapidly vaporize the sample in order to prevent a loss in efficiency from the injection process. Heated detector systems also are used depending on the type of detector, to prevent sample condensation, which inevitably will result in peak broadening and loss of component peaks. Temperature control imparts stability to the detection system, often reducing noise and enhancing the detection limit. When the FID is used, its temperature must be kept high enough to avoid any water or by-products formed during the combustion process.

Detectors

A large variety of detectors have been designed for use in GC. The chromatographic detector, placed at the column exit, constantly monitors the emitted gas, and generates an electrical signal that is amplified and appears as a plot of detector response versus time, i.e., the chromatogram. Detectors may be "universal," which responds to every eluted component (TCD), "selective," which responds only to certain functional or elemental characteristics of the analyte (ECD and FID), or "specific," which provides qualitative information concerning the structure of the eluting component (FPD). However, for classification purposes, GC detectors generally fall into one of two groups: concentration-dependent and mass rate-dependent detectors. The former, which includes the TCD and ECD, produces a signal that is proportional to the concentration of the sample in the carrier gas. In the latter (e.g., FID), the detector signal is dependent on the mass of sample that flows through the detector per unit time (g/s). Some of the most important properties relating to detectors are: (1) their sensitivity, which is a function of the amount of component present in the injected sample; (2) their signal noise, which refers to random, short-term detector response and which combined with sensitivity, determines the detection limit for a given component; and (3) their linearity of response, which indicates the region over which the detector signal is directly proportional to sample concentration or mass flow rate. The dynamic linear range of the detector is the range of sample size for which a signal is detected as a linear function of the sample size. Thus, a wide linear range is useful for quantitative analysis of multi- component mixtures. In contrast to short-term noise, which depends upon electrical factors, temperature sensitivity, or flow variations, long-term noise is manifested by baseline drift in the chromatogram. Detectors commonly used in GC and specified in the USP include FID, alkali FID (NPD, TD), ECD, and TCD. Various other useful detectors for GC include photoionization (PID), flame photometric (FPD), electrolytic conductivity (ELCD), redox (RCD) and sulfur chemiluminescence (SCD), and helium ionization (HID).

In addition to the above, several newer and highly sophisticated detection techniques that involve the coupling of various types of spectrometers with GC have emerged. These "hyphenated" techniques include the on-line interfacing of mass spectrometers (GC–MS), infrared spectrometers that incorporate Fourier transformation techniques (FTIR–GC), and FTIR–GC–MS. Generally, these are considered specific detectors mainly used to obtain qualitative information, although quantitative data can be obtained when operating a GC–MS system in the selected-ion-monitoring mode (SIM). This mode, in contrast to the normal scanning mode used for qualitative purposes, allows a single or a few characteristic ions of an analyte to be monitored and subsequently determined quantitatively. Triple–quadruple MS/MS spectrometers are becoming more prevalent and these are being increasingly coupled to GC's that provide enhanced quantitation capabilities.

Columns

The suitability of a column for a particular use depends on various factors, such as stationary phase, solid support, column tubing material, inside diameter, percent liquid loading, and temperature. Columns may be prepared in various lengths and diameters depending on the particular objective. Preparative columns may range from 0.95 to 10 cm (3/8–4′) in diameter or larger for the collection of quantities of individual components when volumes between 0.5 ml and more are injected. Analytical (or packed) columns generally have outside diameters of 3, 4.7, or 6.25 mm (1/8, 3/16, or 1/4′), and inside diameters of 1–4 mm, while capillary columns with very narrow inside diameters are used for applications that require very high resolution. The inside diameter of the tubing is, in fact, one of the most critical column dimensions in determining the efficiency of separation.

Although packed GC columns may be made from various materials, such as glass, nickel, stainless steel, copper, aluminum, or even Teflon, the USP and BP recommend that glass or stainless steel columns be used for pharmaceutical analyses unless otherwise specified. The advantage of using glass lies in its relative inertness as compared to metal columns, although its fragile nature is certainly a disadvantage. In order to assure further the inertness of glass, silanization of the inside walls with 5–10 vol% dimethyldichlorosilane in toluene is often performed.

Capillary columns are usually fabricated from fused silica, with a polyamide outer coating to impart flexibility and reduce breakage during handling. These columns can be classified into three categories according to the size of the internal diameter. Typical inside diameters are 0.53 mm, 0.32–0.22 mm, and 0.2–0.1 mm for megabore (wide-bore), normal bore (high-resolution), and microbore (high-speed), respectively.

The selection of a stationary phase is extremely important in GC since it is the major controllable variable of selectivity in the separation process. Stationary phases can be non-polar, polar, or of intermediate polarity. Cyclodextrins, cyclic oligosaccharides composed of varying numbers of glucopyranose units, were found recently to be extremely useful for the separation of chiral compounds. Three types of derivatives, 5-hydroxypropyl (hydrophilic), dialkyl (hydrophobic), and trifluoroacetyl (intermediate) have been used, each of these phases having a selected area of specificity.

Capillary columns offer many advantages in terms of speed of analysis, high resolution, and overall very high separation efficiency. New applications that involve the use of capillary columns are included in the USP. In particular, methods for OVI analysis prescribe, almost exclusively, capillary columns, whereas approximately 20% of the other GC methods also prescribe such columns.

Solid supports should be chemically inert and exhibit a large surface area. Support materials used are diatomaceous earths, Teflon, glass beads, and various polymers. Since the surface of the diatomaceous materials consist of silanol (Si—O—H) and siloxane (Si—O—Si) groups, compounds capable of hydrogen bonding (alcohols, acids, amines, etc.) can interact with these media, which results in tailing. This problem may, however, be minimized by silanization following extensive acid washing to remove inorganic impurities. Acid-washed flux-calcined diatomaceous earth is often used for drug analysis.

Specially treated glass beads have been used as supports for high-molecular-weight compounds. The beads are usually etched and silanized prior to coating with the liquid phase. Teflon is a useful support material for the analysis of short chain polar substances, which tail on diatomaceous supports, and is particularly indicated for the analysis of corrosive substances such as halogenated acids.

When a separation can be effected by a purely adsorptive mechanism (GSC), various adsorbants and porous polymers are used. Commercially available adsorbants include silica gel, activated charcoal, and molecular sieve materials. These adsorbants are used mainly for the analysis of gases and low-molecular-weight, low-boiling compounds.

Porous polymers also are useful for gas analyses and for very polar molecules, such as amines, glycols, and acids. Copolymers of styrene and divinylbenzene and others, such as ethylvinylbenzene-divinylbenzene, cross-linked acrylic ester, vinylpyridine, pyrollidone, and ethylene glycol dimethacrylate, are commercially available.

Open tubular columns are simply capillary tubes in which the inside of the column wall is used as the support for the liquid phase. These wall-coated open tubular columns (WCOT) have the stationary phase distributed in the form of a thin film on the inside surface of the open capillary tube, the walls thus serving as the support. In order to reduce the thickness of the liquid phase film, a porous layer may be formed on the inside wall of the capillary tubing and then coated with the liquid phase to produce a support-coated open tubular column (SCOT). Porous-layer open tubular columns (PLOT) are similar to SCOT columns, the difference being that in the former, the stationary phase is deposited on fine crystalline particles or glass powder which is adsorbed onto the walls of the tube. In both cases, the available surface area of the wall is increased, and allows an increased amount of liquid phase to be accommodated in the same length and diameter of tubing. The whisker-walled (WW) column consists of whiskers chemically etched on the surface of the wall, which also result in a significant increase in the available surface area. Wall-coated, porous-layer, and support-coated capillary columns are all available as whisker-walled, i.e., WWCOT, WWPLOT, and WWSCOT, respectively.

The stationary phase film thickness of capillary columns range from about 0.1–10 μm and can be divided into three film thickness ranges. Thin-film columns are usually 0.1–0.2 μm and offer the greatest stability. They have smaller sample capacity as compared to the thicker films but are the best for use with high temperatures. Thick films are usually 0.6–10 μm and allow higher sample loading, better retention for volatile compounds, and a high degree of inertness. Their main drawback, however, is larger bleed at high temperature as compared to the thin film type. The medium film thickness is about 0.3–0.6 μm and is a useful compromise in terms of sample capacity, retention properties, and phase stability.

In addition to the open tubular capillary columns, packed capillaries, and even micropacked capillaries, are commercially available. These columns contain support material, have internal diameters that range from 0.6–1.0 mm, and have the main advantage of being able to handle larger sample loadings. This is useful since direct analysis, as opposed to split-analysis, can be used with very short columns that operate at relatively high efficiency.

Column lengths of 0.3–6.1 m (1–20 ft) are commonly used and configurations can be straight, U-shaped, spiral, or flat coils. Straight and U-shaped columns are purported to be slightly more efficient than the coiled types. However, the dimensions of the GC oven usually dictate the choice. Capillary columns are generally much longer than packed columns and range in lengths from 10–100 m for the open tubular type and 1-6 m for packed type.

Separation Techniques

Gas chromatographic analysis can be performed at constant temperature (isothermal mode) or with the column temperature increasing with time (temperature programming).

Isothermal

In isothermal GC, peak width increases linearly with retention time and retention time increases exponentially with carbon number in a homologous series. In contrast, the peak width remains constant in programmed-temperature gas chromatography (PTGC) and retention times increase only linearly with carbon number in a homologous series.

Gas chromatographic methods for the analysis of impurities in pharmaceutical dosage forms and raw materials generally make use of isothermal techniques where the temperature of the instrument is maintained constant throughout the run. However, when complex mixtures that contain components with widely different boiling ranges need to be analyzed, PTGC is undoubtedly the method of choice. Separation of components in such a mixture may prove difficult if at all possible under isothermal conditions. Using a high temperature for the analysis may result in poor resolution between the rapidly eluting volatile components. On the other hand, operating at a lower temperature could cause excessively long retention times for the less volatile compounds, with resulting peak broadening leading to poor detectability and prolonged running times.

Temperature Programming

The advent in 1952 of PTGC and the subsequent introduction of commercial equipment for temperature programming provided the necessary means to analyze complex mixtures that contained components of widely differing boiling points and solved some of the problems previously described in the section dealing with isothermal separations.

The PTGC technique involves increasing the column temperature at a preset rate during the elution process. This rate may be constant throughout the run, or periods of isothermal operation may be automatically programmed at set times between temperature increases. Generally, the electronically controlled ovens are designed to increase temperature at rates from 0.5–30°C per minute. The initial temperature should be chosen to minimize the retention time for the least retained solute, while the final temperature must be sufficient to elute the least volatile compound in a reasonable time. The instrument then automatically resets the temperature to the initial value in preparation for the next sample.

A major problem with PTGC, however, is that column bleed may cause baseline perturbations as the temperature increases, which results in interference with the analysis. Compensation for this effect is usually accomplished by using a dual column/dual detector system or replacing the liquid stationary phase with another less volatile coating. In the former instance, the output signal from the reference column is used to cancel out the bleed from the analytical column. Electronic compensation using single-column, single-detector systems are also available, as are GC's with electronically controlled programmed gas flows. In the latter case, the carrier flow rate is increased during the analysis, which results in reduced baseline drift by avoiding or reducing column bleed. Since lower temperatures can be used, the analysis of thermolabile compounds is facilitated and a wider range of liquid phases can be used.

Special Techniques

Various compounds do not readily lend themselves to analysis by GC by virtue of several factors, such as non-volatility, instability, elicitation of poor detector response, or high adsorptive properties (presence of polar groups). These problems sometimes can be overcome by the use of pyrolysis or by derivatization. The former technique involves high temperature decomposition of high-molecular-weight, non-volatile substances to lighter, and more volatile compounds.

Derivatization is a valuable aid in GC. Suitable derivatives may be produced using synthetic organic reactions such as esterification, acylation, and silylation. These methods serve to increase thermal stability in unstable compounds, improve detectability in some instances (e.g., derivatives for electron capture detection) and often sensitivity, improve volatility in instances where the parent compound is relatively non-volatile, and mask polar groups to reduce adsorption.

Quantitative and Qualitative Analysis

GC constitutes an analytical technique whereby the separation of components in a mixture and their quantitative and qualitative assessment can be performed simultaneously.

The area under the component elution peak is proportional to the concentration of that particular component. Various methods can be used to measure this area and are based on the assumption that the shape of the peak is Gaussian. Electronic integration is the preferred method since very accurate and precise measurements are obtained this way (RSD $\leq$ 0.5%).

Peak heights may be used but are less reliable since any variability in temperature and/or flow rate will affect this measurement. Peak areas may also be calculated by multiplication of the peak height and the width at half-height. This gives a value equal to 84% of the true area. Triangulation, planimetry, and cutting and weighing also can be used to measure peak areas.

In order to minimize the possibility of errors as a result of variable injection volumes, the internal standard (IS) method should be used. It involves the addition of a compound, the IS, which is not already present in the sample. This is normally a substance that elutes at a position near the sample component of interest and should be well resolved and readily detected under the given chromatographic conditions. The IS is added in constant amount to solutions that contain varying amounts of the analytical standard. Calibration curves are then constructed by plotting the ratio of either the areas or peak heights of the two peaks (analyte/IS) versus amount or concentration of analyte. The amount or concentration of each chromatographed sample can then be obtained by interpolation of the calibration curve. The calibration plot should be a straight line with an intercept of zero. However, non-linear standard curves may result when the linear range of the particular detector is exceeded due to excess analyte concentration. The presence of high background and/or interfering compounds results in plots that have a positive intercept, while negative intercepts are usually indicative of sample loss during handling.

In contrast to the IS method, external standardization may be used in which several standard solutions of varying concentrations of the sample are prepared. Following constant volume injection of each standard solution, a plot of peak area (or height) versus concentration is made, and unknown sample concentrations are obtained from interpolation of the calibration curve. The success of this technique, however, is dependent upon the precision of injection volume, readily accomplished with automatic injection but less so when manual microliter syringes are used.

A further quantitative measure, normalization, is sometimes utilized to determine the proportion of one or more components in a mixture. This involves calculating the ratio of the individual component peak area to the sum of the areas of all component peaks in the chromatogram. It assumes that all the components have identical response factors to the detector. This is a reasonable assumption when all the components of the mixture are chemically similar. When structurally dissimilar components are analyzed, a response factor correction should be used by measuring the peak area for a known quantity of pure material and calculating the respective response factor (F) from:

$$F = \frac{\text{Component amount}}{\text{Peak area}} \qquad \ldots(8)$$

Acquisition of qualitative data may be obtained by using specific detectors such as GC–MS, FTIR–GC, and FTIR–GC–MS, as well as from relative retention times or by the concept of retention index (vide infra).

Headspace Analysis

Specifications for pharmaceutical compounds, in addition to the actual active ingredient itself, include information and limits relating to the intermediates, residual solvents, and other volatile impurities associated with their preparation.

Headspace analysis is a very effective technique for the analyses of volatile compounds, and is particularly valuable when direct injection would ruin the column due to corrosive or highly non-volatile components present in the sample. Headspace analysis obviates extensive sample preparation, eliminates the possibility of unwanted component interference, and avoids degradation of susceptible components in the injection port or on the column.

The liquid or solid sample is placed in a vial, which is sealed with a septum and heated to a predetermined temperature for a period of time. Equilibrium between the sample and vapor phase is then established and a portion of the volatiles in the gas phase (headspace) is subsequently injected onto the column. Several different methods have been used to transfer headspace volatiles into the GC, from manual withdrawal that uses a gas syringe, to sophisticated automatic sampling that involves transfer lines, and valves that lead directly onto the column.

Two main techniques, however, may be used. These are static and dynamic sampling. The static method allows the temperature of the sample container to be held for a sufficiently long period to allow the gas-phase and sample-phase to equilibrate. The dynamic sampling uses an inert gas that is swept over or through the thermostated sample for a period of time sufficient to extract most or all of the volatile components. A general chapter on OVI's, in which five OVI's are specifically mentioned (chloroform, dichloromethane, benzene, trichloroethylene, and dioxane), was introduced into the USP. Previously, the USP included methods II and III, which provided an alternative to direct injection and specified dynamic head- space sampling. These, however, have now been excluded and method IV provides for the general use of static headspace sampling. Method VI, while still included, prescribes analysis by direct injection into a gas chromatograph, but none of the monographs in the USP. or National Formulary (NF) specify use of method VI for OVI testing. The trend, it appears, has been toward using method IV as a replacement for other methods in individual monographs and that monographs that now specify method IV, originally specified method VI. The advantages, sampling techniques, and problems associated with headspace sampling were previously discussed by Hinshaw.

Pharmaceutical Applications

Although HPLC has largely superseded GC as the compendial chromatographic method of choice for the assay of pharmaceuticals, the application of GC continues to be an important and valuable analytical method for monitoring certain impurities and for the determination of various related substances and OVI's in many pharmaceutical dosage forms, as well as in raw materials. GC, furthermore, continue to be a valuable tool for the analysis of drugs in biological fluids for the purposes of therapeutic drug monitoring, pharmacokinetic studies, and in the assessment of bioavailability/bioequivalence. A large number of pharmaceutical compounds can, however, be analyzed by either GC or HPLC. In terms of cost effectiveness, given that the equipment is available, GC often may be preferred due to its advantage of avoiding the use of expensive solvents and associated subsequent disposal problems.

Raw Materials (Bulk Drugs) and Dosage Forms

Both the USP/NF and the BP utilize GC for the following types of determinations:

1. Assay.
2. Chromatographic purity.
3. Identification.
4. Presence of volatile matter, intermediates, and related substances.
5. Water.
6. Presence of isomers, isomeric purity, and racemate ratios.
7. Alcohol content.

Biological Fluids

While it is clearly apparent that packed columns are mainly used for the various compendial tests, the use of capillary columns for the determination of therapeutic agents in biological fluids has become increasingly popular. The high resolution capability of capillary columns often overcomes the problems of interference from the biological sample matrix and, coupled with specificity and increased sensitivity has made possible the quantitative analysis of many, formerly undeterminable drugs in biological fluids. In particular, drugs with very poor ultraviolet (UV) molar absorptivities, as well as drugs which by virtue of their specific physicochemical properties result in extremely low recovery values when extracted from biological fluids, have been successfully determined by GC using capillary columns.

Although the introduction of HPLC has often been perceived as ultimately replacing GC for use in pharmaceutical analysis, perusal of the current literature and new official compendia clearly indicate that GC is "here to stay." The notion of an imminent demise of GC appears unrealistic in the light of innovations and applications that continue to expand. Other innovative quantitative techniques with potential for use in pharmaceutical analysis are certainly looming on the horizon. In particular is the technique of high voltage capillary zone electrophoresis. These newer methods, coupled with the now well-established TLC and HPLC methods, will undoubtedly gain more importance and widespread use in the future. However, all these techniques are unlikely to oust GC, since each have their strengths and weaknesses and together compliment the array of techniques and methods for use in pharmaceutical analysis.

Advances in the manufacture of flexible fused silica WCOT columns will almost certainly extend the applications of GC by virtue of their high-resolution capability, while the advent of sophisticated, computerized detectors forecast the improvement in sensitivity and specificity. The use of chiral stationary phases for the resolution of enantiomers is becoming an increasingly important topic in pharmaceutical analyses. The range and availability of various liquid phases for chiral analysis by GC is bound to make this technique extremely valuable for the assay of pharmaceutical raw materials as well as for use in biological fluids. Multidimensional and multihyphenated techniques may become increasingly useful, particularly for the analysis of drugs in biological fluids where LC–GC interfacing has a great deal of promise with respect to sample cleanup and preparation time. GC–MS applications continue to grow in number from the qualitative structural identification point of view, for quantitative analysis that uses SIM, and for other quantitative applications of GC (in particular, the increasing use of triple-quad MS/MS spectrometers). Thus, it is apparent that GC has firmly established itself as a valuable technique for the qualitative and in particular, quantitative determination of drugs. Its application in monitoring impurities, volatile matter, intermediates, and related substances in pharmaceutical raw materials and dosage forms makes it currently the method of choice in this respect. Meanwhile, its increasing use for the quantitative determination of some "hard-to-measure" drugs and metabolites in biological fluids suggest that it is likely to remain an important tool in this arena in the future.

High Performance Liquid Chromatography

Chromatography is a technique to separate individual components in a mixture. High-performance liquid chromatographic (HPLC) methods are usually preferred over other methods of quantitative analysis. The methods are usually very specific to the analyte or analytes of interest since excellent separation of individual components are easily achieved. HPLC instruments are ubiquitous since the technique finds application in biotechnological, biomedical, clinical, and pharmaceutical analyses. Additionally, HPLC is used in many other fields including chemical, cosmetics, energy, environmental, and food industries. The availability of moderately priced, reliable, efficient, and sophisticated instrumentation has resulted in the use of HPLC as a method of choice in the pharmaceutical analysis, starting from the synthesis or isolation of a potential drug to the final stage of maintaining quality control information on a formulated dosage form.

Since the fundamental theoretical principles of HPLC were established in the 1960s, the development of HPLC instrumentation has been phenomenal. Development in column packing materials led to the development of reverse-phase chromatography in the 1970s. Development of computers and automation in the 1980s led to the ease of use of HPLC. In the 1990s the development of microcolumns, specialized columns, stable detectors, coupled with integrated data acquisition, storage, and retrieval capabilities has vastly increased the speed and efficiency of the HPLC instruments.

Basic Concepts, Definitions, and Chromatographic Theory

Basic Concepts and Definitions

In HPLC for separation of individual components, the sample is introduced into a flowing stream of a liquid (*mobile phase*) and the analytes are allowed to pass through a layer column of packing materials of very small diameters (large surface area), called the *stationary phase*. As the analyte molecules pass through the column, carried by the moving mobile phase, there is constant interaction of the analyte molecules (or solutes) with the stationary phases as well as with the moving mobile phase. This results in a dynamic equilibrium. The differences in the equilibrium processes of the different solute molecules result in the separation of components of the mixture. When such separation is achieved by maintaining a constant composition of all the constituents of the mobile phase, the process is known as *isocratic elution*. If the mobile phase composition is changed continuously with respect to one or more of the solvents in the mobile phase, as a function of time, it is called *gradient elution*. When the *effluent* with mobile phase zones containing the analyte molecules emerges out of the column, it is passed through a *detector*, or a series of detectors. The detector signals respond as function of the solute concentration in the mobile phase zones. These signals are fed into *data processors*, which plot signal responses as a function of time. The graphic display of signals is called a chromatogram and the individual component zones are identified as *chromatographic peaks*. These peaks are characterized by the following parameters: their *peak widths*, *peak areas* or *peak heights*, and the extent of tailing and the retention time of the peaks. The instrumental set up is called a chromatograph.

In HPLC solute molecules are introduced into a moving mobile phase stream. The stream passes through an inlet and emerges through the outlet of the column. Since the particles are extremely small in size (10 μm or less) and the column is fully packed, the moving mobile phase has to be pumped through using high pressure pumps. The solute molecules are only carried by the moving mobile phase. Molecules that interact with the surface of the column will be impeded and the emerging band will elute later than a band of weakly interacting molecules. The relative migration of the solute is dependent on the thermodynamic and kinetic properties of the solute. The extent and quality of separation of two

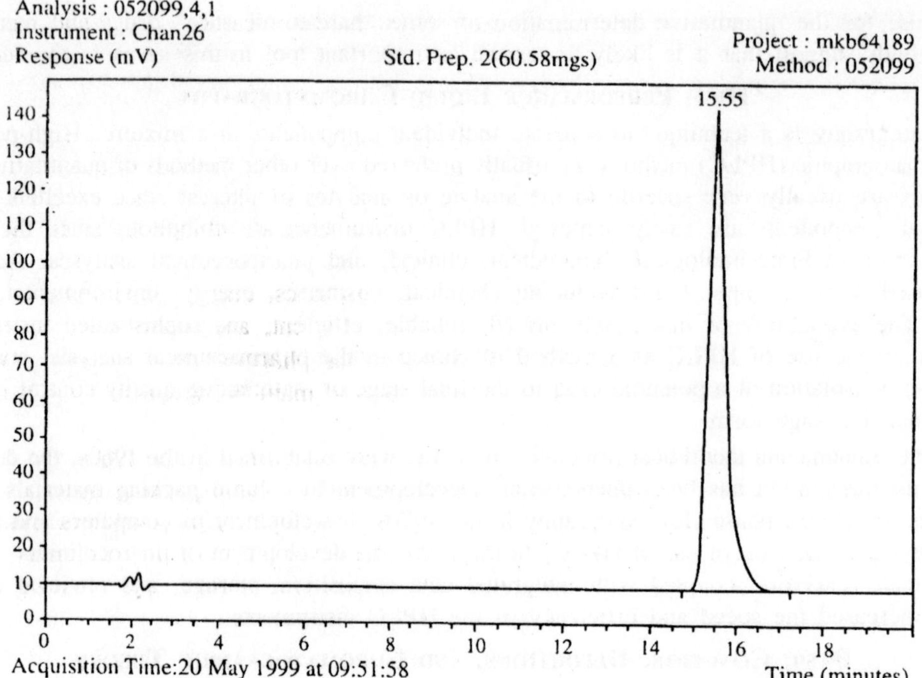

Fig. 14.4. Typical chromatogram.

closely eluting peaks are expressed by retention (or capacity) factor (k'), selectivity factor (α), and the number of theoretical plats (N). Capacity factor is a measure of time that the solute molecules are attached to the column particles, in comparison to that of the mobile phase. Thus greater the value of k', the greater is the interaction with the column particles. The capacity factor is dependent on the nature of the column, the organic or aqueous strength of the mobile phase, and the temperature at which the column is maintained. Experimentally measurable parameter of *relative retention time* with respect to the retention time of an active drug is computed. Under isocratic elution conditions, a value of 2–6 for capacity factor is optimal and normally values between 1 and 10 are acceptable. Greater the value of k', greater is the resolution between adjoining bands. However, as k' increases, there is increase in analysis time, which also results in lower detection limit, because of peak broadening. By using gradient elution these two disadvantages of isocratic elution can be overcome.

The chromatographic separation process is considered *efficient* if all the components are completely separated and the peak width is relatively narrow. Theoretically, when identical molecules enter the column head in a narrow band, the band width should be the same at the outlet. However, since solute molecules can elute at slightly different times because not all molecules will take the same path. These differences are caused by differences in the local surface area, relative physical activity of the interacting surface, the presence of stagnant mobile phase pools in crevices and pores, and minor variations of flow rate of mobile phases through these surfaces. Not all solute molecules traverse the same path and hence they might contribute to peak broadening.

Additionally, the quality of separation is evaluated by measurement of resolution, "R," between two closely eluting peaks.

$$R = 2(t_2 - t_1)/(w_1 + w_2)$$

where w_1 and w_2 are peak widths expressed in the same units as retention times, t_1 and t_2.

The greater the value of R, greater is the separation. For an R value of 1.00, solute purity is about 97.7% if each peak is Gaussian. In practice to attain a peak purity of 99.8% or greater a resolution of 1.50 is required. The efficiency of separation, expressed as theoretical plate number, N, is calculated as follows:

$$N = 16(t_r/w_B)^2 = 5{:}5^4(t_r/w_1/2)$$

where "t_r" is the retention time, w_B, is the peak width at the base, and "w" is the band width at the peak height. A column independent parameter, H [height equivalent to Theoretical Plate, (*HETP*) = L/ N, where L is the length of the column], is more often used.

Column efficiency is inversely proportional to the particle size of the column packing. Thus the efficiency of separation will follow the following order.

$$E3\mu > E5\mu > E10\mu$$

where E is efficiency and the subscripts denote particle size.

HPLC techniques can be used for preparative chemical separations. However, this discussion will be restricted to quantitative analytical separations. For quantitative analysis a known volume of a standard solution of known concentration is injected multiple times (most compendial methods require typically five to six injections). The average peak area of the peak of interest is computed. From a comparison of the peak area of similarly injected and separated analyte with that of the standard, the concentration of the unknown in the analyte is calculated. This procedure is known as *external calibration*. However, sometimes a known compound is added to both the standard and the analyte sample. Then the ratio of the relative peak area (or some times peak height) responses of the peak of interest, and that of the added compound are evaluated. From a comparison of the relative responses of the standard and that of the analyte injections, the concentration of the unknown is computed. This is known as *internal calibration*. Sometimes, peak height is used instead of peak area. The theoretical plates, resolution of two closely eluting peaks, percent relative standard deviation values of multiple injections, and tailing factor (extent of deviation of the chromatographic peak shape from symmetrical Guassian peak) are used as *system suitability parameters*. USP 24, and other monographs provide examples of system suitability requirements and methods of measurement to meet the corresponding requirements.

Columns and Modes of Chromatography

The stationary phase in HPLC is the solid support contained in within a specified column over which the mobile phase flows effecting the separation of the individual components. The HPLC column is normally fabricated using 100- to 300-mm long stainless steel tubes with an internal diameter of 2–5 mm. They are packed with porous, microporous, spherical, or irregularly shaped particles, or particles with specific coatings with the following characteristics. Mean particle sizes of 3–10 μm, surface area between 150 and 400 m^2/g, specific pore volume between 0.2 and 1.5 cm^3 or mL/g, and an apparent density of 0.4–0.6 g/ml. The different modes of chromatography are distinguished based on the differences in the packing materials, coupled with the corresponding compatible mobile phase components and the differences in the nature of the interacting functional groups present in solute molecules. These functional groups selectively and specifically interact with the column support material or mobile phase leading to selectivity and specificity of separation. The stationary phase chemical characteristics are altered by using suitably modified silica particles such that the differences in the functional group properties can be selectively utilized.

Normal Phase Chromatography

In normal phase chromatography, a polar stationary phase and a non-polar mobile phase is used for separation. A modulator, like methanol or acetonitrile, at a suitable concentration can be used to increase the polarity of the mobile phase. Most normal phase chromatographic columns use bare silica

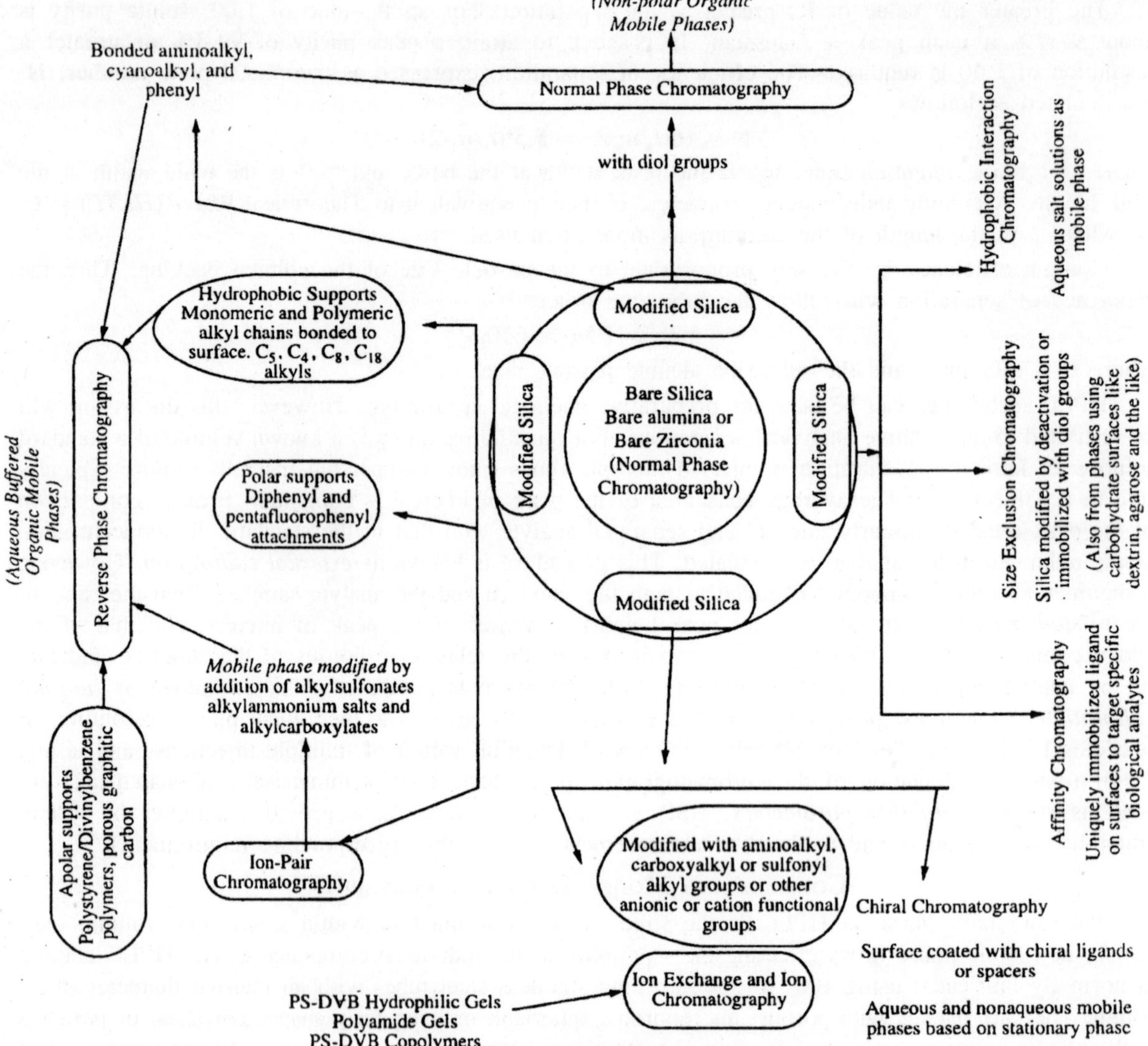

Fig. 14.5. Silica surface and different modes of chromatography.

support, which is acidic and polar. The acidic surface silanol groups, which are hydrophilic, interact differently with different functional groups in the solute molecule. The lipophilicity of the mobile phase also affect the preferential solubility or preferential adsorption on the surfaces. The use of silica support in normal phase chromatography suffers from the following disadvantages: (1) product dependent activity of silica leading to poor separation and variations from column to column and from brand to brand; (2) irreversible adsorption of strong polar solutes on the column support; (3) the necessity to control the water content of the mobile phase; and (4) slow re-equilibration of particles to mobile phase changes. Some of these problems are over come with the use of modified silica stationary phases. The silica surfaces are modified by bonding with appropriate functional groups. Cyanoalkyl or aminoalkyl or phenyl moieties are bonded to these surfaces. Non-polar supports like polystyrene/divinylbenzene copolymers or carbon are also used as column materials. Alumina is polar and acidic while TiO_2, and zirconia are much more neutral. They all have good aqueous stability compared to silica. Normal phase chromatography is restricted to the separation of stereochemical isomers, diastereomers, low molecular weight aromatic compounds and functionalized long chain aliphatic compounds.

Reverse Phase Chromatography

Since many compounds of pharmaceutical interest are generally polar and highly water soluble, reverse phase chromatography is extensively used. In reverse phase chromatography, separation is accomplished by the use of polar mobile phases on non-polar stationary phase. By chemically bonding silanol groups in silica, non-polar stationary phases are obtained. Typically C_3, C_4, C_8, C_{18} alkyl chains are bonded to silica support surfaces. Mobile phases are usually buffered aqueous solutions containing one or more of the organic solvents like methanol, or acetonitrile, or tetrahydrofuran as modulators. The modulators reduce the polarity and decrease retention of solutes. Depending on the organic solvent used selectivity also can be modified. Column designations like octyl (C_8), octadecyl (C_{18}), refers to the length of the carbon chain attached to the silica surface. Amino, cyano, and phenyl columns can also be used in reverse phase chromatography. To increase polarity of the stationary phases diphenyl and pentafluorophenyl columns are also used. Alkylated polystyrene/divinyl benzene polymers also can be used instead of silica based supports.

In reverse phase chromatography separation may be due to either adsorption effects or due to partitioning of the solute between the stationary phase and the mobile phase. More often, separation is probably based on both mechanistic pathways; the relative contribution of each for a specific separation process cannot be estimated. In general, C_{18}-bonded phases yield better retention and better separation compared to C_8-bonded phases because of higher carbon content in the stationary and higher non-polar interaction with the solute.

In isocratic elution, some times compounds are not fully resolved and some compounds are highly retained. The sensitivity of the highly retained compound is reduced considerably due to peak broadening. These drawbacks are overcome when gradient elution is adopted. In gradient elution, the sample is injected when mobile phase has low organic content. The organic fraction is then increased in increments to decrease polarity. These increments are usually linear. Multiple step gradients are also adopted. The capacity factor is dependent on flow rate, slope of the gradient and column dead volume. In linear gradient elution, the bandwidth is generally constant and hence the peak becomes sharper, yielding enhanced sensitivity.

Reverse phase liquid chromatography is very versatile, fast and highly reproducible. Aqueous solutions are normally used and the modifiers used are very cheap and highly pure. Separation is predictable based on the polarity, pH profile, solubility and other physicochemical characteristics of the solute molecules. Analysis time is rather short and re-equilibration is generally fast. Multiple components with minor differences in polarity can be separated by appropriate choice of gradient profiles.

Stationary phases have been modified to

1. Reduce interaction of free silanols.
2. Improve the stability of phases over a wide range of pH.
3. Introduce functional groups on the phases that will enable prediction of selectivity for different solutes.

Only about 50% of the free silanols in silica are bonded in octyl and octadecyl stationary phases. These residual silanols contents is further reduced by a process called *endcapping*, in which hexamethyl and isobutyl groups are additionally introduced into the matrix. Endcapped columns offer better separation and retention in addition to reduced peak tailing. Although endcapped columns offer some advantages, the aqueous instability is still problem. To over come these problems of silica based columns, alternative supports like alumina (Al_2O_3), zirconica (ZrO_2), and titania (TiO_2) have been developed. Alumina columns are stable in the pH range of 2-12, while zirconia columns extend the range from 0 to 14. These are basic oxides and hence silanol-like interactions are eliminated. Different bonded phases can be obtained using zirconia, however, because of poor reactivity such bonded phases are difficult to prepare with alumina supports.

Polydivinylbenzene and polystyrene polymer based stationary phases also eliminate these effects. Porous graphitic carbon provides a highly non-polar surface with excellent chemical stability under acidic and basic conditions, However, they suffer from lower sample loading capacity and lower efficiency than conventional columns. In spite of these efforts, silica based modified columns are still widely used. Many column-manufacturers have introduced quality control procedures for the synthesis and characterization of silica based columns. Therefore, lot to lot variations from the same manufacturers have been considerably reduced. However, identical phases from different manufacturers can yield different separation behaviors of the same analyte under identical instrumental and mobile phase conditions. (Of 13 phenyl columns investigated for an oncolytics, we found only three columns providing similar separation profile for a 13-component impurity mixture.)

Ion-Pair Chromatography

In reverse phase chromatographic separations, ionic compounds, being more water soluble, are not retained in the column. To increase retention and separation a strong counter ion (an organic alkyl or aryl-substituted ion of opposite charge) is added to the mobile phase. Typically alkane sulfonic acid salts or alkyl ammonium salts are added to the mobile phase. These counter ions associate (ion-pairs) with the analyte ion, while displacing the inorganic counter ion like chloride ions. Analyte is retained since the ion-pair partitions into the stationary phase like a large non-polar neutral organic molecule. This technique, also known as *ion-interaction chromatography*, utilizes the effect of pH, ionic strength, mobile phase organic content and temperature to control retention and separation.

Ion-Exchange and Ion Chromatography

Ion-exchange stationary phases consist of solid resin particles that have positive or negative ionic bonding sites incorporated in the stationary phase. The ions of opposite charge in the mobile phase are exchanged with ions on the surface. The ions of opposite charge in the mobile phase are exchanged with ions on the surface. Cation exchange resins contain covalently bound negatively charged functional groups, while anion exchange resins have positively charged functional groups. When the charged functional groups is a sulfonate anion, it is called strong cation exchanger. Week cation exchange resins contain such functional groups as carboxymethyl, phosphate, slulfoalkyl groups. If strongly basic quaternary amines are on the resin, it is called a strong anion exchanger. Weak anion exchangers contain weakly basic groups like aminonethyl, diethyaminomethyl groups. If these functionalities are only on the surface of the stationary phase they are called pellicular particles. When pellicular particles are used, lower eluent concentrations are adequate. When pellicular ion-exchange resins are used, ion-exchange is the only method of separation. When ions are thus separated, particularly in the separation of inorganic ions or small organic acid anions, it is called *ion chromatography*. Most modern ion chromatographic stationary phases use polystyrene divinylbenzene copolymer resins. These stationary phases have very high pH stability and can withstand strong acids and bases.

Using ion chromatographic separation and conductivity detection the inorganic anions like halides, phosphate, nitrite, nitrate, thiocyanate, and sulfate and many cation ions including transition metal ions can be detected. When quantitation of ions are carried out in a solution matrix that is weakly conducting, coductomertric detection and quantitation is possible since the total background conductivity is very small. Examples include the determination of ions in sea water or tap water or from environmental streams. However, if strongly acidic or basic eluents are used, the background conductivity is high. In order to suppress the background conductivity, special suppressor columns are used, which neutralize the acids or bases after elution and before detection. New pulsed amperometric detectors (PAD) are commercially available. With the use of PADs, parts per billion levels of metal ions can be detected. Accurate quantitation of metal ions is possible since ready to use inorganic calibration standards are commercially available. When metal ions are used as counter ions, instead of organic quaternary ammonium ions, in the packing material, the hydroxy (–OH–) functional groups of the carbohydrates and other sugars interact with these metals ion. Pb^{2+}, Ca^{2+}, and Na^{+}, are typical metal ions in the packing material. Depending upon the type of counter ions used, the intensity of the interaction changes and therefore, the retention between different carbohydrates vary. Some of the carbohydrates are also retained because of the size of the molecule under these conditions.

Ion-exchange chromatography is widely used for analyses of proteins, glycoproteins, peptides and other high molecular weight compounds. These organic compounds have considerable surface charge and behave like charged anions. Hence they are amenable to ion exchange separation. To separate nucleotides of similar molecular structures, the differences in the phosphate groups of various nucleotides and the differences in their binding characteristics are used. In addition to silica based resins, acrylic polymer based resins, dextrans, and cellulose bonded phases are used for the separation of proteins. In order to preserve the biological activity during separation, hand poured columns packed with ion-exchange materials are used. Gravity flow of eluent at low temperatures is the norm for separation. Thus, ion exchange chromatography and ion chromatography are no more used synonymously.

Hydrophobic Interaction Chromatography

In hydrophobic interaction chromatography, weakly hydrophobic sorbents are used. Gradient elution with decreasing concentration of salt is used for the separation of large biomolecules, particularly proteins, by this technique. The non-polar functional groups of large bio-polymer molecules (weakly) associate with the hydrophobic ligands in the stationary phase. The stationary phase consists of a highly hydrophobic organic layer. The organic layers contain short alkyl or aryl functional groups attached at the surface. These attached groups are separated with large unattached space in between these attached functional groups. Because of this wider spacing, these "*soft*" stationary phases preserve biological activity without denaturing the proteins. High ionic strength aqueous mobile phases enhance binding between the solute and the stationary phase. Then the salt concentration is decreased to decrease the ionic strength of the mobile phase. The weak mobile phases then reduces the binding and thus separation is effected.

Typical stationary phases include the following: polyvinylpyrrolidone (PVP) coated silica sorbents, monodisperse non-porous silica columns with surface bound amides or ethers and composite agarose and polyacrylamide gels. The eluent normally consists of salts at concentrations greater than 1.0 M. Typical salts include sodium phosphate, sodium sulfate and ammonium sulfate, and organic acid salts like mono-sodium glutamate. Protein retention is stronger with salts that increase surface tension like phosphates, sulfates, citrates, which are solvated in water than with salts such as perchlorates and thiocyanates and the like. Typical biological compounds that are separated by HIC include, cytochrome P-450, enzymes, DNA polymerase, epidermal growth factor, glycoprotein hormones, human immunoglobulins, human recombinant DNA and canine pancreatic juice proteins. Many HIC techniques have been used for large scale purification of proteins.

Affinity Chromatography

This chromatographic technique uses a specific binding agent. The stationary phase is prepared by immobilizing one of a pair of interacting molecules on to particles of support. The immobilized molecule is referred to as a *ligand*. These ligands selectively bind to the interacting second pair in a protein or a biomolecule. For example, an antitransferrin antibody is immobilized on the support. In this example, the antibody is the ligand; the transferrin antigen in the biomolecule will bind to the surface or release out of the surface depending on the mobile phase strength. Therefore, this technique, which utilizes the differences in the affinity of the two specific interacting groups or moieties is called *affinity chromatography*.

Typical ligands may be of biological origin like antibodies, inhibitors, substrates, coenzymes, cofactors, nucleic acids, and the like, or of non-biological origin like triazine dyes, metal chelates, boronate salts, etc. In this technique, sample is injected on to the column using a weak mobile phase called the application buffer. Under these conditions, the only interacting component is bound to the surface and hence retained in the column. The rest are washed out of the column. Then using a stronger mobile phase, called the eluent buffer, the solute of interest is released, eluted from the column, and then quantitated or collected for later use. Elution may involve two separate steps or may be a simple step gradient. This technique is used for the separation of hormones, peptides, proteins, viruses, enzymes, glycopeptides, antibodies, metal binding amino acids, etc. Affinity chromatography is further classified as bioaffinity, bioadsorption, immunoaffinity and the like depending on the nature of the ligand on the support.

Size Exclusion Chromatography

Size exclusion chromatographic (SEC) technique is used for the separation of biomelcules based on their molecular size. Synthetic and many natural polymers like polysaccharides, cellulosics, natural rubber, and some proteins have chains of differing molecular weight components. When such mixed molecular weight species are present it is said to be a *polydisperse* polymer. Otherwise, the monomer is said to be mono- phasic. The SEC chromatographic peak is broad indicative of the elution of the different components of the polydisperse phase. The polydisperse phase is described by up to "3" molecular weight parameters that define the distribution of species. These are (1) number average, M_n; (2) the weight average, M_w; and (3) z-average, M_z, molecular weights. When $M_n = M_w$, the distribution is said to "Monodisperse." M_w/M_n is a measure of the polydispersity of the system. For large biomolecules, M_n and M_w are different since M_w is usually higher, because it is sensitive to the presence of high molecular components in the distribution. M_n, M_w, M_z are defined as follows:

$$M_n = \Sigma N_i M_i / \Sigma W_1$$

$$M_w = \Sigma M_i W_i / \Sigma W_i \text{ and}$$

$$M_z = \Sigma W_i M_i^2 / \Sigma W_i M_i$$

where N_i, is the number of molecules of molecular weight M_i, and W_i refers to the weight (or concentration) of M_i. The ratio of M_w/M_n or M_z/M_w shows the width of the distribution. Size exclusion chromatography is a relative and not an absolute technique.

Gel permeation chromatography (GPC) refers to the technique in which polymers that are soluble in organic solvents are separated. In These cases, more polar organic mobile phases like tetrahydrofuran, toluene, chloroform will be used. Gel filtration chromatography (GFC) is used for separation of water soluble biopolymers. Four different calibration methods are used. If absolute known molecular weight standards are used, it is called *primary calibration method*. In *secondary calibration approach*, poly-dispersity standards of material similar to samples are used. The result is then usually specified as apparent molecular weight distribution. When M_w and M_n are obtained by use of an iteration procedure using a sophisticated software program, it is called broad molecular weight calibration. The iteration procedure uses calibration slopes and intercepts of broad molecular weight standards with known M_n and M_w values. *Universal calibration* is obtained from a plot of log (M_n) vs. Ve, elution volume, where η is the intrinsic viscosity of the polymer measured at the same temperature and in the same solvent as used for the mobile phase. This technique uses on line SEC viscometers in conjunction with universal calibration.

For organosoluble polymers cross linked polystyrene or silica based packings are used. For water soluble polymers various silica based and hydrophobic polymeric packings are used. Pore sizes of the SEC packings may range from 3 to 300 nm. In addition to refractive index detectors, specialized detectors such as on-line SEC detectors and low angle laser light scattering detectors are used for determining the distribution of molecular weights by SEC.

INSTRUMENTATION

Solvent(s) Delivery

Solvent (mobile phase) delivery is achieved usinghigh pressure pumps. There are several types of pumps commercially available for delivêry of mobile phase through the injector, column, detectors and then to the solvent waste container. Since the column head pressure is high, the pumps operate under high pressures (50–300 psi). Most commonly used pumps are reciprocating piston pumps with check valves. These pumps are usually computer controlled. The modern pumps provide flow rate precision which is better than 0.1% in retention time.

For gradient elution at least two solvents has to be pumped and then mixed before it passes through the column. Additionally, the solvent composition is changed in a continuous linear, continuous non-linear, or stepwise fashion. The solvents are mixed with the use of proportioning valves, and the mixed solvents reach the pump. Since solvent mixing occurs before the pump under low pressure conditions, it is called low pressure mixing. This is the most commonly used form of mixing for gradient elution. In high pressure mixing, two or more solvents are individually pumped using different pumps and then they are mixed at high pressures. Pump head leakage is a common problem in such pumps. The pump heads has to be constantly monitored or repaired for leakage.

Dissolved oxygen from mobile phase solvents has to be removed. This is accomplished by passing helium gas through the solvent container or by passing the mobile phases through helium purging units. Currently, computers that control the pumps also control vacuum degassers, which are placed in between the pump and solvent reservoir.

Autosamplers

Autosamplers are used for unattended introduction of samples from vials that are arranged either in a rectangular or circular tray. Autosampler delivers the desired volume of 1–2.5 ml with a precision of less than or equal to 0.5% for injections greater than 10 μl. All autosamplers use mechanized valves. Majority of HPLC autosamplers belong to one of two types. In type I autosamplers the septum cap is pierced using a syringe needle, liquid is displaced into the syringe by gas pressure or plunger action to the inlet port of a six port valve injector. The filled syringe is withdrawn, moved, and the solution deposited into flowing stream of mobile phase by the use of appropriate electromechanical devices. Type 2 autosamplers behave in a very similar way to type I except partial loop volume can be filled and delivered. Additionally, this allows the injection of low volume with high precision compared to type I autosamplers. Both types of autosamplers suffer from carry over problems if appropriate wash cycle and wash solvents are not used between each sampling from the vials.

Detectors

A liquid chromatography detector consists of sensors and an associated electronic device to send signals to a processor. Detectors are classified as bulk property detectors or solute property detectors. Bulk property detectors measure the changes in the property of the combined eluting mobile phase and the eluting solute. For example, the refractive index is characteristic of a liquid. When a solute is dissolved, the refractive index of the solution is different from that of the solvent. These change the property of the bulk solution. Although the change is due to the presence of the solute, the refractive index of the bulk as a whole is different from that of the pure solvent. Refractive index detectors and conductivity detectors are examples of bulk property detectors. Solute property detectors detect the changes in some physical or chemical property of eluting solute component of the mobile phase.

HPLC detector

A HPLC detector should have the following characteristics.

1. Excellent linear response as a function of concentration of the solute.
2. Wide linear dynamic range; the dynamic range over which the response to concentration is linear.
3. High signal to noise ratio. The noise arises as a result of fluctuations or perturbations caused to the signal as a result of temperature, pressure, or flow rate changes in the mobile phase. Noise is also caused by the electronic circuits used in the detector system. All these combined perturbations, called noise, should be low such that very low concentrations of solute can be detected.

Refractive index detectors

The most common Refractive Index (RI) detector uses a differential refractometer, which responds to the deflection of a light beam; the deflection being caused by the differences in the refractive indices of a cell through which eluant passes and that of a reference cell in which the mobile phase is contained. The response of the detector is proportional to the mass concentration irrespective of the nature of solute being analyzed.

Conductivity detector

The conductivity detector measures the conductivity of a solution containing an electrolyte. When current is allowed to pass through two electrodes, there is resistance (or better impedance) to the flow of current through the medium. This impedance decreases if conducting electrolytes are present in the eluant. This detector is mostly used in ion-chromatography. Coupled with ion suppression technology, this has become a versatile detector for low levels of inorganic ion content in analytes of interest.

UV–vis detectors

UV–vis spectophotometric detectors are most commonly used detectors in HPLC, since most organic compounds absorb light in the UV region (190–400 nm) and a few in the visible region (400–750 nm). Fixed wavelength, variable wavelength, and diode array detectors are commercially available. All these operate based on the ability of a solute to absorb light at defined wavelengths based on the chemical structure and functional groups present in the solute molecule. The source of UV light is a deuterium or high pressure xenon lamp while for the visible range it is a simple tungsten lamp.

A beam of light is allowed to pass through a flow cell mounted at the end of the column. As the solute molecules elute from the column and enter the flow cell, they absorb radiation. The differences in the light energy, as a result of absorption, are used as a measure of quantitation. Fixed wavelength detectors operate at a single wavelength, either at 254 or at 280 nm in the UV region. In variable wavelength detector using a monochromator light of a particular wavelength (less than ± 3 nm) can be selected, passed through the sample, and then on to a photocell for detection. Currently available detectors can be programmed to change wavelengths while analysis is in progress to get a spectrum of the eluting species. Otherwise, using appropriate software, the absorbence of the eluate can be monitored simultaneously at two to four different wavelengths. This multi-wavelength detector is less sensitive compared to fixed wavelength detectors (10^{-7} g/ml vs. 5×10^{-8} g/ml).

Photodiode array detectors

Diode array detectors acquire data over the entire range of UV–vis range 190–800nm; in some up to 1100 nm. Two different types of photodiode array detectors are available in the market. In one, to detect over an entire spectrum, light from a continuous source is passed through the cell using a rapidly rotating or vibrating grating, which passes radiation through the cell, one wavelength at a time. The signal of the photodetector is measured as a function of time over the measuring cycle. Then, from the measuring cycle, wavelength is related to time to obtain a plot of wavelength vs. signal. In the second type polychromatic light is passed through the cell and then through a holographic grating. The light dispersed from the grating is arranged to fall on a linear photodiode array. These diode array detectors are very versatile and are used to:

1. Check peak purity using "*peak overlay*" (normalized) methods or by computing peak ratios at two different wavelengths.
2. Identify peaks by spectral matching with accumulated and stored spectral libraries.
3. Generate the spectrum of the eluting peak and determine wavelength of maximum absorption of an unknown or impurity peak.
4. Quantify different peaks at different wave-lengths in a single chromatographic run.
5. Provide graphic 3D or contour plot presentations to regulatory agencies to show the purity of the eluting chromatographic peak.
6. Identify peaks, during method optimization, when the order of elution of the compounds changes.

It should be noted that the sensitivity of these detectors is lower than fixed or variable wavelength detectors. Also, if an overlapping impurity is present either in the fronting or tailing portions of the eluting peak, it can be detected only when the concentration of the impurity is greater than 2.0% relative to that of the major peak.

Fluorescence detectors

Since the fluorescence detector is a highly sensitive, picogram levels of solute can be detected by using this detector. However, this is limited to compounds that naturally fluoresce or can be made to fluoresce by reacting with suitable derivatizing agents. Even this is restricted since appropriate functional groups that undergo such derivatization should be present in the solute molecule. In many HPLC methods where this technique is utilized, the fluorescent agent is added after separation of the components. This has the advantage that the derivatization need not be quantitative. But the reaction should be very rapid, reproducible and proportional to concentration. Because it is an unique property of the solute, it offers selectivity as well as specificity of detection.

Electrochemical detector

This is also a very specific and extremely sensitive detector. The specificity arises from the need to have an electro-oxidizable or reducible functional group present in the solute molecule. Similar to the case of fluorescence detectors, solute molecules can be derivatized to yield compounds containing oxidizable (or rarely, reducible) functional groups. A desired potential is applied between a working electrode and a reference electrode connected to the flow cell. A third electrode known as auxiliary electrode is used to control the potential. As the oxidation takes place at the working electrode surface, the current flow changes. This is monitored, amplified and presented as response using appropriate software and hardware. When the oxidation reaction is allowed to go to completion using a high surface area of working electrode and exhausting all the reactant in the flow cell, it is called a *coulometric* detector. In this case, the total number of coulombs of charge transferred is measured. However, in the most common *amperometric* detector, the solute molecules at the surface and those are very close to the surface are oxidized by maintaining the working electrode at a constant potential. This oxidation process is diffusion controlled and is proportional to concentration. Here the increase in the current flow, "i" is measured, amplified and the signal is presented as a function of time. Glassy carbon electrode is the commonly used electrode for oxidation. Surface coating and the resulting contamination of the surfaces leads to a decrease in sensitivity on constant use. Therefore, this detector has be disassembled, and cleaned very often. Also this requires long equilibration time compared to other detectors. Therefore, it is not an extensively used detector compared to other detectors described in this article. The problem of electrode pollution is overcome in pulsed amperometric detector (PAD). In this technique using a gold or platinum electrode a repeating cycle of potential pulses are applied. Typically, in a one second pulse cycle, three potential pulses are applied. In the initial negative pulse the solute is adsorbed; in the second positive potential pulse the adsorbed compounds are oxidized and the increased current as a result of oxidation is measured. In the third pulse at a high much higher positive, the electrode surface is cleaned by oxidation of the electrode itself. Thus the new surface generated is used for the repeat cycling process. This is very useful in the detection of very low levels of sugars and other polyhydroxy compounds that are otherwise are not easily oxidized.

Evaporative light scattering detector

In this detector, the entire eluate from the column is atomized and evaporated to form small droplets. The solutes finally remaining form particulates suspended in the atomizing gas. When these particles are allowed to pass through a light beam, light is scattered in all directions by the particles. This is known as Rayleigh scattering. However, the light scattered at 45° angle to the incident beam is viewed using appropriate optical filters and the resultant signal is electronically processed. The detector response is sensitive to the mass of the solute particles and hence it is a universal detector. The sensitivity of this detector compares with that of the RI detector.

Computers

The computers are ubiquitous and have become indispensable component of any laboratory. It serves both data processing and process control functions. As a data processor, the computer receives, stores, archives and reprocess the input signals from various detectors. Additionally, as a system processor, the computer monitors the system detectors. The data acquired for each chromatographic run can be processed appropriately to arrive at peak area or peak height or response ratios to an added internal standard. From these it can be used to calculate the concentrations of individual components in an analyte.

Through the use of appropriate software and hardware, the computer can be programmed to do the following: (1) to command injection of the samples; (2) to control and monitor, various parameters of the pump like the flow rate, composition of the mobile phase, column pressure; (3) to monitor and control column oven, and detector temperatures; and (4) to start and stop injectors, detectors and other system units. The computer also can be used to monitor system suitability parameters and reinject samples after adjusting conditions to meet system suitability. A decision tree can be constructed to allow retesting when pre-established system suitability conditions are not met. The computer can be programmed such that if conditions are not met, the system is shut down or paused until it can be attended to. Sample preparation, derivatization and other processes also can be controlled using individual computers. With multiple computers attached to a large computer called the server, data from a number of detectors can be monitored, stored, and archived. The computer is also used as an excellent book-keeper storing all the information regarding samples, their results, and also the conditions under which those results are obtained. The computer has become versatile tool in the highly regulated pharmaceutical industry especially to provide traceability and data integrity to required government and compendial agencies such as FDA, USP, BP, etc.

Method Development and Method Validation

The method development process involves selecting appropriate method conditions for the sample in hand. It is based on prior knowledge of the sample properties, pK_a or pK_b values of functional groups, the polarity and size of solute molecules, UV–vis spectral properties, redox behavior, concentration range, solubility behavior and the like. From a knowledge of these, suitable mode of chromatography, corresponding column(s), mobile phase composition, flow rate, choice of detectors, gradient or isocratic conditions, and the like can be selected. Once the method has been developed with some initial trials, optimization is carried out. Optimization is necessary to accomplish best possible separation of all components within the shortest possible time or in the case of low level detection, conditions have to be optimized such that required level of detection and/or quantitation can be achieved. In general, the system suitability parameters are usually evaluated and specified before method validation is performed.

Method validation is a process by which documented evidence is prepared and provided to show that the method meets the intended need. Highly regulated pharmaceutical analytical laboratories perform method validation and generate data on the following parameters, to comply with the compliance requirements of government agencies such FDA, EPA and/or to provide data for compendial agencies like USP, BP, etc.

The parameters that define validation are accuracy, precision, specificity, linearity, ruggedness, and robustness. Accuracy is a measure of the closeness of the measured value to the true value or an accepted reference value. This is usually measured by spiking known amounts of the analyte to a matrix called the placebo, and computing the recovery of the analyte after sample analysis. Placebo contains all the ingredients of a formulation other than the active ingredient or the ingredient being analyzed. FDA and ICH (International Committee on Harmonization of Technical Requirements for Registration of Pharmaceutical for Human use) guidelines recommend collecting data from nine determinations at (at least) three concentration levels encompassing the range of target analyte concentration.

Precision refers to the degree of repeatability under the stated conditions of the method. It is expressed as percent relative standard deviation (% RSD) for a statistically significant number of analyses of samples. Precision provides a measure of day to day, analyst to analyst and instrument to instrument variation on a routine basis. The precision data provided in support are standard deviation, % RSD, confidence intervals and may also include inter laboratory variations.

Specificity refers to the ability to determine the concentration of the analyte with a high degree of confidence that the other components in the matrix do not interfere with the target analyte. The potential interfering substances include other active and inactive ingredients, impurities, degradation products of the components and active ingredient, and extractables from the container-closure system and the like. Specificity is the currently accepted terminology by regulatory agencies. In the literature selectivity is also used to suggest specificity.

Linearity refers to the linear response of the detector to the analyte concentration within a specified *range*. Range, expressed in the same units as the analytical test results, is the interval between the lower and upper levels of the analyte concentration. To show linearity, a plot of response vs. concentration is provided for at least at five different concentration levels within the range. In addition, the slope and intercept of the regression line with the correlation coefficient are also provided. Normally a single standard is recommended if the intercept is very close to zero. Otherwise, quantitation, based on linear plot of multiple standards, is generally recommended.

Ruggedness is again a measure of precision. ICH guidelines include ruggedness in precision, while USP separates it. Ruggedness according to USP is a measure of the variation in interlaboratory comparison data. It is performed to establish lack of influence of test results based on operational and environmental parameters.

Robustness is a measure of how method parameters like organic content, pH, ionic strength of the mobile phase and column temperature do not affect test results when minor variations are deliberately induced in these parameters. The quality of separation of components, the accuracy and precision of the method and the like should not change as a result of these variations. (It is the belief of the authors that robustness should be part of the method development process regarding the appropriate choice of the column and the mobile phase conditions.)

Two other terms, limit of quantitation (LOQ) and limit of detection (LOD) are used especially in the determination of the analytes at trace levels. The trace level analyte may be impurities or degradation products of ingredients in a sample or it may be a solution of active ingredient at trace levels in rinse or swab samples obtained as part of cleaning validation. LOD refers to the lowest concentration of an analyte that can be detected (but not quantitated), under a given set of chromatographic conditions. Usually, it is expressed as a concentration parameter calculated using a signal to noise ratio of 3:1. LOQ refers to the concentration of the analyte that can be quantified in a sample with a predefined value of variation in precision. Normally accepted signal to noise ratio value for LOQ is 10:1. Generally, LOD and LOQ values are dictated by specific requirements, in order to ascertain reproducibility of LOD and LOQ values. Examples of specific requirements include determination of impurities at 0.05% using a 0.1% surrogate standard, or ppm quantitation or detection requirements based on equipment cleanability and the like. For practical purposes, it is recommended that a control solution at a known concentration of the analyte be prepared such that a peak corresponding to this analyte concentration is always detected (LOD) or quantitated (LOQ). From one of these two parameters, if experimentally obtained, the other can be calculated.

PRACTICAL CONSIDERATIONS

Sample Preparation

For many analyses, sample preparation may simply involve dissolving a known weight or volume of sample and diluting to appropriate concentration for analysis. However, extensive sample preparation may be required, if precolumn derivatization is needed. Precolumn derivatization is carried out to increase sensitivity, to induce specificity, or to separate optical isomers and to reduce or eliminate otherwise complex and expensive clean up procedures. Solid phase extraction using appropriate solid cartridges are normally used in the clean up of biological samples. Solid phase cartridges can also be used to increase the concentration of trace analyte. These purification steps can be done in situ during analysis by appropriate plumbing using six- or ten-port valves and using computer control of the pumps and values. No matter how it is done, attention must be paid for proper sampling and preparation of samples.

Mobile Phase Preparation

Mobile phase should be prepared using HPLC grade solvents and analytical reagent chemicals only. Mobile phases should be filtered using ($\leq$0.5 *mm*) filters to remove any particulate matter from the solvent. To eliminate dissolved air, helium sparging or vacuum degassing is necessary. In gradient elution, in order not to alter solid phase wetting and gelling characteristics, it is advisable to use at least 5% water content instead of pure organic solvents as one of the mobile phases.

System Maintenance

Pumps and columns should be cleaned of with 50:50 methanol–water or acetonitrile–water mixture to eliminate buffers from the system. Pumps, injectors, and detectors should require periodic and scheduled maintenance to keep instruments in good operating conditions. Detector should be calibrated on a regular basis using appropriate calibration standards available from NIST or other sources traceable to NIST. FDA and other regulatory agencies require extensive documentation regarding the "health" of these instruments. Therefore, necessary and appropriate documentation should be maintained regarding details of maintenance. If there is any instrument failure additional documentation is necessary to prove that analytical results were not impacted or compromised because of these failures, if any.

THIN LAYER CHROMATOGRAPHY

Thin layer chromatography (TLC) consists of the sample solution being applied as a spot or band on the origin of a layer spread on a support (the plate). After evaporation of the sample solvent, the plate is placed in a sealed chamber or tank that contains a solvent mixture chosen as the mobile phase. Development occurs as the mobile phase moves up the layer by capillary forces. Instrumental development methods, such as overpressured layer chromatography (OPLC) or automated multiple development (AMD), can provide separations with increased resolution. The plate is removed from the chamber, and the separated zones are detected by physical or chemical methods, identified by comparison of their R_f values (R_f = distance of migration of the sample zone/ distance of the mobile phase front) and colors to standard zones on the same plate, and quantified by visual or instrumental densitometry based on measurement of zone sizes and intensities. Zone identification is confirmed by off- or on-line coupling of TLC with visible/ ultraviolet (UV), Fourier transform infrared (FTIR), Raman, and mass spectrometry (MS). Pharmaceutical applications of TLC include analysis of starting raw materials, intermediates, pharmaceutical raw materials, formulated products, and drugs and their metabolites in biological media.

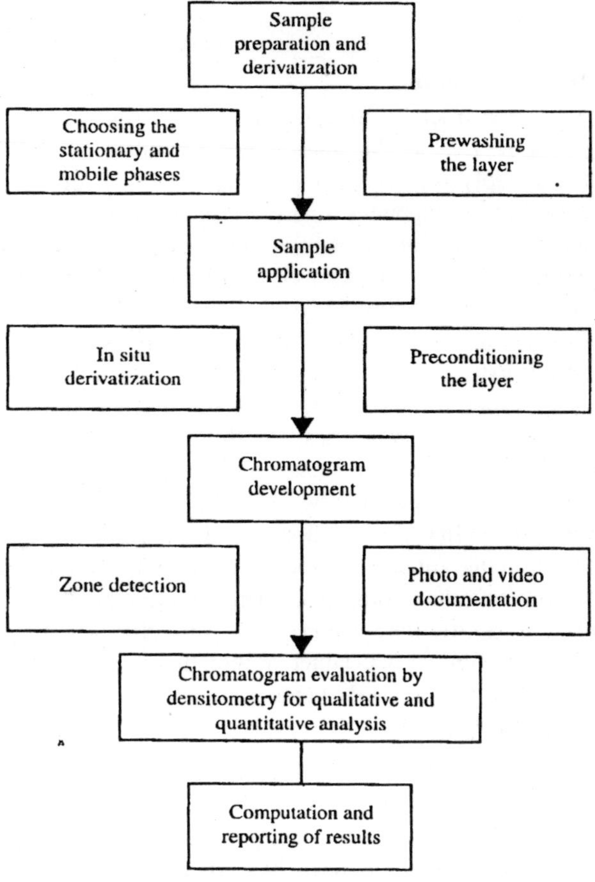

Fig. 14.6. Schematic diagram of the steps in a thin layer chromatographic analysis.

TLC is a flexible, versatile, and economical process in which the various stages are carried out independently. The advantages of this off-line arrangement as compared with an on-line process, such as column high performance liquid chromatography (HPLC), have been outlined and include the following:

1. Availability of a great range of stationary phases with unique selectivities for mixture components.
2. Ability to choose solvents for the mobile phase is not restricted by low UV transparency or the need for ultra-high purity.
3. Repetition of densitometric evaluation can be achieved under different conditions without repeating the chromatography in order to optimize quantification since all sample fractions are stored on the plate.
4. High sample throughput since many samples can be chromatographed simultaneously.
5. Minimal cost of solvent purchase and disposal since the required amount of mobile phase per sample is small.
6. Accuracy and precision of quantification is high because samples and standards are chromatographed and measured under the same conditions on a single TLC plate.
7. Sensitivity limits of analysis are typically at nanogram (ng) to picogram (pg) levels.

Comparative studies have often found that high performance TLC (HPTLC) is superior to HPLC in terms of total cost and time required for pharmaceutical analyses. The Bibliography contains sources of general information on the principles, theory, practice, instrumentation, and applications of TLC and HPTLC.

Experimental Procedures

Sample Preparation

Sample extraction and cleanup procedures for TLC are similar to those for gas chromatography (GC) and HPLC. If the analyte concentration is sufficiently high, pharmaceutical dosage forms can often be simply dissolved in a solvent that will completely solubilize the analyte and leave excipients or extraneous compounds undissolved to yield a test solution that can be directly spotted for TLC analysis. Grinding of the sample and application of heat and/or sonication may be required to assure solubility of the analyte, as well as filtration or centrifugation to remove undissolved excipients. If the analyte is present in low concentration in a complex sample, solvent extraction, cleanup (purification), and concentration procedures usually precede TLC in order to maximize the analyte and minimize interfering extraneous components in the test solution. Since layers are not reused, it is often possible to apply cruder samples than could be injected into a GC or HPLC column, including samples with irreversibly sorbed impurities. Traditional procedures that are still widely used include liquid–liquid partitioning, column chromatography, desalting, and deproteinization, but the newer microwave extraction, solid phase extraction (SPE), and supercritical fluid extraction (SFE) methods are being increasingly applied for isolation and cleanup of samples prior to TLC. Special plates with pre-adsorbent or concentrating zone composed of adsorption-inactive kieselguhr or silicon dioxide may provide sample cleanup by retaining some interfering substances. Assay protocols for samples, such as tablets, usually involve taking multiple tablets (e.g., 10–20), grinding and mixing thoroughly, and weighing a test sample equivalent to one tablet, rather than analyzing only one tablet, so that the sample will be more representative of the batch being sampled.

Stationary Phases

Commercial precoated layers on glass support are used in virtually all analyses. HPTLC uses plates that are smaller (10×10 or 10×20 cm), have a thinner (0.1–0.2 mm) layer composed of sorbent with a finer mean particle size (5–6 μm) and are developed over shorter distances (ca. 3–7 cm), as compared to classical 20×20 cm TLC plates which are generally 20×20 cm with a 0.25-mm layer and developed for 10–12 cm. HP plates provide improved resolution, shorter analysis time, higher detection sensitivity, and improved in situ quantification and are used for industrial pharmaceutical densitometric quantitative analyses. TLC plates are usually used for qualitative identification and purity studies as contained in pharmacopeias.

Normal phase adsorption TLC on silica gel with a less polar mobile phase, such as chloroform-methanol, has been used for more than 90% of reported analyses of pharmaceuticals and drugs. Lipophilic C-18, C-8, C-2; phenyl chemically-modified silica gel phases; and hydrocarbon-impregnated silica gel plates developed with a more polar aqueous mobile phase, such as methanol– water or dioxane-water are used for reversed phase TLC. Other precoated layers that are used include aluminum oxide, magnesium silicate, magnesium oxide, polyamide, cellulose, kieselguhr, ion exchangers (e.g., PEI cellulose anion exchanger), and polar modified silica gel layers that contain bonded amino, cyano, diol, and thiol groups. The polar bonded phases, in which the functional groups are bonded to silica gel by means of a hydrophobic spacer (e.g., *n*-propyl), can function with multimodal mechanisms, depending on the composition of the mobile phase. Silica gel can be impregnated with various reagents to improve separations (e.g., EDTA for tetracycline analysis).

Optical isomer separations that are carried out on a chiral layer produced from C-18 modified silica gel impregnated with a Cu(II) salt and an optically active enantiomerically pure hydroxyproline derivative, on a silica layer impregnated with a chiral selector such as brucine, on molecularly imprinted polymers of alpha-agonists, or on cellulose with mobile phases having added chiral selectors such as cyclodextrins have been reported mostly for amino acids and their derivatives. Mixtures of sorbents have been used to prepare layers with special selectivity properties. Layers are often cleaned by pre-development with the mobile phase or methylene-chloride–methanol (1:1) or immersion in methanol prior to sample application, especially for quantitative TLC.

Mobile Phases

The mobile phase for a particular separation is usually selected empirically using prior personal experience and literature reports of similar separations as a guide. In addition, various computer-assisted mobile phase optimization schemes have been described for selecting the mobile phase components and their relative concentrations, most notably the PRISMA model.

General mobile phases systems that are used based on their diverse selectivity properties are diethyl ether, methylene chloride, and chloroform combined individually or together with hexane as the strength-adjusting solvent for normal-phase TLC, and methanol, acetonitrile, and tetrahydrofuran mixed with water for strength adjustment in reversed phase TLC. Separations by ion pairing on C-18 layers are done with a mobile phase such as methanol–0.1 M acetate buffer (pH 3.5) containing 25 mM sodium pentane-sulfonate (15.5 : 4.5). Specific mobile phases for pharmaceutical and drug analysis are listed in the Applications of TLC in Pharmaceutical and Drug Analysis section.

Application of Samples

The method used for application of sample solutions is determined by whether HPTLC, TLC, or preparative layer chromatography (PLC) and qualitative or quantitative analysis are being performed. Sample volumes of 0.5–5 μl for TLC and 0.1–1 μl for HPTLC are applied manually to the layer origin as spots using fixed volume glass micropipets, such as Drummond Microcaps or selectable volume 10 or 25 μl digital microdispensers. In addition, many manual and automated instruments are available for sample application, especially for quantitative HPTLC.

The partially automated Linomat IV (Fig. 2) can apply 2–99 μl volumes to HPTLC plates (5–490 μl for PLC) as bands of controlled length [1 mm (spot) to 190 mm] by spraying from a glass syringe. This instrument has been used more than any other for densitometric quantification in pharmaceutical analysis. Compact bands are also produced when 1–25 μl samples are applied manually with a digital micro-dispenser to plates that contain a preadsorbent zone. Band application is advantageous for obtaining the highest resolution separations and precise quantitative results by scanning densitometry.

A fully automated, personal computer-controlled spotter, which consists of a stainless steel capillary connected to a dosage syringe operated by a stepper motor, can sequentially apply constant or variable volume samples, chosen from a rack of vials, within the range of 10 nl to 50 μl as spots or bands.

Chromatogram Development

In addition to the stationary and mobile phases, separations obtained in TLC are affected by the vapor phase, which depends on the type, size, and saturation condition of the chamber during development. The interactions of these three phases as well as other factors, such as temperature and relative humidity, must be controlled to obtain reproducible TLC separations. The development process with a single (isocratic) mobile phase is complicated because of progressive equilibration between the layer and mobile phase and separation of the solvent components of the mobile phase as a result of differential interactions with the layer, which leads to the formation of an undefined but reproducible mobile phase gradient.

The important development methods in pharmaceutical and drug analysis include classical linear ascending development, horizontal development, gradient TLC with AMD, OPLC, and two-dimensional (2D) development. These development methods will be described briefly. Other development methods, such as circular, anticircular, continuous, and rotational, will not be covered.

In the classical method of linear, ascending development TLC and HPTLC, the mobile phase is contained in a large volume, covered glass chamber (N-chamber). The spotted plate is inclined against an inside wall of the tank with its lower edge immersed in the developing solvent below the starting line. The solvent begins to rise immediately through the initial zones due to capillary flow. The space inside the tank is more or less equilibrated (saturated) with solvent vapors, depending on the presence or absence of a paper liner and the period of time the tank is allowed to stand before the plate is inserted. Unsaturated chambers can provide different, often higher resolution, separations as compared to saturated chambers with the same mobile phase. The twin trough chamber is an N-chamber modified with an inverted V-shaped ridge on the bottom that divides the tank into two sections. These divisions allow development with low volumes of mobile phase in one and easy pre-equilibration of the layer with vapors of the mobile phase or another conditioning liquid (e.g., a sulfuric acid-water mixture to control humidity) or volatile reagent in the other. A computer-controlled automatic developing chamber offers programmable, reproducible linear ascending development without operator attention.

The use of a horizontal developing chamber (Camag) permits simultaneous development from both ends to the center of up to 70 samples on a 20 × 10 cm HPTLC plate, or 35 samples from one end to the other. The developing solvent, held in narrow troughs, is carried to the layer through capillary slits formed between the trough walls and glass slides. The chamber is covered with a glass plate during pre-equilibration and development, and it can be operated with controlled levels of vapor saturation and relative humidity.

Unidimensional multiple development, in which the layer is developed repeatedly for the same distance with the same solvent system or two different systems, is a manual method for improving the resolution of zones that migrate in the lower half of the layer. Multiple development has been improved by the use of AMD instruments. AMD generally involves 1–25 individual linear ascending developments of an HPTLC plate performed with a mobile phase gradient of decreasing strength (i.e., decreasing polarity for silica gel) over distances that increase by 3–5 mm for each stage. The layer is dried under vacuum and conditioned with the vapor phase of the next batch of fresh solvent before each incremental run. The repeated movement of the solvent front through the chromatographic zones causes compression into narrow bands (width about 1 mm) during AMD, leading to a spot-capacity (the number of zones that can be completely separated in the available layer distance) of more than 50 for an 80-mm run. Typical "*universal gradients*" are produced from the solvents methanol or acetonitrile (polar), methylene chloride, diisopropyl ether, or t-butylmethyl ether (medium polarity), and hexane (non-polar). Mixtures containing compounds with widely different polarities can be separated by AMD on one chromatogram, and migration distances of individual components are largely independent of the sample matrix. AMD is the most promising development method available for modern TLC and will certainly receive increased use in the future for pharmaceutical analysis.

OPLC is a method in which the mobile phase is pumped through a layer that is sandwiched between a rigid support block and a flexible plastic membrane under external pressure of 10 or 25 atm (Chrompres 10 and 25). Mobile phase flows through the layer at a constant linear flow rate velocity in the range of 1–12 ml/min, leading to higher separation efficiency than is possible with capillary flow where the mobile phase velocity is variable. To carry out linear chromatography, the layer must be specially prepared by scraping the edges and treating with a polymer sealant to eliminate leaks during development, and by cutting mobile phase inlet and solvent outlet channels at appropriate positions. A newer OPLC instrument (BS 50) provides linear isocratic or three-step gradient development, on-line or off-line modes, analytical or preparative separations, and ready-to-use pre-sealed 20 × 20 cm or 10 × 20 cm silica gel or C-1 8 TLC and HPTLC layers. Of all TLC methods, OPLC most closely simulates HPLC. Determination of deramciciane by HPTLC-OPLC and forensic and clinical drug screening are examples of applications. In addition to the usual elution-type development, forced flow displacement TLC was reported for pharmaceutical densitometric analysis.

In 2D TLC, the sample mixture is applied to one corner of the TLC plate, which is developed with the first mobile phase, dried, and developed with a second mobile phase that provides different selectivity in a perpendicular direction. Greatly increased spot capacities of 250–400 for capillary flow development and 500–2000 for forced flow have been reported for 2D TLC. The analyses of amphetamine derivatives and thyreostatic drugs by 2D TLC were reported.

Zone Visualization (Detection)

After removal of the mobile phase from the developed plate by heating, zones are detected on the layer by their natural color, natural fluorescence, quenching of fluorescence, or as colored, UV-absorbing, or fluorescent zones after reaction with a reagent (post-chromatographic derivatization). Zones with fluorescence or quench fluorescence are viewed in cabinets that incorporate shortwave (254 nm) and long-wave (366 nm) UV lamps.

Fluorescence quenching occurs on an "F-layer" that contains a fluorescent indicator or phosphor. Compounds that absorb 254 nm UV light, particularly those with aromatic rings and conjugated double bonds, appear as dark violet spots on a green or pale blue background because the absorbing compounds diminish (quench) the uniform layer fluorescence. Many drugs quench fluorescence, and this method is very widely used for detection and quantification by scanning.

Universal or selective chromogenic (dyeing) and fluorogenic detection reagents are applied by spraying onto the layer, dipping the layer into the reagent, exposing the layer to reagent vapors (e.g., iodine), incorporating the reagent in the mobile phase or in the layer, or by pressing an adsorbent polymeric pad soaked with the reagent against the layer (overpressure derivatization). Examples of universal reagents that react with many compound classes are vanillin-sulfuric acid, anisaldehyde, and iodine, while ninhydrin is a selective reagent for detection of amino acids and Dragendorff reagent is widely used to detect alkaloids. Although spray application is most widely used, dipping is more reproducible, especially when carried out in a mechanized chromatogram immersion instrument. Layers must frequently be heated in an oven or on a flat heating plate after applying the detection reagent in order to accelerate the reaction upon which detection is based. Biological-physiological methods of detection, such as bioautography, are also employed for medicinal compounds.

An important advantage of the off-line operation of TLC is the flexibility afforded by the use of multiple methods for zone detection and identification. For example, the layer can be viewed under long- and short-wave UV light, followed by one or more chromogenic, fluorogenic, or biological detection methods.

Documentation of Chromatograms

TLC separations can be documented by photography or video recording. Commercial documentation systems that incorporate standard and instant photographic cameras and charge coupled device (CCD) video cameras are suitable for chromatograms with colored, fluorescent, and quenched zones. The latest approach for copying TLC plates is by use of computer imaging, and a system that incorporates a computer, scanner, and black-and-white or color printer was described. Digital cameras are widely used for photographing TLC plates, but their use for quality control purposes is in question because of the potential for manipulating the file with software.

Quantitative Analysis

Quantification of thin layer chromatograms can be performed indirectly after scraping off the separated zones of samples and standards, and elution of the substances from the layer material with an appropriate solvent. The volumes of the eluates are adjusted and the solutions analyzed by use of a spectrometric method, GC, or HPLC. Scraping and elution are usually performed manually. Although direct quantification has become increasingly important, indirect analysis is still widely used (e.g., for assay of some drugs according to the USP).

Direct quantification is carried out in situ rather than after spot elution. The simplest direct method involves visual comparison of sample zone size and/or intensity (color) variation according to concentration against reference standards developed on the same plate. This qualitative/semi-quantitative approach is specified in various pharmacopeias for the purity analysis of active raw materials and formulated products. These pharmacopeial methods are designed for analyses at several levels: (1) simple detection of impurities as additional spots; (2) detection and identification of impurities by comparison to the R_f values distances of standards; or (3) detection, identification, and estimation of amounts of impurities by comparing intensities between samples and standard dilutions of the same compounds.

Most modern HPTLC quantitative analyses are performed in situ by measuring the zones of samples and standards using a chromatogram spectrophotometer (usually called a densitometer or scanner) with a fixed sample light beam in the form of a rectangular slit. A tungsten or halogen lamp is used as the source for scanning colored zones (visible absorption) and a deuterium lamp is used for scanning UV-absorbing zones directly or as quenched zones on F-layers. Of all possible densitometric modes, most quantitative pharmaceutical assays have been carried out by UV absorption scanning of fluorescence-quenched zones. The monochromator is a prism or, more often, a grating, and the detector is a photomultiplier or photodiode. For normal fluorescence scanning, a high intensity xenon or mercury lamp would be used as the source and a cutoff filter would be placed between the plate and detector to block the exciting UV radiation and transmit the visible emitted fluorescence. Zig-zag, dual wavelength reflection scanning with a point source also has been used for pharmaceutical analysis.

Many modern scanners have a computer-controlled motor-driven monochromator that allows automatic recording of in situ absorption and fluorescence excitation spectra. These spectra can aid compound identification by comparison of unknown spectra with stored standard spectra obtained under identical conditions or spectra of standards measured on the same plate. The spectral maximum determined from the in situ absorption spectrum is usually the optimal wavelength for scanning standard and sample areas for quantitative analysis. The densitometer is usually connected to a computer with software designed specifically for data handling and automation of the scanning process in modern instruments. With a fully automated system, the computer can perform the following: (1) data acquisition; (2) automated peak searching and optimization of scanning for each fraction located; (3) multiple wavelength scanning; (4) baseline location and correction; (5) computation of peak areas and/or heights of samples and co-developed standards, calculation of calibration curves by linear or polynomial regression, interpolation of sample concentrations, statistical analysis of reproducibility, and presentation of a complete analysis report; and (6) storage of data on disk. In general, external standardization is employed for quantification with a calibration curve generated from a series of standards that covers the full concentration range of the analysis. Although the internal standard method is sometimes used, it is not normally needed, unless losses during the sample preparation steps are anticipated, since samples and standards are run on the same plate under essentially identical conditions.

Image processing with a video densitometer is an alternative for colored or fluorescence-quenched zones to the use of a slit-scanning densitometer. A video scanner consists of a transilluminator system for totally lighting the plate, CCD camera, computer and printer, and chromatogram evaluation software. Video densitometers cannot measure UV-absorbing zones or fluorescent zones directly; cannot scan a layer with uniform, monochromatic light of selectable wavelength; and are not as accurate, precise, or sensitive as slit scanning densitometers in their present state of development. One of their advantages as compared to slit-scanning densitometers is for quantification of 2D chromatograms. TLC with video technology is being used successfully for fingerprint analysis of herbal supplements and medicines.

Special Techniques

Transfer of mobile phases to HPLC

An important application of TLC is to serve as a pilot method for HPLC, the most widely used analytical method for pharmaceutical analysis. If the stationary phases are similar, TLC can predict solute retention behavior and suitability of a particular mobile phase through correlation of log k' in HPLC and R_f data in TLC. Particularly useful is detection of compounds that migrate minimally in the mobile phase and can contaminate the HPLC column during subsequent runs.

Determination of lipophilicity

The determination of the lipophilicity of drugs is extremely important because the biological activity of a molecule can generally be correlated with its ability to penetrate the different hydrophobic barriers (membranes) (i.e., with its lipophilicity or hydrophobicity). One of the best ways to determine lipophilicity is by measurement of retention characteristics [R_M values, $R_M = (1 - R_f - 1)$] of the compounds of interest by reversed phase TLC on a silica gel layer impregnated with paraffin oil or a C-18 chemically bonded silica gel layer. The study of anti-inflammatory drugs is an example of an application.

Preparative layer chromatography

Analytical TLC differs from PLC in that larger weights and volumes of samples are applied as a band across the entire layer width to thicker (0.5–2 mm) and sometimes larger layers, the purpose of which is the isolation and purification of 10–1000mg of sample for further analysis. Multiple development of the plate is commonly used, and the separated substances are detected by a non-destructive method (e.g., under UV light and iodine vapors), and recovered by extraction from scraped layer material. PLC can be used to isolate sufficient pure drug compounds for confirmation by spectrometry in cases where analytical TLC is not adequate for identification. Examples of pharmaceutical applications of PLC include a new sesquiterpene trimer and phenylpropanoid glycosides.

Combined TLC–spectrometry methods

Compound identification is initially made by comparing sample and standard zones based on R_f values and colors produced by selective detection reagents. Identification is confirmed by off- or on-line combination of TLC and spectrometric methods such as visible/UV, fluorescence, FT-Raman, FTIR, solid state (NMR), MS, and MS–MS. HPTLC coupled on-line with spectrometric methods has been proposed as a reference method in clinical chemistry for identification prior to quantitative analysis. This is particularly important for unequivocal diagnosis as the basis for further clinical therapeutic measures.

Thin layer radiochromatography

Location and quantification of radioisotope-labeled substances on a thin layer requires the use of autoradiography, zonal analysis with scintillation counting, or direct scanning with a digital autoradiograph or a bio-imaging analyzer. Thin layer radiochromatography is widely used for metabolism studies of pesticides and drugs in plant, animal, and human samples, and in quality control and development of radiopharmaceuticals.

Method Validation

Validation procedures are performed according to the recommendations of regulatory agencies, such as the Committee for Proprietary Medicinal Products (CPMP) of the European Economic Community (EEC) and with consideration for the special features of the TLC procedure. The following validation parameters are typically monitored: (1) selectivity; (2) stability before, during, and after TLC development; (3) linearity of the calibration graph; (4) range of levels within which the analyte can be quantified; (5) limits of detection and accurate and precise quantification; and (6) accuracy (indication of systematic errors), precision (indication of random errors), sensitivity (ability to measure small variations in concentration), and ruggedness (results of the method when used by different analysts in a variety of locations). Each step of the analysis must be validated through error analysis and a suitability test, and includes sample preparation, application of samples, TLC separation, detection procedures, and quantification. Definitions, general principles, and practical approaches for validation of pharmaceutical TLC analysis are described by Szepesi and Nyiredy. Benchmarking studies of the assay and purity testing of phospholipids by silica gel HPTLC with copper (II) sulfate-phosphoric acid detection reagent and scanning of the brown-violet zones at 365 nm showed that HPTLC provided a cost reduction of 1: 2.5 as compared to HPLC.

Applications of TLC in Pharmaceutical and Drug Analysis

Gas chromatography, HPLC, and TLC are complimentary methods with their own advantages and disadvantages for pharmaceutical and drug analysis. Regular reviews of the TLC literature have shown that applications to pharmaceuticals and drugs are more prevalent than for any other class of compounds.

Applications of TLC include analysis of the following sample types:

1. Starting raw materials (plant extracts, extracts of animal origin, fermentation mixtures).
2. Intermediates (crude products, reaction mixtures, mother liquors and secondary products).
3. Pharmaceutical raw materials (identification, purity testing, assay, separation of closely related compounds, stability testing).
4. Formulated products (identification, purity testing, assay, stability testing under storage and stress, content uniformity test, dissolution test).
5. Drugs and their metabolites in biological media such as urine, plasma, or gastric fluid (pharmacological, toxicological, pharmacokinetic, metabolic, bioequivalence, forensic, and compliance and pharmacodynamic studies).

TLC analyses are performed in a wide variety of laboratories, including government, pharmaceutical manufacturer, hospital, police, and contract testing laboratories dealing with illicit drug detection in sports, horse racing, and employment screening. For identification of known compounds and impurities, purity testing, and obtaining impurity profiles in bulk raw materials and formulations, R_f values and spot sizes/intensities between samples and reference materials developed on the same plate are compared by non-instrumental or instrumental methods using TLC systems that can separate compounds from different classes or closely related compounds within a single class. Confirmation of identity often requires use of an on-line or off-line ancillary method, such as IR, NMR, or mass spectrometry, GC, or HPLC. The following eight general, standardized TLC systems are recommended for the analysis of drugs:

For basic drugs: Silica gel layer dipped in 0.1 M KOH and dried; mobile phases: (1) methanol–ammonia (100:1.5); (2) cyclohexane-toluene-diethylamine (75:15:10); (3) chloroform–methanol (9:1); and (4) acetone.

For acidic and neutral drugs: Silica gel layer; mobile phases: (1) chloroform-methanol (4:1); (2) ethyl acetate–methanol–ammonia (85:10:5); (3) ethyl acetate; and (4) chloroform–methanol (9:1)

Migration data for many drugs in these systems have been tabulated. Retention data for 443 drugs were reported for four other standardized silica gel systems: (1) ethyl acetate-methanol-30% ammonia (85:10:15); (2) cyclohexane–toluene–diethylamine (65:25:10); (3) ethyl acetate–chloroform (1:1); and (4) acetone. The plate was dipped in KOH solution before development with acetone. The following screening system (UniTox) employs three mobile phases for normal and reversed phase TLC:

For acidic and neutral drugs: (1) methanol–water (65:35), C-18 silica gel.

For basic, amphoteric, and quaternary drugs: 1) toluene–acetone–ethanol–conc. ammonia (45 :45: 7:3), silica gel and (2) methanol–water–conc. HCl (50:50:1), C-18 silica gel.

The USP 24/NF 19, section 201, contains a general TLC identification test that involves a non-high-performance silica gel layer with fluorescent indicator, chloroform–methanol–water (180:15:1) mobile phase, and detection under 254 nm UV light for verification of the identities of compendial drugs in dosage form test solutions prepared according to the individual monographs. Section 621 of the USP 24/NF 19 presents brief information on the equipment and procedures of classical ascending and continuous development TLC.

Analytical information and data were presented on the TLC analysis of the most widely prescribed human and animal drugs as well as illicit drugs. In addition, applications of quantitative TLC in pharmaceutical analysis were described. Biennial reviews of TLC typically contain more than 75 references that describe applications to drug and pharmaceutical analysis.

The following are brief descriptions of TLC analyses of drugs in pharmaceutical dosage forms and biological samples that were selected as typical examples.

Analysis of Biological Fluids Using Visual Zone Comparison

Clenbuterol and salbutamol residues in animal urine

1. *Sample preparation*. Solid phase extraction on C-18 column, elution with 0.1% triethylamine in methanol.
2. *TLC*. Silica gel 60 layer with concentrating zone, ethyl acetate-methanol-acetic acid (8: 1: 1) mobile phase.
3. *Detection*. N-chlorination with chlorine vapors and detection of the N-chloro derivatives as blue spots with iodide-o-tolidine solution.
4. *Qualitative screening and semiquantitative analysis*. Based on Rf value and color brightness comparison between samples and standards.

Analysis of Biological Fluids Using Fluorescence Densitometry

Cortisol in plasma and urine

1. *Sample preparation*. Extraction with dichloromethane.
2. *TLC*. Extracts and standards applied in 3–6mm bands with a Linomat IV to an aluminum-backed silica gel 60 layer, chloroform–methanol (9:1) mobile phase.
3. *Detection*. Layer dipped into isonicotinic acid hydrazide reagent for 20s and then into chloroform-liquid paraffin (9:1) to enhance and stabilize fluorescence.
4. *Quantification*. Scanning with 366 nm excitation and 460 nm emission wavelengths.
5. *Validation*. Limit of detection 1 ng, RSD 1.4–6.3%, comparison of results to a TLC-radio-immunoassay method gave correlation coefficients of 0.97 and 0.98.

Sulfamethazine in pork tissue

1. *Sample preparation*. Sulfabromomethazine added to tissue as an internal standard, extraction with water, centrifugation, and cleanup and concentration by a series of solid phase extractions using C-18 bonded silica, acidic alumina, and AG MP-1 anion exchange microcolumns.

2. *TLC*. Samples and standards applied in 6 mm bands with a Linomat IV to a silica gel 60 layer, ethyl acetate–toluene (1:1) mobile phase.
3. *Detection*. Layer dipped into fluorescamine solution.
4. *Quantification*. Fluorescence scanning of analyte and internal standard zones at 366 nm or 400 nm.
5. *Validation*. Limit of detection 0.25 ppb, average recovery over analysis range (0.54–2.18 ppb) was 95.6% (standard deviation 29.4%, $n = 54$).

Analysis of Pharmaceutical Preparations Using Visual Zone Comparison

Purity test for allylestrenol bulk drug substance and tablets

1. *Sample preparation*. Drug substance was dissolved in chloroform; tablets were powdered and sonicated in acetone.
2. *TLC*. 2.5 and 5 μl aliquots of sample and allylestrenol and impurity standard solutions were manually applied in 8mm bands to HPTLC silica gel plates, which were developed by OPLC with cyclohexane–butyl acetate–chloroform (90:12:2) mobile phase.
3. *Detection*. Spray with 10% ethanolic sulfuric acid and heat at 120°C for 2 min.
4. *Assay*. Visual comparison of sample and standard zones under 366 nm UV light.

Analysis of Pharmaceutical Preparations Using Visible Densitometry

S-*Carboxymethylcysteine in syrups used to treat respiratory diseases*

1. *Sample preparation*. Syrup diluted with 96% alcohol–ammonia (4:1).
2. *TLC*. Samples and standards applied with a Nanomat III to a silica gel 60, 1-butanol–glacial acetic acid–water (3:1:1) mobile phase, development in a twin-trough chamber.
3. *Detection*. Plate dipped into ninhydrin reagent and heated for 3–4 min at 100°C.
4. *Quantification*. Zones scanned at 487 nm.
5. *Validation*. Detection limit 15 ng/spot, RSD 0.99–1.6%, recoveries from adult and children's syrup 100.0 and 99.5%, respectively.

Analysis of Pharmaceutical Preparations Using UV Densitometry

Salbutamol sulfate and bromhexine hydrochloride in formulations

1. *Sample preparation*. Sample solutions were prepared in methanol at concentrations of 200–800 ng/μl.
2. *TLC*. Standards and samples applied with a Linomat IV to precoated alumina-backed silica gel 60 F layer, methanol–chloroform– triethylamine (5.5:4.5:0.05) mobile phase, development in a twin-trough chamber.
3. *Quantification*. Fluorescence quenched zones of samples and standards scanned at 276 nm.
4. *Validation*. Calibration curves linear over the range 20–580 ng/μl; RSDs ranged from 1.1 to 1.6% and recoveries from 98.8 to 99.6% for assay of the compounds in a syrup and tablet.

Diphenhydramine hydrochloride in tablet, gelcap, and capsule antihistamine pharmaceuticals

1. *Sample preparation*. Ground powder or gel dissolved in ethanol.
2. *TLC*. HPTLC silica gel 60 F layer, samples and standards applied as 6 mm bands with Linomat IV, ethyl acetate–methanol–conc. ammonia (85:10:15) mobile phase, development in twin-trough chamber.
3. *Quantification*. Fluorescence-quenched zones scanned at 260 nm.
4. *Validation*. Precision ranged from 1.7 to 1.9% RSD and errors in recovery analyses of spiked samples were 0.81 and 0%.

Betamethasone valerate and miconazole nitrate in cream preparations

1. *Sample preparation.* Creams were ultrasonicated with 96% ethanol, and insoluble material was removed by centrifugation and filtration.
2. *TLC.* 4 μl aliquots of samples and standards applied using a Nanomat III to a silica gel 60 F layer, development in a twin-trough chamber with chloroform–acetone–glacial acetic acid (34:4:3).
3. *Quantification.* Fluorescence-quenched zones of scanned at 233 nm.
4. *Validation.* Recoveries from laboratory-made cream were 100.1 and 100.5%, respectively, and RSD ranged from 0.68 to 1.67% (n = 6).

Pyridoxine hydrochloride and doxylamine succinate in tablets

1. *Sample preparation.* Tablets were powdered, sonicated in methanol, and the solution filtered.
2. *TLC.* 5 μl aliquots of samples and standards applied as 6 mm bands to HPTLC silica gel 60 F layer with the Linomat IV, acetone–chloroform–methanol–25% ammonia (7:1.5:0.3:1.2) mobile phase.
3. *Quantification.* Fluorescence-quenched zones scanned at 269 nm.
4. *Validation.* Linearity range 0.5–2.0 μg/spot; RSD 0.73 and 1.93%, and recoveries 99.3–103% and 97.7–101%, respectively.

Analysis of Pharmaceutical Preparations Using Fluorescence Densitometry

Amlodipine besylate in tablets

1. *Sample preparation.* Tablets powdered, dissolved in methanol, and filtered.
2. *TLC.* Samples and standards applied to a silica gel 60 F layer with a Linomat IV, developed with chloroform–acetic acid–toluene–methanol (8:1:1:1) mobile phase in a twin-trough chamber.
3. *Quantification.* Fluorescent zones scanned at 233 nm.
4. *Validation.* Minimum detectable limit 0.2 ng; recovery from pre-analyzed tablet spiked with three different levels of the drug standard was 100.1%.

Analysis of Pharmaceutical Preparations Using Scraping and Elution of Zones

Sulfur in topical acne medications

1. *Sample preparation.* Liquid and cream samples dissolved by boiling with acetone or chloroform.
2. *TLC.* Samples and standards applied as 2 cm bands, silica gel G layer, petroleum ether mobile phase.
3. *Detection.* Iodine vapor.
4. *Quantification.* Bands scraped and extracted with chloroform, UV absorption spectrometry at 265 nm.
5. *Validation.* Recovery from three spiked samples containing 3–5% sulfur averaged 99.2 ± 2%, 100 ± 2%, and 101 ± 1% for five replicates each.

15

CAPILLARY SEPARATION TECHNIQUES

Capillary electrophoresis (CE) is a modern analytical method that is being extensively applied to the characterization of biotechnology-derived products like peptides and proteins. Due to its ease of automation and facilitating the development of reproducible routine analysis, CE seems to be well suited for the quality control of biotechnological products, including process monitoring, purity assessments, and stability studies. Moreover, the high-resolution capacity of CE offers great potential for the analysis of hetero geneous protein products such as glycoproteins and polymer-conjugated proteins. Recently, the importance of CE in protein analysis is enhanced, with efforts being made to learn more about the compositions and functions of proteins. As the field of proteomics becomes more important, the thousands of new proteins and peptides will be discovered, which will lead to the developments of many new pharmaceutical drugs.

Recently, CE has emerged as a powerful tool because it has many advantages over the conventional protein separation techniques such as polyacrylamide gel electrophoresis (PAGE) and high-performance liquid chromatography (HPLC). Compared with PAGE, CE is faster, easier, simpler, quantitative, and has automation capability. Like HPLC, CE has various different separation modes and is applicable to a wide range of analytes. CE requires a very small sample amount (nanoliters) and limited quantities of reagents (microliters of buffer), compared with HPLC that requires microliters of sample and milliliters of solvent. The main advantage of CE over PAGE and HPLC is the ability to produce a higher number of theoretical plates. The efficient separations result from the application of high electric fields (100–500 V/cm) and flat flow generated by the electro-osmotic flow (HPLC generates the pressure-driven parabolic flow). The high electrical resistance of a capillary and its favorable surface area-to-volume ratio, permitting efficient heat dissipation, enables the application of high electric fields without causing detrimental heat generation. Furthermore, the mild separation conditions of CE, which use mostly aqueous buffer solutions, present the compatibility to protein studies in native state, which can be important especially in the characterization of pharmaceutical proteins. The main disadvantage of CE is the low concentration limits of detection due to the short path length and the limited introduction of sample volume. The enhancements in this issue have been achieved by the advent of several preconcentration methods and highly sensitive detection methods such as laser-induced fluorescence and mass spectrometry.

This chapter introduces the fundamental principles of CE and its application to the separation and characterization of peptides and proteins. One major characteristic of CE is the availability of various separation modes with different separation mechanisms based on the differences in charge-to-mass ratio (capillary zone electrophoresis), molecular size (capillary gel electrophoresis), isoelectric point (capillary isoelectric focusing), and hydrophobicity (micellar electrokinetic capillary chromatography and capillary electrochromatography). In the principles of CE, the instrumentation, theory, separation modes, and detection methods are described focusing on the analysis of peptides and proteins. In applications, CE methods for identification, purity assessment, heterogeneity characterization, and stability of peptide and protein products are highlighted with the characterization of Poly(ethylene glycol) (PEG)ylated biomolecules. Finally, the role of CE in proteomics research is discussed with the recent approaches.

Principles of Capillary Electrophoresis

Instrumentation

The main components of a CE system are a high-voltage power supply, a capillary, inlet and outlet buffer vials, a detector, and a data output and handling device such as an integrator or computer. A variety of commercial instruments are available with different capabilities, including injection methods, detectors, capillary cooling systems, and software. CE is performed by filling inlet and outlet vials and the capillary with an electrolyte, usually an aqueous buffer solution. Electrodes connected to a high-voltage power supply are then immersed in the vials. Very small amounts of sample are introduced into one end of the capillary, and these are driven electrophoretically down the lumen of the capillary toward the opposite electrode. The species that migrate through the capillary are detected by an online optical detector near the capillary outlet, and these data are displayed as an electropherogram, in which separated compounds appear as peaks with different migration times.

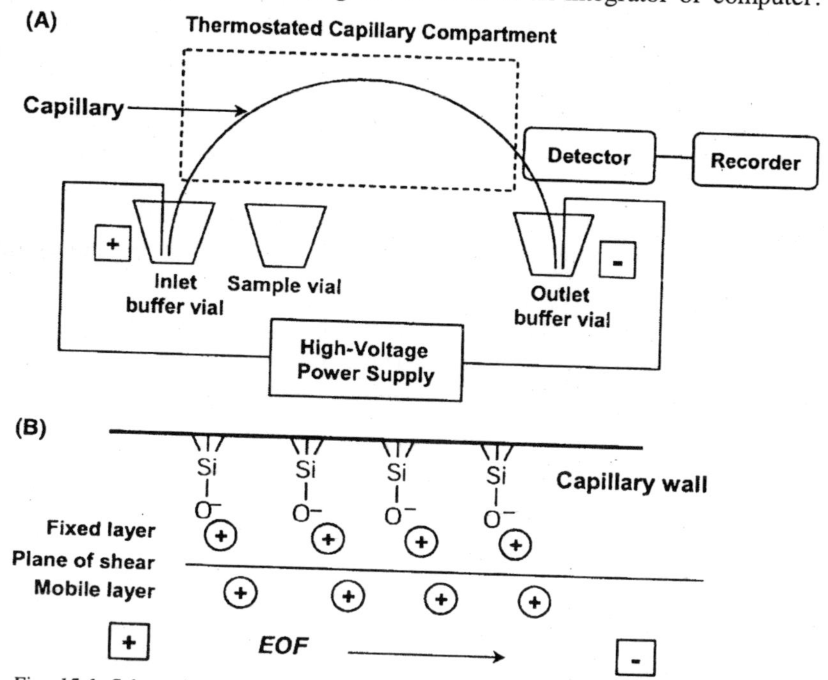

Fig. 15.1. Schematic diagram of a capillary electrophoresis system (A) and electro-osmotic flow (EOF) (B).

Fused silica capillaries of length of 20–100 cm and inner diameters of 50–100 μm are typically used. The outer surface of capillary is coated with polyimide, which is strongly ultraviolet (UV) absorbent. A detection window can be made by simply burning or scraping off a small section of the polyimide outer capillary coating. This section of the capillary is then placed in the light path of the detector, and thus solutes are detected while in the capillary. Most commercial instruments have a capillary cartridge, which retains the capillary, provides mechanical support, and allows the capillary to be consistently aligned at the optical center of the detector. Cartridges are used in conjunction with cooling systems, which maintain capillary temperatures using coolant or cooled air.

Only a few microliters of sample are required for CE because usually only 1–50 nanoliters of sample are injected into a capillary. For example, a 50-μm inner diameter capillary 50 cm long has a volume of only ca. 1 μL. Samples are injected into capillaries using different techniques, such as hydrodynamically or electrokinetically. Hydrodynamic injection can be performed by pressure or siphoning. Pressure injection is performed by either pressurizing the sample vial or by applying a vacuum to the outlet vial. Siphon injection is performed by raising the sample vial, which causes the sample to be siphoned into the capillary. In electrokinetic injection, an electric field is applied to the sample vial, causing the sample components to migrate into the capillary. Most commercially available instruments have autosamplers into which several sample vials can be loaded. The samples are then automatically injected into capillaries using one or more of the techniques above.

A variety of detectors have been used for CE, including UV absorbance, fluorescence, laser-induced fluorescence, and mass spectrometry. The most widely used is the UV absorbance detector. In some cases, two or more detectors are connected in series. The power supply provides an electric field across the capillary with voltages up to 30 kV, currents up to 300 μA, and power up to 6 W. Most instruments can be operated in either constant voltage, constant current, or constant power mode and have a reverse applied polarity facility. The constant voltage mode is most commonly used. It is necessary to have a stable voltage, as any variations in voltage will cause changes in migration times. Most CE systems are controlled by an external computer that controls all instrumental functions. The operating parameters for each analysis are programmed by computer. The electropherograms obtained are plots of detector response versus time; thus, they resemble familiar HPLC or gas chromato graphy (GC) chromatograms, which means that familiar data handling systems can be used. In addition, electronic integrators or computers are used for qualitative identification and quantitation, as in HPLC or GC.

Theory

Electrophoresis is the phenomenon whereby ionic species in a conductive aqueous medium moves under the influence of an electric field. Thus, ionic molecules are separated due to differences in their electrophoretic mobilities. The electrophoretic mobility (μ) of a spherical ion is given by

$$\mu = q/6\pi\eta r$$

where q is the charge of the ion, η is the viscosity of the solution, and r is the hydrodynamic radius of the ion. This equation demonstrates the positive relation between charge-to-mass ratio (q/r) and electrophoretic mobility. The electrophoretic migration velocity (v) depends on the electrophoretic mobility (μ) and the applied electric field (E):

$$v = \mu E$$

Besides the electrophoretic migration, a fundamental electrophoretic phenomenon occurring in CE is the electro-osmotic flow (EOF), which essentially is an electrical field-driven bulk solution flow from the anode to the cathode. This flow occurs because acidic silanol groups on the inside of fused-silica capillary are ionized when in contact with buffer solution. At pH above 3, these silanol groups are deprotonated and form an electric double layer. When an electric field is applied, the net positively charged solution in a capillary moves toward the cathode. EOF is highly dependent on buffer pH; i.e., it increases on raising pH and plateaus at about pH 8, but it is not significant below pH 4. At neutral and higher pH, the EOF is sufficiently strong to allow all molecules, regardless of charge, to move toward the outlet and pass the detector. EOF can be effectively controlled by changing several experimental conditions, including separation buffer pH, ionic strength, addition of organic solvents, and buffer additives. The apparent migration velocity of the analyte depends on their electrophoretic mobility (μ_e), electroosmotic mobility (μ_{eo}), the applied voltage (V), and capillary length (L):

$$v = (\mu_e + \mu_{eo})V/L$$

The electrophoretic mobility of peptides and proteins was first described by Offord, who proposed the following equation, which relates the mobility (μ) with valence (Z) and molecular mass (M):

$$\mu = kZM^{-2/3}$$

where k is an empirical constant. This equation states that frictional forces opposing electrophoretic migration are proportional to the surface areas of the species concerned. This implies that the electrophoretic mobility would be proportional to $1/r^2$ ($1/M^{2/3}$), rather than $1/r$ ($1/M^{1/3}$), which is suggested by the Stoke's model. This relationship was later confirmed and modified by several researchers in the CE field. Janini et al. presented the electrophoretic mobilities of 58 peptides that varied in size from 2 to 39 amino acids and in charge from 0.65 to 7.82. The electrophoretic data were used to test existing theoretical models that correlate electrophoretic mobility with physical parameters. The best fit of the experimental data was obtained with the Offord model that correlates electrophoretic mobility with the charge-to-size parameter $q/M^{2/3}$.

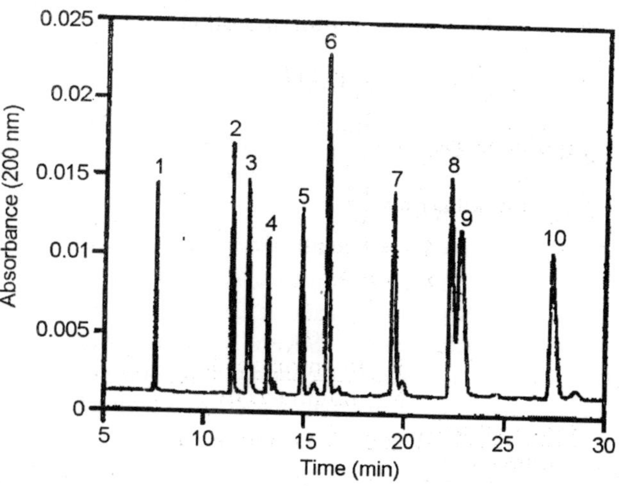

Fig. 15.2. Electropherogram of a mixture of bioactive peptides separated at pH 2.5.

Separation Modes

As HPLC has different separation modes of chromatography, including adsorption, partition (normal and reversed phase), ion-exchange, size-exclusion, and affinity, CE also has various separation modes, e.g., capillary zone electrophoresis (CZE), capillary gel electrophoresis (CGE), capillary isoelectric focusing (CIEF), micellar electrokinetic capillary chromatography (MEKC), and capillary electro-chromatography (CEC). Moreover, these different CE separation modes can be used to complement each other, and thus, they greatly enhance the versatility of the technique. In many cases, it seems that no single method can separate peptides and proteins because these biomolecules are diverse and complex in terms of structure and composition. Therefore, different optimal strategies involving different CE separation modes are often used to solve the separation problems.

Capillary zone electrophoresis (CZE)

CZE is a widely used CE technique and separates peptides and proteins based on differences in their charge-to-mass ratios. Separations occur in a capillary filled with a buffer of constant composition. For CZE, the run buffer choice is extremely important because it determines the charge on the analyte molecule and its migration rate. Thus, the type of buffer, its ionic strength, and its pH are optimized for particular separation problems. Buffers based on sodium phosphate, citrate, acetate, or combinations thereof with concentrations ranging from 10 to 200 mM are frequently used.

Proteins contain both positively and negatively charged functional groups. The positively charged moieties in proteins, such as the guanidinium group of arginine residues, the amino groups of lysine residues and N-termini, and histidine residues, interact with negatively charged silanol groups on capillary walls at pH values above 3. These interactions between proteins and capillary walls (protein adsorption) lead to sample loss, peak broadening, poor resolution, and longer migration times.

Many strategies devised to overcome protein–wall interactions have focused either on selecting separation buffer conditions that reduce protein binding sites or on treating capillary surfaces to reduce interaction sites. By using separation buffers with extreme pH values (e.g., below pH 2~3 or above pH 10), protein adsorption can sometimes be reduced. At pH values below around 2, the silanol groups of the capillary are fully protonated and surface charge approaches zero, whereas at pH values above

10, capillary surfaces are completely deprotonated and highly anionic. In these situations, protein adsorption is significantly reduced because of electrostatic repulsion. However, operations at extreme pH conditions can be problematic in finding suitable separation conditions due to reduction of differences of analytes in effective electrophoretic mobility. At low pH, EOF is negligible, making separations slow, and at high pH, EOF is generally high and resolutions are reduced. Additional problems encountered under extreme pH conditions include the effect on protein conformational changes. Unfolding or aggregation of proteins may occur, resulting in irreproducible data, often reduced efficiency, and a loss of biological activity. Therefore, the use of this approach is limited to a few selected applications.

To optimize separation conditions at moderate pH conditions, surface modifications of capillary can be helpful. Such modifications can decrease protein–surface interactions by reducing the surface charge of the silica material. Several approaches have been proposed for modifying the inner walls of capillaries, such as chemical coating with bonded/cross-linked polymers, physical adsorption coating with cationic polymers, and dynamic coating with adsorbed surfactants. The most popular coating method is to covalently bind polymers such as polyacrylamide or poly(vinyl alcohol) to capillary walls. Chemically coated capillaries are widely used and are available commercially. The preparations of this capillary type often involve several chemical reactions that may cause large variances between capillaries. In addition, these coatings are usually stable in restricted pH ranges and have limited lifetimes. Noncovalent capillary coatings are simply formed by treating the capillary with one or more charged polymers that are physically adsorbed onto internal walls. Initially, positively charged monolayer coatings of polybrene, polyethyleneimine, or poly(diallyldimethylammonium chloride) were used. More recently, noncovalently bilayer-coated capillaries prepared by add anionic polymer to cationic polymer-coated capillary have been reported to be long-lived and to have an EOF that is stable over wide pH ranges (2–11). Katayama et al. reported on the use of a polymeric bilayer of polybrene and dextran sulfate for the separation of some model proteins. Catai et al. demonstrated the use of capillaries coated with a bilayer of polybrene and poly(vinyl sulfonate) for the fast, highly reproducible, and efficient analysis of peptides and proteins. Another way of coating capillaries is to add the coating agents (usually low-molecular-weight compounds such as amines and surfactants) to the separation buffer for the dynamic coating of the inner capillary surface.

Sodium dodecyl sulfate-capillary gel electrophoresis (SDS–CGE)

SDS–CGE is a capillary-based version of SDS–polyacrylamide gel electrophoresis (SDS–PAGE) in the slab gel format, with advantages of shorter analysis times, ease of automation, and online detection and quantitation. In SDS–CGE, replaceable sieving polymers, such as linear polyacrylamide, poly(ethylene oxide), dextran, or pullulan, are used to achieve reproducible separations. These polymers permit the replacement of a separation matrix for each sample, thereby eliminating cross-contamination between samples and improving reproducibility. Best results are often obtained using chemically or dynamically coated capillaries.

For SDS–CGE, proteins are denatured and complexed with SDS before analysis. These SDS–protein complexes are then separated based on their sizes. The molecular mass of an unknown protein can be estimated by running protein standards as well. This assumes that migration is dependent on relative mass, on the basis of the following two assumptions. First, all SDS–protein complexes have the same charge-to-mass ratio in the presence of excess SDS (~1.4 g of SDS/1 g of protein). Second, the SDS–protein complexes have similar shapes, and thus, their sizes are linearly related to their molecular masses. However, these assumptions are not valid for some classes of proteins, e.g., basic proteins, hydrophobic membrane proteins, and glycoproteins, because deviations from predicted charge-to-mass ratio are often observed for their SDS–protein complexes. For example, basic proteins have lower charge-to-mass ratios because of the presence of positively charged amino acids, whereas hydrophobic membrane proteins have larger charge-to-mass ratios. Moreover, in the case of glycoproteins, the carbohydrate moieties do not bind with SDS, and this lowers the charge-to-mass ratio, leading to a decreased migration and overestimation of molecular mass. The SDS–CGE result for ricin toxin purified from the seeds of the castor bean (*Ricinus communis*), in which two peaks of ricin toxin were partially separated, while only a single band appeared in the SDS–PAGE gel. Two peaks were identified to be ricin glycoform isomers with identical protein sequences but with different carbohydrate contents. When the molecular masses of two peaks were determined with a calibration curve made by protein standards (MW 14–200 kDa), they were significantly higher than those measured by matrix-assisted laser desorption/ionization time-of-flight mass spectrometry (MALDI–TOF MS). This shows the slower electrophoretic migration of glycoproteins in SDS-based gel electrophoresis compared with that of standard proteins. However, the presence of carbohydrate may improve the resolution between glycoforms in SDS–CGE.

In addition to the estimation of protein molecular mass, SDS–CGE is also the common choice for checking the presence of other proteins, protein aggregates, or protein degradation products during characterization, purity, or stability studies.

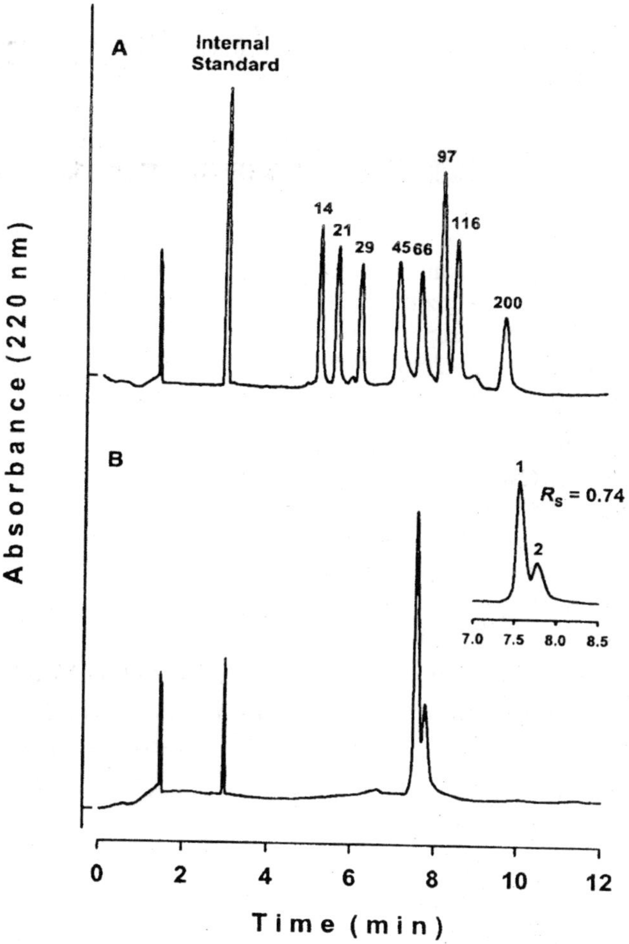

Fig. 15.3. SDS-CGE electropherograms of molecular weight standard marker (A) and ricin toxin glycoprotein under nonreducing conditions (B).

Capillary isoelectric focusing (CIEF)

CIEF separates peptides and proteins according to isoelectric point (p*I*) differences. Proteins that differ by 0.0 05 p*I* units or even less have successfully been separated by CIEF. The sample is normally mixed with ampholytes (zwitterionic compounds), which have slightly different p*I* values spanning the desired pH range and act as a strong buffer at their p*I* values and then the capillary is filled with this mixture. The capillary inlet is placed in a vial containing acidic solution (anolyte) and the capillary outlet in a basic solution (catholyte), before applying an electric field. A pH gradient is quickly formed by the ampholytes ranging from low to high pH along the entire capillary length. According to their electrophoretic mobilities, proteins migrate to their p*I*s in the capillary where they are focused into very sharp zones. The overall focusing process can be monitored by observing current changes, which approach zero when ion movement inside a capillary stops. The CIEF process can be performed in one or two steps. One-step CIEF is performed in an uncoated capillary and usually employs polymers such as hydroxypropyl methyl cellulose or hydroxyl ethyl cellulose in order to reduce but not eliminate EOF. At this point, either migration past a detection window or whole-column imaging is needed to visualize the separation. In two-step CIEF, proteins are first focused in a coated capillary to eliminate EOF and then mobilized by adding a salt (sodium chloride) to the catholyte or by applying pressure to the capillary inlet (anolyte). In general, the two-step method is preferred because it provides a much higher reproducibility. As CIEF is usually run from positive to negative polarity, the most basic proteins pass the detector first. Absorbance must be monitored at UV 280 nm to avoid the strong absorption of ampholytes at lower wavelengths. The use of a coated capillary is required for high resolution because EOF interferes with maintenance of focused zones. The estimation of p*I* in CIEF needs appropriate p*I* markers. Synthetic peptide and oligopeptide p*I* markers for CIEF with UV absorption detection have been developed. Shimura et al. proposed a set of 16 synthetic oligopeptides as p*I* markers for CIEF that are fully compatible with UV detection. CIEF produces the best resolution for proteins and peptides among the CE separation modes, and it is a powerful tool for resolving modified proteins, for characterizing microheterogeneity, and for identifying glycoforms. CIEF has also been found to be a powerful tool in proteomics studies.

Micellar electrokinetic capillary chromatography (MEKC)

MEKC separation is based on the partition of analytes between micelles and the surrounding aqueous phase. This technique can be considered a type of chromatography where the stationary phase is essentially mobile and the mobile phase is electro-osmotically pumped. The micellar phase is composed of a surfactant added to the buffer above its critical micellar concentration (CMC). The most commonly used surfactants are SDS, bile salts, and hydrophobic chain quaternary ammonium salts. In general, neutral or alkaline buffer solutions are used to create a strong EOF that moves even anionic micelles in the capillary toward the cathode.

MEKC has been applied with great success to the analysis of a variety of small molecules. However, relatively few protein applications have been found for MEKC, which may be because most proteins (>MW 5000) are too large to partition into the hydrophobic core of micelles. However, proteins can associate with micelles through hydrophobic, hydrophilic, and electrostatic mechanisms, and these interactions have been exploited to manipulate protein separation using MEKC. By manipulating these protein–micelle interactions using the variables, such as surfactant concentration, pH, ionic strength, and the addition of an organic modifier, MEKC has been demonstrated to resolve proteins with minor structural variations and to allow the quantitative analysis of proteins present in complex matrices.

Capillary electrochromatography (CEC)

Capillary electrochromatography (CEC) is a hybrid technique of CE and HPLC that is generally carried out using packed capillary columns by the electro-osmostically driven mobile phase at high electric field strength. CEC has been rapidly developed in recent years as it has combined advantages of both techniques, i.e., the high selectivity of HPLC and the high efficiency of CE, with minimum consumption of both reagents and samples, and good compatibility with mass spectrometry. The separation mechanism involved is based on chromatographic retention, and for charged analytes, on a combination of this and electrophoretic mobility. Initially, CEC was mainly used to separate neutral compounds such as polyaromatic hydrocarbons. Recently, the successful development of CEC column technology and improvements in instrumentation have encouraged research on CEC for peptide and protein separations. Various capillary columns have been used for peptide and protein analysis, including packed capillaries, open-tubular capillaries, and monolithic columns. In addition to the use of octadecylsilane (ODS) as a stationary phase, sulfonated poly(styrene-divinylbenzene), poly(2-sulfoethylaspartamide) -silica, open tubular silica, porous styrenic sorbents and octadecylsilica, pentofluorophenylsilica, trycontysilica, octadecylsilica, acrylate-based porous monoliths, and wide-pore stationary phases have been recently investigated. CEC separations using monolithic columns are being actively investigated because the stationary phases are easily prepared and supporting frits are unnecessary. In monolithic columns, the stationary phase is covalently bound to inner capillary walls. CEC separations of peptides and proteins in monolithic columns are usually performed in counter-directional mode; i.e., peptides and proteins migrate electrophoretically in a direction opposite to the EO.

Recently, a great deal of interest has been shown in the combination of CEC and mass spectrometry (MS) because CEC is considered to overcome many of the limitations of other CE techniques. When combined with electrospray ionization (ESI)–MS, CZE is limited to a small number of buffer systems and suffers from low sample loading capacity. MEKC has relatively poor selectivity and difficult compatibility with MS because it requires the use of high surfactant concentrations. In contrast, CEC has good compatibility with MS, selectivity, sample loading capacity, and general applicability.

Detection

In the CE system, peptides and proteins are typically detected by UV absorbance, laser-induced fluorescence (LIF), or MS. UV absorbance is the most widely used detection method, but when higher sensitivity is required, LIF or MS are preferred. Recently, MS is being increasingly used to detect peptides and proteins separated by CE with the improvement of proteomics research.

UV absorbance

UV detection of peptides and proteins is mostly performed at 200–220 nm, where the absorption is proportional to the number of peptide bonds, but sometimes around 254 or 280 nm, where the detection is based on the absorbance of the aromatic residues such as tryptophan, tyrosine, and phenylalanine. This detection method is most commonly used, but it has low sensitivity, which is a major disadvantage for the detection of analytes present at low concentrations. In CZE, UV detection is limited to micromolar or submicromolar concentrations for peptides and proteins. Several capillaries have been designed to improve the sensitivity in CE: (1) a rectangular capillary extended in the direction of the light path, (2) a Z-shaped capillary, and (3) a bubble cell capillary with an locally enlarged diameter in the detection region. These capillaries help somewhat to improve sensitivity, but practical difficulties of availability and implementation into existing instruments remain.

Laser-induced fluorescence (LIF)

Fluorescence is inherently a sensitive detection method with lower detection limits than UV absorbance detection. In addition, fluorescence detectors are selective because only fluorescing molecules are detected. Typical detection limits of fluorescence detection lie in the range 10^{-7}–10^{-9} M. The light sources used are usually deuterium, tungsten, or xenon lamps. Lasers are also good sources of high-intensity radiation and are used for LIF detection. LIF is the most sensitive detection method in CE. Detection limits of LIF have been reported to fall in the range 10^{-18}–10^{-21} M. A variety of lasers have been employed for the detection of peptides and proteins, which include Nd:YAG, argon ion, helium–cadmium, and helium–neon lasers. As proteins containing aromatic amino acid residues (tryptophan, tyrosine, and phenylalanine) have native fluorescence around 310 nm, the intrinsic fluorescence has been directly measured using Nd:YAG at 266 nm or helium-cadmium at 320 nm as a laser source. However, these systems are expensive and the helium–cadmium lasers have a problem of short lifetimes. The most popular lasers for the detection of peptides and proteins are argon lasers at 488 and 514 nm and helium–neon lasers at 544, 593, and 633 nm that are relatively inexpensive, stable, and compact. However, they are often not suitable for exciting most proteins to induce native fluorescence. To overcome this disadvantage, the labeling of the molecules with a suitable fluorescent dye is required via pre-column, on-column, or post-column. Several fluorescence-labeling reagents are commercially available and conveniently used for peptides and proteins. Rhodamine, solvatochromic dyes, and Albumin Blue 580 have been used to form stable and highly fluorescent complexes with proteins.

Mass spectrometry (MS)

MS is an important and powerful detection tool for the characterization of peptides and proteins by CE,as evidenced by recent developments of CE–MS methodology and its applications. MS detection considerably enhances the utility of CE by providing information about the identity of the separated molecules. The availability of CE–MS is also highly desirable for purity and stability studies of peptide and protein drugs. Especially, in proteomics, peptidomics, and peptide mapping, the importance of both on- and offline coupling of MS with CE separations of peptides and proteins is greatly growing.

The introduction of soft ionization techniques such as ESI and MALDI brought tremendous progress in on- and offline characterization of electrophoretically separated peptides and proteins by MS. Combination of CE with MS techniques allows not only high-accuracy molecular mass determination of peptides and proteins separated by CE, but also it provides important structural data on amino acid sequence, the sites of posttranslational modifications, peptide mapping, and the noncovalent interactions of peptides and proteins.

ESI forms gaseous ions by applying a strong electric field to a fine spray of their liquid solutions. It allows the generation of multiply charged ions, which enables the detection of very large molecules even with instruments having a low mass range. The multiply charged peaks can be transformed into a singly charged peak by mathematical deconvolution, which enables the determination of the molecular weight of the original species. ESI is the preferred mode for online coupling CE with MS because molecules can be transferred directly from the capillary to the mass spectrometer via an interface. Three types of interfaces, i.e., sheathless, liquid–junction, and coaxial liquid sheath-flow, have been constructed for CE–ESI–MS coupling. In MALDI, the analyte is cocrystalized with the matrix (small organic compounds having strong absorbance in the laser wavelength) and a laser beam is directed onto this crystal, causing vaporization of the matrix and desorption of the ions. The main advantage of MALDI is the generation of predominantly single- charged molecular ions of even macromolecules with a molecular mass up to 300 kDa with the exact determination of molecular mass with accuracy of $\pm 0.1\%$. Therefore, the MALDI–MS is a more attractive option for the characterization of heterogeneous samples. The MALDI–MS is combined with CE separations of peptides and proteins more in an offline mode than with an online liquid sample delivery connection. In offline mode, fractions separated from the CE are collected and deposited on a MALDI target in the form of spots for MS analysis. Recently, approaches for the online coupling of CE with MALDI–MS have been developed to minimize sample handling and potential losses.

Applications

In pharmaceutical biotechnology, the development of analytical procedures to validate identity, strength, quality, and purity of biopharmaceutical products is one of the most important issues for the production of highly specialized biotechnology products, as described in the U.S. Food and Drug Administration's (FDA's) current Good Manufacturing Procedures (cGMP) requirements for drugs. In this chapter, we discuss the use of CE to assess the identity, purity, heterogeneity, and stability of peptides and proteins, and its applications of CE in proteomics research.

Identity Determination

The identity of peptides and proteins can be determined by specific activity assays, determination of amino acid composition and sequence, and assessment of such physico-chemical parameters as molecular mass and p*I*. Several CE techniques have been used for the identity of peptides and proteins, which include peptide mapping by CZE or CEC, CIEF for the determination of protein's p*I*, SDS–CGE for the determination of relative molecular masses of proteins, and CE–MS for direct molecular mass assignment of peaks separated by CE.

Traditionally, IEF and SDS–PAGE in slab gel systems have been routinely used to confirm the identity of the proteins. CE formats, CIEF and SDS–CGE, offer fast and reproducible separations and direct online detection without the need of staining and destaining procedures used in slab gel techniques. As a typical example, Hunt et al. showed CIEF and SDS–CGE methods for the qualitative analysis of recombinant humanized monoclonal antibody HER2 (rhuMAbHER2). The CIEF separated five charged isoforms of rhuMAbHER2 with estimated p*I* values in the range of 8.6–9.1. These results agreed well with the p*I* values determined on slab gel IEF. In SDS–CGE, the expected molecular masses of intact rhuMAbHER2 under nonreduced conditions and its heavy-chain and light-chain fragments under reduced conditions were identified with good correlation with SDS–PAGE analysis. This study demonstrated the feasibility of replacing the slab gel techniques with CE methods in a quality control environment.

CE–MS

In SDS–PAGE, the molecular mass of proteins is estimated based on comparison with reference proteins with relatively poor accuracy of ±5–10%. When proteins are extracted from slab gels and subsequently transferred to ESI–MS or MALDI–MS, the mass accuracy somewhat improves, but the methodology still suffers from the interferences originated from gel. Frequently, accurate molecular mass determination is necessary especially for the identification of unambiguous peptides and proteins. Since its introduction in 1987 by Olivares et al., CE coupled to MS has gained increasing attention in peptide and protein research because of the CE ability to separate analyte from complex mixtures with high efficiency and minimal sample consumption. In CZE–ESI–MS, mass accuracies down to 0.0008% have been realized for model mixtures of proteins.

Tsuji et al. reported CZE–ESI–MS for the analysis of recombinant bovine and porcine somatotropins (rbSt and rpSt). The average molecular masses of rbSt and rpSt were determined to be 21,812.6 and 21,798.3, which were nearly identical to the theoretical values of 21,812.0 and 21,797.9, respectively. Yeung et al. reported on the CE–E SI–MS method for the analysis of high-mannose glycoproteins, ribonuclease B, and recombinant human bone morphogenetic protein-2. CE separations were performed with 50-mM beta-alanine buffer (pH 3.5) in a polyacrylamide-coated capillary and a coaxial sheath–liquid interface was used for CE–MS coupling. The identities of glycoform peaks separated by CE were determined by the combination of UV and MS detection data without the need of oligosaccharide release or derivatization treatments.

Na et al. reported on an offline combination of CZE and MALDI–TOF MS for the identification of salmon calcitonin (sCT) acylation products formed in the degrading poly(lactic-co-glycolic acid) (PLGA) microsphere formulations. The peptides extracted from sCT microspheres incubated in drug release medium were analyzed by both CZE with UV detection (200 nm) and MALDI–TOF MS. After the incubation, the additional peak was observed in CE and mass peaks of m/z 3491.15 and 3549.16 except the intact sCT were presented in MALDI–TOF MS spectrum. The identities of two peaks separated in CE were confirmed by reanalysis of each peak fraction using MALDI–TOF MS, which was also used for the quantitation of peptide loaded into microsphere formulations.

Peptide mapping

Peptide mapping is an important tool for protein identif-ication, primary structure determination, the detection of posttranslational modifications, the identification of genetic variants, and the determination of glycosylation and/or disulfide sites. For these reasons, peptide mapping is widely used for quality control and for the characterization of recombinant DNA-derived products. Moreover, the high resolution of CE makes it a powerful peptide mapping technique.

Rush et al. (1993) reported on the CE-based peptide mapping of recombinant human erythropoietin (EPO) derived from Chinese hamster ovary (CHO) cells. Using 100-mM heptanesulfonic acid in 40-

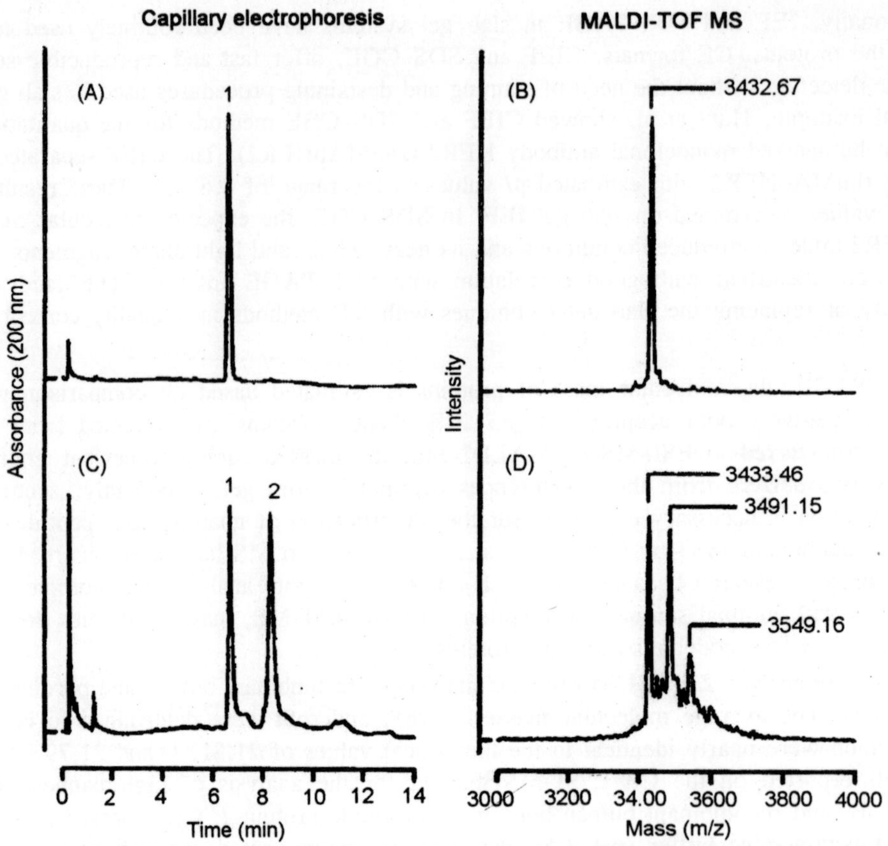

Fig. 15.4. CZE and MALDI-TOF MS analysis of sCTs extracted from microsphere at 0 day (A and B) and 21 days (C and D) of incubation in release medium at 37°C.

mM sodium phosphate buffer (pH 2.5) as a separation buffer, this technique showed a baseline separation of 16 tryptic-digested peptides with one partial separation of two peptides. This peptide map demonstrated the structural differences between the glycosylated form expressed in CHO cells and the non-glycosylated form expressed in *E. coli*, and it provided information on the heterogeneity in glycoforms of EPO. Zhou et al. presented the results of the CE–ESI-MS analysis of tryptic digests of EPO, and they found that the technique is complementary to HPLC–ESI-MS. Boss et al. reported on an evaluation of CE–MS for the peptide mapping of EPO. In this study, tryptic-digested peptides were first separated by reversed-phase (RP)–HPLC and collected fractions were analyzed by offline and online CZE–MS experiments employing a capillary coated with Polybrene in the presence of polyethylene glycol and 0.67-M formic acid as a separation buffer.

Despite the impressive ability of CE to separate peptides, a complete separation of all digested peptides is unlikely to be achieved because of the highly complex natures of the peptide maps of large proteins. Recently, multidimensional separations, such as two-dimensional (2D) electrophoresis, HPLC–CZE, HPLC–MS, CZE–MS, and HPLC–CZE–MS, have been applied for complete resolution of highly complex peptide mixtures. A sequential offline combination of RP–HPLC and CZE was used for the peptide mapping of pepsin isoenzymes, recombinant human tissue plasminogen activator, cytochrome c, and myoglobulin. Kang et al. presented unique "*fingerprint*" peptide maps of two closely related proteins, β-lactoglobulins A and B, by combining CZE separations performed in four different channels and MEKC separations performed in two different channels in a 96-capillary array. He et al. developed a novel multiplex CE system for the high- throughput comprehensive peptide mapping of proteins. By using multiple separation conditions using six CZE buffers and two MEKC buffers in a 20-capillary array, the peptide fragments of proteins digested by three different enzymes were readily resolved and showed unique fingerprints. These 20 capillaries were monitored simultaneously at 214 nm using a single photodiode array detector, and the overall analysis time from reaction to detection was about 40 min.

Purity Control

Purity control is necessary on peptide and protein products for process and quality control purposes. Minor amounts of impurities and degradation products must be determined in the presence of much larger quantities of primary components. These components may be structurally very similar to the main component. CE can be applied as a sensitive control method for such determinations because it provides rapid and accurate qualitative and quantitative data on peptide and protein preparations.

Peptide purity

Peptide purity checks have been routinely performed by RP–HPLC. Recently, CE has increasingly been used as a versatile technique for the analysis of peptide drugs in the pharmaceutical industry. Because of the different separation mechanisms, CZE is recognized as an excellent complementary tool to RP-HPLC. CZE separates the peptide based on differences in mass-to-charge ratios, whereas RP–HPLC separation is per-formed based on hydrophobicity differences. Peptides with similar hydrophobicities, which are difficult to be separated by RP–HPLC, can often be resolved based on charge-to-mass ratio differences. Therefore, peaks that appear pure by RP–HPLC are often resolved in multiple peaks by CZE. Moreover, CZE requires only nanoliter quantities of sample so that almost all of the sample can be used for subsequent sequence analysis.

Ridge and Hettiarachchi reported on CZE separations of bradykinin and its impurities using phosphate buffers at various pH values (pH 2.5, 3.5, and 4.5), which were not fully resolved by HPLC. When buffer pH was increased from 2.5 to 4.5, several impurities were well separated from the major peak of bradykinin. In purity checks of peptide, the similar superiority of CZE over RP–HPLC is also found in publications by Chen et al., Hettiarachchi et al., and Moumakwa et al.

Protein purity

During the production of recombinant proteins, process monitoring is required to assure purity levels required in every step. The recovery and purification of product from fermentation broth typically involve various procedures, such as filtration, centrifugation, and chromatography. After each purification and final step, constituent levels must be determined to ensure that the desired levels of purity have been achieved. In addition to its control function, this purity information is also frequently used to further optimize purification processes. CZE and SDS–CGE can be mostly used for the purity checks of protein products.

Several CZE methods were reported for the purity determinations of recombinant human insulin. Human insulin consists of two peptide chains, A (21 amino acids) and B (30 amino acids), which are connected by two disulfide bonds. To determine the purity of insulin, two main degradation products, acidic and neutral desamido-insulin (desamidated at positions A-21 or A-21 and B-3, respectively), should be separated from the main compound. According to U.S. Pharmacopoeia (USP), the relative amount of desamido insulin must not exceed 3% of the total amount of insulin and desamido insulin.

A CZE method for the separation of insulin and its deamidation products with untreated fused-silica capillaries using a run buffer containing 2-(*N*-cyclohexylamino) ethanesulfonic acid (CHES), triethylamine, and 10% acetonitrile has been reported. This system separated acidic and neutral desamido-insulin in formulated human insulin with the relative standard deviation (RSD) of the migration times ≤1%, whereas RP–HPLC coeluted the neutral desamido -insulin with insulin. Sergeev et al. described an analytical scheme for monitoring recombinant human insulin during the various steps of its production. The CZE method has been included, together with narrow-bore HPLC and MALDI–TOF MS, in the analytical scheme for monitoring the production of recombinant human insulin. Combinations of these complementary techniques allowed us to obtain unambiguous information about the purity and primary structure of all intermediates of recombinant human insulin production, and they enabled the optimization of some process parameters. This CZE analysis showed the presence of several impurities from the preparation (Arginsulin) and degradation (unidentified desamido-insulins) in the isolated insulin. SDS–CGE provides an overall composition of a protein sample based on the molecular mass, even if it is less suited for the analysis of subtle changes in a protein. Thus, SDS–CGE is mainly used to check for the presence of other proteins, protein aggregates, or protein degradation fragments in the purity checks.

Hunt and Nashabeh showed the SDS–CGE method with LIF detection for the analysis of humanized recombinant IgG_1-monoclonal antibody (MAb). For LIF detection, the MAb was first derivatized with a 5-carboxytetramethylrhodamine succinimidyl ester. The derivatized sample was then incubated with SDS, and the SDS–MAb complexes were separated by SDS–CGE using a hydrophilic polymer as a sieving matrix. The capabilities of SDS–CGE using UV detection or LIF detection after derivatization were compared. Under reducing conditions, the light and heavy chains originating from the original MAb were well separated, and the results of SDS–CGE under both reducing and nonreducing conditions generally showed good agreement with band profiles obtained by silver-stained SDS–PAGE. SDS–CGE using LIF detection allowed the detection of MAbs at a low-nanomolar concentration (~9 ng/mL), which was comparable with silver-stained SDS–PAGE and was a 140-fold increase over SDS–CGE using UV detection. This improved sensitivity also allowed the detection of low-level impurity peaks, which were not detected by UV detection. Repeated analysis showed that RSD values for the migration time were below 1%, and the RSD of the area of the main peak was lower than 0.6%. These applications demonstrate the usefulness of SDS–CGE–LIF for detecting manufacturing inconsistencies in recombinant protein production.

Heterogeneity Characterization of Glycoproteins

Glycoproteins produced from mammalian expression systems consist of a population of glycosylated variants (glycoforms). Glycosylation is one type of posttranslational modification that requires monitoring because variation in the carbohydrate composition may significantly alter the properties of a protein such as biological activity, pharmacokinetic properties, solubility, and stability. Several CE methods have been used for analyzing the intact glycoproteins and monitoring their production. Because of simplicity and high resolving capacity based on the charge-to-mass ratio, CZE has been routinely used for characterizing the heterogeneity of glycoproteins. In addition, CIEF has been increasingly used for separation of the glycoforms.

Erythropoietin (EPO)

EPO is a glycoprotein produced primarily by the kidney and the main regulator of red blood cell production. Human EPO consists of 165 amino acids that are heavily glycosylated (one O-linked and three N-linked carbohydrate chains corresponding to 40% of the molecular mass). Several glycoforms of human EPO exist with different degrees of glycosylation and sialic acid residue numbers. Several reports are available on the application of CE for the separation of EPO glycoforms, involving different CE modes. Among them, CZE and CIEF are the most successful CE modes in this respect. A CZE method for the characterization of the glycoform patterns of pharmaceutical EPO is included in the 2002 European Pharmacopoeia, as a substitute for the conventional isoelectric focusing test. EPO was resolved with high resolution into its glycoforms using a separation buffer containing putrescine (1,4-diaminobutane) and urea. Individual peaks correspond to multiple glycoforms with similar overall mass-to-charge ratios. At pH 5.5, sialic acid residues are negatively charged and migrate against the EOF, and thus the glycoforms are considered to elute in the order of increasing number of sialic acid residues. The addition of putrescine to the separation buffer leads to a reduction in EOF and solute interaction with the capillary wall. Urea is used to inhibit protein aggregation by preventing the formation of intermolecular hydrogen bonds and disrupting hydrophobic and noncovalent interactions. Sanz-Nebot et al. described the CZE separation of a novel erythropoiesis-stimulating protein (NESP), which is a recently approved hyperglycosylated analog of human EPO with a long-lasting effect. As NESP, due to its two extra *N*-linked oligosaccharide chains, has a higher sialic acid content than EPO, its glycoforms are expected to carry a higher overall negative charge at pH 5.5. NESP glycoforms migrated slower than EPO glycoforms at pH 5.5 and the peaks corresponding to NESP glycoforms were only partially resolved. The peak resolution was improved at lower pH condition, which may be due to the lower p*I* of NESP compared with EPO. At pH 4.5, the seven peaks of NESP glycoforms were resolved to baseline.

CIEF is an important technique for analyzing the charged variants of EPO glycoforms on the basis of sialic acid content differences. Cifuentes et al. showed that EPO glycoforms could be resolved by using a mixture of broad and narrow pH-range ampholytes and by adding urea to the EPO sample. The separation and quantification of seven EPO glycoforms with apparent p*I* values of 3.78–4.69 was accomplished using an optimized hydrodynamic mobilization method. Compared with conventional gle-IEF, better resolution was obtained in a shorter time. Lopez-Soto-Yarritu et al. described an improved CIEF method for the separation of EPO glycoforms with neutral-coated capillaries using ampholytes in the pH range 2–10 and bovine β-lactoglobulin-A as an internal standard. CIEF analysis of EPO glycoforms was achieved with a migration time reproducibility of 0.05% and peak area reproducibility better than 3.4%.

Monoclonal antibodies

Monoclonal antibodies (MAbs) are being in-creasingly used for a variety of diagnostic and therapeutic applications. As is the case for most recombinant proteins, preparations of MAbs often show considerable heterogeneity due to posttranslational modifications involving glycosylation. CIEF has been widely used for the separation of charged isoforms of several MAbs.

Hunt et al. reported validation of CIEF method for recombinant MAb C2B8. CIEF separated four isoforms of MAb C2B8. Among them, three peaks were identified as charge isoforms present due to incomplete C-terminal lysine processing and represent MAb C2B8 with 2, 1, and 0 C-terminal lysines, respectively. The CIEF method was validated in accordance with International Conference on Harmonization (ICH) guidelines, and the result demonstrated that it is accurate, precise, linear, and highly specific for the determination of identity and charge distribution of MAb C2B8.

Tang et al. performed a systematic study on the routine analysis of a recombinant immunoglobulin G (IgG) by CIEF. The method used a dimethyl siloxane-coated capillary (DB-1) and a separation matrix of 2% ampholytes in 0.4% methylcellulose. The composition of various IgG samples with respect to isoform content was analyzed and compared quantitatively with gel-IEF. The reproducibility of the method was examined with the quantitative analysis of IgG sample in replicate over 3 days. The RSD of peak areas was below 2% intraday and 8% interday. The RSD for the mobilization times was below 1% intraday and 3% interday. Separation variability was examined over 150 runs. During this period, reproducible migration times and good resolution without peak shape deterioration were observed. This type of robustness demonstrates the potential of the CIEF method as a useful routine analysis tool.

Kats et al. employed the MEKC method to separate isoforms of chimeric MAb BR96. In the range from pH 2 to 12, MAb BR96 was separated into one to five isoforms by MEKC using a 12-mM borate buffer (pH 9.4) containing 25-mM SDS in uncoated capillary. Kats et al. further applied MEKC to separate structurally similar isoforms of a single-chain immunotoxin fusion protein BR96-sFV-PE40 using a 12-mM borate buffer (pH 9.6) containing 16-mM cholic acid.

Stability Study

Peptides and proteins are complex molecules containing many functional groups, which can undergo a variety of degradation reactions, such as oxidation, reduction, deamidation, hydrolysis, arginine conversion, β-elimination, and racemization of amino acids. Proteins further undergo physical changes in the secondary, tertiary, and quaternary structures. These degradation reactions can alter the conformation, size, charge, and hydrophobicity of the peptides and proteins, thereby affecting the biological activity or even leading to formation of toxic compounds. As is recognized by the ICH guidelines for stability testing of biotechnological products, the monitoring of the stability of pharmaceutical peptides and proteins is of the utmost importance in the aspects of quality control and safety. CE has been used as a powerful tool for monitoring of stability and degradation of peptides and proteins in various conditions.

The high resolving power of CZE could be used for monitoring the stability and degradation reactions of peptide and protein products. Hoitink et al. applied CZE–MS for a stability study of goserelin, a luteinizing hormone-releasing hormone analog. Using a 10% acetic acid as running buffer, high-resolution separation was obtained. In a stability study of goserelin at pH 5 and 9, the degradation of the C-terminal semi-carbazide group was observed. Lai et al. used CZE for the separation of asparagines-containing hexapeptide and its deamidation products and applied this method to a peptide stability study in the presence of polymers. The offline CZE/MALDI–TOF MS combination has been used to monitor the stability of sCT, human parathyroid hormone 1-34 (PTH), and leuprolide in biodegradable PLGA microsphere formulations. CZE separations were performed using a 100-mM phosphate buffer (pH 2.5) in polyacylamide-coated capillary with UV detection at 200 nm. During the *in vitro* drug release study, intact sCT peak rapidly decreased, whereas the additional peaks predominantly appeared after 28 days of incubation. MALDI–TOF MS data supported CE results with good correlation.

SDS–CGE can be also a useful stability-indicating method because it detects changes in fragmentation of proteins. Hunt et al. demonstrated that SDS–CGE could detect peaks resulting from the fragmention and aggregation of MAb HER2 when incubated at 37°C for 27 days . Hunt and Nashabeh showed the potential of SDS-CGE for the separation and detection of proteolytic and deglycosylated fragments generated from MAbs.

Characterization of PEGylated Peptides and Proteins

The covalent attachment of PEG, PEGylation, is a well-established technique of overcoming several problems associated with the therapeutic uses of proteins. This technique has demonstrated reduced immunogenicity, extended circulating half- life, and improved stability for these therapeutic agents.

In general, the PEGylation process results in molecular heterogeneity with respect to the distribution in terms of number and positions of attached PEG molecules as well as the inherent polydispersity of PEG itself. Therefore,

PEGylated molecules are among the most challenging products in analytical biochemistry, and their characterizations are becoming more important because these heterogeneities may confer different biological properties. When developing PEGylated biomolecules as therapeutic agents, various points should be considered, including the characterization of starting materials (i.e., proteins and PEG molecules), the determination of PEGylation sites, and the stoichiometry of PEG attachment. The consistency of each preparation should also be established. For well-characterized PEGylated biomolecules, it is important to develop and validate suitable analytical techniques that enable consistent manufacturing processes to be established.

Cunico et al. described a charge-reversed CZE method for the analysis of PEGylated proteins. A removable coating using ethylene glycol was applied to allow the negative capillary surface charge to be made positive, to prevent the protein adsorption to the capillary wall. Using this coated capillary, six different PEGylated molecules were characterized. Bullock et al. characterized PEGylated superoxide dismutase (SOD) by CZE using a low-pH separation buffer (pH 2.05). At low pH, protein molecules are completely protonated and the charge differences between individual PEG-mers (i.e., mono-, di-, or tri-PEGmers) are minimized due to neutralization of lysine residues modified by PEG attachment. This results in a predominantly size- based separation of PEGylated proteins. Under low pH conditions, PEG–SOD conjugates were size-dependently separated and the separation pattern was very similar to the MALDI–TOF MS spectrum.

Li et al. used a semi-aqueous phosphate buffer (pH 2.5) of acetonitrile-water (1:1, v/v) to improve the resolution of PEGylated proteins. They found that acetonitrile was mainly responsible for the good resolution observed, and this was attributed to reduced protein adsorption to the inner wall of the silica capillary used. Na et al. determined PEGylation sites in three positional isomers of mono-PEGylated salmon calcitonins (mono-PEG-sCTs) using CZE-based peptide mapping analysis. The resistance of PEGylation sites to proteolytic degradation resulted in different CE electropherogram patterns for tryptic digested mono-PEG–sCT isomers, and PEGylation sites were assigned accordingly and confirmed by MALDI–TOF MS. Na and Lee reported on the characterization of PEGylated human parathyroid hormone (PEG–PTH) using CZE. The CZE was used to optimize reaction conditions by monitoring the effects of reaction pH and the molar ratios of reactants on the PEGylation of PTH. The CZE method also allowed for determination of the extent of positional isomers in mono-PEG–PTH as well as for the identification of PEGylation sites.

Na et al. applied SDS–CGE to characterize PEGylated interferon alpha (PEG-IFN). The method well resolved the PEG–IFN species as well as the native IFN. Four PEGylated IFNs (i.e., mono-, di-, tri-, and tetra-PEGylated IFNs) were detected and completely separated by SDS–CGE. The distribution of PEGylation reaction mixture in the SDS–CGE was found to be almost identical with that obtained by SDS–PAGE with Coomassie blue staining, although no band corresponding to tetra-PEGylated IFN was visualized. SDS–CGE was also useful for monitoring PEGylation reaction to optimize the reaction conditions such as the reaction molar ratio. This study demonstrated the potential of SDS–CGE for the characterization of PEGylated proteins with the advantages of speed, minimal sample consumption, and high resolution.

Proteome Analysis

Analysis of the proteome through the detection and identification of proteins from biological samples is gaining importance in the postgenomic era. The most traditional way to analyze proteome consists of protein separations by 2D gel electrophoresis (2-DE) and identifications by MS employing ESI or MALDI ionization. However, the 2-DE–MS approach remains difficult for the detection of proteins expressed at extremely low levels or having extreme p*I* values or molecular masses and sensitivity. In view of the limitations of 2-DE-based techniques, a considerable effort has been focused on the development of liquid phase-based analytical techniques, such as HPLC and CE, enabling the rapid, broad, and sensitive analysis of complex proteomic samples through the combination with MS or tandem MS analysis. Various CE-based techniques have been widely used for proteome analysis, as has been described in numerous recent review articles. In addition to the complexity of protein samples, the large variation of the protein relative is one of the great challenges to the proteome analysis. For the broad proteome analysis, including the identification of lower abundance proteins, developments in capillary separations capable of providing extremely high resolving power and selective analyte enrichment are being highlighted. As the resolving power of one-dimensional separation systems is generally not adequate for highly complex mixtures, multidimensional separations are becoming increasingly important for the comprehensive proteome analysis. Chen et al. developed an online combination system of CIEF with capillary RP–HPLC (CRPLC) using a microinjector as the interface for 2D separations of complex protein mixtures. The resolving power of a combined CIEF–CRPLC system was demonstrated with tryptic digests of proteins from *Drosophila* salivary glands. The overall peak capacity was estimated to be around approximately 1800 over a run time of less than 8 hours.

Mohan and Lee developed a 2D CE separation system for proteomics by combining CIEF with transient capillary isotachophoresis (CITP) –CZE. 2D separation of proteolytic peptides was applied to analyze tryptic digests of model proteins, including cytochrome c, ribonuclease A, and carbonic anhydrase II. Maximum peak capacity was estimated to be around 1600. Ramsey et al. have combined MEKC with CZE, using switching of applied voltages to control fraction transport between the separation dimensions. In analysis times of less than 15 min, 2D separation of tryptic digests of bovine serum albumin produced a peak capacity of 4200 (110 in the first dimension and 38 in the second dimension). The system was used to identify peptides from a tryptic digest of ovalbumin using standard addition and to distinguish between tryptic digests of human and bovine hemoglobin.

In biopharmaceutical analysis, CE is becoming the method of choice for the separation and characterization of peptide and protein pharmaceuticals. The application of CE in this area has significantly increased during the past decade. The high efficient separation capability of CE provides an alternative and complementary technique to conventional analytical methods that are currently used to characterize biopharmaceuticals. Diverse separation modes of CE have been applied for the identity determination, purity control, heterogeneity characterization, stability study, and process consistency of biopharmaceuticals. In particular, CE has been recognized as a highly valuable tool for the efficient separation and characterization of the heterogeneous and complex protein products such as glycoproteins and PEGylated proteins. Recently, as the field of proteomics is becoming increasingly important, the role of CE in the strategy of protein analysis increases, with an emphasis on multidimensional separation and the combination of mass spectrometric techniques.

16

ELECTROANALYTICAL METHODS

Voltammetry is a term that encompasses all measurements based on controlled electrolysis at a microelectrode. Polarography, first introduced by the Czech electrochemist Jaroslav Heyrovsky in 1922, is voltammetry at a special form of mercury microelectrode, the dropping mercury electrode (DME). Mercury electrodes can only be driven to negative potentials because otherwise, the metal dissolves in aqueous solutions as Hg^{2+}. Consequently, polarography is an electroanalytical method based on the cathodic reduction of electroactive species, either metal cations or electroreducible organic species, in an electrically conducting solution. By contrast, voltammetry is based on electroanalysis involving anodic oxidation, preferably in a flowing system in which a self-cleaning action prevents fouling of the solid electrode surface by the products of the electrochemical reaction, thereby leading to non-reproducible current/voltage curves.

HISTORICAL BACKGROUND OF POLAROGRAPHY AND VOLTAMMETRY

The determination of electrocapillary curves for mercury, a phenomenon attributable to changes in the surface tension of the liquid metal as a function of applied potential in an electrolyte solution, was known from the beginning of the 20th century. An electrode consisting of mercury dropping from a fine glass capillary was devised for this purpose. However, secondary maxima appeared at certain points on the electrocapillary curves. The origin of these distortions to the electrocapillary curve was unknown at that time, and it was this phenomenon that Heyrovsky originally sought to investigate and explain. He noted that when certain cations were added to an electrolyte solution, kinks appeared on the electrocapillary curves at potentials close to the values for known electrochemical processes at the DME. The applied voltage between the DME and a mercury pool formed at the bottom of a cell containing an aqueous metal ion solution was gradually increased. Under these conditions, the resulting current had a small initial value that began to rise rapidly in a reproducible manner as the voltage scan progressed. The point at which this rapid rise in current occurred, the threshold potential, depended only on the species of metal ion present in the test solution. The rapid current rise increased linearly with an increasing applied voltage until the current eventually became constant again. This constant current value, which was found to be proportional to the concentration of metal ion in solution, forms the quantitative basis of polarographic/voltammetric analysis. The method by which Heyrovsky obtained the current voltage curve at the DME involved gradually increasing the applied external voltage (the voltage scan), measuring the corresponding mean current, and plotting this current against the applied voltage. This method constitutes analytical polarography, sometimes referred to as classic or direct current (d.c.) polarography to distinguish it from more modern variants. Heyrovsky was awarded the Nobel Prize in 1959 for his work on the discovery and development of polarographic analysis.

Classic d.c. polarography was limited in its development by the unreliability of early polarographs (instruments used to record current versus applied voltage curves), and the difficulties inherent in operating what were, at that time, relatively complex instruments. Although the method was suitable for metal cations, analytical applications in the field of electroactive organic compounds were restricted by the problem of the higher electrical resistance of non-aqueous solvent systems. Thus, only a water or water-alcohol system could be used with a conventional polarographic cell making up a two-electrode system of DME and reference electrode. Furthermore, determination of metals could be achieved at great sensitivity with spectroscopic methods such as flame emission and atomic absorption spectroscopy. This situation generally remained unchanged until the late 1950s, when modified polarographic techniques, such as square-wave, pulse, and a.c. polarography, began to appear, facilitated by the development of solid-state electronics. The development of a three-electrode system, linked to an electrical circuit known as a potentiostat, overcame the high resistance associated with the use of non-aqueous systems and widened the analytical applicability of the polarography. These developments, which form the basis of modern polarographic and voltammetric analysis, including their applications to the pharmaceutical sciences, have been referred to as the "*renaissance*" in polarography.

THEORY OF POLAROGRAPHY AND VOLTAMMETRY

In a simple electrolysis experiment in which an electrolyte solution is electrolyzed between two platinum plate electrodes, an anode and a cathode, efficient stirring of the solution is necessary to drive ions toward the electrodes. When the potential difference between the two electrodes, which is a function of the applied external voltage, is sufficiently high, ions are discharged at the electrode surfaces. Such electrodes are working electrodes. The current flowing caused by ion discharge is an electron transfer or faradaic current, i.e., a current attributable to transfer of electrons to the electrode (anodic oxidation) or gain of electrons from the electrode (cathodic reduction). This faradaic current continues to flow until all of the electroactive species is consumed by electrolysis. Replacement of a platinum plate electrode with a platinum wire microelectrode and use of a quiet (unstirred) solution result in the electrolysis current reaching a limiting value.

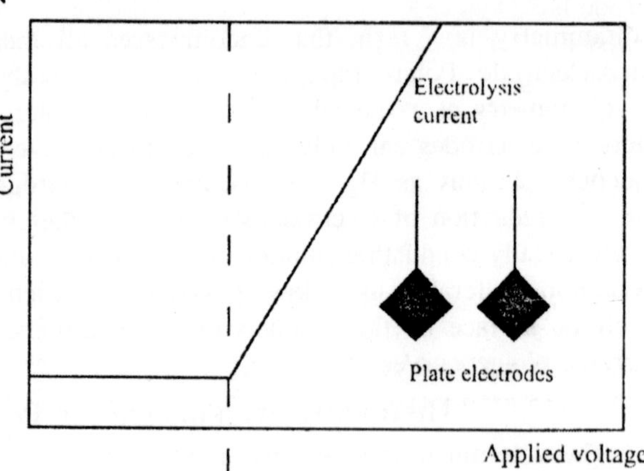

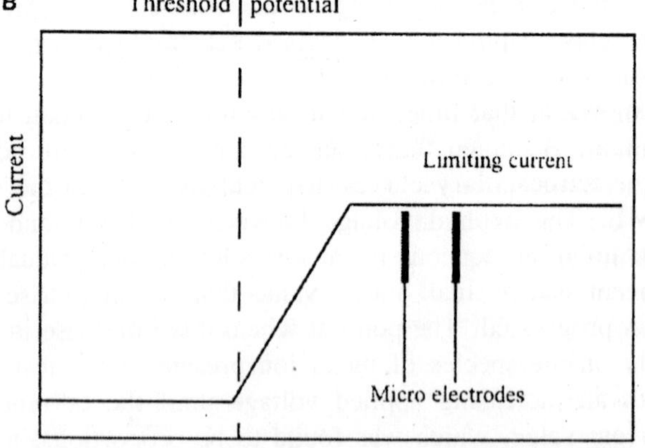

Fig. 16.1. Comparison between electrolysis are limiting currents. A–A faradaic electrolysis current between platinum plate electrodes at an applied voltage beyond the threshold potential of the electroactive species. B–Effect of replacing the platinum plate electrodes with platinum wire microelectrodes.

The current interest in polarography is attributable to electron transfer between the electrode and the electroactive species. Therefore, the limiting current must be proportional to the concentration of the electroactive species in the bulk solution. This remains true provided the electroactive species can only reach the electrode surface by diffusion along a concentration gradient. The concept of a limiting diffusion current is central to quantitative analysis by polarography or voltammetry. However, the magnitude of this limiting current is non-reproducible because the electrode surface becomes fouled easily by the products of the electrochemical reaction. To overcome this problem, a microelectrode with a renewable surface is required. Use of a microelectrode ensures that an infinitesimally small proportion of the bulk electroactive species is consumed in a single polarographic run, making the technique essentially non-destructive of the analate. Suitable working electrodes for voltammetry are those that can be driven to take up a new potential in response to an applied external voltage, a process known as electrode polarization. Reduction or oxidation of an electrochemically active species at a working electrode results in depolarization of the electrode. The word depolarizer is therefore sometimes used to describe an electrochemically active species. In voltammetry, the working electrode may be fabricated from metals such as gold or platinum, various forms of carbon, or metallic mercury.

The use of mercury dropping from the tip of a fine glass capillary (the DME) as the polarizable electrode has certain specific advantages. Most important, however, the electrode surface is reproducibly renewed as each succeeding drop is formed at the capillary tip. Electrical connection to the DME can be made using a brass post projecting through the glass capillary and contacting the liquid mercury column. The primary disadvantages of mercury as an electrode relate to environmental and safety concerns, difficulties in using mercury in flowing systems (although this is now possible to some extent), and its restriction to electroactive species amenable to cathodic reduction rather than to anodic oxidation. Problems of safety and practicality can be solved through the use of a multimode electrode polarographic/ voltammetric electrode assembly. This replaces the classic DME and can also generate a hanging mercury drop electrode (HMDE.) for use in stripping analysis, in addition to the intermediate static mercury drop electrode (SMDE). Multimode electrodes also offer replacement electrode assemblies for non-DME voltammetric applications in both quiet and stirred solutions. Rotating electrode designs can also be accommodated. For mercury electrodes, the multimode electrode is compact and does not require the gravitational force of the mercury column to extrude the drop. Rather, the drop is formed pneumatically, using nitrogen gas pressure. The mercury is hermetically sealed, an important safety consideration, and only a few milliliters are required for up to 200,000 drops without the need for refilling.

Classic d.c. Polarography

In classic polarography at the DME, as with classical electrolysis, the electrochemical reduction occurs when the applied potential becomes sufficiently negative, i.e., when the applied potential exceeds the threshold value for a given depolarizer. The applied potential is in the form of a linearly increasing voltage ramp with a typical slope of between 2 and 10 mVs^{-1}. Unlike electrolysis, however, the current resulting from application of the ramp voltage does not continue to increase indefinitely until all the electroactive material is consumed. This current is limited because when the applied potential is sufficiently negative, the rate of electron transfer becomes instantaneous and exceeds the rate of supply of the depolarizer to the electrode surface. Because the depolarizer can reach the electrode surface only by diffusion along a concentration gradient, the process is said to be diffusion-limited, and the resulting electron-transfer current is the limiting diffusion current, i_d. The limiting diffusion current is directly proportional to the analyte concentration in the bulk solution.

The electroactive species can also reach the electrode surface by migration under the influence of the electrical field between the electrodes. This gives rise to a migration current that is not diffusion- and, therefore, concentration-dependent. This migration current must be eliminated by providing an excess of charge carriers in the solution that are not discharged within the working potential range of the experiment. Various salt solutions may be used for this purpose. More conveniently, because electrochemical reactions are often pH-dependent, a buffer solution may be used. This solution is variously referred to as the base, inert, or supporting electrolyte. Therefore, although the ions of the supporting electrolyte will move through the solution and carry charge, no current will flow in the external circuit because no faradaic process will occur in the absence of a depolarizer.

The electroactive species can also reach the electrode surface by convection, giving rise to a convection current that is, again, non-concentration-dependent. Convection effects are attributable to stirring of the solution or, less frequently, to thermal currents. Thus, polarography and voltammetry are carried out in quiet (unstirred) solutions.

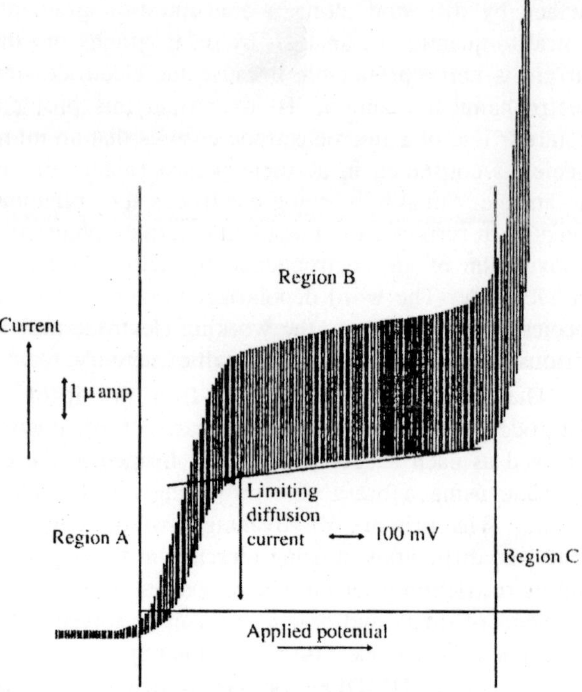

Fig. 16.2. Classic d.c. polarogram of diazepam (20 mg ml⁻¹) in 0.1 sulfuric acid as the supporting electrolyte.

The concentration-dependent mass transport process, when other mass transport processes have been eliminated, is diffusion of the electroactive species toward the electrode surface along a concentration gradient. As the electroactive species approaches the surface of the DME, it will be electrochemically reduced. Thus, in a narrow solution layer, the diffusion layer, immediately adjacent to the drop surface, there will be a lower concentration of the electroactive species than that present in the bulk solution, giving rise to the concentration gradient. It may be shown from Fick's law of diffusion that for an electroactive species diffusing across a thin diffusion layer of thickness d, the diffusion current, i_d, will be given by Eq. (1).

$$i_d = n \cdot F \cdot A \cdot D \cdot (C - C_i)/d \quad \ldots(1)$$

where D is the diffusion coefficient of the electroactive species, F is Faraday's Constant, A is the drop surface area, n is the number of electrons transferred per molecule of depolarizer, C is the bulk concentration of the depolarizer, and C_i is its concentration in the diffusion layer.

As C_i approaches zero, the rate of diffusion becomes proportional to the concentration of depolarizer in the bulk solution. Beyond the threshold potential, the electron transfer reaction will be initiated, and, as the potential is gradually increased, the rate of this reaction will continue to increase until it exceeds the rate of supply of the depolarizer to the electrode surface by diffusion, with all other mass transport processes having been suppressed. Under these conditions, the diffusion process becomes the rate-limiting step, and the resulting faradaic current, id, is now said to be the limiting diffusion current. Because id is measured over many individual drop lifetimes, it is properly described as the average limiting diffusion current and is given by Eq. (2), where i_d and C are the only variables.

$$i_d = n \cdot F \cdot A \cdot D \cdot C/d \quad \ldots(2)$$

The limiting diffusion current is described quantitatively by the Ilkovic equation Eq. (3).

$$i_d = 708 \cdot n \cdot D^{1/2} \cdot m^{2/3} \cdot t^{1/6} \cdot C \quad \ldots(3)$$

where m is the rate of flow of mercury from the DME in mg s^{-1} and t is the drop lifetime in seconds. D has units of $cm^2\ s^{-1}$, C is expressed as mMl^{-1}, and i_d is expressed in mA.

Electrical Double Layer

When only the inert electrolyte is present in the polarographic cell a residual current will still flow. This current, which is non-faradaic, is attributable to the formation of an electrical double layer in the solution adjacent to the electrode surface. At all applied potentials, a current flows to develop this double layer, and the process may be considered analogous to the charging of a parallel plate capacitor. Therefore, the charging current is a capacitance current and varies during the drop lifetime, i.e., with the size of the mercury drop. When the drop surface area is increasing rapidly from the start of the drop lifetime, the capacitance current is a maximum, falling to a minimum near the end of the drop lifetime when the drop size is at amaximum and the surface area of the drop is momentarily constant. The magnitude and direction of the capacitance current vary with the applied potential because of the variation in the surface tension of mercury with electrode potential. When the mercury drop is at its maximum surface tension, there is effectively no electrical double layer at the drop surface and, therefore, no capacitance current, a point known as the electrocapillary maximum. Beyond this potential, the capacitance current changes direction as the double layer is reversed, with the mercury drop now possessing a negative charge. The practical consequence of this is to impose the familiar serrated pattern on the polarographic wave.

Mechanisms of Electrode Processes

The shape of the polarographic wave is further influenced by the nature of the electrode process occurring at the drop surface. Polarographic waves may be reversible, irreversible, or quasireversible. The overall electrode process comprises the diffusion, electron transfer, and electrochemical reaction steps.

Reversible processes are those that attain thermodynamic equilibrium at every instant of the drop life owing to rapid electron transfer. Reversible processes give rise to well-defined d.c. polarograms, and diffusion control is always the determining factor. Irreversible processes are so slow that equilibrium is not attained during the drop lifetime, and d.c. polarograms dependent on such processes often show poor definition. The rate-controlling step may be either the electron transfer process or the subsequent chemical reaction. Many organic reductions at the DME, however, fall into an intermediate category, quasireversible processes. Whereas the rate constant for the reverse reaction will be negligible for a wholly irreversible reaction, it has an intermediate value for quasireversible reactions. Such reactions are normally seen only with longer drop times of at least 3 s. The reversibility, or otherwise, of an electrode process is best investigated using the technique of cyclic voltammetry, in which a rapid

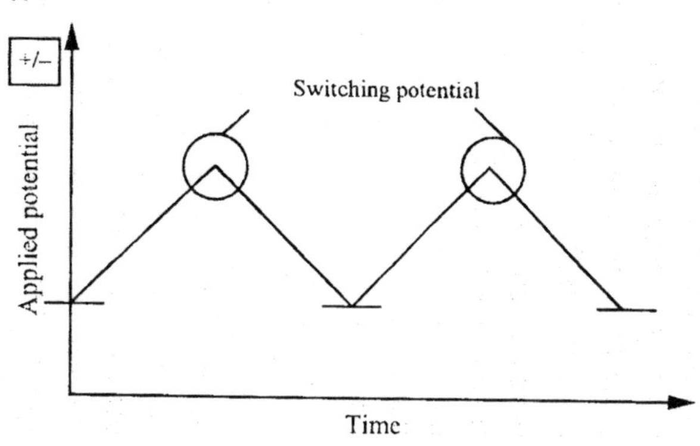

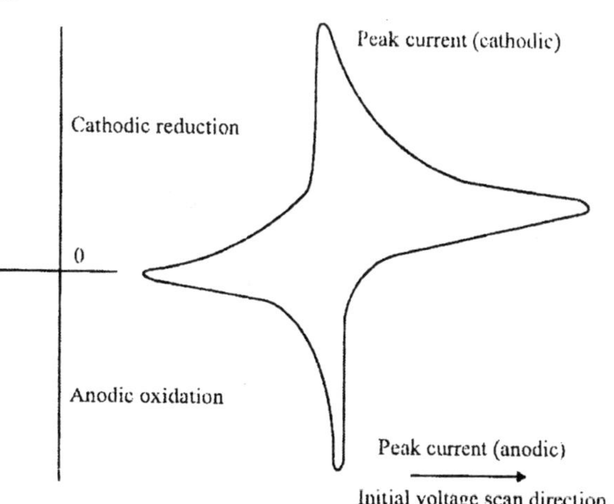

Fig. 16.3. Cyclic voltammetry. A–Voltage waveform showing the rapid forward and reverse voltage sweeps. B–Typical cyclic voltammogram for completely reversible system.

forward and reverse voltage ramp is applied in triangular form to interact with both the electroactive substance and its reduction product that, for quasi- or fully reversible processes, may be oxidized back to the starting material. The separation between anodic and cathodic peaks indicates whether the electrode process is quasi- or fully reversible. Additional mechanistic investigations can also be made in respect to the number of electrons involved per molecule in the electron transfer process, a factor that can be determined by controlled-potential coulometry.

Effect of Oxygen in Polarography

In polarography, but not in anodic voltammetry, it is necessary to provide a facility for removing oxygen from the electrolyte solution in the polarographic cell. This is normally achieved by bubbling oxygen-free nitrogen through the solution for 10 min before starting the voltage scan. The surface of the solution is then blanketed by oxygen-free nitrogen during the polarographic run to prevent ingress of additional oxygen from the atmosphere. Removal of oxygen is necessary because the dissolved gas is polarographically active and can mask the analytical signal of interest in certain potential regions.

Modern Polarographic and Voltammetric Methods

In classic d.c. polarography, the actual current measured comprises the limiting diffusion current, together with current components, because of background electrical signals and, more important, the current charging the double layer capacitor at the electrode surface. Classic d.c. polarography is in many ways best suited to the elucidation of electrode processes. It lacks sensitivity for modern analytical purposes, and the sigmoidal current/voltage curves are difficult to measure. Modern polarographic and voltammetric methods are now available in which these problems have generally been resolved, producing an analytical technique with much enhanced sensitivity and a more easily interpretable current–voltage waveform.

Current-Sampled d.c. Polarography

Current-sampled polarography is a modern variant of the original tast polarography, a method that involved the measurement of the polarographic current only at a fixed time interval during each drop lifetime. This was originally accomplished by the use of a mechanical touching contact but is achieved in modern instruments using a digital approach in which the current is electronically sampled at a precise moment, typically 20 ms, near the end of the drop lifetime when the area of the drop is effectively constant. For this purpose, the drop lifetime is precisely and mechanically controlled by the instrument rather than being gravity-dependent, a feature shared by other modern methods. Current-sampled polarography produces a smooth polarogram by elimination of the current variation during the

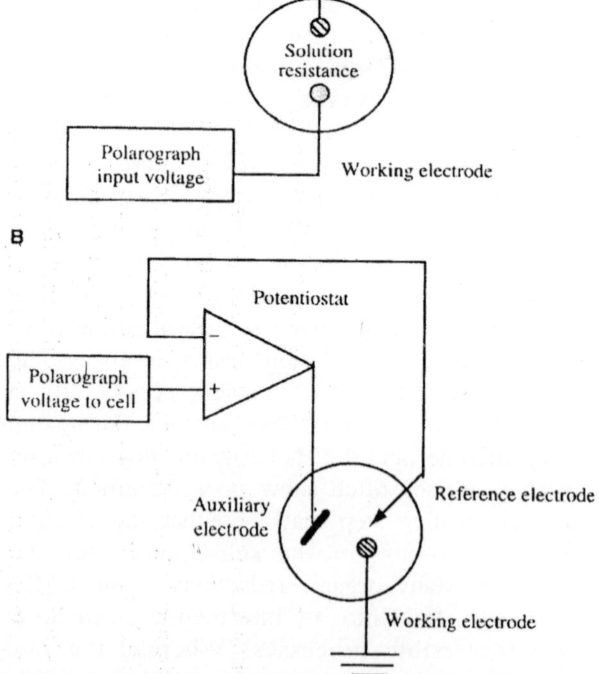

Fig. 16.4. Electrical circuitry for polarography/voltammetry. A–A simple two-electrode system. B–Illustrates a modern three-electrode system incorporating a potentiostat circuit.

drop lifetime. However, although the typical serrations of the classic polarogram are gone, a slight staircase pattern can still be discerned on the current- sampled polarogram, a feature shared with many other modern voltammetric methods. The staircase pattern is attributable to the sampled current being held in the memory of the instrument and its value fed out continuously to the recording device until the next sampling period. Current-sampled polarography offers only a marginal improvement on the sensitivity of the classic method because there is a more favorable faradaic-to-charging-current ratio at the end of the drop time when the drop is almost stationary. Thus, its only real benefit over the classic method is the clearer polarogram obtained.

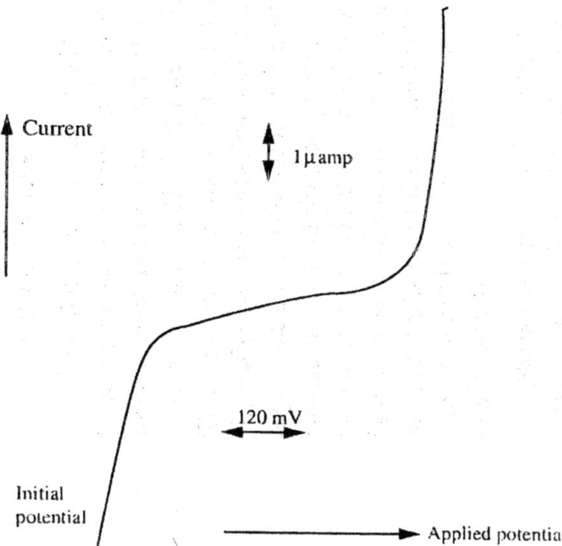

Fig. 16.5. A typical current-sampled polarogram. Note the staircase pattern indicating the individual current sampling periods.

Pulse Polarography

For routine quantitative analysis, pulse polarography and voltammetry are perhaps the most useful of the modern variants on the classic method. Unlike d.c. and current-sampled polarography, the applied voltage is not a simple d.c. ramp but has a more complex format involving periodic application of the potential during short time intervals. There are two major pulse methods: normal (integral) pulse and differential pulse polarography/voltammetry, although many variations of these are now available.

The primary advantage of pulse methods is its significantly more favorable faradaic-to-charging-current ratio and, in the case of differential pulse methods, a more conventional Gaussian-shaped waveform for the current potential plot. In pulse methods, the initial charging current is increased when the pulse is applied, effectively giving a pulse charging current. If the pulse falls on the rising (faradaic) portion of the polarogram/voltammogram, there will be a large increase in current, over and above the value of the pulse charging current. Provided the pulse has been applied at the end of the drop lifetime, when the drop surface area of the DME is briefly constant, or if a solid electrode is used, then both currents will decay from the point of the initial pulse application, the current decay being a function of time. However, the charging current component of the total measured current decays much more rapidly than does the faradaic component. Thus, if the current is measured (sampled) at the end of the pulse application period, it will consist primarily of the faradaic component, thus yielding a marked sensitivity increase over d.c. methods. Sensitivity is also greater because the boundary diffusion layer at the electrode-solution interface is narrower than is that when the potential is applied continuously. Therefore, the rate of diffusion of the electroactive species toward the electrode is increased, with a concomitant increase in the diffusion current.

Normal (Integral) Pulse Polarography/Voltammetry (NPP/NPV)

In NPP/NPV, the voltage is applied in a series of increasing voltage pulses from a baseline voltage selected by the analyst. Between pulses, the baseline voltage is restored. The pulse amplitude increases linearly with time, depending on the conditions set by the operator. The voltage pulse is applied at the end of the drop lifetime in polarography. Although precise timings vary with different instruments, typically the voltage pulse is applied for the last 60 ms of the drop. As with current-sampled polarography, the resulting current is sampled over only the final 20 ms of the drop lifetime, producing a polarogram/voltammogram identical in appearance to that of the current-sampled technique but with a greater current yield. The appearance of the polarogram is perceived to be the primary disadvantage of NPP/NPV because analysts tend to prefer a more conventional Gaussian-shaped graphic output of data, the sigmoidal shape being difficult to quantify.

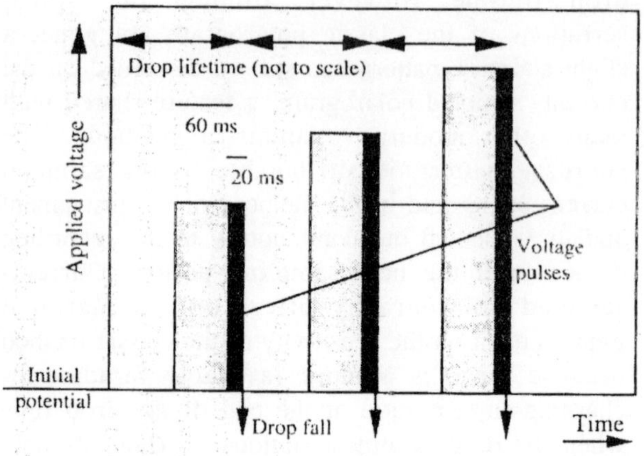

Fig. 16.6. Applied voltage waveform for normal pulse polarography.

Differential Pulse Polarography/Voltammetry (DPP/DPV)

DPP and DPV are probably the most analytically useful of all the voltammetric methods. DPP and DPV produce current-potential plots in the typical peak form familiar to, and readily interpretable by, the analyst. DPP and DPV result from a variation in the pattern of the applied voltage. In DPP/DPV, a small fixed voltage pulse of between 5 and 100mV is superimposed on a slow linear voltage ramp. When the ramp voltage coincides with the faradaic process, a faradiac current occurs continuously, along with the charging current. When the small pulse voltage is applied, in addition to the ramp voltage, at a given time, then both a new faradaic and a new charging current will be generated. As with NPP/NPV, the faradaic component decays during the pulse application, which, for polarography, is at the end of the drop lifetime. The charging current owing to the pulse also decays, but much more rapidly than the faradaic component so that if the current is sampled at the end of the pulse application, there is maximum separation between faradaic and charging currents and, thus, maximum sensitivity. In fact, in DPP/DPV the current is sampled twice, typically for 20 ms immediately before application of the pulse and again for the last 20 ms of the pulse application. The differential signal thus recorded results from the small increase in current (di) because of the small increase in the applied voltage pulse (dE). This further reduces the charging current contribution before the pulse and leads to an additional sensitivity increase over NPP/NPV. Effectively, it is the derivative (di/dE) of the classic polarographic wave that is produced. This quantity, when plotted against the applied potential, yields a peak-shaped output because the change in the faradaic component when the constant voltage pulse is applied reaches a maximum on the steepest part of the polarogram and falls to almost zero in the baseline and plateau regions.

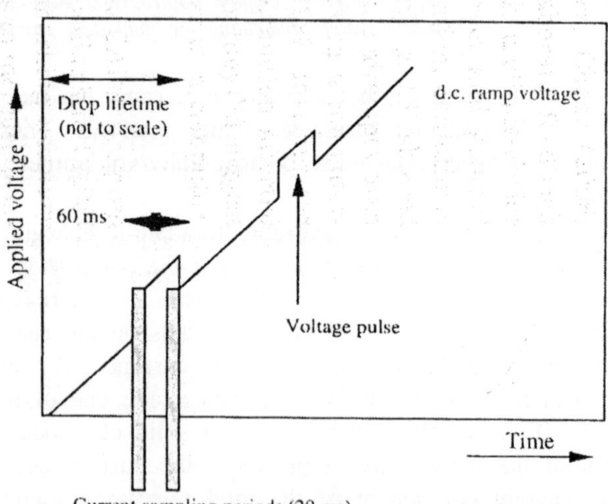

Fig. 16.7. Applied voltage waveform for differential pulse polarography.

The sensitivity of DPP/DPV exceeds even that of the normal pulse method by approximately a single order of magnitude, being approximately equivalent to that of gas chromatography with F.I.D. (approximately 10^{-8} M). It may, therefore, be used for the determination of drugs in biological matrices. In addition, DPP and DPV have excellent resolving power, being able to differentiate peaks, which are no more than 50 mV apart, owing to different electroactive species in the same solution. Both normal and differential pulse techniques are suitable for use with solid working electrodes such as glassy carbon. The various instrumental timings remain the same even though the constraint imposed by the variable area of the DME has been removed. The $E_{1/2}$ value is, of course, not discernible from DPP/DPV and is replaced by the near-identical quantity E_p, the peak potential.

The magnitude of the peak current (i_p) in DPP/ DPV is given by Eq. (4).

$$i_p = \frac{n^2F^2}{RT} \cdot \Delta E \cdot A \cdot C \cdot \frac{D}{\sqrt{\pi t}} \cdot \frac{\exp(E - E_{12} + 0.5E) \cdot CnF/RT}{\{1 + [\exp(E - E_{1/2} + 0.5E) \cdot nF/RT]\}^2} \qquad \ldots(4)$$

where n is the number of electrons transferred in the electrode reaction, F is Faraday's constant, R is the universal gas constant, T is the absolute temperature, ΔE is the pulse amplitude or modulation, A is the electrode surface area, C is the concentration of the electroactive species, D is the diffusion coefficient of the electroactive species, t is the time elapsed from pulse application to current measurement, E is the ramp potential just before application of the pulse, and $E_{1/2}$ is the half-wave potential.

Eq. (4) indicates that a linear relationship exists between peak current in DPP/DPV and peak potential and that the peak current will increase with pulse amplitude. However, the charging current also increases with pulse amplitude so that the value for ΔE must be chosen to maximize i_p but must not be too large; otherwise, resolution of the peak will be diminished. Typical values for ΔE are 50 or 100 mV.

Linear Sweep Voltammetry (LSV)

Linear sweep voltammetry involves the application of a rapid voltage scan, 100 mV s^{-1} or higher, to a stationary electrode such as the HMDE or a solid electrode such as glassy carbon. The theoretical treatment is based on the Randles-Sevcik equation. At slow scan rates, the magnitude of the concentration gradient across the diffusion layer is governed by the rate of depletion of the electroactive species across this layer. With the fast scan rates used in LSV, the diffusion layer is narrower, the concentration gradient is consequently larger, and the resulting diffusion current is greater. As the depolarizer is used up by reaction at the electrode surface, the diffusion layer widens as it extends further into the bulk solution, and, unlike the DME, equilibrium conditions are not periodically restored by the stirring effect of the falling drop. Thus, there is a gradual decay in the diffusion current, giving a peak-like appearance to the LSV output. The rapidly increasing potential in LSV results in non-equilibrium conditions at the electrode surface throughout the period of the voltage scan.

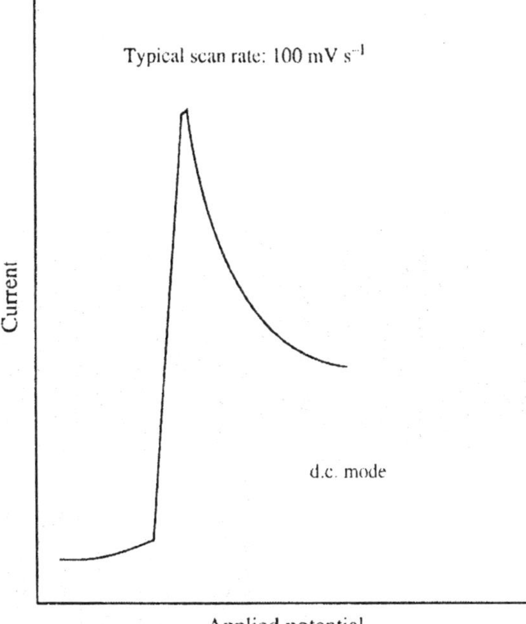

Fig. 16.8. Typical appearance of a linear sweep voltammogram at a fast-scan rate of 100 mV s^{-1}.

Alternating Current Polarography/Voltammetry (ACP/ACV)

Alternating current polarography and voltammetry encompass a wide range of polarographic and voltammetric modes characterized by a periodic applied voltage waveform, such as a square-wave, pulsed, or saw-tooth pattern. The production of such waveforms may require a voltage function generator in addition to the normal polarograph, although some instruments have the function generator built in and can therefore perform ACP/ACV as a standard technique. The most common applications of ACP/ACV involve the application of a small-amplitude sinusoidal alternating potential superimposed onto a ramp voltage. The resulting current is an alternating current, the d.c. component being filtered out by use of a phase-sensitive current detector. This is possible because the faradaic and charging components of the current, respectively, have phase angles of 45 and 90° with reference to the applied sinusoidal potential. The detector rejects the 90° component and measures only the faradaic current.

The applied sinusoidal voltage has a typical amplitude range of ±50 mV, and the polarogram is a plot of the fundamental harmonic alternating current (a.c.) against the ramp voltage. Because the d.c. current component is filtered out, the current values before and after the rising portion of the d.c. polarogram are close to zero in the a.c. mode, and therefore, the resulting polarogram has a peak shape that approximately follows the rising portion of the d.c. wave. The use of a fast voltage scan, analogous to LSV, is possible with ACV at a solid (stationary) electrode. The special case of square-wave voltammetry (SWV) is worth noting separately from other alternating current techniques because it is both more rapid and more sensitive than DPP/DPV. In SWV, the applied potential waveform is a staircase with constant step height on which is superimposed an asymmetrical forward and reverse voltage pulse of constant amplitude and very short duration, typically less than 10 ms. Thus, the entire polarogram may be run in about approximately 1 s, with the enhanced sensitivity of the method owing to sampling of the current at the end of both the forward and reverse directions of the pulse.

Stripping Voltammetry

This is an ultrasensitive technique most widely used in the trace determination of metals and, increasingly, for organic compounds, including pharmaceuticals. The outstanding sensitivity of the method is due to an initial pre-concentration (accumulation) step that can result in a 1000-fold increase in the available analyte concentration compared with the bulk solution. The most commonly used working electrode design for stripping analysis has a single mercury drop hanging from the electrode tip during the course of the stripping experiment. Such an electrode is the HMDE, although other designs such as the mercury film electrode (MFE), in which the mercury is supported as a thin film on a carbon electrode support, and SMDE have become increasingly important. The SMDE allows faster stirring rates during the deposition step than are possible with the HMDE, the limiting factor in the latter case being the dislodgement of the mercury drop by vigorous stirring. In addition to mercury, non- plated solid electrodes fabricated from a noble metal (gold or platinum) or from carbon (glassy carbon, carbon paste) have also been used for stripping analysis, typically for the determination of metals that are insoluble in mercury that have very positive redox potentials. For most pharmaceutical applications of stripping analysis that involve organic compounds, mercury electrodes are used. Stripping analysis can then be performed using a conventional modern polarograph linked to a specific working electrode suitable for the chosen analysis.

Stripping analysis for compounds of pharmaceutical interest consists of two steps. First, the electroactive material is deposited onto a mercury electrode, thus concentrating the analate by extracting it from the bulk solution. This controlled deposition, which may be electrolytic, is carried out for a defined time period, with constant stirring of the bulk solution because, in this case, it is necessary to drive the analyte toward the electrode surface as efficiently as possible. Second, there is the stripping step. This involves stripping (removing) the analyte from the electrode surface back into the solution by application of a suitable potential. This second step is the measurement step, the resulting faradaic current being quantitative in respect to the amount of analate present in the bulk solution. The applied potential can be a simple ramp voltage, pulse, or periodic waveform. Thus, most of the modern polarographic modes can be coupled to the stripping step to give additional increases in both sensitivity and selectivity. Fast stripping steps such as the use of the semidifferential mode have become increasing popular, although differential pulse and linear sweep modes remain prevalent.

Anodic stripping voltammetry (ASV) has been the most widely used stripping variant, typically for the trace analysis of metals in solution. Thus, an electrolytic deposition step onto a mercury cathode, possibly lasting several minutes, is followed by an anodic stripping step in which the potential scan goes toward positive values. The deposition step itself results in the formation of a metal amalgam. As with all stripping variants, hydrodynamic parameters (stirring rate, deposition time, solution composition, electrode location) must be carefully controlled and reproducible to obtain a quantitative response to changing bulk concentrations. The process may be summarized as:

Cathodic deposition : $M^{n+} + ne \rightleftarrows M(Hg) \downarrow$

Anodic stripping $M(Hg) \rightarrow M^{n+} + ne + Hg$

Cathodic stripping voltammetry (CSV) may be considered the reverse of ASV in that the electrolytic deposition step is carried out at a positive (anodic) applied potential, the deposited analate then being stripped by application of a cathodic voltage scan. CSV has been used for the determination of various anions and for certain drug molecules such as organosulfur compounds. CSV may be summarized as:

Anodic deposition: $2Hg \rightleftarrows Hg^{2+} + 2e$

$Hg_2^{2+} + \rightleftarrows 2A^- Hg_2A_2\downarrow$

Cathodic stripping: $Hg_2A_2 + 2e$ ® $2Hg + 2A^-$

Adsorptive stripping voltammetry (AdSV) is of increasing importance in trace determinations of pharmaceutical compounds. In this method, the preconcentration step is adsorptive rather than electrolytic, resulting in an adsorbed film of the analate on the electrode surface. The stripping step typically uses LSV or the differential pulse mode in either the cathodic or anodic direction, as required. The HMDE is typically used for cathodic reductive stripping, whereas carbon or noble metal electrodes are used in the adsorptive mode.

Factors affecting the adsorptive process in AdSV include the solvent, solution pH, mass-transport processes, stirring rate, deposition time, and applied potential. The sensitivity advantage of AdSV over conventional polarography/voltammetry using an equivalent mode may be up to 100-fold. However, the primary advantage of AdSV is its ability to simplify sample preparation when the analyte is in a complex matrix, such as the determination of a drug or its metabolite in body fluids. Having adsorbed the analyte to the electrode directly from the complex medium, the electrode with the adsorbed analate film may then be transferred to a blank electrolyte solution before the stripping step. This method, known as medium exchange, has considerable potential, particularly in a flow analysis mode for both pharmaceutical and clinical analyses. Its value is perhaps not yet fully realized because of a preference for, and greater familiarity with, chromatographic methods.

Electrochemical Detection for High-Performance Liquid Chromatography (ELCD) and Flow-Injection Analysis (ED-FIA)

Pharmaceutical analysts often have no experience in direct polarographic or voltammetric methods, but almost all will have used high-performance liquid chromatography (HPLC) for the determination of drugs and/or metabolites in biological matrices or drugs and/ or their degradation products in pharmaceutical formulations. Spectroscopy (ultraviolet and fluorescence) is the most common detection method in HPLC, but for molecules that do not possess a suitable chromophore or when increased sensitivity or specificity is required, electrochemical detection offers a suitable alternative. ELCD is applicable to any molecular species capable of electrochemical oxidation or reduction at an electrode. Most detectors are based on solid electrodes, notably carbon paste and, particularly, glassy carbon. These detectors are best operated in the anodic mode, but they can also be used for reductive processes. Alternatively, mercury films on a noble metal electrode can be used for cathodic reduction.

The principle of ELCD has been addressed in detail by Stulik and Pacakova. The detector is set to an applied voltage large enough to cause the electrochemical reaction of interest to occur, i.e., the applied voltage is on the plateau of the polarographic wave. Thus, when the species of interest is eluted from the column, a faradaic current is produced in the detector and results in the usual chromatographic signal. This is an example of amperometric detection because an electrical current is responsible for the analytical signal. With a solid electrode, the detector may be described as a voltammetric detector. Various detector cell designs are available. The most common configuration is the wall-jet cell, in which the eluent is sprayed against an internal wall of the detector cell. The wall is fabricated from glassy carbon, a highly polished and impermeable material. The flowing eluent spray ensures that any products from the electrochemical oxidation reaction are removed from the electrode surface, thus ensuring signal reproducibility.

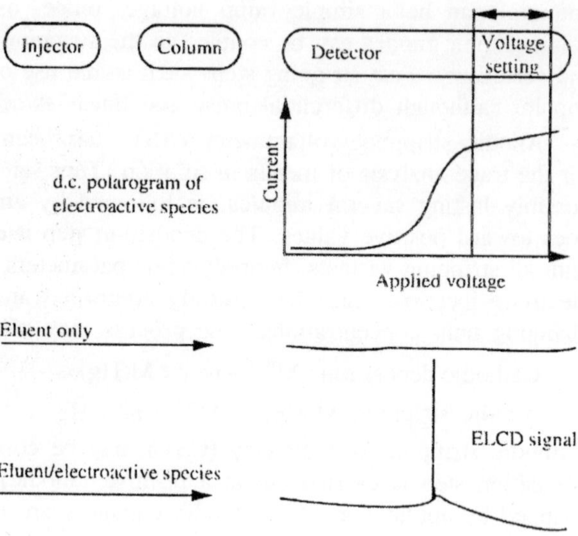

Fig. 16.9. Principle of electrochemical detection for HPLC.

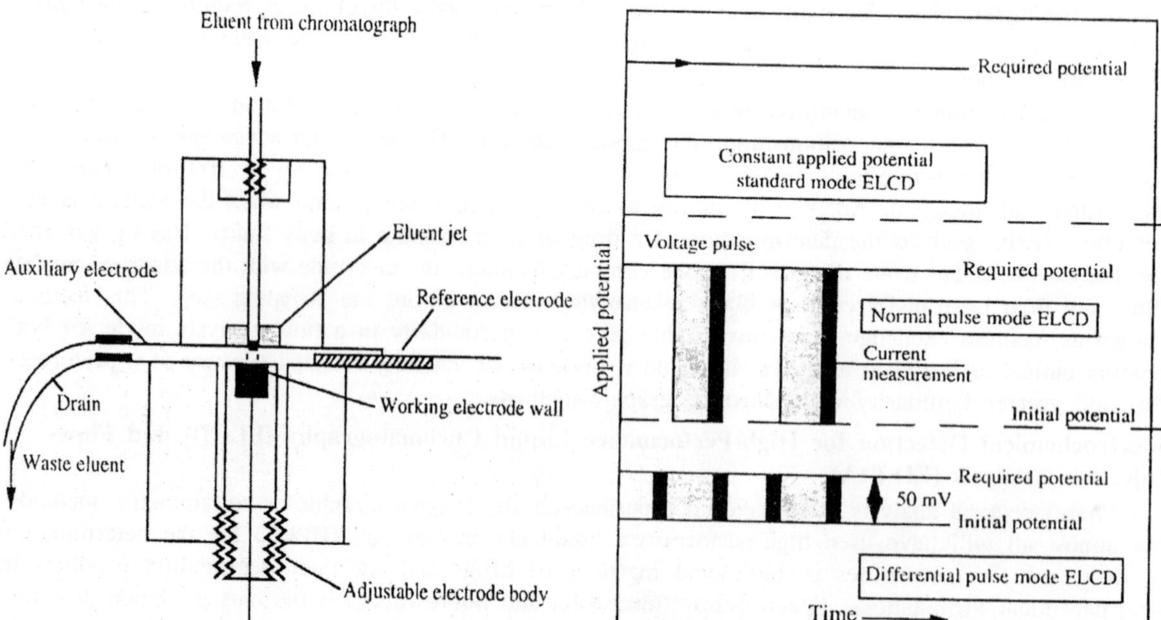

Fig. 16.10. Wall-jet electrochemical detector cell for HPLC.

Fig. 16.11. Applied voltage waveforms for various models of electrochemical detection in HPLC.

In conjunction with the various designs of electrochemical detector cells, a range of applied voltage waveforms may be used for ELCD. The differential pulse mode is particularly suited to ELCD because it can further enhance the separability of components by selectively setting the detector to the peak potential of an individual component in a mixture. Additional information can also be obtained using a rapid-scan square-wave detector. As the name implies, this mode uses very fast voltage scans so that a three-dimensional output can be obtained. In effect, many voltammograms are run of a component as it elutes from the column, giving an output of current vs. applied potential vs. time. Thus, peak purity can be checked, and the device is analogous in its applications to the better known diode array spectrophotometric detector. Voltammetric detectors may also be used in a flow-injection mode,[17] effectively omitting the chromatographic step, for drug analysis. Again, a wide range of detector cell designs and polarographic/voltammetric modes are available.

The availability of a wide range of modern polarographic and voltammetric modes, together with the use of ELCD and stripping analysis, offers the analyst powerful analytical tools for performing drug assays. The decision as to whether an electroanalytical method should be used for a given assay and the selection of a particular polarographic/voltammetric technique will depend on the drug of interest, the analytical matrix, and the type of data that are required. Given the advances in analytical instrumentation, polarography/voltammetry may now be used with confidence, when necessary, by all pharmaceutical analysts.

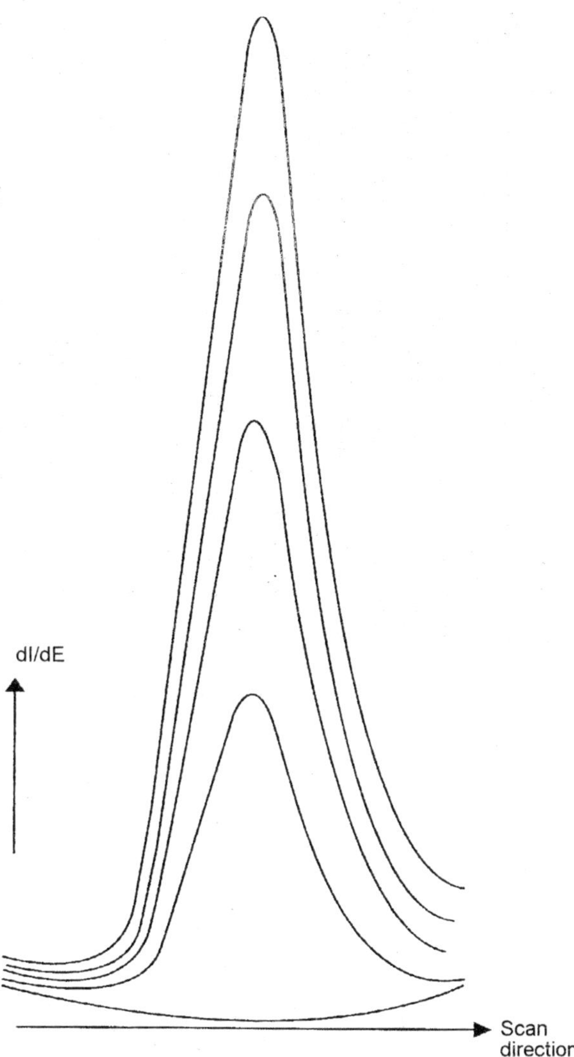

Fig. 16.12. Differential pulse voltammogram of pyridoxine hydrochloride at the glassy carbon electrode obtained by adding successive aliquouts of an aqueous solution of the vitamin to pH 4 citric acid as the supporting electrolyte.

17

Electrical Power Systems

Electrical power systems that serve pharmaceutical equipment must be safe, reliable, functional, predictable, flexible, clean, and sometimes validated. The electrical power systems have voltages ranging from 120 to 69,000 V. Pharmaceutical plants in the United States and Canada can purchase 3 phase, 60 Hz electric power from utility companies that is more reliable than the power they could generate in house. Whereas in other countries, electric power is purchased at 3 phase, 50 Hz, and may not be as reliable as power that is generated in the plant.

This article is meant to convey a basic understanding of various power distribution system configurations and familiarize the reader with the electrical distribution equipment that are commonly installed within pharmaceutical plants in the United States. It will help in the evaluation of both new and existing electrical power distribution systems that serve pharmaceutical equipment.

Electrical Power Sources

Electricity can be purchased from an energy provider or can be generated in the pharmaceutical plant. Usually, purchased electricity is cheaper than on-site generated electricity. Large plants have many options when purchasing electricity. A thorough understanding of these options can significantly reduce the electrical operating cost and will increase the reliability of the electrical power system. All plants and especially small- and medium-size plants must accurately determine their current and future normal electrical power loads and normal/emergency power loads when deciding how to purchase electricity and how to install a reliable electrical power system.

The pharmaceutical plant's electrical loads can be divided into four categories:

1. Normal loads—Loads that can be turned off for a period of time without creating a hazardous condition or causing a substantial loss of product or research.
2. Standby loads—Loads that if they lose electricity will cause a hazardous condition or cause a substantial loss of product or research but which can sustain a power interruption of 60 sec.
3. Standby non-interruptible load—Loads that cannot sustain any interruption in power.
4. Emergency loads—Legally required emergency and egress lighting and other loads classified as such by governmental agencies and locally adopted building codes.

Loads can be further divided into groups based on their utilization voltage, category, type, and location within the plant. Typical utilization voltages within pharmaceutical plants include 480/277 and 208/ 120 V. Categories include linear and non-linear loads. Linear loads typically include incandescent lamps and induction motors that are not controlled by a variable frequency drive (VFD). Non-linear loads include all loads that have switching power supplies or silicon control rectifiers such as VFDs, uninterruptible power supplies, and electronic ballasts on 480/277 V systems and personal computers, copy machines, faxes, electronic devices, and instruments on 208/120 V systems. Types include continuous loads such as lighting that stay on all day and non-continuous loads that will not operate for more than 3 hr at a time. The areas in the plant should be divided into locations based on the function or process performed in the area and based on whether or not the area being classified is a current good manufacturing practices (cGMP) area. The load projections should be based on a minimum of 7 years. To obtain the group demand for each group of loads, multiply the connected load for the group by a diversity factor that reflects the proportion of load that will operate at any one time to the total connected load. The sum of the group demands will equal the plant's maximum demand. After determining the maximum demand, consult with the local public utility company for assistance in determining the optimum voltage and configuration for the electrical service entrance for the plant.

The ampacity or rated current carrying capacity of the electrical service entrance conductors that connect the utility company's lines to the plant's service entrance equipment must be a minimum of 125% of the calculated maximum demand for continuous loads plus 100% of the maximum calculated demand for non-continuous loads. Service entrance conductors and equipment with higher ratings or provisions to increase the rating of the service entrance conductors are recommended. Large plants, which have a central utility plant (CUP) with chiller motors rated above 200 hp, should consider purchasing and in some instances distributing electricity at primary voltage levels such as 4160 V and 13,800 V. An emergency generator should have a rating that is 25% and possibly 100% higher than the sum of the total calculated standby and emergency demand for the plant. Alternately, provisions for a future emergency generator should be provided as part of the initial installation. Discuss the type of fuel required for the generator's engine with the local authority having jurisdiction. The National Electrical Code, NFPA 70 (NEC), requires that the fuel be on site if the generator provides power for emergency loads. However, exceptions to this requirement have been permitted where reliable natural gas service is available.

Electrical Power System Utility Services

Primary services are typically installed for medium and large pharmaceutical plants and can be purchased as a single service, a dual service, or a regular-reserve service. The utility company will install two separate power lines to the plant for a dual service and for a regular-reserve service. Each dual service power line will normally serve half of the loads in the plant but each will be capable of serving all of the loads in the plant. Regular-reserve service power lines are connected to a common bus with only the regular power line normally serving all of the plant's loads. Secondary services are typically installed for small- to medium-size pharmaceutical plants. They are available at the utilization voltages of 277/480 or 120/208 V. Secondary services are less expensive to install and maintain than primary services. However, the kilowatt- hour cost for electrical power supplied by a secondary service is higher.

Secondary Configurations

The following items should be considered when planning an electrical power system's secondary, less than 1000 V, configuration.

1. The utility company will provide and own the transformer that will supply secondary voltage for the service to the plant. This transformer should be dedicated to the pharmaceutical plant and should have a grounded wye secondary. Sharing a utility-owned transformer with other utility customers will reduce the quality and the reliability of the electric service to the plant.
2. The size of the utility company's transformer will affect the rating of the service entrance equipment and the starting of large motors. If the transformer rating is low, reduced voltage starting will be

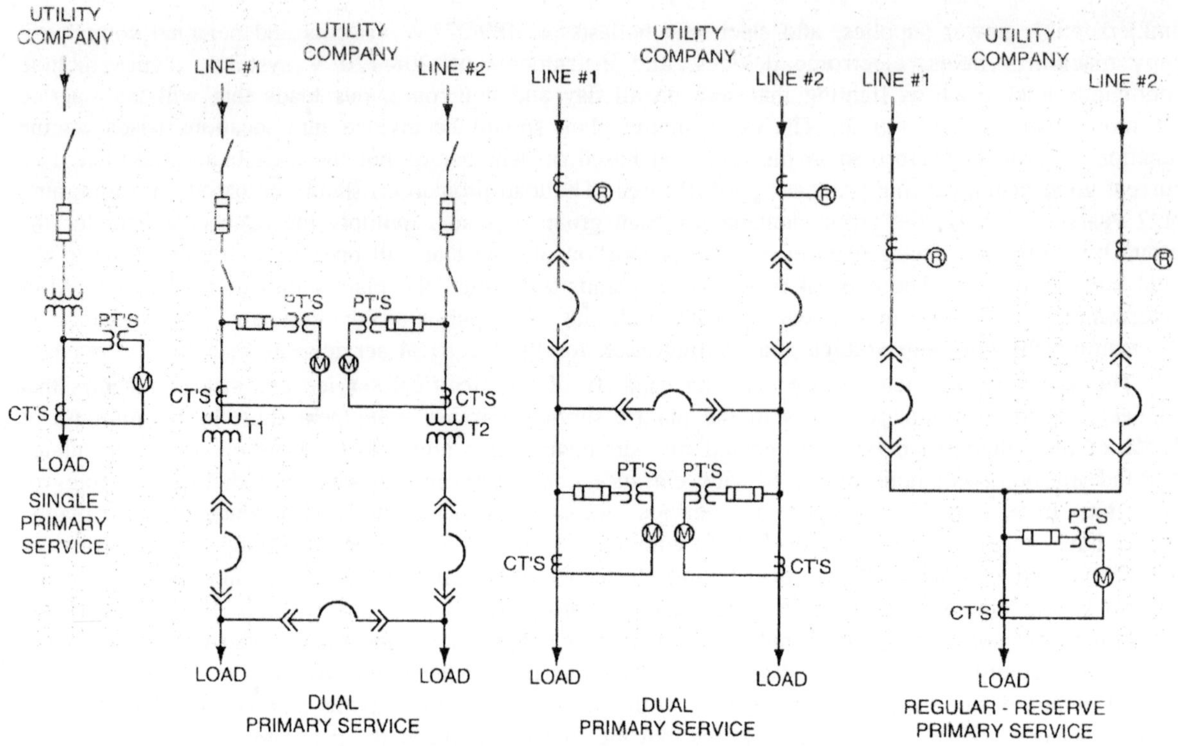

Fig. 17.1. Typical primary electric service arrangements.

required for starting large motors. If the transformer rating is high, service entrance equipment will require a high symmetrical short-circuit (IAC) rating. The utility company will provide the maximum available symmetrical short-circuit current available at the secondary of their transformer.

3. Service entrance equipment must have a current rating equal to or greater than the present and future service entrance conductors' ampacity. Moreover, this equipment must have an IAC current rating that is higher than the available short circuit current at the utility company's transformer. Spare service entrance conduits should be installed for future service entrance conductors. The service entrance equipment should include spaces for future feeder circuit breakers to supply future loads. All incoming service entrance conductors must be 3 phase, 4 wire and should be installed in underground metal conduit.
4. Service entrance equipment should be installed in an indoor electrical room whenever possible. The equipment should include one to six main service entrance power circuit breakers or load break disconnect switches and feeder circuit breakers for loads within the plant. Circuit breakers and disconnect switches for 480/277 V systems that are rated at 1000 A or more must include ground fault protection. Feeder circuit breakers will typically be molded case. Integrally fused circuit breakers are available with very high short circuit IAC ratings for both power and molded case circuit breakers. Fuses and current limiters for integrally fused circuit breakers must be stored within the electrical room.
5. Fuses should not be used to protect secondary voltage feeders. The time current characteristics of fuses above 100 A will not coordinate with the ground fault pickup currents and time delays of the main overcurrent protection (circuit breaker or fused disconnect switch) ground fault protection. A main load break disconnect switch can be equipped with current-limiting fuses to reduce the

available short-circuit current from the utility and should have a three-phase voltage relay for single-phase protection.

6. Ground fault protection, including circuit breakers or relays, should be set as low as possible without causing nuisance tripping. The ground fault pickup and time delay for the main overcurrent protection should coordinate with the trip characteristics of the largest feeder circuit breaker that does not have ground fault protection and must be less than the maximum current permitted by the NEC.
7. If fuses are used in the power distribution system, three-phase motor starters should have solid-state overload devices that include single- phase protection.
8. Two (2) to six (6) separate service entrance cables connected to the secondary side of one utility owned transformer can connect to separate main circuit breakers or main load brake fused disconnect switches that are mounted next to each other. The sum of the ampacity of all of the service entrance conductors must have a current rating equal to or greater than the present and future maximum demand for the plant. This approach can reduce the cost of the service entrance installation but will not provide the additional level of protection provided by having one main circuit breaker or one main fused disconnect switch. Therefore it is not as reliable.
9. A maintenance program should document all tests, inspections, and faults cleared by a main and feeder circuit breaker. Lack of such a program will reduce the reliability of the electrical equipment. Molded case circuit breakers require no internal maintenance. They should be inspected for broken casing and loose connections after they operate to clear a fault and should be replaced after they have operated to clear two faults. Feeder circuit breakers, especially older circuit breakers, should be exercised (repeatedly opened and closed) whenever possible. Part of the initial commissioning of an electrical power system must include testing of the ground fault protection.
10. The secondary selective circuit arrangement is recommended for all critical loads. It requires the installation of double-ended switch-gear or a variation thereof. Double-ended switchgear includes two main circuit breakers that serve separate feeder buses with a tie circuit breaker in the middle. Each feeder bus has its own set of feeder or branch circuit breakers. The load should be evenly split between each of the feeder buses.
11. Important loads can be connected to redundant feeder circuit breakers, one on each side of the double-ended switchgear, by connecting the load sides of the circuit breakers together with a feeder cable. This approach should be used with caution. Another approach is to connect the redundant feeder circuit breakers to a time-delayed automatic transfer switch.

Primary Configurations

The following items should be considered when planning an electrical power distribution system's primary configuration.

1. A single primary service can have one to six primary service entrance circuit breakers or fused disconnect switches. These overcurrent devices will protect primary feeders that distribute power to distribution unit substations located in electrical rooms throughout the plant, to primary voltage motor starters in the CUP, and sometimes to generator switchgear when the generator system is designed for momentary or continuous operation in parallel with the utility line.
2. Double-ended unit substations provide economical, reliable, pre-engineered, and factory- tested configuration for obtaining secondary selective circuit arrangements at utilization voltage of 480/277 or 120/208 V and for installing a primary selective circuit arrangements. Double-ended unit substations include one or two main primary circuit breakers or fused disconnect switches on both sides that are connected to transformers that are connected to the feeder circuit breaker sections.

Each feeder circuit breaker section has a main secondary circuit breaker that protects the internal bus, which connects to the feeder circuit breaker, and is connected to the other feeder circuit breaker section through a secondary tie circuit breaker. Each transformer should be rated to carry at least 125% of the maximum present and future connected load for the entire double-ended substation.

3. A dual service will have two main service entrance circuit breakers and a service entrance tie circuit breaker and may have additional primary feeder circuit breakers. A regular-reserve service will have two main service entrance circuit breakers and may have additional primary feeder circuit breakers. In very large pharmaceutical plants, the primary feeder circuit breakers will connect to outdoor substation transformers that will provide 4160 V for the CUP and 13,800 V for distribution unit substations.
4. Unit substations, each consisting of a primary fused disconnect switch or circuit breaker, a dry transformer, and secondary switchgear should be in a central location near their loads. Unit substation transformers should be sized to carry at least 125% the maximum present and future connected load.
5. Primary selective circuit arrangements utilize two primary selectable feeders for each transformer. These feeders are either connected to the line side of two interlocked primary non- fused disconnect switches that have a common load side fuse or to the line side of two interlocked primary fused disconnect switches.
6. Dry-type transformers are typically installed indoors and include ventilated, sealed, or gas filled, totally enclosed non-ventilated, and cast coil types. Cast coil transformers are the most expensive and they have the highest overload capability. Transformers should be sized based on their air to air (AA) rating. Provisions for future automatic fans that will provide a higher force air (FA) rating and an alarm that indicates when the fans are operating due to the temperature within the transformer should be provided.
7. If installed outdoors, pad mounted liquid filled transformers up to 2500 KVA are available with mineral oil or less flammable silicon liquids. Outdoor liquid-filled transformers sometimes have an advantage over outdoor dry-type transformers, which present a relatively difficult lightning protection problem because of their lower basic impulse levels (insulation level). Substation transformers with ratings above 2500 KVA are utilized for higher secondary voltages, including 4160V for large motors and 13,800 V for medium voltage feeders.
8. All configurations described herein are based on radial feeders. Radial feeders provide power to feeders for panel-boards and other electrical distribution equipment within the pharmaceutical plant. Branch circuits connect to feeders and provide power to the electrical loads.

Feeders and Branch Circuit Arrangements

Feeders originating in switchgear, panelboards, and motor control centers provide power to electrical distribution equipment within the pharmaceutical plant. Branch circuits originating in panelboards and motor control centers provide power to pharmaceutical equipment, lighting, motors, and other equipment.

1. Three phase, 3 wire or 3 phase, 4 wire power and lighting panelboards having current ratings from 100–1600 A may have a main circuit breaker or may have main lugs only. They will have feeder circuit breakers for other electrical equipment and/or branch circuit breakers for pharmaceutical equipment, lighting fixtures, etc. The panelboards should have an IAC rating greater than the available short-circuit current calculated at the transformer serving the panel- board. Four-wire switchgear, panelboards, and motor control centers should have a separate neutral bus and a separate ground bus. The secondary neutral of a separately derived 4 wire system should be bonded

to ground at one point ahead of the main secondary circuit breaker, ideally in the transformer and not in the panel- board. Panelboard schedules and nameplates must be installed and maintained for reliability and to comply with the NEC.

2. Separately derived systems that originate at the secondary of two winding transformers including single-phase and three-phase delta-wye transformers and at the output of a wye connected generators should be connected to the power distribution system with a 4 pole automatic transfer switch (ATS) when the neutral conductor is installed in the feeder to the ATS. This will avoid circulating ground currents that can trip ground fault relays and effect sensitive electronic equipment.
3. Secondary unit substations (120/208 V) and transformers need to be distributed throughout the pharmaceutical plant to provide 120 and 208 V branch circuits to pharmaceutical equipment. Because of their lower voltage, the length of these branch circuits should be short.
4. AC motors 1 hp and larger should be 3 phase, 460 V. Smaller motors can be 120V, single phase. If the plant purchases power at 208/ 120V, 3 phase or 240V, 3 phase, all motors 1 hp and larger should be 200 or 230 V, 3 phase motors.
5. Motor control centers (MCCs) are typically 480 V, 3 phase, 3 wire or 277/480 V, 3 phase, 4 wire with current ratings from 600–2500 Å. Motor control centers should be a type that have been designed for industrial applications rather than commercial applications and must have IAC ratings greater than the available short-circuit current calculated at the transformers serving the MCCs. New MCCs that are designed to incorporate intelligent starters, protective equipment, network communication, and 24 V control circuits should be considered for future pharmaceutical process applications.
6. Individual motor controllers are sometimes connected to the main switchgear when they serve large motors but are more often connected to motor branch circuits originating in the distribution panelboards or MCCs. Individual motor controllers can be full voltage non-reversing or full voltage reversing, reduced voltage, and solid state. Reduced voltage and solid state motor controllers are used when the load requires a soft start or when there is insufficient let through (short circuit) current to start the motor without causing a severe voltage drop. When controlling a piece of critical pharmaceutical equipment within a cGMP area or process, the operation of the motor controller and all of its control circuits should be part of the qualification and validation process.
7. Variable frequency drives are special types of motor controllers. They are almost always used with 480 V motors and sometimes for motors greater than 200 hp because they require less line current to deliver the same amount of torque as compared to reduced voltage starters. They are complex and require a clean, cool, ventilated environment to properly operate. Variable frequency drives vary the speed of motors, which if continuously run at a slow speed may need supplemental cooling. Motors, designed to be controlled by VFDs, should be specified. Variable frequency drives generate harmonics on their input (line side) and output (load side) motor branch circuits. Capacitors cannot be installed on the load side of VFDs. Capacitors installed on the line side of VFDs at the switchgear or MCC must have a KVAR rating that will not cause a resonant circuit at any of the harmonic current frequencies generated by the VFDs. Variable frequency drives require many parameter settings, most of which can remain at the factory default settings and all of which should be recorded. When controlling a piece of critical pharmaceutical equipment within a cGMP area or process, the operation of the VFD, its parameter settings, and all of its control circuits should be part of the qualification and validation process.
8. Custom-built control cabinets are provided for various types of pharmaceutical equipment, usually by the equipment manufacturer. These control cabinets should be UL listed or labeled, otherwise

all of the wire and electrical equipment in them are subject to the requirements of the NEC. The functions controlled by these control cabinets and sometimes the equipment within the control cabinets and all of its control circuits should be part of the qualification and validation process.

9. Uninterruptible power supplies (UPSs) must be installed for all standby non-interruptible loads. Smaller UPSs that are dedicated to individual pieces of pharmaceutical equipment are usually better than a single large UPS. Because of the amount of non-linear loads within pharmaceutical distribution systems, UPSs are the only source of clean electricity that does not contain harmonics generated by other non-linear loads. Uninterruptible power supplies usually have parameter settings and alarms. When providing power to a piece of critical pharmaceutical equipment within a cGMP area or process, the operation of the UPS, its parameter settings, and alarms should be part of the qualification and validation process for the piece of equipment.
10. Automatic transfer switches (ATSs) are commonly used to transfer emergency and standby loads from a normal source of power to an emergency source of power. Automatic transfer switches are available at different voltages, with three or four poles, with contacts to start an emergency generator, with time delays when part of a priority load shedding circuit, with controls that will permit bumpless transfer between the normal and emergency power system, and with integral battery chargers for the emergency generator starting batteries. They can be simple or complex and are critical parts of a reliable power distribution system. Automatic transfer switches are a latent single point of failure within normal/emergency circuits and therefore must be inspected and tested as often as possible.

Generators and Emergency Power Sources

A pharmaceutical plant can obtain emergency or standby electrical power from generators, rechargeable batteries, and in rare cases from a separate utility service. Uninterruptible power supplies, central storage battery system, and unit equipment all use rechargeable batteries for their emergency source of power.

1. Unit equipment (self-contained battery packs with integral or remote lamps) provide the lowest initial cost for emergency egress lighting and exit signs but require considerable maintenance.
2. Emergency generators can provide emergency power for egress lighting and exit signs and standby loads. The 1996 NEC introduced a requirement that all legally required emergency loads must be supplied by a dedicated ATS with dedicated feeders and branch circuits. Therefore installations after 1996 must have two or more ATSs when serving both emergency and standby loads. Emergency generators typically have a standby rating and sometimes have a lower prime rating. The standby rating should be used unless the generator is intended to run for weeks at a time. Standby generators can deliver 100% of their rated KW output for short periods of time to linear loads. Non-linear loads will reduce the rating of the emergency generator. Outdoor emergency generators can be purchased with subbase double-wall fuel tanks and can be installed in walk-in enclosures in sizes up to 1600 KW.

When the entire pharmaceutical plant or a large portion thereof requires emergency power, two or more generators are recommended. These generators should have a priority load shedding circuit that turns off the non-critical loads before critical and legally required loads. Emergency generators that can be synchronized with each other can also synchronize with one of the utility lines if approved and designed in accordance with the requirements of the utility company.

Harmonics

Non-linear loads have a distorted periodic wave form. Any periodic wave shape can be broken into or analyzed as a fundamental wave and a set of harmonics. Fundamental wave, 60Hz, and harmonics currents exist within the branch circuits and feeders that serve non-linear equipment. The highest magnitudes of currents exist at the 3rd, 5th, 7th, 9th, 11th, and 13th harmonics.

1. The triplet harmonics, including the 3rd, 9th, and 15th, exists only in circuits that have a neutral conductor such as computer circuits and lighting circuits. The triplet harmonics that exist on the secondary side of a Δ-Y transformer will not be transformed to the primary side of the transformer. Transformers with K ratings of 4–50 are specifically designed to handle these harmonic currents.
2. Variable frequency drives generate harmonic other than the triplets, the highest of which are the 5th, 7th, 11th, and 13th harmonic currents, on the three-phase circuits that feed them. Drive transformers have been specifically designed for VFD loads.

A harmonic analysis should be performed before installing capacitors on a power distribution system that has a significant non-linear load.

Grounding

Grounding for any electrical distribution system can be divided into two areas: system grounding and equipment grounding. These two areas are kept separate from each other except at the point where the system receives its source of power, namely the service equipment or a separately derived system (*D* - Y transformer or generator). Grounding the neutral conductor at more than one point will cause circulating ground currents that could trip ground fault relays and circuit breakers with ground fault detection and can cause noise in the electronic equipment whose enclosures are required to be solidly grounded to the electrical systems equipment ground.

Pharmaceutical plants will become more dependent on reliable electrical power because of technological advances in pharmaceutical equipment and other loads associated with cGMP areas within plant. A reliable electrical power system is not something that just happens. It requires adequate and knowledgeable planning, engineering, design, installation, testing, and maintenance. A failure to provide any one of these will lesson the reliability of the electrical power system and could leave the plant without electricity. A pharmaceutical plant without electricity is very dark, very quite, and very unsafe.

18

Components for Pharmaceutical Industry

The primary function of elastomeric components used by the pharmaceutical industry, which includes both drugs and medical devices, is to protect and deliver. Elastomeric components are typically primary packaging components; that is, they are or may be in direct contact with the dosage form. They must neither interact with the dosage form nor allow the ingress or egress of materials. Elastomeric or rubber components typically provide the means for sealing parenteral containers of varying size and shape because of their unique physical properties. Elasticity particularly permits intimate contact between the closure and the relatively rigid surfaces of container openings. No other material known today has this same unique property. This property is primarily responsible for the ability of the closure to be pierced with a sharp device, such as a hypodermic needle, and then to reseal. This is an example of the delivery function of elastomeric components. Rubber closures are an essential component of the primary package for most parenteral or injectable products. In order to understand how rubber performs its unique "protect and deliver" function, it is necessary to know how rubber is compounded and manufactured.

Rubber Compounds

Rubber, like all other primary packaging materials, is not inert. Any material used in the compounding of the rubber component may be leached into and/or chemically react with the dosage form. These materials, and the amounts used, are significantly different from those that may be used in industrial rubber belts, tires, and hoses where heat, abrasion, and solvent resistance are typically the main concern. More than one type of each material may be used in a rubber compound. For example, compounds containing two elastomers, such as isoprene and chlorobutyl rubber, and two pigments, such as titanium dioxide and carbon black, are very common. Compounds used for parenteral closures consist of an elastomer as the base material combined chemically and physically with other necessary rubber chemicals.

The elastomer determines most of the physical and chemical characteristics of a rubber compound. Typical elastomers are natural elastomers such as natural rubber (NR), sometimes called crepe, and synthetic elastomers such as butyl (including chlorobutyl and bromobutyl), ethylene propylene diene monomer (EPDM), and styrene butadiene rubber (SBR).

In the pharmaceutical industry, natural rubber and its synthetic analog, isoprene rubber, are normally used in products that require good physical strength or that must be able to withstand multiple punctures while maintaining seal integrity. Due the "*latex sensitivity*" issue, the use of natural rubber is declining. This issue is discussed in a later section. Neoprene, a halogenated form of polyisoprene, is typically used for oil-based pharmaceutical products, such as mineral oil or vegetable oil. SBR and nitrile rubber (NBR), which issued primarily for oil-based products, are specialty elastomers that are not as commonly used. Butyls and halobutyls comprise the largest segment of pharmaceutical rubber compounds, having properties that make them applicable for the packaging of many products, especially those requiring protection from moisture vapor or oxygen. Most lyophilized and powdered products require this protection, and some liquid products require protection from oxygen. EPDMs are less commonly used, though they have been selected for large intravenous (IV) stoppers. Silicones also are not often used due to their permeability to moisture vapor and oxygen as well as their relatively high cost.

Curing (or vulcanizing/cross-linking) agents are chemicals used to cross-link elastomer chains into the three-dimensional (3D) network required to give a rubber component the desired elasticity. The term "vulcanization" indicates that heat is employed in the manufacturing or molding process. Common curing agents are sulfur, thiurams, zinc oxide, peroxides, resins, and amines. A desirable property of pharmaceutical rubber formulations is "cleanliness," that is, that they contain materials that neither leach nor volatilize into the packaged pharmaceutical. Sulfur-cured rubber, because it requires other chemicals to effect an efficient cure, is not usually as clean as resin-, metal oxide-, or peroxide-cured formulations. The demands of the pharmaceutical industry and regulatory agencies are such that these relatively clean cure systems are becoming more common.

Accelerators reduce the cure time considerably by increasing the cure rate. They are not catalysts because they are chemically altered and, in many cases, also react as curing agents. Common sulfur-cure accelerators are amines, dithiocarbamates, sulfenamides, thiazoles, and thiurams. Some accelerators, because of their reactivity, may form toxic compounds, such as 2-(2-hydroxyethylmercapto)benzothiazole from mercaptobenzothiazole (2-MCBT), residues of which may be extractable. Accelerators that are secondary amines may form toxic nitrosamines. Activators, which affect the efficiency of accelerators, are commonly added. Normally these are metal oxides, such as zinc oxide or stearic acid.

Antioxidants are classified as antidegradants or age resistors. Chemically, antioxidants protect the reactive (sensitive) sites of the rubber chains against oxygen attack. Typical antioxidants are chemicals such as hindered phenols and amines. Unsaturated elastomers, such as natural rubber, require antioxidants for protection against oxidation, which causes surface cracking and loss of elasticity. Saturated elastomers, such as silicones and fluoroelastomers, are resistant to oxidation and usually require no added antioxidants. Some antioxidants are classified as antiozonants, which are designed to provide protection when high levels of reactive ozone are likely to be in the environment.

Plasticizers are used in rubber compounds to assist in the mixing or molding of the rubber, to soften the final vulcanized rubber, or to add surface lubricity to the surface of the rubber component. Examples are paraffinic wax, silicone oil, paraffinic and naphthenic oils, phthalates, and organic phosphates. Silicone oil is commonly used in syringe pistons that must slide freely within a glass or plastic barrel; it also reduces the coring or fragmentation tendency of vial stoppers.

Fillers are materials that modify rubber characteristics (e.g., hardness) and improve its physical characteristics (e.g., tensile strength), in addition to reducing costs. Rubber is sometimes compounded without the use of fillers; the resultant product is called "gum rubber." Typical fillers are calcined and hydrated clays, magnesium silicate (talc), magnesium oxide, and silicas. Carbon black, a common filler used to increase the heat resistance in industrial components such as tires, is not used as a filler in pharmaceutical components but it is used in smaller amounts as a black pigment. Polynuclear aromatic (PNA) hydrocarbons are a concern with carbon blacks but the grades used by manufacturers of pharmaceutical components contain very low concentrations.

The pigments used are inorganic salts and oxides, carbon black, or organic dyes that are used for aesthetic or functional purposes (e.g., identification, designating a dosage, etc.). Typical pigments are carbon black, titanium dioxide, and iron oxide. With these three pigments white, black, red, and many shades of gray and pink can be produced. These pigments are chemically pure and stable, non-toxic, and relatively inexpensive. Other pigments such as phthalocyanines and ultramarine blue can be used for blues and greens, but their color fastness in not as good as the aforementioned pigments.

In terms of percentage by weight, the elastomer and filler are the chief materials used, accounting typically for over 90% of a compound. However, the other "minor" materials are quite necessary in order for the compound to have the necessary chemical, physical, and toxicological properties required for a functional packaging component. For example, without the curing agent the compound would remain a physical mixture of materials that would have the consistency of chewing gum. On the other hand, materials such as pigments may be omitted from the compound with only minor consequences—i.e., the loss of the desired color.

Selection of Compound Materials

Many materials may be used in a rubber compound; however, only a fraction of materials are acceptable in components used for the drug industry. A source of acceptable materials is the U.S. Code of Federal Regulations (CFR). Since the CFR has no list for drug contact, the drug industry uses the CFR list designated for foods. Applicable sections of 21 CFR are as follows:

Section 175—Indirect Food Additives

Sections 177 and 178—Indirect Food Additives Polymers

Sections 182, 184, 185—Generally Regarded as Safe (GRAS) Lists

Section 177.2600—Rubber Articles Intended for Repeated Use

There are some cautions with the CFR lists. First, manufacturers may not always submit materials to the Food and Drug Administration (FDA) for listing in the CFR. They may not want to take the time or incur the costs if they see only a limited market for their material in the pharmaceutical or food market. Second, some materials, such as 2-MCBT, which is not permitted by the FDA, are listed but are strongly discouraged. Finally, some materials listed in the CFR, such as food, drug, and cosmetic dyes, are really not applicable for rubber compounds used for pharmaceuticals. Many of these dyes are water-soluble and are not applicable for rubber formulations that come in contact with aqueous solutions, since the dyes could be extracted from the rubber and discolor the drug. Component manufacturers may use materials not listed in the CFR provided that acceptable toxicity data is available to the reviewing health authority.

Types of Rubber and the Manufacturing Process

Elastomeric closures for parenteral products are made from two types of elastomers or rubbers. Thermoset rubber, the most common, undergoes a chemical reaction during the molding or component-forming processing. In this chemical reaction cross-links, or bonds are inserted between the long polymer chains to form a resilient 3D network. Without these cross-links elastomeric closures would have properties resembling those of chewing gum, which is an uncross-linked rubber blended with sugar, flavors, and food coloring. The cross-linking process is not reversible. Once a closure is molded it cannot be remolded into another shape or size. Addition of heat only causes degradation or reversion of the rubber.

Another type of rubber that is used frequently is thermoplastic rubber. Components are fabricated in a process that is similar to that used for common hard plastics, such as polyethylene or polystyrene, but the final product is an elastic material with properties otherwise equivalent to those of thermoset rubbers. No chemical reactions are involved in the processing of a thermoplastic rubber. The fabrication process consists of heating the rubber compound until it liquefies, injecting the liquid into a mold, cooling the mold, and finally removing the closure from the mold. The process is reversible. Closures can be remelted and remolded into different shapes or sizes as desired. Cross-linking in this case is not a chemical process but a physical intertwining of polymeric chains. The resulting intertwined 3D network gives thermoplastic elastomers their elasticity and resiliency.

Currently, thermoplastics account for less than 5% of the elastomeric closures for parenterals. Their limited resistance to heat deformation under stress during autoclave sterilization is the main reason for this limited use. However, thermoplastics have two advantages over thermosets. First, they are chemically less complex and therefore less prone to interact with par- enteral medications, and second, they may be manufactured by a simpler and more automated process. Thermoplastic elastomers have found use in baby bottle nipples and dropper bulbs that are not typically heat sterilized under compression. The manufacturing of rubber components for pharmaceutical applications is a multistep process with controls on each step. Fully validated processes are now common.

There are generally three molding processes used for manufacturing pharmaceutical closures: compression molding, injection molding, and transfer molding. The choice of molding method usually depends on the necessary final dimensional tolerances of the item being molded. Injection molding gives the best dimensional tolerances; however, it is usually the most expensive technique, especially as compared to compression molding. Thermoset rubbers are commonly compression or transfer molded, while thermoplastic rubbers are typically injection molded. Sheets of molded components vary in shape from round to rectangular, and in size from 12 in. in diameter to 36 × 36 inches square, and may contain 50–10,000 components. A recent trend in rubber component manufacturing is the production of "preprocessed" components. Components are prepared for shipment in either one of two states:

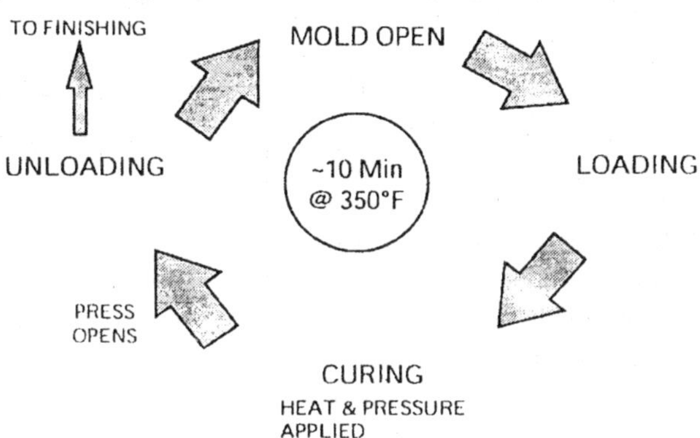

Fig. 18.1. Compression modeling cycle.

1. *Ready to sterilize* (RtS): Typically components are washed, then rinsed with Water For Injection (WFI) to reduce bioburden and endotoxin levels, lubricated with silicone oil, and finally packaged in a classified area (Classes 100–10,000) in Tyvek bags that can be steam sterilized by the drug or device manufacturer before use. Alternately polyethylene bags may be used if the end user is utilizing gamma radiation for sterilization.
2. *Ready to Use* (RtU): The process is identical to that used for RtS components except that the component manufacturer takes responsibility for component sterilization and the sterilized components are received by the drug or device manufacturer. No additional component processing is required before use.

Both processes typically require extensive validation by the component manufacturer, a description of the process in a Drug Master File (DMF), quality audits by customers, and perhaps FDA approval before RtS or RtU components are utilized. Nevertheless, RtS and RtU are trends that are moving rapidly; most major rubber component manufacturers now market RtS components.

Sterilization of Rubber Components

Heat, radiation, and sterilizing gases may be used to sterilize rubber components. However, components, especially vial stoppers, are most frequently sterilized by pressurized steam (autoclaving), a highly effective method and probably the most reliable of available methods when an F_0 value of at least 8 min is reached. However, the poor thermal conductivity of rubber and the relatively large mass of wet stoppers placed in a stainless steel container for sterilization require a careful validation of the process. Assurance must be obtained that the moist heat penetrates throughout the mass of stoppers so that every stopper receives a dose equivalent to a minimal F_0 of 8 min. However, rubber closures subjected to elevated temperatures or extended heating even at moderate temperatures degrade or revert, which is most frequently evidenced by stickiness. Therefore, the application of moist heat must be controlled because this degradation is most likely to be greatest at the outer layers of the mass of stoppers.

This undesirable effect can be markedly reduced by distributing the stoppers in a shallow tray or otherwise reducing the mass, thus making it possible to reduce the thermal cycle time and the applied heat. Cycle times of 121°C for 30–60 min are usually well tolerated by rubber components made from butyl or halobutyl rubbers. Natural and isoprene rubbers are less tolerant. Increasing the sterilization temperature above 121°C or the time above 60 min is not recommended unless components have been tested to assure that no significant degradation will take place. Dry heat sterilization or drying of components above 105°C is also not recommended without prior testing. Testing may include inspection of the surface for cracks or tackiness, swelling studies to determine state of cure, functional tests such as coring and reseal, and chemical tests such as the United States Pharmacopoeia (USP) protocol or extraction studies performed before and after the sterilization cycle.

Under the usual autoclaving conditions, moist heat does not destroy pyrogens. For closures to be pyrogen-free, a final rinse with WFI before sterilization is necessary. Ethylene oxide, a sterilizing gas, may be used to sterilize rubber components when they are part of a medical device; however, the gas is readily absorbed by the rubber and sufficient time must be allowed after sterilization for the concentration of residual ethylene oxide to dissipate to acceptable levels.

Radiation sterilization, by either gamma or e-beam, also may be utilized to sterilize rubber components. However, some elastomers, such as butyl, chlorobutyl, and bromobutyl, do not tolerate high doses of radiation, while others, such as natural, isoprene, neoprene, and nitrile rubbers are readily radiation- sterilized without degradation. The challenge with radiation sterilization of rubber components in bulk (i.e., cartons or bags) is to obtain a uniform dose of radiation throughout the entire package—enough of a dose to assure the desired sterility assurance level (SAL), usually 10^{-6}, without degrading the components, especially those nearest the radiation source. There are generally two approaches that can be followed. One is to target a uniform dose of 25 kGy, which is generally accepted to assure sterility, while the other is to follow the ANSI/AAMI/ISO 11137: 1994 standard and target a dose of radiation that is dependent on the bioburden of the components. The first approach is usually overkill but may be acceptable for radiation-resistant rubbers. The second approach usually results in lower doses applied, which may be critical with butyl and other rubbers that are not so radiation resistant. There are several necessary steps if the ANSI/AAMI/ISO standard is used. These are:

1. Selection of the SAL, usually 10^{-6}
2. Determination of the average bioburden from samples taken from three consecutive production lots
3. Establishment of the Verification Dose. This is the dose in kGy of the standard that will give a SAL of 10^{-2}
4. Confirmation of the Verification Dose by irradiating 100 components and testing each for sterility. No more than two positives are permitted
5. Establishment of the Sterilizing Dose

6. Dose mapping, using dosimeters, on a shipping container filled with components. Irradiate and determine the maximum and minimum doses (D_{max} and D_{min}) received in the container
7. Calculation of the Target Dose by multiplying the Sterilizing Dose by the ratio, D_{max}/D_{min}. The Target Dose is typically increased 6% or more to account for dosimeter error and to add additional sterility assurance.

Tests and Standards

In-Process Tests

Several tests may be performed on unvulcanized rubber or on standard-shaped test specimens to measure the properties of a rubber compound. These include the following:

1. *Rheometer measurements* measure cure and cure rate characteristics of the rubber. The component manufacturer performs this test on unvulcanized rubber. The rheometer measures the viscosity of the rubber as a function of time at a constant temperature. As time increases, the degree of cure or cross-linking increases and thus the viscosity increases.
2. *Durometer hardness* is measured on tests specimens that meet specific standards for shape and thickness. Durometer hardness is usually measured using the Shore A scale, which measures relative hardness on a scale of 0 to 100 units. Most rubber components for medical use are found in the 35–60 range with 40–50 typical for rubber vial stoppers. Durometer Hardness may be measured on some actual components if they have a sufficiently large flat surface and thickness, i.e., 28–32 mm IV stoppers.
3. *Compression set* is commonly used as a measure of the dimensional recovery of a rubber compound after compression at a defined level, usually 25%, at a specified time and temperature, usually 24 h at 70°C. High compression set values are associated with rubber that "takes a set" or loses its ability to spring back after compression. Low compression set is important for rubber closures and syringe plungers that are heat sterilized while under compression and remain under compression for long periods of time before use but must remain elastic and resilient to maintain seal integrity. Compression Set is measured on dimensionally defined test specimens.
4. *Tensile*, *modulus*, and *elongation* are measures of the strength of a rubber compound. They are measured on bow tie-shaped specimens that are clamped in a tensile measuring apparatus and stretched.
5. *Water vapor* and *oxygen transmission* (WVT and O_2T) are commonly measured on thin-film specimens. Butyl and halobutyl compounds have very low WVT and O_2T rates, while rates for natural and isoprene rubbers are higher and for silicone even higher.

Finished Component Tests

Finished component tests may be divided into three categories: those used as routine identity and/or quality control tests, those tests recommended or mandated by government, standards, and compendial groups, and those test that are part of the larger rubber component acceptance and drug/device approval process. In many instances, a test may fall into more than one category.

Identity and quality control tests

1. *Percentage ash* is a measure of the non-volatile materials in a rubber formulation, such as clays and other fillers.
2. *Specific gravity* is a measure of the type and quantity of fillers in a formulation.
3. An *infrared spectrum* of a compound pyrolysate identifies the elastomer qualitatively (natural, butyl).
4. An *ultraviolet (UV) spectrum* of an aqueous rubber extract identifies and quantifies the antioxidants, curing agents, accelerators, and other UV-absorbing species extracted from the compound.

5. *Percentage swelling* in an organic solvent is a measure of the degree and consistency of cure or cross-linking that determines the physical and functional properties of a component.

These five tests may be used to characterize a rubber formulation or serve, either individually or in combinations, as quality control tests.

Compendial, standard, and government tests

The most influential of these test protocols are the USP, the *European Pharmacopoeia* (EP), the Pharmacopoeia of Japan (JP), the Organization for International Standardization (ISO), and the Parenteral Drug Association (PDA). USP<381>, Elastomeric Closures for Injections, contains five chemical tests and two biological tests. Closures must meet the biological requirements but there are no current specifications for the chemical tests. All USP chemical tests are commonly performed on aqueous extracts but isopropyl alcohol and the drug product vehicle are also permitted. A brief description of the USP<381> tests follows.

1. *Turbidity*. The clarity of the closure extract is measured with a nephelometer with appropriate standards. Turbidity is a measure of the insoluble extractables from a closure and is affected by the type and amounts of ingredients in a formulation, pretreatments such as washing, extractions, sterilizations, and degree of cure.
2. *Reducing agents*. Organic extractables oxidizable by iodine are determined in this procedure. It is affected by the same variables as turbidity.
3. *Heavy metals*. Extractable lead as well as other metals, such as zinc and cadmium, are determined colorimetrically or by atomic absorption.
4. *pH change*. The pH of the extract is a measure of the acidic and alkaline water-soluble extractables from a compound.
5. *Total extractables*. The sum of the inorganic, organic (non-volatile), soluble, and insoluble extractables is measured in this test. The weight of total extractables is an indication of the "cleanliness" of a formulation.
6. *Biological tests*. USP 24 lists two levels of biological tests—the in vitro tissue culture test and the in vivo systemic injection and intracutaneous tests. A parenteral closure must pass either type of test to meet USP requirements.

The application of numerical specifications to the USP <381> chemical tests is under discussion and probably will become effective in USP 24 via a supplement. Not all pharmacopeias and standards groups designate the same tests; therefore, it is important to consult a wide spectrum of references to design a test protocol for specific applications and geographical submissions. Of the four protocols compared, the JP is the most stringent in terms of limits for extractables.

The USP, EP, and ISO test protocols are based on a specific closure "area" per volume of water in the extraction step. The JP test protocols, on the other hand, are based on a specific "weight" of closures per volume of water. This difference makes it more difficult for smaller closures than for larger closures in the same rubber compound to meet JP specifications; i.e., 13-mm closures will be less likely to meet JP specifications than 20-mm closures, and 20-mm closures are less likely than 28-mm closures to meet JP specifications.

Although packaging components, such as vial closures, syringe plungers, and needle shields, may meet all compendial and accepted standards, this does not mean that they will be acceptable for use with any specific drug or device. Specific evaluation tests must be performed for that purpose. Compendial and standard tests should be regarded as the first necessary but not sufficient hurdle in the race to gain approval of a component for use with a drug or device.

Specific tests for component evaluation and regulatory approval

There are three requirements for a rubber component:

1. Compatible with the drug
2. Meets functional requirements
3. Provides closure-container seal integrity

Many factors influence the choice of a rubber compound for a particular drug, the most important of which is the solvent vehicle. If the solvent vehicle is an aqueous material, then a butyl, natural, or EPDM may be used. If the solvent vehicle is an oil, then a neoprene or nitrile is utilized.

Configuration is also important and is determined by the required function. A lyophilization stopper, designed to keep out moisture, almost certainly requires a butyl formulation, while a vial stopper for aqueous-based solutions could be formulated from isoprene rubber.

Some preservatives are especially reactive with rubber. Bromobutyl rubbers, but not chlorobutyls, are recommended for drug formulations that contain chlorobutanol. A pH that is either very low or very high affects rubber formulations more than a pH in the range of 5–8. Buffer systems may also affect the choice of rubber formulations. Materials such as phosphates not only attack the rubber at high pHs but also may attack glass as well.

Metallic sensitivities affect compatibility, as drug formulations that are sensitive to divalent cations, such as calcium, zinc, or iron, may not be able to use certain rubber compounds that are cured or pigmented with these materials. An obvious factor is the need for oxygen or moisture vapor protection. A butyl-based compound is normally chosen whenever protection from materials transmitted either into or from a drug product is required. When it comes to color preference, most rubber manufacturers of closures used for drugs prefer to use three pigments: iron oxide to produce reds, carbon black for blacks, and titanium dioxide for whites; combinations of these are used for pinks and grays. Organic materials used as pigments are not generally acceptable since they are not very heat stable and are generally more toxic than the three pigments mentioned.

Choice of sterilization method is extremely important in choosing a rubber formulation. Many heat-sensitive drugs, such as proteins, are packaged aseptically; that is, the rubber closure, the vial, and drug are sterilized separately, and then all three items are brought together in a sterile environment to form the final package. The FDA, however, encourages terminal sterilization. In this method, the three materials are brought together and then the entire package, the drug in contact with the vial and closure, is sterilized by heat. This method is much more demanding on the closure than aseptic processing.

Radiation (Co-60) is used to sterilize many rubber items, especially those used in devices. The effect of gamma radiation on rubber closures is a function of the elastomer, dose, and post-irradiation time. NR and isoprene are much more resistant to irradiation effects than butyl.

To give the drug manufacturer a high degree of assurance that the closures being investigated for a possible package will be acceptable, a prescreening procedure is commonly used by component suppliers. In this procedure, information and a sample of the drug are obtained from the drug manufacturer. Then three to five possible closures, along with an inert control stopper (a Teflon plug or coated closure), are used to package vials of the drug. The closures are put onto the drug-containing vials using an exaggerated closure area-to-volume ratio (2× to 3× the normal ratio). Vials are stored at higher and/or lower temperatures than the drug package will normally experience in the upright, inverted and on-side positions.

An inert control stopper should be used since a drug may be stable against glass but not against uncoated rubber. Only when an inert control is used will it be possible to determine whether the rubber and/or glass vial is the cause of the drug instability. Ampoules do not make good controls for the prescreening of drugs in vials since the glass for vials may be different from that used for ampoules.

These factors along with the functional and seal integrity requirements can be used to write specifications for components. The packaging engineer, as with the rubber compounder, faces the challenge of choosing a compound that best meets the overall requirements but, only at best, provides a balance of all the actual chemical and functional needs. For example, an engineer may choose an isoprene vial closure because multiple punctures with a large cannula are required. Isoprene will provide the low coring and excellent reseal required. But the engineer may give up some shelf life since isoprene is a poor oxygen barrier. Choosing a butyl closure would give additional shelf life due to its better barrier properties, but coring and reseal would not be acceptable. Closure compound choice is always a give-and-take proposition where drug/device requirements must be prioritized before the choice of a rubber compound can be made. There are four general types of closure–drug interactions:

1. Adsorption occurs when a drug is concentrated at the surface of a closure or vial.
2. Absorption occurs when a drug material is dispersed in the closure matrix.
3. Permeation is the transmission of a drug ingredient through a closure into the atmosphere or transmission of an outside material into the container.
4. Leaching is the process by which closure ingredients are extracted into the drug product.

All four of these interactions commonly occur. No rubber compound is absolutely inert to a drug. In many cases, the extent of the particular interaction is extremely small and may not be measurable, but generally all four are occurring, albeit at a low rate. With proteins, adsorption can be a problem. Many proteinaceous materials made by the biotechnology industry are highly adsorbent onto rubber surfaces and their potency may be readily lost. Other drugs products, especially ones that are very acidic or basic, may attack the stopper and cause the extraction of rubber compound ingredients. Common leachables from rubber closures include low molecular weight elastomer fragments, metal ions, antioxidants, plasticizers, lubricants, curing agents, and accelerators. The rate and relative importance of these four interactions determines the degree of compatibility or incompatibility of a stopper with a drug product.

In May 1999, the FDA issued an updated guidance entitled "Container Closure Systems for Packaging Human Drugs and Biologics—Chemistry, Manufacturing and Controls Documentation," that listed in tables the packaging information that should be submitted in an application. The guidance divides the information into four sections:

1. *Description*. Overall general description of the container-closure system plus specific information on suppliers, materials of construction, and postmanufacturing treatments.
2. *Suitability*. This section prescribes that tests must be done to assure protection of the drug product, safety of the packaging component material, compatibility of the component with the drug product, and performance of the component.
3. *Quality control*. The rubber component manufacturer's release criteria and drug packager's acceptance are found in this section. Also recommended is a method to monitor the consistency in composition of elastomeric components such as periodic extraction profiles.
4. *Stability*. Testing of the drug product using the packaging component is required. Unlike compendial tests that utilize water for extraction studies of the packaging component, the complete drug product is utilized in these stability studies.

This guideline advocates more information on rubber extractables and the proper use of DMFs. Knowledge of extraction data from elastomeric components refers not only to the broad (and usually non-specific) type of extractable data generated in USP<381> testing, but also to the identification and quantification, where necessary, of specific extractable species. Example of non-specific extractables include turbidity, reducing agents, heavy metals, pH change, and total extractables-; They all measure broad types of extractables. Specific extractables include inorganics, such as zinc or lead and organics, such as PNA, stearic acid, nitrosamines, tetramethylthiuram disulfide, or 2,6-di-tert-butyl-4-sec-butyl phenol. Both liquid (HPLC) and gas chromatography (GC) are well suited for this purpose. Drug/ device producers who utilize elastomeric packaging components require information from their suppliers on extractables (extractable profiles), including test methods, that are generated in water at various pH values (i.e., 3, 7, and 10) and in organic solvents such as isopropanol. Armed with this information, they can look for extractables in their drug products.

Confidential packaging component information, such as the compound recipe, may be placed in a Type III DMF so that the FDA can review the information when it reviews the drug application (IND, NDA, ANDA, or BLA). Most elastomeric compounds are filed at the request of a pharmaceutical manufacturer who has chosen to use the rubber closure in one or more drug packages or devices applications. The name of a rubber compound is associated with a precise recipe that designates specific ingredients and quantities. Once a rubber compound is filed in a DMF, no changes can be made in that compound without changing the DMF and notifying all customers on whose behalf the DMF was accessed and reviewed by the FDA. Since changes in a supplier's DMF may require additional stability studies by the drug manufacturer, changes are infrequent.

Recent Issues and Developments

Latex Sensitivity

There are medical and regulatory issues surrounding the use of "*latex rubber*" due to allergic reactions that have resulted in medical emergencies. Even deaths have been noted. There are two broad types of rubber—natural and synthetic. Several synthetic rubbers or elastomers are used for pharmaceutical components. However, there is only one type of commercial NR, which is derived from the rubber tree Hevea Brasiliensis. "*Latex sensitivity*" is associated only with NR and not with the synthetics, although other types of allergic reactions can result from contact with synthetic rubbers. NR is processed and used in two forms—liquid or latex rubber and solid or dry rubber, often referred to as crepe, SMR, and SIR. Specific proteins that are contained in both the latex and dry types cause the sensitivity to NR. Thus, the medical community and regulatory authorities have used the term "latex" for both forms of NR when "*latex sensitivity*" is discussed. Latex reactions reported in the literature have thus far been attributed to contact with components made from liquid rubber but not from dry rubber. Components made from liquid rubber are made by a dipping process that is best suited for thin-walled items such as gloves, condoms, and catheters. None of the typical rubber packaging components made from latex rubber; they are all made from dry rubber via a molding process. Many studies have been published regarding the allergic properties of latex and dry rubber and further studies are in progress to determine if exposure to these dry rubber components can cause allergic latex reactions.

There is a great deal of regulatory activity in an attempt to protect the public from unexpected latex reactions. In 1996, the USP proposed a change in section <381> that would prohibit the use of NR in elastomeric closures; however, it rescinded this change in April 1997, stating that closure manufacturers should instead devise latex protein limits. A test for the water-soluble protein content of elastomers, based on an ASTM test, was published as USP <836> but no specifications or limits were proposed. At the same time, the FDA published a final rule that made it mandatory to provide labeling statements on medical devices and packaging components that contain NR. This rule was later amended to exclude combination drug/device and biologic/device products such as rubber stoppers and plungers for prefilled syringes. The uncertainty about the allergic risk from dry NR components and pending regulations have significantly reduced the use of NR in packaging for new drugs and in devices. Substitutes such as isoprene and SBR rubbers are finding increased use.

Preprocessed Components

Preprocessed closures, commonly referred to as RtS or Ready for Sterilization and RtU or Ready for Use, are an unstoppable trend in pharmaceutical packaging. Information on the manufacturing of these products was described previously in this review. The purpose of preprocessed closures is to reduce total processing costs and improve closure characteristics. Typical RtS closure characteristics are as follows:

Endotoxin Level:	<1 EU/closure
Bioburden Level:	<2 cfu/closure
Silicone Level:	10–40 μg/closure
Visible Particulate:	<20 particles in 25 to 50-μ
Matter:	range; <2 particles in 50 to 100-μ range; <1 particle over 100 μ

Coating and Surface Treatments

Although the material science of rubber compounds has greatly improved, drug-closure-interactions and surface lubricity are problematic for packaging engineers. Surface modifications of closures are frequently necessary to meet acceptance standards set by the USP, EP, JP, and ISO as well as the expectations of regulatory authorities. In practice, both liquids and solids are applied to closure surfaces to minimize interactions and improve lubricity. Although these coating and surface treatments may add significantly to the purchase price of closures they often reduce the total drug product cost by providing the following benefits:

1. Increased lubricity, which allows faster processing speeds
2. Decreased drug–closure interactions, which permits the marketing of some products not compatible with uncoated rubber and better quality and longer shelf life for others
3. Decreased particulate matter, which reduces the number of units rejected for visible particulate matter

Container-Closure Seal Integrity

The FDA Guidance on Container Closure Systems lists sterility or container integrity as an important parameter to be considered in the section on Protection. Seal integrity tests can be done by both physical and microbial methods, but historically, sterility testing alone has been used. A 1998 FDA draft guidance discusses the replacement of the sterility test with an appropriate container- closure integrity test in the stability protocol, permitting an alternative to sterility testing for proving the continued capability of containers to maintain sterility. Kirsch et al. published a series of four papers that studied mass spectrometry-based helium leak detection, microbial ingress, and vacuum decay and the correlation between these methods. The PDA also published an updated technical report that provides guidance for evaluating pharmaceutical package integrity, and Guazzo has published an excellent review article that outlines the advantages and limitations of current methods.

Rubber packaging and device components are an important part of the overall medical delivery system. Without innovative packaging systems, modern drugs would not be available today. Advances in drug development have initiated research in new packaging and delivery systems while the availability of innovative packaging has led to the introduction of new drug therapies. Innovation, while containing costs and conforming to regulations, is the challenge for the 21st century.

INDEX